T0320774

Oxford Textbook of

Neuro-Oncology

Oxford Textbooks in Clinical Neurology

Oxford Textbook of
Neuro-Oncology

Edited by

Tracy T. Batchelor

Count Giovanni Auletta Armenise-Harvard Professor of Neurology,
Harvard Medical School, Executive Director, Stephen E. and Catherine Pappas Center
for Neuro-Oncology, Massachusetts General Hospital; Associate Clinical Director,
Massachusetts General Hospital Cancer Center; Co-Leader, Neuro-Oncology
Program, Dana-Farber/Harvard Cancer Center, Boston, MA, USA

Ryo Nishikawa

Professor and Chair, Department of Neurosurgery, Head,
Department of Neuro-Oncology, Comprehensive Cancer Center,
International Medical Center, Saitama Medical University, Saitama, Japan

Nancy J. Tarbell

CC Wang Professor of Radiation Oncology, Dean for Academic and Clinical Affairs,
Harvard Medical School, Boston, MA, USA

Michael Weller

Professor and Chairman, Department of Neurology, University Hospital
and University of Zurich, Zurich, Switzerland

Series Editor

Christopher Kennard

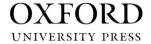

OXFORD
UNIVERSITY PRESS

UNIVERSITY PRESS

Great Clarendon Street, Oxford, OX2 6DP,
United Kingdom

Oxford University Press is a department of the University of Oxford.
It furthers the University's objective of excellence in research, scholarship,
and education by publishing worldwide. Oxford is a registered trade mark of
Oxford University Press in the UK and in certain other countries

© Oxford University Press 2017

The moral rights of the authors have been asserted

First Edition published in 2017

Impression: 1

Published in the United States of America by Oxford University Press
198 Madison Avenue, New York, NY 10016, United States of America

British Library Cataloguing in Publication Data
Data available

Library of Congress Control Number: 2017937403

ISBN 978–0–19–965187–0

Printed in Great Britain by
Bell & Bain Ltd., Glasgow

Foreword

During my 50 years of laboratory research and caring for patients with central nervous system (CNS) tumours, I have witnessed and participated in many developments that at first seemed promising, but dead-ended in disappointing blind alleys; fortunately, others resulted in greater knowledge and clarity about CNS diseases as well as improved outcomes.

Over the years, books published on CNS cancer and its treatment were met with mixed reviews by small audiences, but, nonetheless, helped educate multiple generations of physicians and scientists. When I began my career, I was one of very few in the world willing to focus on CNS cancer research and treatment. Learning from books and experts in other fields helped in that process. Book chapters, being less constrained than articles, can provide more contextual information for the reader than a single article can provide. In my view, a book is frequently the best vehicle for educating others. After moving to Houston, Texas, United States, to become Chair of the Department of Neuro-Oncology at The University of Texas MD Anderson Cancer Center, I wanted to write a textbook, which became *Cancer in the Nervous System* (1996, 2002, Oxford University Press), to educate a new generation of neuro-oncologists and address problems in treatment as well as concerns about symptom management for tumour- and treatment-related effects.

We are now at another crossroads in information because of the explosion of molecular and genetic studies that affect the way we classify tumours and, in turn, how we treat the considerable number of rare benign and malignant tumours of the CNS. I believe this novel paradigm was why so many senior international authors from the multiple specialties essential to our field took the time to create this well-structured and highly informative book. This book brings together the changing neuropathology landscape, important molecular–genetic drivers of these tumours, and provides thoughtful discussions by experts on how best to treat and manage patients afflicted with these rare tumours. Each generation must strive to educate the next generation of clinicians and scientists if we are to make progress in the care of our patients. This requires a book, such as the *Oxford Textbook of Neuro-Oncology*, to bring together the relevance of pathology, molecular–genetic associations, prospective clinical trials, and the experiential insights gained by experts who have treated the very rare tumours absent from formal clinical trials. This panoply of knowledge is well conveyed in this textbook. Taken together, it informs and affects how these tumours are understood today and how best to approach their diverse treatments.

This 21-chapter book, modeled after the World Health Organization classification of central nervous system tumors, takes a 'meet the professor' approach. It provides a framework to assist the reader prepare to understand how we treat and inform patients with respect to treatment options and prognosis when new molecular–genetic knowledge is revealed. Is this textbook the last word? Certainly not, but it is the current word and, as such, deserves a special place in the library of those who care for individuals with CNS tumours and those who research possibilities for improving their survival.

Victor A. Levin, M.D.
Emeritus Professor, Department of Neuro-Oncology,
The University of Texas,
MD Anderson Cancer Center, Houston, TX, USA
Clinical Professor, Department of Neurosurgery, University of
California San Francisco, San Francisco, CA, USA

Preface

The practice of neuro-oncology entails the management of many different types of tumours of the nervous system by a multidisciplinary team of healthcare providers. These tumours represent a diverse spectrum of underlying molecular biological subtypes, prognostic categories, age distributions, and treatment recommendations. The World Health Organization (WHO) classification of central nervous system tumours is the foundation for the categorization and, by extension, clinical management and treatment of patients with all types of nervous system tumours. The WHO classification has traditionally been based on light microscopic description of the cellular elements of tumours in the brain, spinal cord, nerves, and meninges. The 2016 WHO classification of central nervous system tumours for the first time incorporates molecular markers into the categorization of some types of nervous system tumours, particularly gliomas. This revised classification will serve as the basis for future clinical trials and, ultimately, management recommendations for these newly recognized pathological-molecular subsets of central nervous system tumours. Current management guidelines are derived, however, from clinical trials and studies utilizing earlier versions of the WHO classification system. This book is intended for clinicians as a complement to the WHO classification system with a focus on clinical management of nervous system tumours in adults and children. Each chapter is co-authored by a multidisciplinary, international group of leading authorities in adult and paediatric neuro-oncology. The book is organized according to the 2007 WHO classification of central nervous system tumours and each chapter follows a similar framework. The introductory chapter reviews the 2016 revision of the WHO classification of central nervous system tumours and how these changes may influence future clinical trials, clinical practice, and subsequent editions of this book.

Tracy T. Batchelor
Ryo Nishikawa
Nancy J. Tarbell
Michael Weller

Contents

Abbreviations

5-ALA	5-aminolevulinic acid
AED	antiepileptic drug
ASCT	autologous stem cell transplantation
CBTRUS	Central Brain Tumor Registry of the United States
CBV	cerebral blood volume
CCG	Children's Cancer Group
CHOP	cyclophosphamide, doxorubicin, vincristine, and prednisone
CI	confidence interval
CNS	central nervous system
COG	Children's Oncology Group
CPC	choroid plexus carcinoma
CPP	choroid plexus papilloma
CPT	choroid plexus tumour
CR	complete response
CSF	cerebrospinal fluid
CSI	craniospinal irradiation
CSRT	craniospinal radiotherapy
CT	computed tomography
DI	diabetes insipidus
DIA	desmoplastic infantile astrocytoma
DIG	desmoplastic infantile ganglioglioma
DIPG	diffuse intrinsic pontine glioma
DLBCL	diffuse large B-cell lymphoma
DNET	dysembryoplastic neuroepithelial tumour
EANO	European Association for Neuro-Oncology
EBRT	external beam radiotherapy
ED	Erdheim–Chester disease
EFS	event-free survival
EGFR	epidermal growth factor receptor
EMA	epithelial membrane antigen
EOR	extent of resection
EORTC	European Organization for Research and Treatment of Cancer
ESCC	epidural spinal cord compression
ETMR	embryonal tumour with multilayer rosettes
FAP	familial adenomatous polyposis
FLAIR	fluid-attenuated inversion recovery
GC	gangliocytoma
GFAP	glial fibrillary acidic protein
GG	ganglioglioma
GH	growth hormone
GTR	gross total resection
HAART	highly active antiretroviral therapy
HAR	hyperfractionated accelerated radiotherapy
HDT	high-dose therapy
HFRT	hyperfractionated radiotherapy
HIV	human immunodeficiency virus
HL	Hodgkin's lymphoma
HNPCC	hereditary nonpolyposis colorectal cancer
IARC	International Agency for Research on Cancer
IDH	isocitrate dehydrogenase
IELSG	International Extranodal Lymphoma Study Group
iGCT	intracranial germ cell tumour
IPCG	International PCNSL Collaborative Group
ISCM	intramedullary spinal cord metastasis
JXG	juvenile xanthogranuloma
KPS	Karnofsky performance score
LDD	Lhermitte–Duclos disease
LEAT	long-term epilepsy-associated tumour
MB	medulloblastoma
MGMT	O^6-methylguanine-DNA methyltransferase
MPNST	malignant peripheral nerve sheath tumour
MRI	magnetic resonance imaging
MRS	magnetic resonance spectroscopy
mTOR	mammalian target of rapamycin
NCCN	National Comprehensive Cancer Network
NF	neurofibromatosis
NGGCT	non-germinomatous germ cell tumour
NHL	non-Hodgkin's lymphoma
NIH	National Institutes of Health
NK	natural killer
NM	neoplastic meningitis
NOA	Neuro-Onkologische Arbeitsgemeinschaft/German Neuro-Oncology Group
NSCLC	non-small cell lung cancer
NSE	neuron-specific enolase
ONG	optic nerve glioma
ONSM	optic nerve sheath meningioma
OS	overall survival
PA	pilocytic astrocytoma
PCNSL	primary central nervous system lymphoma
PCV	procarbazine, CCNU (lomustine), and vincristine
PET	positron emission tomography
PFS	progression-free survival
PNET	primitive neuroectodermal tumour
PPT	primary parenchymal tumour
PTEN	phosphatase and tensin homologue

PXA	pleomorphic xanthoastrocytoma	SIOP	International Society of Paediatric Oncology
RDD	Rosai–Dorfman disease	SRS	stereotactic radiosurgery
RGNT	rosette-forming glioneuronal tumour	SRT	stereotactic radiotherapy
RTOG	Radiation Therapy Oncology Group	TSC	tuberous sclerosis complex
SBRT	stereotactic body radiotherapy	UKCCSG	United Kingdom Children's Cancer Study Group
SEER	Surveillance, Epidemiology and End Results	VAD	ventricular access device
SEGA	subependymal giant cell astrocytoma	VPS	ventriculoperitoneal shunt
SFOP	Société Française d'Oncologie Pédiatrique/French Pediatric Oncology Society	WBRT	whole-brain radiotherapy
SFT	solitary fibrous tumour	WHO	World Health Organization

Contributors

Oussama Abla, Staff Oncologist, Division of Haematology/Oncology, Department of Paediatrics, The Hospital for Sick Children, Toronto, ON, Canada; Associate Professor of Paediatrics, University of Toronto, ON, Canada

Claire Alapetite, Institut Curie, Radiation Oncology Department, Paris & Proton Therapy Center, Orsay, France

Jeffrey Allen, Otto and Marguerite Manley and Making Headway Foundation Professor of Pediatric Neuro-Oncology, Department of Pediatrics; Professor, Department of Neurology, NYU Langone Medical Center, New York, USA

Tracy T. Batchelor, Count Giovanni Auletta Armenise-Harvard Professor of Neurology, Harvard Medical School, Executive Director, Stephen E. and Catherine Pappas Center for Neuro-Oncology, Massachusetts General Hospital, Associate Clinical Director (Academic Affairs), Massachusetts General Hospital Cancer Center, Co-Leader, Neuro-Oncology Program, Dana-Farber/Harvard Cancer Center, Boston, MA, USA

Glenn Bauman, Department of Oncology, Western University and London Regional Cancer Program, London, ON, Canada

Brigitta G. Baumert, Department of Radiation Oncology and Clinical Cooperation Unit Neurooncology, MediClin Robert Janker Clinic & University of Bonn Medical Center, Bonn, Germany

Martin J. van den Bent, Neuro-oncology Unit, The Brain Tumor Center at Erasmus MC Cancer Institute, Rotterdam, The Netherlands

Mitchell S. Berger, Professor and Chairman, Department of Neurological Surgery, Bethold and Belle N. Guggenheim Endowed Chair, Director, Brain Tumor Research Center, University of California, San Francisco, CA, USA

Jaclyn A. Biegel, Chief, Division of Genomic Medicine, Director, Center for Personalized Medicine, Department of Pathology and Laboratory Medicine, Children's Hospital Los Angeles, Professor of Clinical Pathology (Clinical Scholar), USC Keck School of Medicine, Los Angeles, CA, USA

Eric Bouffet, Professor of Paediatrics, Director, Brain Tumour Program, The Hospital for Sick Children, Toronto, ON, Canada

Michael Brada, University of Liverpool, Department of Molecular & Clinical Cancer Medicine and Department of Radiation Oncology, Clatterbridge Cancer Centre, Wirral, UK

Alba A. Brandes, Chair, Medical Oncology Department, AUSL-IRCCS Institute of Neurological Sciences, Bologna, Italy

Paul D. Brown, Department of Radiation Oncology, Mayo Clinic, Rochester, MN, USA

Marc C. Chamberlain, University of Washington, Department of Neurology and Neurological Surgery, Division of Neuro-Oncology, Fred Hutchinson Research Cancer Center, Seattle Cancer Care Alliance, Seattle, WA, USA

Zhong-ping Chen, Professor and Chairman, Department of Neurosurgery and Neuro-oncology, Sun Yat-Sen University Cancer Center, Guangzhou, China

Stephanie E. Combs, Institute of Innovative Radiotherapy (IRT), Department of Radiation Sciences (GAS), Helmholtz Zentrum München, Oberschleißheim, Germany

Peter B. Crino, Professor and Chairman, Department of Neurology, University of Maryland School of Medicine, Baltimore, MD, USA

Frederic Dhermain, Department of Radiation Oncology, Gustave Roussy University Hospital, Cancer Campus Grand Paris, France

Hugues Duffau, Department of Neurosurgery, Gui de Chauliac Hospital, Montpellier, Montpellier, France

D. Gareth Evans, Department of Genomic Medicine, MAHSC, University of Manchester, Division of Evolution and Genomic Medicine, St Mary's Hospital, Manchester, UK

Carolyn Freeman, Professor of Oncology and Pediatrics and Mike Rosenbloom Chair of Radiation Oncology, Department of Radiation Oncology, McGill University Health Centre, Montreal, QC, Canada

Takamitsu Fujimaki, Professor, Department of Neurosurgery Saitama Medical University, Japan

Mark R. Gilbert, Director, Neuro-Oncology Branch, National Cancer Institute and National Institute of Neurologic Disorders and Stroke, National Institutes of Health, Bethesda, MD, USA

Samar Issa, Consultant Haematologist, Clinical Head, Lymphoma Services, Founding Chair, Lymphoma Network of New Zealand, Member, Scientific Advisory Committee, Auckland Regional Tissue Bank, Honorary Academic, Department of Molecular Medicine & Pathology, University of Auckland School of Medicine, Middlemore Hospital, Auckland, New Zealand

Rakesh Jalali, Professor of Radiation Oncology, Tata Memorial Hospital, Mumbai, India

M. Yashar S. Kalani, Department of Neurosurgery, University of Utah School of Medicine, Salt Lake City, UT, USA

Hiroshi Kanno, Department of Neurosurgery, International University of Health and Welfare Atami Hospital, Atami, Japan

Paul Kleihues, Medical Faculty, University of Zurich, Zurich, Switzerland

Douglas Kondziolka, NYU Langone Medical Center, NYU Neurosurgery Associates, New York, USA

Rolf-Dieter Kortmann, Department of Radiation Oncology, Leipzig, Germany

Edward R. Laws, Jr, Department of Neurosurgery, Brigham and Women's Hospital and Harvard Medical School, Boston, MA, USA

Jay S. Loeffler, Joan and Herman Suit Professor of Radiation Oncology, Departments of Neurosurgery and Radiation Oncology, Chair, Department of Radiation Oncology, Massachusetts General Hospital and Harvard Medical School, Boston, MA, USA

Stephen Lowis, MacMillan Consultant in Paediatric and Adolescent Oncology, Department of Paediatric Haematology, Oncology and BMT, Bristol Royal Hospital for Children, Bristol, UK

David Malkin, Professor, Department of Paediatrics, University of Toronto, Senior Oncologist, Division of Haematology/Oncology, Senior Scientist, Genetics and Genome Biology Program, The Hospital for Sick Children, Toronto, ON, Canada

Robert L. Martuza, William and Elizabeth Sweet Professor in Neuroscience, Harvard Medical School, Department of Neurosurgery, Massachusetts General Hospital, Boston, MA, USA

Minesh P. Mehta, Deputy Director and Chief of Radiation Oncology, Miami Cancer Institute, Miami, FL, USA

Ryo Nishikawa, Professor and Chair, Department of Neurosurgery; Head, Department of Neuro-Oncology, Comprehensive Cancer Center, International Medical Center, Saitama Medical University, Saitama, Japan

Brian P. O'Neill, Professor of Neurology, Department of Neurology, Mayo Clinic, Rochester, MN, USA

Hiroko Ohgaki, Molecular Pathology Section, International Agency for Research on Cancer (IARC), Lyon, France

Barry L. Pizer, Consultant Paediatric Oncologist, Alder Hey Children's Hospital; Honorary Professor, Institute of Translational Medicine, University of Liverpool, UK

Scott R. Plotkin, Professor of Neurology, Associate Director, Stephen E. and Catherine Pappas Center for Neuro-Oncology, Massachusetts General Hospital and Harvard Medical School, Boston, MA, USA

Matthias Preusser, Department of Medicine I and Comprehensive Cancer Center, Medical University of Vienna, Vienna, Austria

Roberta Rudà, Division of Neuro-Oncology, Departments of Neuroscience and Oncology, University and San Giovanni Battista Hospital, Turin, Italy

Elisabeth Rushing, Institute of Neuropathology, University Hospital Zurich, Zurich, Switzerland

Maria Santos, Neurosurgery Department, University Hospital of Santa Maria, Lisbon, Portugal

Sith Sathornsumetee, Associate Professor and Director of Neuro-Oncology Program, Department of Medicine (Neurology), Faculty of Medicine Siriraj Hospital, Mahidol University, Bangkok, Thailand

Gabriele Schackert, Department of Neurosurgery, University of Dresden, Germany

David Schiff, Departments of Neurology, Neurological Surgery, and Medicine (Hematology-Oncology), University of Virginia, Charlottesville, VA, USA

Jonathan Sherman, Department of Neurological Surgery, George Washington University, Washington, DC, USA

Soichiro Shibui, Department of Neurosurgery, Teikyo University Hospital, Tokyo, Japan

Dennis C. Shrieve, Huntsman Cancer Institute Chair in Cancer Research, Professor and Chair, Department of Radiation Oncology, University of Utah School of Medicine, The Huntsman Cancer Hospital, Salt Lake City, UT, USA

Riccardo Soffietti, Department of Neuro-Oncology, University and City of Health and Science Hospital, Turin, Italy

Mark M. Souweidane, Professor of Neurological Surgery, Weill Cornell Medical College, New York, NY, USA

Joachim P. Steinbach, Dr. Senckenberg Institute of Neuro-Oncology, Department of Neurology, Frankfurt University Hospital, Frankfurt, Germany

Walter Stummer, Department of Neurosurgery, University of Münster, Albert-Schweitzer Campus, Münster, Germany

Nancy J. Tarbell, CC Wang Professor of Radiation Oncology, Dean for Academic and Clinical Affairs, Harvard Medical School, Boston, MA, USA

Roger E. Taylor, Professor of Clinical Oncology, College of Medicine, Swansea University, Swansea, UK; Honorary Consultant Clinical Oncologist, South West Wales Cancer Centre, Singleton Hospital, Swansea, UK

Charles Teo, Centre for Minimally Invasive Neurosurgery, Sydney, NSW, Australia

Joerg-Christian Tonn, Department of Neurosurgery, Ludwig Maximilian University Muenchen, Munich, Germany

Michael A. Vogelbaum, Professor of Surgery (Neurosurgery), The Robert W. and Kathryn B. Lamborn Chair for Neuro-Oncology, Cleveland Clinic Lerner College of Medicine of Case Western Reserve University, Associate Director, Rose Ella Burkhardt Brain Tumor and Neuro-Oncology Center, Cleveland Clinic, Cleveland, OH, USA

David Walker, Department of Paediatric Oncology, Nottingham, UK

Colin Watts, Reader in Neurosurgical Oncology, University of Cambridge, Department of Clinical Neurosciences, Division of Neurosurgery, Addenbrooke's Hospital, Cambridge, UK

Howard Weiner, Chief of Neurosurgery, Texas Children's Hospital, Houston, TX, USA

Michael Weller, Professor and Chair, Department of Neurology, University Hospital and University of Zurich, Zurich, Switzerland

Patrick Y. Wen, Professor of Neurology, Harvard Medical School, Director, Center For Neuro-Oncology, Dana-Farber Cancer Institute, Boston, MA, USA

Wolfgang Wick, Chairman and Professor, Neurology Clinic, Heidelberg University Medical Center, Clinical Cooperation Unit Neurooncology, German Cancer Research Center, Heidelberg, Germany

Tai-Tong Wong, Division of Pediatric Neurosurgery, Taipei Veterans General Hospital, National Yang Ming University School of Medicine, Taipei, Taiwan, China

Whitney W. Woodmansee, Division of Endocrinology and Metabolism, Brigham and Women's Hospital, Harvard Medical School, Boston, MA, USA

Takaaki Yanagisawa, Professor, Division of Paediatric Neuro-oncology, Department of Neurosurgery, Jikei University School of Medicine, Tokyo, Japan

CHAPTER 1

The 2016 revision of the WHO classification of tumours of the central nervous system

Paul Kleihues, Elisabeth Rushing, and Hiroko Ohgaki

Introduction

Uniform classification and nomenclature of human cancers are a prerequisite for epidemiological studies of cancer causation, comparison of clinical trials, and the validation of novel cancer therapies. In 1957, the World Health Organization (WHO) established a worldwide network of collaborating centres to establish uniform histological criteria for the diagnosis of human neoplasms. The first edition of the *Histological Typing of Tumours of the Central Nervous System* was edited by K.J. Zülch and published in 1979 (1). Considering the highly divergent views held in the Americas, Asia, and Europe, this classification and grading scheme was a remarkable achievement, although some misclassifications were soon recognized. These were eliminated in the second edition published in 1993, mainly due to the introduction of more sophisticated diagnostic methods, in particular immunohistochemistry (2, 3). A further refinement in the typing of brain cancers was achieved with the addition of genetic profiling, reflected in the title of the third edition: *Pathology and Genetics of Tumours of the Nervous System* (4, 5). A revision of the 2007 fourth edition (6, 7) has been published in 2016 and comprises several newly recognized tumour entities (8). Some of these are histologically recognized, but an ever increasing fraction of CNS neoplasms are now defined by their genetic profile (Table 1.1).

The *WHO Classification of Tumours of the Central Nervous System* has become the internationally accepted nomenclature for brain neoplasms. Cancer registries worldwide now routinely assign the morphology code of the International Classification of Diseases for Oncology (ICD-O) to each tumour entity (9), which facilitates the generation of population-based, epidemiological data on brain tumour incidence and mortality. The WHO grading system assigns a malignancy grade to each neoplasm that is widely used in clinical practice, particularly for gliomas.

Glial and glioneuronal neoplasms

New tumour entities

IDH-wildtype and IDH-mutant glioblastoma

The 2016 *WHO Classification of Tumours of the Central Nervous System* contains important, newly defined subtypes of glioblastoma, primary glioblastoma IDH-wildtype and secondary glioblastoma IDH-mutant. They are histologically largely indistinguishable, but develop in different age groups and carry a significantly different prognosis (10–19) (Table 1.2).

IDH-wildtype glioblastomas develop very rapidly, with a short clinical history. At a population-based level, approximately 90% of all glioblastomas fall into this group (12). They typically develop in older patients (median age 62 years), and are genetically characterized by *TERT* promoter mutations, *EGFR* amplification, and *PTEN* mutations (Table 1.2). The synonymous designation primary glioblastoma IDH-wildtype indicates that this glioblastoma typically arises *de novo*, with no recognizable lower-grade precursor lesion. The prognosis is very poor. Median overall survival of patients with standard treatment with surgery, radiotherapy, and temozolomide is 15 months (17).

IDH-mutant glioblastomas (~10% of all glioblastomas) develop through progression from an antecedent diffuse astrocytoma (WHO grade II) or anaplastic astrocytoma (WHO grade III) and are therefore designated as secondary glioblastoma (8, 10). Patients are younger (median, 44 years), tumours have a lesser degree of necrosis, and are preferentially located in the frontal lobe (Table 1.2). Early genetic alterations already present in their precursor lesions include IDH, *TP53*, and *ATRX* mutations. The presence of an IDH mutation is associated with a hypermethylation phenotype. IDH-mutant glioblastomas carry a significantly better prognosis than IDH-wildtype glioblastomas. Reported overall survival following standard therapy is 31 months (17). Despite similar histological features, primary and secondary glioblastomas are distinct tumour entities that eventually may require different therapeutic approaches.

Diffuse midline glioma, H3 K27M-mutant

This tumour was first introduced as diffuse intrinsic pontine glioma (DIPG). Patients are typically young children with brainstem symptoms and signs of cerebrospinal fluid obstruction that rapidly develop within a few months. On magnetic resonance imaging (MRI), DIPGs often present as a large pontine mass, which may encase the basilar artery. Contrast enhancement is usually focal. Infiltration of neighbouring structures has frequently been

Table 1.1 2016 WHO classification of tumours of the central nervous system

Diffuse astrocytic and oligodendroglial tumours	
Diffuse astrocytoma, IDH-mutant	9400/3
Gemistocytic astrocytoma, IDH-mutant	9411/3
Diffuse astrocytoma, IDH-wildtype	9400/3
Diffuse astrocytoma, NOS	9400/3
Anaplastic astrocytoma, IDH-mutant	9401/3
Anaplastic astrocytoma, IDH-wildtype	9401/3
Anaplastic astrocytoma, NOS	9401/3
Glioblastoma, IDH-wildtype	9440/3
Giant cell glioblastoma	9441/3
Gliosarcoma	9442/3
Epithelioid glioblastoma	9440/3
Glioblastoma, IDH-mutant	9445/3*
Glioblastoma, NOS	9440/3
Diffuse midline glioma, H3 K27M−mutant	9385/3*
Oligodendroglioma, IDH-mutant and 1p / 19q-codeleted	9450/3
Oligodendroglioma, NOS	9450/3
Anaplastic oligodendroglioma, IDH-mutant and 1p/19q-codeleted	9451/3
Anaplastic oligodendroglioma, NOS	9451/3
Oligoastrocytoma, NOS	9382/3
Anaplastic oligoastrocytoma, NOS	9382/3

Other astrocytic tumours	
Pilocytic astrocytoma	9421/1
Pilomyxoid astrocytoma	9425/3
Subependymal giant cell astrocytoma	9384/1
Pleomorphic xanthoastrocytoma	9424/3
Anaplastic pleomorphic xanthoastrocytoma	9424/3

Ependymal tumours	
Subependymoma	9383/1
Myxopapillary ependymoma	9394/1
Ependymoma	9391/3
Papillary ependymoma	9393/3
Clear cell ependymoma	9391/3
Tanycytic ependymoma	9391/3
Ependymoma, *RELA* fusion−positive	9396/3*
Anaplastic ependymoma	9392/3

Other gliomas	
Chordoid glioma of the third ventricle	9444/1
Angiocentric glioma	9431/1
Astroblastoma	9430/3

Choroid plexus tumours	
Choroid plexus papilloma	9390/0
Atypical choroid plexus papilloma	9390/1
Choroid plexus carcinoma	9390/3
Melanotic schwannoma	9560/1
Neurofibroma	9540/0
Atypical neurofibroma	9540/0
Plexiform neurofibroma	9550/0

Neuronal and mixed neuronal-glial tumours	
Dysembryoplastic neuroepithelial tumour	9413/0
Gangliocytoma	9492/0
Ganglioglioma	9505/1
Anaplastic ganglioglioma	9505/3
Dysplastic cerebellar gangliocytoma (Lhermitte–Duclos disease)	9493/0
Desmoplastic infantile astrocytoma and ganglioglioma	9412/1
Papillary glioneuronal tumour	9509/1
Rosette-forming glioneuronal tumour	9509/1
Diffuse leptomeningeal glioneuronal tumour	
Central neurocytoma	9506/1
Extraventricular neurocytoma	9506/1
Cerebellar liponeurocytoma	9506/1
Paraganglioma	8693/1

Tumours of the pineal region	
Pineocytoma	9361/1
Pineal parenchymal tumour of intermediate differentiation	9362/3
Pineoblastoma	9362/3
Papillary tumour of the pineal region	9395/3

Embryonal tumours	
Medulloblastomas, genetically defined	
Medulloblastoma, WNT-activated	9475/3*
Medulloblastoma, SHH-activated and *TP53*-mutant	9476/3*
Medulloblastoma, SHH-activated and *TP53*-wildtype	9471/3
Medulloblastoma, non-WNT/non-SHH	9477/3*
Medulloblastoma, group 3	
Medulloblastoma, group 4	
Medulloblastomas, histologically defined	
Medulloblastoma, classic	9470/3
Medulloblastoma, desmoplastic/nodular	9471/3
Medulloblastoma with extensive nodularity	9471/3
Medulloblastoma, large cell/anaplastic	9474/3
Medulloblastoma, NOS	9470/3
Embryonal tumour with multilayered rosettes, C19MC-altered	9478/3*
Embryonal tumour with multilayered rosettes, NOS	9478/3
Medulloepithelioma	9501/3
CNS neuroblastoma	9500/3
CNS ganglioneuroblastoma	9490/3
CNS embryonal tumour, NOS	9473/3
Atypical teratoid/rhabdoid tumour	9508/3
CNS embryonal tumour with rhabdoid features	9508/3

Tumours of the cranial and paraspinal nerves	9560/0
Schwannoma	
Cellular schwannoma	9560/0
Plexiform schwannoma	9560/0

Table 1.1 Continued

Perineurioma	9571/0
Hybrid nerve sheath tumours	
Malignant peripheral nerve sheath tumour	9540/3
Epithelioid MPNST	9540/3
MPNST with perineurial differentiation	9540/3

Meningiomas

Meningioma	9530/0
Meningothelial meningioma	9531/0
Fibrous meningioma	9532/0
Transitional meningioma	9537/0
Psammomatous meningioma	9533/0
Angiomatous meningioma	9534/0
Microcystic meningioma	9530/0
Secretory meningioma	9530/0
Lymphoplasmacyte-rich meningioma	9530/0
Metaplastic meningioma	9530/0
Chordoid meningioma	9538/1
Clear cell meningioma	9538/1
Atypical meningioma	9539/1
Papillary meningioma	9538/3
Rhabdoid meningioma	9538/3
Anaplastic (malignant) meningioma	9530/3

Mesenchymal, non-meningothelial tumours

Solitary fibrous tumour/haemangiopericytoma	
Grade 1	8815/0
Grade 2	8815/1
Grade 3	8815/3
Haemangioblastoma	9161/1
Haemangioma	9120/0
Epithelioid haemangioendothelioma	9133/3
Angiosarcoma	9120/3
Kaposi sarcoma	9140/3
Ewing sarcoma/PNET	9364/3
Lipoma	8850/0
Angiolipoma	8861/0
Hibernoma	8880/0
Liposarcoma	8850/3
Desmoid-type fibromatosis	8821/1
Myofibroblastoma	8825/0
Inflammatory myofibroblastic tumour	8825/1
Benign fibrous histiocytoma	8830/0
Fibrosarcoma	8810/3
Undifferentiated pleomorphic sarcoma/ malignant fibrous histiocytoma	8802/3
Leiomyoma	8890/0
Leiomyosarcoma	8890/3
Rhabdomyoma	8900/0
Rhabdomyosarcoma	8900/3
Chondroma	9220/0
Chondrosarcoma	9220/3
Osteoma	9180/0
Osteochondroma	9210/0
Osteosarcoma	9180/3

Melanocytic tumours

Meningeal melanocytosis	8728/0
Meningeal melanocytoma	8728/1
Meningeal melanoma	8720/3
Meningeal melanomatosis	8728/3

Lymphomas

Diffuse large B-cell lymphoma of the CNS	9680/3
Immunodeficiency-associated CNS lymphomas	
AIDS-related diffuse large B-cell lymphoma	
EBV-positive diffuse large B-cell lymphoma, NOS	
Lymphomatoid granulomatosis	9766/1
Intravascular large B-cell lymphoma	9712/3
Low-grade B-cell lymphomas of the CNS	
T-cell and NK/T-cell lymphomas of the CNS	
Anaplastic large cell lymphoma, ALK-positive	9714/3
Anaplastic large cell lymphoma, ALK-negative	9702/3
MALT lymphoma of the dura	9699/3

Histiocytic tumours

Langerhans cell histiocytosis	9751/3
Erdheim−Chester disease	9750/1
Rosai−Dorfman disease	
Juvenile xanthogranuloma	
Histiocytic sarcoma	9755/3

Germ cell tumours

Germinoma	9064/3
Embryonal carcinoma	9070/3
Yolk sac tumour	9071/3
Choriocarcinoma	9100/3
Teratoma	9080/1
Mature teratoma	9080/0
Immature teratoma	9080/3
Teratoma with malignant transformation	9084/3
Mixed germ cell tumour	9085/3

Tumours of the sellar region

Craniopharyngioma	9350/1
Adamantinomatous craniopharyngioma	9351/1
Papillary craniopharyngioma	9352/1
Granular cell tumour of the sellar region	9582/0
Pituicytoma	9432/1
Spindle cell oncocytoma	8290/0

Metastatic tumours

The morphology codes are from the International Classification of Diseases for Oncology (ICD-O) (9). Behaviour is coded /0 for benign tumours; /1 for unspecified, borderline, or uncertain behaviour; /2 for carcinoma in situ and grade III intraepithelial neoplasia; and /3 for malignant tumours.

*These new codes were approved by the IARC/WHO Committee for ICD-O.

Reproduced from Louis DN, Ohgaki H, Wiestler OD, Cavenee WK, Ellison DW, Figarella-Branger D, Perry A, Reifenberger G, Von Deimling A (Eds), *World Health Organization Classification of Tumours of the Central Nervous System*, Fourth Edition Revised, Copyright (2016), with permission from IARC Publications.

Table 1.2 Key characteristics of IDH-wildtype and IDH-mutant glioblastoma in adults

	IDH-wildtype glioblastoma	IDH-mutant glioblastoma	References
Synonym	Primary glioblastoma, IDH-wildtype	Secondary glioblastoma, IDH-mutant	10
Precursor lesion	Not identifiable; develops *de novo*	Diffuse astrocytoma Anaplastic astrocytoma	11
Proportion of glioblastomas	~90%	~10%	12
Median age at diagnosis	~62 years	~44 years	12–15
Male-to-female ratio	1.42:1	1.05:1	12, 13, 16
Mean length of clinical history	4 months	15 months	12
Median overall survival Surgery + RT Surgery + RT + chemotherapy	9.9 months 15 months	24 months 31 months	12 17
Location	Supratentorial	Preferentially frontal	16
Necrosis	Extensive	Limited	16
TERT promoter mutations	72%	26%	10, 18
TP53 mutations	27%	81%	12
ATRX mutations	Exceptional	71%	19
EGFR amplification	35%	Exceptional	12
PTEN mutations	24%	Exceptional	12

RT, radiotherapy.

Source data from Louis DN, Ohgaki H, Wiestler OD, Cavenee WK, Ellison DW, Figarella-Branger D, Perry A, Reifenberger G, Von Deimling A (Eds), *World Health Organization Classification of Tumours of the Central Nervous System*, Fourth Edition Revised, Copyright (2016), IARC Publications.

observed. Histopathologically, these tumours are diverse, although commonly show how a uniform population of cells resembling neoplastic astrocytes. Necrosis and vascular proliferation are also seen in some cases.

Heterozygous mutations at position K27 in the histone coding genes *H3F3A*, *HIST1H3B*, and *HIST1H3C* are found in approximately 80% of cases. However, it was then shown that this mutation is present in a larger spectrum of midline gliomas, particularly in the thalamus (~50%) and spinal cord (~60%) (20–25).

Extrapontine lesions typically affect older children and occasionally adults. Since most cases contain the typical mutational profile, the term proposed by the WHO Working Group is diffuse midline glioma, H3 K27M-mutant (8).

Ependymoma, RELA fusion-positive

This subtype of ependymoma accounts for approximately 70% of childhood supratentorial ependymomas (26), but may also develop in adults (27). The histopathological spectrum is variable and does not allow a diagnosis. The defining genetic alteration is a fusion of the *RELA* gene, mostly the *C11orf95-RELA* fusion, which forms in association with chromotrypsis from which oncogenic gene products such as RELA fusion can emerge (26–29). *L1CAM* is typically expressed in tumours with a RELA fusion, which can be identified by immunohistochemistry (26). The prognosis is poor (27).

Anaplastic pleomorphic xanthoastrocytoma

Pleomorphic xanthoastrocytoma (PXA) is a rare glioma that typically manifests in young adults in a preferential superficial location,

often in the temporal lobe (30, 31). Due to its location, seizures are a common clinical feature. On MRI, the tumours present as a supratentorial, peripherally located mass, often with a cystic component (8). PXAs are histologically characterized by neoplastic spindled astrocytes, some of which are exceptionally large and multinucleated, and an admixture of neuronal elements. Despite the pleomorphic appearance, the clinical course is relatively benign (WHO grade II) (8).

The 2016 WHO classification has added anaplastic PXA as a distinct new entity, histologically defined by the presence of more than five mitoses per ten high-power fields (30, 32). Patients have a significantly worse prognosis (8).

Both types of PXA contain the *BRAF* V600E mutation as a genetic signature, which appears to be somewhat more frequent in PXA (50–78% of cases) than in anaplastic PXAs (47–75%) (32, 33). The absence of IDH mutations strongly supports the diagnosis.

Diffuse leptomeningeal glioneuronal tumour

Beck and Russell were the first to describe this entity in 1942, which they reported as oligodendrogliomatosis of the cerebrospinal pathway. Relatively few cases have been added to the literature since then. This rare tumour occurs chiefly but not exclusively in childhood (median age of 5 years), with very few patients older than 18 years. Males are more frequently affected than females. As the name implies, diffuse leptomeningeal glioneuronal tumour is an intracranial and intraspinal tumour that grows largely in the leptomeninges with frequent extension along

Virchow–Robin spaces. Tumour growth is most conspicuous in the posterior fossa, especially along the brainstem and base of the brain. Some examples show an additional intraparenchymal component consisting of well-defined, single or multiple solid or cystic tumour nodules, with intramedullary spinal localization more commonly reported (34–36). Microscopically, tumours closely resemble oligodendroglioma, with sheets or small clusters of uniform, round cells embedded in a desmoplastic stroma. Rarely, ganglion cells in a delicate neuropil background and myxoid change may be seen. Mitotic activity is inconspicuous. Histological evidence of anaplasia such as high mitotic activity (greater than four mitoses per ten high-power fields), vascular proliferation or necrosis is infrequent, and when encountered, more often in recurrences. Immunohistochemically, tumour cells stain strongly and diffusely with OLIG2, and to a slightly lesser extent with S100 protein and glial fibrillary acidic protein (GFAP). The neuronal component is synaptophysin positive. Epithelial membrane antigen (EMA), NeuN, and mutant IDH are consistently negative (34). Molecular profiling typically reveals *KIAA1549-BRAF* gene fusions accompanied by either solitary 1p deletion or 1p19q co-deletions (37). *IDH1* and *IDH2* mutations have not been detected (38), whereas *RAF1* and *BRAF* V600E point mutations have been reported, each in a single patient (39). Despite the presence of disseminated disease, the clinical course of most tumours documented thus far is indolent, albeit marked by considerable morbidity (34, 38).

Newly recognized variants and patterns

Epithelioid glioblastoma
This tumour has been added to the 2016 classification as a provisional variant of glioblastoma IDH-wildtype (8). It occurs preferentially in the cerebral hemispheres and in the diencephalon of young adults and children (8). On MRI, it presents as a contrast-enhancing mass, often with haemorrhages and signs of leptomeningeal spread (40–42). Tumour cells show epithelioid features with distinct cell membranes and an eosinophilic cytoplasm. The cell density is high and foci of necrosis are frequently encountered. Palisading tumour necrosis and vascular proliferation are usually absent. About 50% of cases contain a *BRAF* V600E mutation (40, 41). Since IDH mutations are absent, this lesion is considered a rare variant of IDH wildtype glioblastoma, although typical genetic alterations present in primary IDH-wildtype glioblastomas (*EGFR* amplification, *PTEN* mutation, *CDKN2* homozygous deletion) are infrequent. The prognosis is very poor (40, 43, 44).

Glioblastoma with primitive neuronal component
Primary glioblastoma IDH-wildtype covers a wide spectrum of histological features. Well known is the small cell pattern, which is genetically characterized by a high percentage of *EGFR* amplifications (8). The 2016 classification lists an additional pattern, the glioblastoma with primitive neuronal component (8), first described by Perry et al. (45). This otherwise typical glioblastoma contains sharply delineated foci of increased cellularity and features of primitive neuroectodermal tumours (PNETs), including Homer Wright rosettes and immunoreactivity for neuronal markers such as synaptophysin. In these foci, astrocytic differentiation (GFAP expression) is lost while the mitotic index is higher than

in neighbouring tumour areas (8). The genetic signature is similar to other IDH-wildtype glioblastomas (45). However, approximately 40% of glioblastoma with primitive neuronal component show *MYC* amplification, which is found only in the primitive-appearing nodules (45).

Some examples of this subtype are IDH-mutant secondary glioblastomas. Foci of abrupt transition from low-grade or anaplastic astrocytoma to glioblastoma have been previously described in secondary glioblastomas (46). Again, the proliferation rate was higher and GFAP expression lost but Homer Wright rosettes were absent. These foci have been interpreted as emerging new tumour clones during malignant progression with increased genetic instability. Most foci displayed LOH at one or two flanking markers of *PTEN* but lack *PTEN* mutations (46).

Multinodular and vacuolating neuronal tumour of the cerebrum
Although extremely rare, with fewer than 20 cases reported, multinodular and vacuolating neuronal tumour of the cerebrum deserves separate consideration because of its characteristic histological picture and benign behaviour. Due to the small number of reported cases, it is not included as a distinct entity in the 2016 WHO classification. It occurs chiefly in adults and has a predilection for the temporal lobe. Clinical manifestations reflect location, with seizures as the most common presentation (47–50). These tumours lack contrast enhancement and show a particularly characteristic nodularity and superficial localization on T2 and FLAIR-weighted MRI (47). The microscopic features have a characteristic appearance when seen at low power. Multiple discrete nodules confined to the cortex or subcortical regions are accompanied by marked stromal and intracellular vacuolization. Closer inspection reveals bland-appearing, small- to medium-sized neuroepithelial cells lacking obvious dysmorphic features, and there is virtually no mitotic activity. Immunohistochemical confirmation can be accomplished using a panel of markers such as synaptophysin, OLIG2, and ELAV3/4, which are expressed by the tumour cells, coupled with NeuN, chromogranin, IDH1, and GFAP, which are typically negative (47, 48). In addition, tumour cells display strong immunoreactivity for alpha-internexin, a neuronal intermediate filament (50, 51) and show nuclear labelling with HuCHuD neuronal antigens (47). CD34-positive cells can be encountered in the adjacent cortex (47). Consistent genetic alterations have not been identified, with a *MAP2K1* point mutation reported in a single case; *BRAF* V600E mutations have not been detected (47).

Diagnostic terms deleted from the WHO classification

Gliomatosis cerebri
In previous versions of the WHO classification (6), gliomatosis cerebri was listed as distinct astrocytic tumour, characterized by extensive infiltration of at least three cerebral lobes, usually with bilateral involvement of the cerebral hemispheres and frequent extension into the basal ganglia and infratentorial space. Macroscopy and imaging show large swollen regions without foci of necrosis. There is no primary focus recognizable from which the tumour cells could have spread. Genetic analyses showed that tumours with these stringent criteria were IDH-wildtype and thus a

variant of primary glioblastoma, whereas cases with a solid tumour portion were frequently *IDH1*-mutant (52). A more recent study of 25 cases showed a variable genetic profile (53). Accordingly, the WHO Working Group has recommended to delete this entity from the classification, arguing that glioblastomas can manifest at initial clinical presentation with a gliomatosis cerebri pattern of extensive involvement of the CNS.

Oligoastrocytoma

This tumour is characterized by a conspicuous mixture of two distinct cell types morphologically resembling neoplastic astrocytes and oligodendrocytes (6). The histological diagnosis has been a problem for many years since their response to therapy is largely unpredictable. Genetic analyses showed they carry an IDH mutation in about 80% of cases. However, those with a predominant astrocytic phenotype often have an additional *TP53* mutation, while those with prominent oligodendroglial features have a 1p/19q deletion (54, 55). The problem is that morphologically there is extensive overlap, which often resulted in large differences in incidence between neuropathological laboratories.

The 2016 classification strongly discourages the designation oligoastrocytoma and recommends using genetic analysis for a correct diagnosis of either diffuse astrocytoma or oligodendroglioma (8). The WHO Working Group considered deleting the diagnostic term altogether but rare cases have been reported that carry both a *TP53* mutation and 1p/19q deletion.

Cellular ependymoma

This variant of ependymoma was previously defined as being more common in an extraventricular location and characterized by increased cellularity and mitotic activity. Typical histological features such as perivascular and ependymal rosettes were rare or absent. The WHO Working Group considered these features insufficient for the definition of a variant and recommended deleting it from the WHO classification.

Mesenchymal and nerve sheath tumours

Brain invasive atypical meningioma

Relatively modest changes have been introduced in the meningioma category. In the previous WHO edition, brain invasion as such was not listed as a separate criterion for the diagnosis of atypical meningioma. Instead, the recommendation was made to consider meningiomas with brain invasion, whether histologically benign or atypical, as prognostically equivalent to WHO grade II. Because data derived from large studies have indicated that brain invasion is associated with a greater likelihood of recurrence, the justification for this sometimes confusing definition has gradually eroded (56). Accordingly, the WHO 2016 edition has simplified this task by defining brain invasion as another criterion of atypia, essentially equivalent to increased mitotic activity.

Solitary fibrous tumour and haemangiopericytoma

The concept of solitary fibrous tumour/haemangiopericytoma (SFT/HPC) has undergone significant change over the past decade. For many years the diagnosis has been based on a combination of histopathological and immunohistochemical (variable CD34, CD99, and bcl2 immunoexpression) features (57, 58). The histopathological picture of the classic HPC phenotype is dominated by haphazardly disposed, tightly packed, round to fusiform tumour cells interrupted by ramified and dilated vessels. In contrast, SFT contains abundant, brightly eosinophilic wire-like collagen bands that separate the tumour cells. Identification of a common gene inversion at the 12q13 locus, fusing the *NAB2* and *STAT6* genes, which leads to *STAT6* nuclear expression, clearly supports the contention that these morphologically distinctive neoplasms are closely related (59, 60). The STAT6 nuclear fusion can be demonstrated using routine immunohistochemical methods (61). Similar to their non-meningeal counterparts, fusion variants are recognized, which may correlate with distinct morphological patterns (62, 63). SFT and HPC are now considered to form two ends of a morphological spectrum. In all non-meningeal sites, SFT has become the preferred designation. Whereas most SFTs outside the CNS are clinically benign, meningeal tumours with the haemangiopericytoma phenotype have a higher rate of recurrence (75% >10 years) and 20% are associated with extracranial metastases (64). Accordingly, a separate, three-tiered grading system has been implemented for CNS tumours: a hypocellular, highly collagenized tumour of the SFT phenotype corresponds to grade I, tumours with an HPC phenotype and fewer than five mitoses per ten high-power fields correspond to grade II and HPCs with greater than five mitoses per ten high-power fields, grade III (65, 66). During this transitional period, the recommendation has been made to retain the SFT/HPC designation for CNS tumours, pending further adjustments based on larger clinical studies.

Hybrid nerve sheath tumours

The taxonomic dilemma of assigning a benign peripheral nerve tumour with features of more than one conventional type (neurofibroma, schwannoma, perineurioma) has been resolved with the introduction of the category of hybrid nerve sheath tumour. Combined nerve sheath tumours, which often arise in cutaneous sites and only rarely involve cranial or spinal nerves, have a tendency to occur multifocally, indicating a genetic predisposition. With the exception of hybrid schwannoma/perineurioma, which occurs sporadically (67), hybrid neurofibroma/schwannoma presents in the setting of either schwannomatosis, neurofibromatosis type 1 (NF1) or type 2 (NF2) (68), and hybrid neurofibroma/perineurioma tumours with NF1 (69, 70). The clinical features are dependent on the anatomical site and indistinguishable from other nerve sheath tumours. Microscopically, the dominant component of hybrid schwannoma/perineurioma closely resembles schwannoma with strong S100 and SOX10 positivity, whereas the more subtle perineurioma component is best revealed by EMA, claudin, and GLUT1 immunohistochemistry (71). On the other hand, the two components of hybrid neurofibroma/schwannoma tend to be sharply delineated, although the relative amounts may vary. The immunoprofile of the neurofibroma component reflects the diverse cellular elements with Schwann cells expressing S100 and SOX10, and perineurial cells, EMA and GLUT1. The presence of mosaic SMARCB1 (INI1) immunoexpression suggests that a schwannoma may be associated with neurofibromatosis, especially NF2 and schwannomatosis (72, 73). Rare examples of hybrid neurofibroma/perineurioma have been reported in the setting of NF1, with extensive areas of plexiform neurofibroma blending imperceptibly with perineurioma (69).

Melanotic schwannoma

Melanotic schwannoma is an uncommon, distinctive neural tumour that contains abundant melanin-bearing cells that account for its heavily pigmented gross appearance. Most tumours, which can either be psammomatous or non-psammomatous, arise from spinal or autonomic nerves during adulthood, albeit a decade earlier than conventional schwannomas. Approximately half of patients with psammomatous tumours have evidence of Carney complex, an autosomal dominant disorder, which comprises cardiac myxomas, endocrine overactivity, and lentiginous pigmentation. Patients with Carney complex show allelic loss of the *PRKAR1A* region on 17q (74), which can be detected with a commercially available antibody (75). A genetic signature has not been identified for non-psammomatous tumours, which harbour complex karyotypes with recurrent monosomy of chromosome 22q (76). These tumours deserve special mention because about 10% of melanotic schwannomas follow an aggressive course (75). Although well delineated, tumours are not surrounded by a true capsule. In further contrast to conventional schwannomas, nests of polygonal to spindled-shaped tumour cells, rather than individual cells, are surrounded by laminin and collagen IV. Not surprisingly, tumour cells express melanocytic immunomarkers such as S100, Melan-A, tyrosinase, and HMB-45 (75). Ultrastructurally, tumour cells resemble Schwann cells with elaborate interdigitating processes and are accompanied by melanosomes in different phases of maturation (77).

Embryonal tumours

Since publication of the 2007 WHO classification, the stratification of medulloblastomas has undergone extensive changes. There are now five subtypes based on genetic and expression profiles (Tables 1.3 and 1.4), which correspond to the histological subtypes only to a very limited extent.

Histological stratification of medulloblastomas according to the 2007 WHO classification (6) has indeed limited prognostic value, although it has long been recognized that the desmoplastic and extensive nodularity variants carry a better (7) and the large cell anaplastic variants a worse prognosis. Also, the degree of anaplasia correlates significantly with clinical outcome (78).

Medulloblastoma with extensive nodularity is closely related to the desmoplastic/nodular medulloblastoma (6). It occurs in infants and children below the age of 5, and differs from the desmoplastic variant by exhibiting a markedly expanded lobular architecture. The reticulin-free zones are unusually large and rich in neuropil-like tissue. Such zones contain a population of small cells resembling central neurocytoma and exhibit a streaming pattern. The internodular reticulin-rich component, which dominates in the desmoplastic/nodular variant, is markedly reduced (7). Following radiotherapy or chemotherapy, or both, medulloblastomas with extensive nodularity occasionally undergo maturation to tumours dominated by ganglion cells (79).

DNA sequencing and expression array analysis have led to the identification of five distinct subgroups that greatly differ in clinical outcome (80, 81) (Tables 1.3 and 1.4). The most benign course is seen in medulloblastomas with activation of the WNT pathway, as determined by nuclear β-catenin accumulation, and the presence of *CTNNB1* mutations in most cases (82). This is typically associated with loss of chromosome 6 (83). The affected are mostly children and adults, rarely infants. Immunohistochemistry using an antibody to DKK1, an inhibitor of the WNT pathway, appears to reliably define this group. The WNT subtype shows classic medulloblastoma histology and cannot be identified morphologically. The outcome after standard

Table 1.3 Medulloblastoma subtypes characterized by combined genetic and histological parameters

Genetic profile	Histology	Prognosis
Medulloblastoma, WNT-activated	Classic	Low-risk tumour; classic morphology found in almost all WNT-activated tumours
	Large cell/anaplastic (very rare)	Tumour of uncertain clinicopathological significance
Medulloblastoma, SHH-activated, TP53-mutant	Classic	Uncommon high-risk tumour
	Large cell/anaplastic	High-risk tumour; prevalent in children aged 7–17 years
	Desmoplastic/nodular (very rare)	Tumour of uncertain clinicopathological significance
Medulloblastoma, SHH-activated, TP53-wildtype	Classic	Standard-risk tumour
	Large cell/anaplastic	Tumour of uncertain clinicopathological significance
	Desmoplastic/nodular	Low-risk tumour in infants; prevalent in infants and adults
	Extensive nodularity	Low-risk tumour of infancy
Medulloblastoma, non-WNT/non-SHH, Group 3	Classic	Standard-risk tumour
	Large cell/anaplastic	High-risk tumour
Medulloblastoma, non-WNT/non-SHH, Group 4	Classic	Standard-risk tumour; classic morphology found in almost all Group 4 tumours
	Large cell/anaplastic (rare)	Tumour of uncertain clinicopathological significance

Source data from Louis DN, Ohgaki H, Wiestler OD, Cavenee WK, Ellison DW, Figarella-Branger D, Perry A, Reifenberger G, Von Deimling A (Eds), World Health Organization Classification of Tumours of the Central Nervous System, Fourth Edition Revised, Copyright (2016), IARC Publications.

Table 1.4 Characteristics of genetically defined medulloblastomas

| | WNT- activated | SHH-activated | | Non-WNT/non-SHH | |
		TP53-wildtype	TP53-mutant	Group 3	Group 4
Predominant age(s) at presentation	Childhood	Infancy Adulthood	Childhood	Infancy Childhood	All age groups
Male-to-female ratio	1:2	1:1	1:1	2:1	3:1
Predominant pathological variant(s)	Classic	Desmoplastic/nodular	Large cell/anaplastic	Classic Large cell/ anaplastic	Classic
Frequent copy no. alterations	Monosomy 6	PTCH1 deletion 10q loss	MYCN amplification GLI2 amplification 17p loss	MYC amplification Isodicentric 17q	MYCN amplification Isodicentric 17q
Frequent genetic alterations	CTNNB1 mutation DDX3X mutation TP53 mutation	PTCH1 mutation SMO mutation (adults) SUFU mutation (infants) TERT promoter mutation	TP53 mutation	PVT1-MYC GFI1/GFI1B structural variants	KDM6A GFI1/GFI1B structural variants
Genes with germline mutation	APC	PTCH1 SUFU	TP53		

Source data from Louis DN, Ohgaki H, Wiestler OD, Cavenee WK, Ellison DW, Figarella-Branger D, Perry A, Reifenberger G, Von Deimling A (Eds), *World Health Organization Classification of Tumours of the Central Nervous System, Fourth Edition Revised*, Copyright (2016), IARC Publications.

therapy is remarkably good and dose de-escalation has been suggested for future trials (84).

The SHH type is biologically characterized by activation of the sonic hedgehog signalling pathway, which in about one-third of cases is caused by a mutation in the *PTCH* gene (85). Infants and adults are the preferred age groups. Depending on the *TP53* status, two types are recognized (Tables 1.3 and 1.4). SHH-activated *TP53*-mutant medulloblastomas usually have a large cell/anaplastic histology, affect predominantly children aged 7–17 years, and are clinically high-risk tumours, while SHH-activated *TP53*-wildtype medulloblastomas often show the desmoplastic/nodular phenotype, which is associated with a relatively favourable prognosis (Tables 1.3 and 1.4).

There are two subtypes that are neither WNT- nor SHH-activated (non-WNT/non-SHH medulloblastomas; Group 3 or Group 4 medulloblastomas). They are listed as provisional entities since they are less clearly separable by clinical and genetic criteria (8). Non-WNT/non-SHH tumours account for approximately 60% of all medulloblastomas and typically have classic histopathological features. Most non-WNT/non-SHH tumours present in childhood; they are relatively uncommon in infants and adults. Overexpression of *MYC* is a cardinal feature of Group 3 medulloblastomas, and *MYC* amplification (often associated with *MYC-PVT1* fusion) (86) is common in Group 3 medulloblastomas. *MYC* amplification is found in up to one-quarter of Group 3 tumours, (87, 88). Group 4 tumours are characterized by recurrent alterations in *KDM6A* and *SNCAIP* genes.

This genetically based classification is a great step forward and a valuable basis for future clinical trials.

Embryonal tumour with multilayered rosettes

The nomenclature not only of medulloblastoma but also of other embryonal tumours has undergone significant revision in the WHO 2016 classification. Old classification schemes utilizing separate terms such as medulloepithelioma, ependymoblastoma, and embryonal tumour with abundant neuropil and true rosettes have been replaced with the rubric embryonal tumour with multilayered rosettes (ETMR) (89). The presence of a common molecular signature with alterations (amplifications and fusions) in the *C19MC* locus 19q.13.42 provides convincing evidence that all three morphological patterns are related (90). In fact, any CNS embryonal tumour with alterations in the *C19MC* locus is now considered an ETMR, even when typical morphological features are lacking. Virtually all patients are children under 4 years, most commonly less than age 2 years. There does not seem to be any gender predilection. ETMR is distributed in both supratentorial and infratentorial compartments, although preferentially in the cerebral hemispheres. Tumours tend to be large when first detected and show contrast enhancement on MRI (91–94). The histological hallmark is the presence of distinctive multilayered rosettes, which is featured in the three morphological subtypes of ETMR. Tumours showing the *medulloepithelioma* pattern replicate the appearance of embryonic neural tube with ribbons of primitive pseudostratified, mitotically active cells displaying obvious epithelial features. In the *ependymoblastoma* variant, the outer cell layer of the multilayered rosettes blends into a patternless proliferation of closely packed, small- to medium-sized, undifferentiated cells. *Embryonal tumour with abundant neuropil and true rosettes* is another morphologically distinctive variant in which multilayered rosettes are distributed in a neuropil-rich stroma populated by mature neurocyte-like cells. Immunohistochemically, the primitive neuroepithelial component consistently expresses vimentin and nestin, with strongest expression along the abluminal surface of the multilayered rosettes. In the small cell component, tumour cells show immunoreactivity for synaptophysin, NFP, and NeuN (91, 92). Helpful in the diagnosis of ETMR is the diffuse cytoplasmic immunolabelling with LIN28A, a highly conserved RNA-binding protein

Table 1.5 WHO grades of selected CNS tumours

Diffuse astrocytic and oligodendroglial tumours			Papillary glioneuronal tumour	I
Diffuse astrocytoma, IDH-mutant	II		Rosette-forming glioneuronal tumour	I
Anaplastic astrocytoma, IDH-mutant	III		Central neurocytoma	II
Glioblastoma, IDH-wildtype	IV		Extraventricular neurocytoma	II
Glioblastoma, IDH-mutant	IV		Cerebellar liponeurocytoma	II
Diffuse midline glioma, H3 K27M-mutant	IV		**Tumours of the pineal region**	
Oligodendroglioma, IDH-mutant and 1p/19q-codeleted	II		Pineocytoma	I
Anaplastic oligodendroglioma, IDH-mutant and 1p/19q-codeleted	III		Pineal parenchymal tumour of intermediate differentiation	II or III
			Pineoblastoma	IV
Other astrocytic tumours			Papillary tumour of the pineal region	II or III
Pilocytic astrocytoma	I		**Embryonal tumours**	
Subependymal giant cell astrocytoma	I		Medulloblastoma (all subtypes)	IV
Pleomorphic xanthoastrocytoma	II		Embryonal tumour with multilayered rosettes, C19MC-altered	IV
Anaplastic pleomorphic xanthoastrocytoma	III		Medulloepithelioma	IV
Ependymal tumours			CNS embryonal tumour, NOS	IV
Subependymoma	I		Atypical teratoid/rhabdoid tumour	IV
Myxopapillary ependymomas	I		CNS embryonal tumour with rhabdoid features	IV
Ependymoma	II		**Tumours of the cranial and paraspinal nerves**	
Ependymoma, *RELA* fusion–positive	II or III		Schwannoma	I
Anaplastic ependymoma	III		Neurofibroma	I
Other gliomas			Perineurioma	I
Angiocentric glioma	I		Malignant peripheral nerve sheath tumour (MPNST)	II, III or IV
Chordoid glioma of third ventricle	II		**Meningiomas**	
Choroid plexus tumours			Meningioma	I
Choroid plexus papilloma	I		Atypical meningioma	II
Atypical choroid plexus papilloma	II		Anaplastic (malignant) meningioma	III
Choroid plexus carcinoma	III		**Mesenchymal, non-meningothelial tumours**	
Neuronal and mixed neuronal-glial tumours			Solitary fibrous tumour/haemangiopericytoma	I, II or III
Dysembryoplastic neuroepithelial tumour	I		Haemangioblastoma	I
Gangliocytoma	I		**Tumours of the sellar region**	
Ganglioglioma	I		Craniopharyngioma	I
Anaplastic ganglioglioma	III		Granular cell tumour	I
Dysplastic gangliocytoma of cerebellum (Lhermitte–Duclos)	I		Pituicytoma	I
Desmoplastic infantile astrocytoma and ganglioglioma	I		Spindle cell oncocytoma	I

Adapted from Louis DN, Ohgaki H, Wiestler OD, Cavenee WK, Ellison DW, Figarella-Branger D, Perry A, Reifenberger G, Von Deimling A (Eds), World Health Organization Classification of Tumours of the Central Nervous System, Fourth Edition Revised, Copyright (2016), with permission from IARC Publications.

involved in many biological processes (93, 95, 96). However, it should be noted that *LIN28A* is expressed in other CNS tumours including ATRT and even gliomas (93, 97). The outlook for patients with ETMR is grave, with survival averaging 12 months despite multimodal therapy (91, 93, 94).

WHO grading of central nervous system tumours

In many organ sites, the histological grading of tumours is an important criterion for therapeutic decisions, in particular, whether or not adjuvant radio-chemotherapy is likely to improve clinical outcome. The WHO grading is based on a four-tier system, although there is no brain tumour that actually occurs over this entire range. Some brain neoplasms only manifest as a single grade, for example, pilocytic astrocytoma, subependymoma, subependymal giant cell astrocytoma, myxopapillary ependymoma, and most glioneuronal tumours (6–8) (Table 1.5). Accordingly, WHO grading is best defined as a malignancy scale across a large number of diverse neoplasms.

From a clinical point of view, the relevance of tumour grades may not be as significant as before. There are new, genetically defined entities, for example, the secondary glioblastoma IDH-mutant, which clearly has a better prognosis than primary glioblastoma IDH-wildtype. It remains to be shown whether this justifies the assignment of WHO grade III for secondary glioblastoma IDH-mutant. On the other hand, IDH-mutant diffuse astrocytomas WHO grade II and anaplastic astrocytomas WHO grade

III show insignificant differences in survival (17). This is probably due to a contamination of anaplastic astrocytomas with IDH-wildtype gliomas, in particular, primary glioblastomas. Similarly, the response to therapy of grade II and III oligodendrogliomas is comparable and generally better if defined by 1p/19q co-deletion and IDH mutation (17). Medulloblastomas are all assigned grade IV, although the prognosis of patients with WNT-activated medulloblastoma is excellent; with current surgical approaches and adjuvant therapy regimens, overall survival is close to 100% (82, 98). A lower grade cannot be assigned since grading reflects the inherent malignancy of a tumour and does not change with therapeutic progress.

References

1. Zulch KJ. *Histological Typing of Tumours of the Central Nervous System.* Geneva: World Health Organization, 1979.

2. Kleihues P, Burger PC, Scheithauer BW. *Histological Typing of Tumours of the Central Nervous System. World Health Organization International Histological Classification of Tumours* (2nd edn). New York: Springer Verlag, 1993.

3. Kleihues P, Burger PC, Scheithauer BW. The new WHO classification of brain tumours. *Brain Pathol* 1993; 3(3):255–268.

4. Kleihues P, Cavenee WK. *Pathology and Genetics of Tumours of the Nervous System.* Lyon: International Agency for Research on Cancer, 1997.

5. Kleihues P, Louis DN, Scheithauer BW, et al. The WHO classification of tumors of the nervous system. *J Neuropathol Exp Neurol* 2002; 61(3):215–225.

6. Louis DN, Ohgaki H, Wiestler OD, et al. (eds). *WHO Classification of Tumours of the Central Nervous System.* Lyon: International Agency for Research on Cancer, 2007.

7. Louis DN, Ohgaki H, Wiestler OD, et al. The 2007 WHO Classification of Tumours of the Central Nervous System. *Acta Neuropathol (Berl)* 2007; 114(2):97–109.

8. Louis DN, Ohgaki H, Wiestler OD, et al. (eds). *WHO Classification of Tumours of the Central Nervous System* (revised 4th edn). Lyon: International Agency for Research on Cancer, 2016.

9. Fritz A, Percy C, Jack A, et al. *ICD-O International Classification of Diseases for Oncology* (3rd edn). Geneva: World Health Organization, 2000.

10. Ohgaki H, Kleihues P. The definition of primary and secondary glioblastoma. *Clin Cancer Res* 2013; 19(4):764–772.

11. Ohgaki H, Kleihues P. Genetic pathways to primary and secondary glioblastoma. *Am J Pathol* 2007; 170(5):1445–1453.

12. Nobusawa S, Watanabe T, Kleihues P, et al. IDH1 mutations as molecular signature and predictive factor of secondary glioblastomas. *Clin Cancer Res* 2009; 15(19):6002–6007.

13. Bleeker FE, Atai NA, Lamba S, et al. The prognostic IDH1(R132) mutation is associated with reduced NADP+-dependent IDH activity in glioblastoma. *Acta Neuropathol* 2010; 119(4):487–494.

14. Ichimura K, Pearson DM, Kocialkowski S, et al. IDH1 mutations are present in the majority of common adult gliomas but rare in primary glioblastomas. *Neuro Oncol* 2009; 11(4):341–347.

15. Reuss DE, Mamatjan Y, Schrimpf D, et al. IDH mutant diffuse and anaplastic astrocytomas have similar age at presentation and little difference in survival: a grading problem for WHO. *Acta Neuropathol* 2015; 129(6):867–873.

16. Lai A, Kharbanda S, Pope WB, et al. Evidence for sequenced molecular evolution of IDH1 mutant glioblastoma from a distinct cell of origin. *J Clin Oncol* 2011; 29(34):4482–4490.

17. Yan H, Parsons DW, Jin G, et al. IDH1 and IDH2 mutations in gliomas. *N Engl J Med* 2009; 360(8):765–773.

18. Nonoguchi N, Ohta T, Oh JE, et al. TERT promoter mutations in primary and secondary glioblastomas. *Acta Neuropathol* 2013; 126(6):931–937.

19. Liu XY, Gerges N, Korshunov A, et al. Frequent ATRX mutations and loss of expression in adult diffuse astrocytic tumors carrying IDH1/IDH2 and TP53 mutations. *Acta Neuropathol* 2012; 124(5):615–625.

20. Buczkowicz P, Hoeman C, Rakopoulos P, et al. Genomic analysis of diffuse intrinsic pontine gliomas identifies three molecular subgroups and recurrent activating ACVR1 mutations. *Nat Genet* 2014; 46(5):451–456.

21. Fontebasso AM, Papillon-Cavanagh S, Schwartzentruber J, et al. Recurrent somatic mutations in ACVR1 in pediatric midline high-grade astrocytoma. *Nat Genet* 2014; 46(5):462–466.

22. Schwartzentruber J, Korshunov A, Liu XY, et al. Driver mutations in histone H3.3 and chromatin remodelling genes in paediatric glioblastoma. *Nature* 2012; 482(7384):226–231.

23. Taylor KR, Mackay A, Truffaux N, et al. Recurrent activating ACVR1 mutations in diffuse intrinsic pontine glioma. *Nat Genet* 2014; 46(5):457–461.

24. Wu G, Broniscer A, McEachron TA, et al. Somatic histone H3 alterations in pediatric diffuse intrinsic pontine gliomas and non-brainstem glioblastomas. *Nat Genet* 2012; 44(3):251–253.

25. Wu G, Diaz AK, Paugh BS, et al. The genomic landscape of diffuse intrinsic pontine glioma and pediatric non-brainstem high-grade glioma. *Nat Genet* 2014; 46(5):444–450.

26. Parker M, Mohankumar KM, Punchihewa C, et al. C11orf95-RELA fusions drive oncogenic NF-kappaB signalling in ependymoma. *Nature* 2014; 506(7489):451–455.

27. Pajtler KW, Witt H, Sill M, et al. Molecular classification of ependymal tumors across all CNS compartments, histopathological grades, and age groups. *Cancer Cell* 2015; 27(5):728–743.

28. Pietsch T, Wohlers I, Goschzik T, et al. Supratentorial ependymomas of childhood carry C11orf95-RELA fusions leading to pathological activation of the NF-kappaB signaling pathway. *Acta Neuropathol* 2014; 127(4):609–611.

29. Zhang CZ, Leibowitz ML, Pellman D. Chromothripsis and beyond: rapid genome evolution from complex chromosomal rearrangements. *Genes Dev* 2013; 27(23):2513–2530.

30. Giannini C, Scheithauer BW, Burger PC, et al. Pleomorphic xanthoastrocytoma: what do we really know about it? *Cancer* 1999; 85(9):2033–2045.

31. Kepes JJ, Rubinstein LJ, Eng LF. Pleomorphic xanthoastrocytoma: a distinctive meningocerebral glioma of young subjects with relatively favorable prognosis. A study of 12 cases. *Cancer* 1979; 44(5):1839–1852.

32. Ida CM, Rodriguez FJ, Burger PC, et al. Pleomorphic xanthoastrocytoma: natural history and long-term follow-up. *Brain Pathol* 2015; 25(5):575–586.

33. Schmidt Y, Kleinschmidt-DeMasters BK, Aisner DL, et al. Anaplastic PXA in adults: case series with clinicopathologic and molecular features. *J Neurooncol* 2013; 111(1):59–69.

34. Rodriguez FJ, Perry A, Rosenblum MK, et al. Disseminated oligodendroglial-like leptomeningeal tumor of childhood: a distinctive clinicopathologic entity. *Acta Neuropathol* 2012; 124(5):627–641.

35. Cho HJ, Myung JK, Kim H, et al. Primary diffuse leptomeningeal glioneuronal tumors. *Brain Tumor Pathol* 2015; 32(1):49–55.

36. Gardiman MP, Fassan M, Orvieto E, et al. Diffuse leptomeningeal glioneuronal tumors: a new entity? *Brain Pathol* 2010; 20(2):361–366.

37. Rodriguez FJ, Schniederjan MJ, Nicolaides T, et al. High rate of concurrent BRAF-KIAA1549 gene fusion and 1p deletion in disseminated oligodendroglioma-like leptomeningeal neoplasms (DOLN). *Acta Neuropathol* 2015; 129(4):609–610.

38. Preuss M, Christiansen H, Merkenschlager A, et al. Disseminated oligodendroglial-like leptomeningeal tumors: preliminary diagnostic and therapeutic results for a novel tumor entity [corrected]. *J Neurooncol* 2015; 124(1):65–74.

39. Dodgshun AJ, SantaCruz N, Hwang J, et al. Disseminated glioneuronal tumors occurring in childhood: treatment outcomes and BRAF alterations including V600E mutation. *J Neurooncol* 2016; 128(2):293–302.

40. Broniscer A, Tatevossian RG, Sabin ND, et al. Clinical, radiological, histological and molecular characteristics of paediatric epithelioid glioblastoma. *Neuropathol Appl Neurobiol* 2014; 40(3):327–336.

41. Kleinschmidt-DeMasters BK, Aisner DL, Birks DK, et al. Epithelioid GBMs show a high percentage of BRAF V600E mutation. *Am J Surg Pathol* 2013; 37(5):685–698.

42. Tanaka S, Nakada M, Nobusawa S, et al. Epithelioid glioblastoma arising from pleomorphic xanthoastrocytoma with the BRAF V600E mutation. *Brain Tumor Pathol* 2014; 31(3):172–176.

43. Chen SC, Lin DS, Lee CC, et al. Rhabdoid glioblastoma: a recently recognized subtype of glioblastoma. *Acta Neurochir (Wien)* 2013; 155(8):1443–1448.

44. Kleinschmidt-DeMasters BK, Alassiri AH, Birks DK, et al. Epithelioid versus rhabdoid glioblastomas are distinguished by monosomy 22 and immunohistochemical expression of INI-1 but not claudin 6. *Am J Surg Pathol* 2010; 34(3):341–354.

45. Perry A, Miller CR, Gujrati M, et al. Malignant gliomas with primitive neuroectodermal tumor-like components: a clinicopathologic and genetic study of 53 cases. *Brain Pathol*, 2009; 19(1):81–90.

46. Fujisawa H, Kurrer M, Reis RM, et al. Acquisition of the glioblastoma phenotype during astrocytoma progression is associated with LOH on chromosome 10q25-qter. *Am J Pathol* 1999; 155(2):387–394.

47. Huse JT, Edgar M, Halliday J, et al. Multinodular and vacuolating neuronal tumors of the cerebrum: 10 cases of a distinctive seizure-associated lesion. *Brain Pathol* 2013; 23(5):515–524.

48. Bodi I, Curran O, Selway R, et al. Two cases of multinodular and vacuolating neuronal tumour. *Acta Neuropathol Commun* 2014; 2:7.

49. Fukushima S, Yoshida A, Narita Y, et al. Multinodular and vacuolating neuronal tumor of the cerebrum. *Brain Tumor Pathol* 2015; 32(2):131–136.

50. Yamaguchi M, Komori T, Nakata Y, et al. Multinodular and vacuolating neuronal tumor affecting amygdala and hippocampus: a quasi-tumor? *Pathol Int* 2016; 66(1):34–41.

51. Nagaishi M, Yokoo H, Nobusawa S, et al. Localized overexpression of alpha-internexin within nodules in multinodular and vacuolating neuronal tumors. *Neuropathology* 2015; 35(6):561–568.

52. Seiz M, Tuettenberg J, Meyer J, et al. Detection of IDH1 mutations in gliomatosis cerebri, but only in tumors with additional solid component: evidence for molecular subtypes. *Acta Neuropathol* 2010; 120(2):261–267.

53. Herrlinger U, Jones DT, Glas M, et al. Gliomatosis cerebri: no evidence for a separate brain tumor entity. *Acta Neuropathol* 2016; 131(2):309–319.

54. Ohgaki H, Kleihues P. Genetic profile of astrocytic and oligodendroglial gliomas. *Brain Tumor Pathol* 2011; 28(3):177–183.

55. Kim YH, Nobusawa S, Mittelbronn M, et al. Molecular classification of low-grade diffuse gliomas. *Am J Pathol* 2010; 177(6):2708–2714.

56. Perry A, Stafford SL, Scheithauer BW, et al. Meningioma grading: an analysis of histologic parameters. *Am J Surg Pathol* 1997; 21(12):1455–1465.

57. Perry A, Scheithauer BW, Nascimento AG. The immunophenotypic spectrum of meningeal hemangiopericytoma: a comparison with fibrous meningioma and solitary fibrous tumor of meninges. *Am J Surg Pathol* 1997; 21(11):1354–1360.

58. Rajaram V, Brat DJ, Perry A. Anaplastic meningioma versus meningeal hemangiopericytoma: immunohistochemical and genetic markers. *Hum Pathol* 2004; 35(11):1413–1418.

59. Robinson DR, Wu YM, Kalyana-Sundaram S, et al. Identification of recurrent NAB2-STAT6 gene fusions in solitary fibrous tumor by integrative sequencing. *Nat Genet* 2013; 45(2):180–185.

60. Chmielecki J, Crago AM, Rosenberg M, et al. Whole-exome sequencing identifies a recurrent NAB2-STAT6 fusion in solitary fibrous tumors. *Nat Genet* 2013; 45(2):131–132.

61. Schweizer L, Koelsche C, Sahm F, et al. Meningeal hemangiopericytoma and solitary fibrous tumors carry the NAB2-STAT6 fusion and can be diagnosed by nuclear expression of STAT6 protein. *Acta Neuropathol* 2013; 125(5):651–658.

62. Fritchie KJ, Jin L, Rubin BP, et al. NAB2-STAT6 gene fusion in meningeal hemangiopericytoma and solitary fibrous tumor. *J Neuropathol Exp Neurol* 2016; 75(3):263–271.

63. Yuzawa S, Nishihara H, Wang L, et al. Analysis of NAB2-STAT6 gene fusion in 17 cases of meningeal solitary fibrous tumor/hemangiopericytoma: review of the literature. *Am J Surg Pathol* 2016; 40(8):1031–1040.

64. Guthrie BL, Ebersold MJ, Scheithauer BW, et al. Meningeal hemangiopericytoma: histopathological features, treatment, and long-term follow-up of 44 cases. *Neurosurgery* 1989; 25(4):514–522.

65. Mena H, Ribas JL, Pezeshkpour GH, et al. Hemangiopericytoma of the central nervous system: a review of 94 cases. *Hum Pathol* 1991; 22(1):84–91.

66. Bouvier C, Metellus P, de Paula AM, et al. Solitary fibrous tumors and hemangiopericytomas of the meninges: overlapping pathological features and common prognostic factors suggest the same spectrum of tumors. *Brain Pathol*, 2012; 22(4):511–521.

67. Hornick JL, Bundock EA, Fletcher CD. Hybrid schwannoma/perineurioma: clinicopathologic analysis of 42 distinctive benign nerve sheath tumors. *Am J Surg Pathol* 2009; 33(10):1554–1561.

68. Harder A, Wesemann M, Hagel C, et al. Hybrid neurofibroma/schwannoma is overrepresented among schwannomatosis and neurofibromatosis patients. *Am J Surg Pathol* 2012; 36(5):702–709.

69. Kacerovska D, Michal M, Kuroda N, et al. Hybrid peripheral nerve sheath tumors, including a malignant variant in type 1 neurofibromatosis. *Am J Dermatopathol* 2013; 35(6):641–649.

70. Inatomi Y, Ito T, Nagae K, et al. Hybrid perineurioma-neurofibroma in a patient with neurofibromatosis type 1, clinically mimicking malignant peripheral nerve sheath tumor. *Eur J Dermatol* 2014; 24(3):412–413.

71. Yang X, Zeng Y, Wang J. Hybrid schwannoma/perineurioma: report of 10 Chinese cases supporting a distinctive entity. *Int J Surg Pathol* 2013; 21(1):22–28.

72. Patil S, Perry A, MacCollin M, et al. Immunohistochemical analysis supports a role for INI1/SMARCB1 in hereditary forms of schwannomas, but not in solitary, sporadic schwannomas. *Brain Pathol* 2008; 18(4):517–519.

73. Plotkin SR, Blakeley JO, Evans DG, et al. Update from the 2011 International Schwannomatosis Workshop: from genetics to diagnostic criteria. *Am J Med Genet A* 2013; 161A(3):405–416.

74. Stratakis CA. Mutations of the gene encoding the protein kinase A type I-alpha regulatory subunit (PRKAR1A) in patients with the 'complex of spotty skin pigmentation, myxomas, endocrine overactivity, and schwannomas' (Carney complex). *Ann N Y Acad Sci* 2002; 968, 3–21.

75. Torres-Mora J, Dry S, Li X, Binder S, Amin M, Folpe AL. Malignant melanotic schwannian tumor: a clinicopathologic, immunohistochemical, and gene expression profiling study of 40 cases, with a proposal for the reclassification of 'melanotic schwannoma'. *Am J Surg Pathol* 2014; 38(1):94–105

76. Koelsche C, Hovestadt V, Jones DT, et al. Melanotic tumors of the nervous system are characterized by distinct mutational, chromosomal and epigenomic profiles. *Brain Pathol* 2015; 25(2):202–208.

77. Di BC, Declich P, Assi A, et al. Melanotic schwannoma of the sympathetic ganglia: a histologic, immunohistochemical and ultrastructural study. *J Neurooncol* 1997; 35(2):149–152.

78. Giangaspero F, Wellek S, Masuoka J, et al. Stratification of medulloblastoma on the basis of histopathological grading. *Acta Neuropathol (Berl)* 2006; 112(1):5–12.

79. de Chadarevian JP, Montes JL, O'Gorman AM, et al. Maturation of cerebellar neuroblastoma into ganglioneuroma with melanosis. A histologic, immunocytochemical, and ultrastructural study. *Cancer* 1987; 59(1):69–76.

80. Kool M, Korshunov A, Remke M, et al. Molecular subgroups of medulloblastoma: an international meta-analysis of transcriptome, genetic aberrations, and clinical data of WNT, SHH, Group 3, and Group 4 medulloblastomas. *Acta Neuropathol* 2012; 123(4):473–484.

81. Taylor MD, Northcott PA, Korshunov A, et al. Molecular subgroups of medulloblastoma: the current consensus. *Acta Neuropathol* 2012; 123(4):465–472.

82. Ellison DW, Onilude OE, Lindsey JC, et al. β-Catenin status predicts a favorable outcome in childhood medulloblastoma: the United Kingdom Children's Cancer Study Group Brain Tumour Committee. *J Clin Oncol* 2005; 23(31):7951–7957.

83. Clifford SC, Lusher ME, Lindsey JC, et al. Wnt/Wingless pathway activation and chromosome 6 loss characterize a distinct molecular sub-group of medulloblastomas associated with a favorable prognosis. *Cell Cycle* 2006; 5(22):2666–2670.

84. Ramaswamy V, Northcott PA, Taylor MD. FISH and chips: the recipe for improved prognostication and outcomes for children with medulloblastoma. *Cancer Genet* 2011; 204(11):577–588.

85. Schwalbe EC, Lindsey JC, Straughton D, et al. Rapid diagnosis of medulloblastoma molecular subgroups. *Clin Cancer Res* 2011; 17(7):1883–1894.

86. Northcott PA, Shih DJ, Peacock J, et al. Subgroup-specific structural variation across 1,000 medulloblastoma genomes. *Nature* 2012; 488(7409):49–56.

87. Ellison DW, Kocak M, Dalton J, et al. Definition of disease-risk stratification groups in childhood medulloblastoma using combined clinical, pathologic, and molecular variables. *J Clin Oncol* 2011; 29(11):1400–1407.

88. Lamont JM, McManamy CS, Pearson AD, et al. Combined histopathological and molecular cytogenetic stratification of medulloblastoma patients. *Clin Cancer Res* 2004; 10(16):5482–5493.

89. Korshunov A, Jakobiec FA, Eberhart CG, et al. Comparative integrated molecular analysis of intraocular medulloepitheliomas and central nervous system embryonal tumors with multilayered rosettes confirms that they are distinct nosologic entities. *Neuropathology* 2015; 35(6):538–544.

90. Korshunov A, Remke M, Gessi M, et al. Focal genomic amplification at 19q13.42 comprises a powerful diagnostic marker for embryonal tumors with ependymoblastic rosettes. *Acta Neuropathol* 2010; 120(2):253–260.

91. Gessi M, Giangaspero F, Lauriola L, et al. Embryonal tumors with abundant neuropil and true rosettes: a distinctive CNS primitive neuroectodermal tumor. *Am J Surg Pathol* 2009; 33(2):211–217.

92. Korshunov A, Sturm D, Ryzhova M, et al. Embryonal tumor with abundant neuropil and true rosettes (ETANTR), ependymoblastoma, and medulloepithelioma share molecular similarity and comprise a single clinicopathological entity. *Acta Neuropathol* 2014; 128(2):279–289.

93. Spence T, Sin-Chan P, Picard D, et al. CNS-PNETs with C19MC amplification and/or LIN28 expression comprise a distinct histogenetic diagnostic and therapeutic entity. *Acta Neuropathol* 2014; 128(2):291–303.

94. Horwitz M, Dufour C, Leblond P, et al. Embryonal tumors with multilayered rosettes in children: the SFCE experience. *Childs Nerv Syst* 2016; 32(2):299–305.

95. Korshunov A, Ryzhova M, Jones DT, et al. LIN28A immunoreactivity is a potent diagnostic marker of embryonal tumor with multilayered rosettes (ETMR). *Acta Neuropathol* 2012; 124(6):875–881.

96. Hennchen M, Stubbusch J, Abarchan-El Makhfi I, et al. Lin28B and Let-7 in the control of sympathetic neurogenesis and neuroblastoma development. *J Neurosci* 2015; 35(50):16531–16544.

97. Weingart MF, Roth JJ, Hutt-Cabezas M, et al. Disrupting LIN28 in atypical teratoid rhabdoid tumors reveals the importance of the mitogen activated protein kinase pathway as a therapeutic target. *Oncotarget* 2015; 6(5):3165–3177.

98. Thompson MC, Fuller C, Hogg TL, et al. Genomics identifies medulloblastoma subgroups that are enriched for specific genetic alterations. *J Clin Oncol* 2006; 24(12):1924–1931.

CHAPTER 2

Astrocytic tumours: pilocytic astrocytoma, pleomorphic xanthoastrocytoma, and subependymal giant cell astrocytoma

Brian P. O'Neill, Jeffrey Allen,
Mitchell S. Berger, and Rolf-Dieter Kortmann

Definitions (histology)

The following definitions are taken from the *WHO Classification of Tumours of the Central Nervous System*, fourth edition (1).

- *Pilocytic astrocytoma (PA) (World Health Organization (WHO) grade I)*: a relatively circumscribed, slow-growing, often cystic astrocytoma occurring in children and young adults, histologically characterized by a biphasic pattern with varying proportions of compacted bipolar cells associated with Rosenthal fibres and loose-textured multipolar cells associated with microcysts and eosinophilic granular bodies. Most PAs are localized, macrocystic, and only marginally infiltrative. However some PAs, such as those arising in the optic pathways, are rarely cystic and may have an extensive infiltrative pattern but within a neuroanatomical pathway.

- *Pleomorphic xanthoastrocytoma (PXA) (WHO grade II)*: an astrocytic neoplasm with a relatively favourable prognosis, typically encountered in children and young adults, with superficial location in the cerebral hemispheres and involvement of the meninges; characteristic histological features include pleomorphic and lipidized cells expressing glial fibrillary acidic protein and often surrounded by a reticulin network as well as eosinophilic granular bodies.

- *Subependymal giant cell astrocytoma (SEGA) (WHO grade I)*: a benign, slow-growing tumour typically arising in the wall of the lateral ventricles and composed of large ganglioid astrocytes. It is the most common central nervous system (CNS) neoplasm in patients with tuberous sclerosis.

Epidemiology

Much of the epidemiological data in this section is derived from the Central Brain Tumor Registry of the United States (CBTRUS) Statistical Report for 2005–2009 (2). CBTRUS is a research organization that provides quality statistical data on population-based primary brain and CNS incident tumours in the United States. CBTRUS works in partnership with a public surveillance organization, the National Program of Central Registries (NPCR) (3), from which data are directly received under a special agreement. This agreement permits transfer of data through the Case Submission Specifications (NPCR-CSS) mechanism, the system utilized for collection of central (state) cancer data (4). CBTRUS combines the NPCR data with data from the National Cancer Institute (NCI) Surveillance, Epidemiology and End Results (SEER) Program (5).

A major limitation of the CBTRUS is that it is histology based: patients with suspected primary brain tumours are not registered. This practice excludes most children with a diagnosis of an optic pathway glioma, diffuse infiltrative pontine glioma, tectal glioma, or other indolent brainstem tumours that are clinically diagnosed such as those that arise in children with neurofibromatosis type 1 (NF1). The majority of these patients probably have some form of low-grade glioma (LGG), such as a PA. Another limitation is that NF1-associated tumours are not differentiated, impacting epidemiological data and interpretation. Given the relative infrequency of PXA and SEGA, precise epidemiological data is scant and likely not reliable. Nevertheless, recent incidence data suggests that the diagnosis of low-grade astrocytoma (LGA) is distributed rather evenly throughout childhood (6).

Another confounding contemporary variable is the increasing awareness of brain lesions suggestive of incidentally diagnosed LGA encountered with the liberal use of screening magnetic resonance imaging (MRI) for such indications as headache disorders, minor head injuries, and a baseline MRI prior to instituting growth hormone therapy in children with idiopathic short stature. Such presumably asymptomatic lesions are rarely biopsied but may represent early manifestations of LGGs that could become symptomatic later in life.

Age, race, and gender

The overall distribution of primary brain tumours for all ages by major histological group is shown in Fig. 2.1. Fig. 2.2 displays the distribution in children and adolescents, and Fig. 2.3 shows the distribution of primary brain and CNS tumours by histology in young adults (ages 20–34 years) (2).

Within these distributions, PAs represent approximately 5–6% of all gliomas and have an overall incidence of 0.37 per 100,000 persons per year (7). Because their discovery is often in the first three decades, the distributions are respectively 0.750, 0.671, and 0.121 per 100,000 person-years for the first, second, and third decades respectively (8). There is no gender preference.

Incidence data by race are shown in Fig. 2.4 (1). In many epidemiological studies of glioblastoma, incidence rates by race varied about three- to four-fold, with the highest among non-Hispanic white people followed by Hispanic white people, black people, Asian/Pacific Islanders, and American Indians/Alaskan Natives (9). These figures may be skewed by the fact that glioblastomas occur in older adults and thus incidence is affected by mortality figures for the population studied. For example, the incidence of glioblastoma in parts of Africa may be obscured by the reduced life expectancy of black people there versus North America.

Comparable studies of LGGs by race tend to consider LGG as a group rather than report data on histological subtypes such as PA, PXA, and SEGA. Furthermore, comparisons of glioblastoma and 'non-glioblastoma' incidence by race did not differentiate between the subtypes; the 'non-glioblastoma' category included those forms usually considered as WHO grades II and III but was not further subdivided nor was there a differentiation between those associated

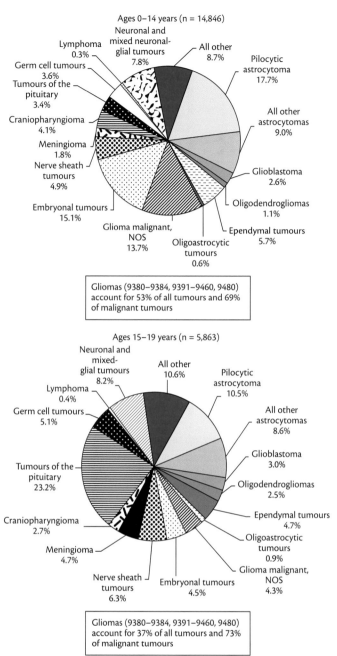

Gliomas (9380–9384, 9391–9460, 9480) account for 53% of all tumours and 69% of malignant tumours

Gliomas (9380–9384, 9391–9460, 9480) account for 37% of all tumours and 73% of malignant tumours

Fig. 2.2 Distribution of primary brain and CNS tumours by major histological group in children and adolescents.

with NF1 and those not associated (10). As with glioblastoma, rates for non-glioblastoma were highest among non-Hispanic white people followed by Hispanic white people, with rates among black people, Asian/Pacific Islanders, and American Indians/Alaskan Natives each about 40% of the rates among non-Hispanic white people. The difference in race/ethnic variation between glioblastoma and non-glioblastoma was highly significant among both males and females (P-value for heterogeneity <0.0001 in each sex) (10).

Anatomical distribution

In all age groups combined, the cerebellum (43%) and supratentorial structures (37%), excluding the optic pathway and hypothalamus,

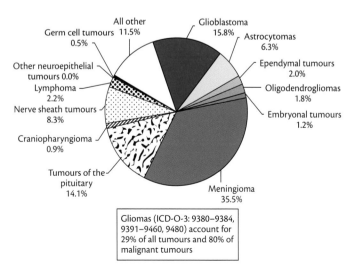

Gliomas (ICD-O-3: 9380–9384, 9391–9460, 9480) account for 29% of all tumours and 80% of malignant tumours

Fig. 2.1 Overall distribution of primary brain tumours for all ages by major histological group.

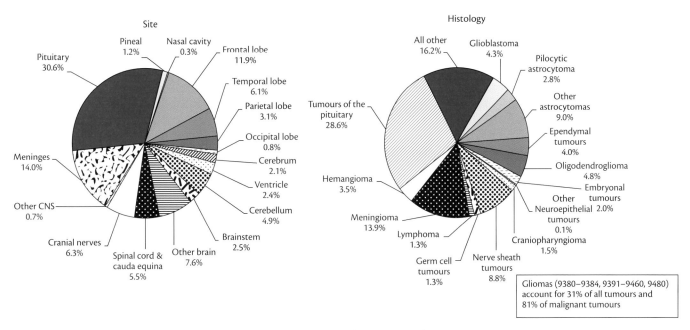

Fig. 2.3 Distribution of primary brain and CNS tumours by histology in young adults (ages 20–34 years).

were affected at a similar frequency. There is a significant age factor, however. In a population-based study of PAs from the canton of Zurich (Switzerland) (11), the majority of PAs in children, in whom histological material was available, were located in the cerebellum (67%); whereas those in adults most frequently involved supratentorial structures (55%) (Fig. 2.5). However, it is customary not to biopsy clinically diagnosed optic pathway gliomas, especially those arising in patients with NF, with the assumption that the vast majority represent PAs.

The 'optic nerve glioma syndrome' in NF children is somewhat unpredictable, and precise clinical criteria justifying chemotherapy intervention are evolving (12). Approximately 20% of unselected children under 5 years of age with NF1 will have an abnormality on MRI suggestive of an optic nerve glioma, but less than half of these children will develop clinical symptoms (13). Some children may have clear MRI features of an optic nerve glioma without any visual loss of optic atrophy; and in a small minority, these MRI features may improve and even normalize over time without any intervention. For those who are treated with some form of chemotherapy, only one-third will experience improvement in visual function, whether or not improvement is documented on MRI (14). The selection of chemotherapy alternatives for children with NF1 is more limited since there is a conscientious attempt to avoid alkylating agents such as CCNU in patients with tumour suppressor gene syndromes, and radiation therapy is employed as a last resort after most chemotherapy options have been explored.

Variations by geography

There is little support for specific geographic loci of increased prevalence. According to data from the CBTRUS, PAs amounted

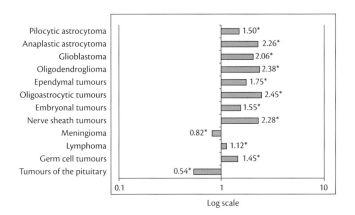

Fig. 2.4 Incidence data by race.
* Incidence rate ratio is statistically significantly different in white and black populations.

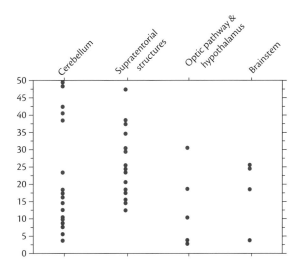

Fig. 2.5 Graph showing patient age in years (*y*-axis) and location of PAs. In children and adolescents, the cerebellum is most frequently affected; in adults the supratentorial location prevails. In no patient younger than 12 years of age did PAs develop in the basal ganglia, thalamus, or cerebral hemispheres. Each *circle* corresponds to one patient.

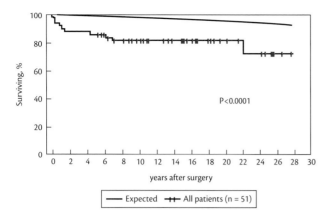

Fig. 2.6 Survival curves for 51 patients with supratentorial pilocytic astrocytomas and expected survival of age- and sex-matched people from the general population. Vertical lines represent the length of follow-up for patients still alive at last follow-up.

to 1.9% of all CNS tumours in all age groups in the United States (2) between 1970 and 2000. Similar data reported by Suh et al. were shown based on 3221 CNS tumours from the files of 13 pathology institutes in Korea between 1997 and 1998 (15). Of 1014 glioma cases entered in the Tohoku Brain Tumor Registry in Japan between 1979 and 1990, 41 (4%) were PAs (16). Neither study analysed their data by NF1 association.

Natural course

The natural course of these astrocytoma subtypes is variable and may relate to certain host and tumour factors such as age at diagnosis, presence of NF1, location, and histology. For example, infants with PAs have a shorter PFS than older children following similar chemotherapy interventions (17). NF1 children with optic nerve glioma are less likely to experience tumour progression; and when progression occurs, their optic nerve glioma responds more favourably and for a longer duration than children without NF1 (18), lack of surveillance, or observational studies specifically addressing the natural history of LGA for whom an intervention such as surgery, chemotherapy, or radiation has been deferred. It seems evident that juvenile PAs or their variants have a very low probability of undergoing malignant transformation unless they are irradiated, and their growth rate may attenuate over time (19).

The closest 'natural course' data is shown in Fig. 2.6, which displays Kaplan–Meier plots for 51 patients (median age at diagnosis: 15 years) with supratentorial PA compared to sex- and age-matched controls (20). In this series, patients with PA were typically managed with surgery alone; and the favourable course for PA is reflective of their successful surgical management. This is further discussed in the section on surgery. More recently, Qaddoumi and colleagues reviewed the outcomes and prognostic features in 6212 cases of paediatric gliomas seen at St. Jude's Research Hospital (21). This study also did not separate out subtypes and did not factor in NF.

Aetiology and pathogenetic mechanisms

Most of what is known regarding tumourigenesis of the astrocytoma subtypes comes from studies of those tumours occurring in the context of cancer predisposition syndromes such as NF1 and tuberous sclerosis.

Pilocytic astrocytoma

Unique mutational configurations confined primarily to the MAPK pathway differentiate PAs from fibrillary astrocytomas (22). *BRAF* gene duplications are the most frequently observed alteration arising in over 70% of samples (23). There is usually a tandem duplication and fusion of this oncogene with another gene, *KIAA1549*, that results in constitutive activation of the MAPK pathway. Since this oncogene can also induce senescence, it is also most likely responsible for the relatively slow growth rate and low incidence of malignant transformation. Recent evidence suggests that alterations of the *NF1* tumour suppressor gene can also activate the MAPK/ERK pathway independently of BRAF (24).

PAs are the most frequent CNS neoplasms associated with NF1. Optic nerve involvement, especially when bilateral, is the classic finding; but other anatomical sites such as the tectum and brainstem, sometimes multiple, may also be affected. Approximately 30% of PAs arise in NF1 patients; and approximately 10–15% of patients with NF1 develop PA, particularly of the optic pathways (25). Conversely, up to one-third of patients with a PA at that location have NF1 (26). While most are classic PA, some are difficult to classify and have been termed 'low-grade astrocytoma subtype indeterminate' (27). These latter tumours exhibit peculiar morphologies including plump cytoplasmic processes and macronucleoli. Differential expression of neuronal-related genes and increased mammalian target of rapamycin (mTOR) activation may underlie phenotypic variations in NF1-associated LGAs (28). In anaplastic PA, PI3K/AKT and MAPK/ERK signalling pathways perturbations appear to correlate with biological aggressiveness in PA (29).

Pleomorphic xanthoastrocytoma

Pleomorphic xanthoastrocytoma shares some similar genetic features to PA (i.e. alteration of the *BRAF* gene); but as opposed to *BRAF* duplication, the most common mutation involves the *BRAF* V600E point mutation (30). In one study, 42 of 64 (66%) PXA specimens had a point mutation in the *BRAF* oncogene (V600E) (31). Giannini and colleagues reviewed 71 cases with sufficient clinical, pathological, and treatment data from the Mayo Clinic and Johns Hopkins Hospital (32). They concluded that PXA is a generally favourable astrocytoma subtype and that gross tumour resection appears to be the main predictor of relapse-free survival and overall survival. PXAs may recur and, when they do, often demonstrate aggressive clinical behaviour with a mortality rate between 15% and 20%. A surprising feature of the pattern of failure in PXA is its tendency to have leptomeningeal spread at tumour progression, sometimes with minimal local recurrence. Occasional patients have presented with meningeal spread with a uniformly poor prognosis (33).

Subependymal giant cell astrocytoma

This tumour arises almost exclusively in patients with tuberous sclerosis complex (TSC), usually in a subependymal location adjacent to the foramen of Monro. The tumours may be unilateral but are frequently bilateral. They arise in over 90% of TSC patients, usually by the second decade, and may cause hydrocephalus. The majority of these tumours have activating mutations in the *TSC1* (hamartin) or *TSC2* (tuberin) genes whose function appears to inhibit the mTOR pathway (34). As a result, there is constitutive activation of this growth-regulating pathway. There are many other less well-understood phenomena about this syndrome such as the unique localization of these tumours and the predisposition to cortical dysplasia and epilepsy. Nevertheless, drugs that inhibit the mTOR pathway have had a remarkable ability to reduce tumour size in this syndrome (35).

Clinical presentation

In general, a brain tumour's clinical presentation varies with histology, patient age, and location. Each astrocytoma subtype will be discussed separately in the following sections.

Pilocytic astrocytoma

The more common sites of origin include the cerebellar hemisphere, optic nerve/optic chiasm and optic tracts, the hypothalamus, cerebral cortex, midbrain, and medulla. The majority occur in children and adolescents, but up to 25% occur in adults. In the paediatric population, more tumours arise in the infratentorial region, and the opposite is true in adults. The most common supratentorial site for PA is in the hypothalamic/optic pathways followed by the diencephalic region. PAs of the spinal cord constitute less than 10% of all PAs in children (7). Large diencephalic and midbrain lesions may obstruct cerebrospinal fluid flow. In patients with NF1, the sites of involvement are similar; but the distribution and frequency are different. In NF1 the most common site for PA is the optic nerve/chiasm complex whereas this site is less in sporadic cases. Sporadic optic gliomas present with impaired vision more frequently and are more aggressive than NF1 optic gliomas (36).

PAs produce local neurological deficits appropriate to the anatomical site or non-localizing signs such as headache, endocrinopathy, or increased intracranial pressure due to mass effect or ventricular obstruction. Seizures are uncommon since the lesions infrequently involve the cerebral cortex. Given their slow rate of growth, the clinical presentation of pilocytic tumours is generally that of an evolving lesion. PAs of the optic pathways often produce visual loss. Proptosis may be seen with intraorbital tumours. As part of NF1 screening, suspected optic nerve glioma may be detected radiographically, presymptomatically, and these and some symptomatic ones may spontaneously regress. Hypothalamic pituitary dysfunction, including obesity, can arise in diencephalic and optic nerve gliomas. PAs of the thalamus generally present with signs of CSF obstruction or neurological deficits such as hemiparesis or movement disorders due to pyramidal and extrapyramidal tract compression. Cerebellar PAs usually present in the first two decades with clumsiness, worsening headache, nausea, and vomiting. Brainstem examples, especially those that arise in the tectum of the midbrain, present with macrocrania and signs and symptoms of raised intracranial pressure. PAs arising dorsally in the medulla or cervicomedullary region may obstruct outflow of the fourth ventricle or cause medullary or upper spinal cord dysfunction.

Pleomorphic xanthoastrocytoma

Pleomorphic xanthoastrocytomas typically present with a focal seizure disorder. Age at diagnosis varied considerably in the largest case series published with mean age of 26 ± 16 years (32). Imaging usually identifies a large and cortically based tumour in the frontal or temporal lobes with heterogeneous gadolinium enhancement and occasional intratumoural cysts and calcifications. They may also have focal signs consistent with their anatomical position.

Because they extend to the meninges, they may occasionally present with meningeal signs and symptoms (33). They are usually amenable to radical resection.

Subependymal giant cell astrocytoma

Subependymal giant cell astrocytomas occur most commonly in the first two decades of life with mean age at presentation of 11 years. Although these tumours are generally benign and classified as WHO grade I, more aggressive lesions can infiltrate the thalamus, hypothalamus, and basal ganglia and produce obstructive hydrocephalus and mass effect (34). SEGAs originate within the wall of the lateral ventricle, most frequently in the region of the foramen of Monro. Because of this location, SEGAs typically result in obstructive hydrocephalus and symptoms of elevated intracranial pressure. SEGAs are often 2–3 cm at the time of presentation. Sudden death from acute hydrocephalus can occur with the risk directly proportional to tumour volume. Surgical resection has been the standard treatment for SEGAs and is generally curative with gross total excision. Endoscopic resections are becoming more common, especially for the smaller tumours (37). Stereotactic radiosurgery, primarily with the Gamma Knife®, has been used for primary management on a case-by-case basis but is not the primary treatment (38). Recently, inhibitors of the mTOR pathway have been shown to produce significant responses in TSC patients, and long-term therapy is relatively safe and tolerable (39, 40). When an mTOR inhibitor such as sirolimus (rapamycin) or everolimus is stopped, the tumour usually recurs. Decision-making regarding surgery, radiosurgery, mTOR inhibitors, and their combinations are usually made on a case-by-case basis.

Imaging

A particular challenge of diffuse astrocytomas is their stealthy imaging characteristics. All clinicians have had the experience of seeing a patient who presents with their first seizure and has 'normal' imaging only to later receive the report that a faint hypodensity with variable mass effect has emerged thus indicating the possibility of a neoplasm. This was particularly the case with computed tomography (CT) and has become less so with MRI (41). The 'false-negative' rate with current standard MRI scanning is hard to come by but is probably in the 15–20% range, although in one series it was 39% (42).

PAs, PXAs, and SEGAs have distinct almost pathognomonic imaging features. In contrast to diffuse astrocytomas, CT scanning is nearly equivalent to MRI in terms of diagnostic accuracy—although calcification, an imaging marker of slow growth, is much more easily identified with the former. The following sections address imaging characteristics of PAs, PXAs, and SEGAs.

Pilocytic astrocytoma

PAs are well circumscribed, often cystic masses, and usually exhibit homogeneous enhancement except when they arise in certain locations such as the tectum, optic pathways, and medulla (43). Only a minority are calcified. Anterior optic pathway tumours involving the optic nerve are somewhat restrained in their outward expansion by the optic sheath and usually grow as a fusiform, tortuous intraorbital mass often producing proptosis (Fig. 2.7). In contrast, optic pathway tumours involving the chiasm and tracts appear to respect anatomical pathways as they spread to involve the optic

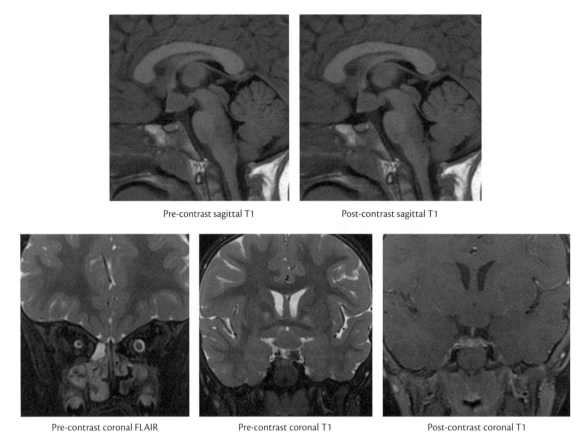

Pre-contrast sagittal T1   Post-contrast sagittal T1

Pre-contrast coronal FLAIR   Pre-contrast coronal T1   Post-contrast coronal T1

Fig. 2.7 Optic nerve glioma in a 4-year-old with NF1.

radiations (Fig. 2.8). Cyst formation is often location dependent. For example, cerebellar PAs are often comprised mostly of large tumoural cysts with enhancing mural nodules (Fig. 2.9) whereas cysts are less common in optic nerve or tectal gliomas.

Pleomorphic xanthoastrocytoma

These tumours typically present in late adolescence/early adulthood. They are usually located in temporal or parietal lobes and extend to the pial surface where they present a characteristic imaging appearance (Fig. 2.10). Presumably because of their superficial location the majority of patients present with seizures. More than half of these tumours have a cystic component, and in most instances, the solid component enhances avidly. A distinguishing feature of PXA is that some tumour cysts will have mural nodules projecting into the cavity, and the nodule may be calcified.

Subependymal giant cell astrocytoma

These tumours are usually identified in patients with TSC where as many as 20% of patients may have imaging evidence for SEGA. As such, the imaging may display other characteristic imaging features of the TSC such as subcortical tubers. SEGAs may be found in patients without evidence of TSC. Imaging features of the tumours in sporadic and TSC cases are similar. On axial T2-weighted and fluid-attenuated inversion recovery (FLAIR) MRI, a SEGA is usually identified near the foramen of Monro with heterogenous, somewhat hyperintense signal compared to white matter. Intense homogeneous enhancement is seen on contrast-enhanced axial and coronal T1-weighted images (Fig. 2.11). Subependymal nodules may be

seen along the lateral ventricles. Occasionally SEGAs may be bilateral (44). Multiple foci of increased signal are seen on FLAIR images in the subcortical regions representing parenchymal tubers.

Treatment

The cornerstone for all three astrocytoma subtypes is surgery with the goal being gross total resection. This goal is usually achievable when the primary tumour arises in the cerebrum, cerebellum, and occasionally in the spinal cord. It is difficult to achieve in hypothalamus, thalamus, or brainstem and is not possible in the optic nerves or chiasm. A gross total resection not only relieves symptoms, provides internal decompression, and establishes the histological diagnosis—it serves as a curative procedure in the majority of patients. Even patients with partial resections may ultimately experience prolonged stabilization.

In progressive disease, chemotherapy is increasingly used especially in younger patients and in children with NF1. Currently there is insufficient data on the efficacy of specific chemotherapy regimens for each subtype of LGG, and they are all treated in a similar fashion. The first choice of chemotherapy is usually carboplatin and vincristine. Gnekow et al. reported the long-term follow-up of the HIT-LGG-1996 study for LGG in children and described a 10-year progression-free survival of 44% in 137 patients with three-quarters of surviving patients not requiring radiotherapy (50). As more is learned about the molecular specificity and vulnerability of LGG, molecular-targeted therapy may assume a more important role.

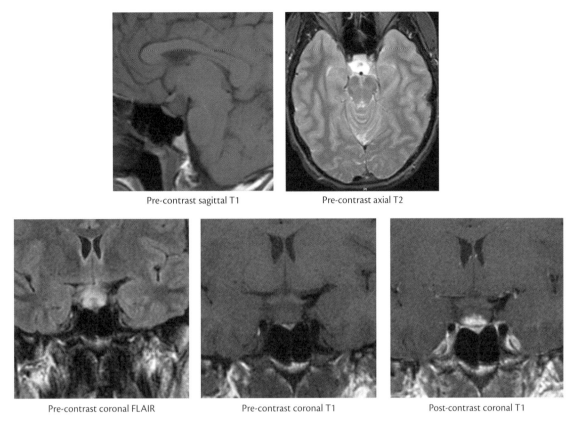

Pre-contrast sagittal T1   Pre-contrast axial T2

Pre-contrast coronal FLAIR   Pre-contrast coronal T1   Post-contrast coronal T1

Fig. 2.8 Optic nerve pilocytic astrocytoma in a 6-year-old without NF1.

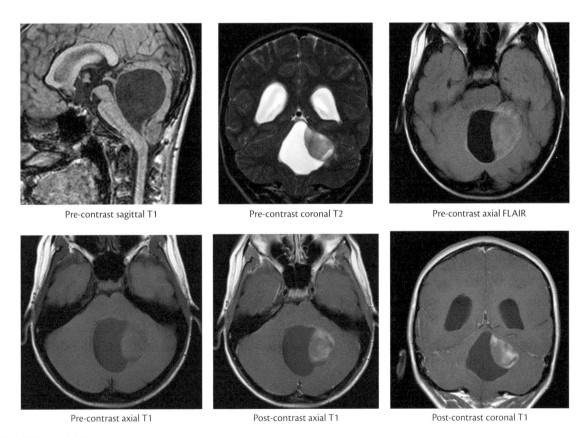

Pre-contrast sagittal T1   Pre-contrast coronal T2   Pre-contrast axial FLAIR

Pre-contrast axial T1   Post-contrast axial T1   Post-contrast coronal T1

Fig. 2.9 Classic infratentorial pilocytic astrocytoma.

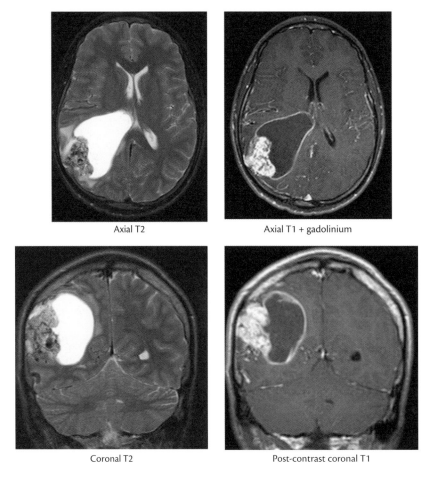

Fig. 2.10 Anaplastic pleomorphic xanthoastrocytoma.

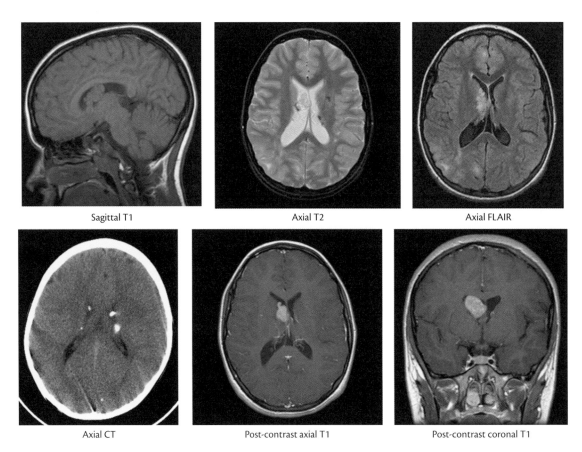

Fig. 2.11 Subependymal giant cell astrocytoma.

Radiotherapy is reserved for older children and when chemotherapy has failed (51, 52). Modern three-dimensional conformal radiotherapy is increasingly used in PA (Table 2.1). In the series of Merchant et al., a 5- and 10-year event-free survival of 87.4% or 74.3% was achieved. The corresponding overall survival was 98.5% and 95.9%, respectively (53). The Boston group treated 81 children with fractionated stereotactic convergence therapy and achieved an 8-year progression-free survival of 65% (51). In the prospective multicentre HIT-LGG-1996 trial, 117 patients underwent radiation therapy. The 5- and 10-year progression-free survival after external fractionated radiation therapy was 76%. The 10-year overall survival was 97%. Disease progression was not influenced by gender, NF1, tumour location, age, or prior chemotherapy (52)

Brachytherapy is a useful option. It seems that small, circumscribed tumours with a diameter of less than 4 cm in locations other than the optic nerve and chiasm are preferred cases for interstitial brachytherapy. A 15-year progression-free and overall survival of 65% and 82% could be reached in one series (59). Proton therapy might possess an advantage mainly in normal tissue preservation; its use, however, is still experimental.

Table 2.1 Recent series in external fractionated radiotherapy in childhood low-grade glioma using modern treatment technologies

Author (reference)	Dose prescription	Patients	Results	Follow-up
Debus et al., 1999 (54)	Median 52.4 Gy/1.6–2.0 Gy Margin: 7 mm	10	5-year PFS: 90%, 5-year OS: 100% No acute toxicities	12–72 months
Saran et al., 2002 (55)	Median 50–55 Gy/30–33 fractions Margin: 5–10 mm	14	3-year PFS: 87%, 3-year OS: 100% 1 relapse within GTV	33 months
Hug et al., 2002 (56)	Protons 50.4–63.0 CGE 1.8 Gy Margin: no data	27	Local control survival Hemispheric 71% 86% Diencephalic 87% 93% Brainstem 60% 60%	3.3 years
Marcus et al., 2005 (51)	Stereotactic Convergence technique Median 52.2 Gy/1.8 Gy Margin: 2 mm	81	5-/8-year PFS: 82.5%/65% 5-/8-year OS: 97.8%/82% 6 local relapses All within field	6.9 years
Combs et al., 2005 (57)	3D conformal RT Median 52.2 Gy/1.8 Gy Margin: 5 mm	15	3-/5-year PFS: 92%/72% 5-year OS: 90%	97 months
Merchant et al., 2009 (53)	3D conformal RT Median 54 Gy/1.8 Gy Margin: 15 mm	78	5-/10-year EFS: 87.4%/74.3% 5-/10-year OS: 98.5%/95.9% 13 relapses (8/13 within PTV) (1/13 margin) (4/14 CNS metastases)	89 months
Paulino et al., 2013 (58)	IMRT 45–60 Gy Margin: 5–10 mm	39	8-year EFS/OS: 78.2%/93.7% 7/7 failures in field	n.a.
Müller et al., 2013 (52)	Conventional/3D planning Median 54 Gy/1.8 Gy Margin: 1–2 cm	75	Pilocytic astrocytoma 5/10 y. PFS: 76.5% 5/10 y. OS: 96.2% Relapse pattern: n.a.	8.4 years

CGE, cobalt Gray equivalent; EFS, event-free survival; IMRT, intensity-modulated radiotherapy; n.a., not applicable; OS, overall survival; PFS, progression-free survival; PTV, planning target volume; RT, radiotherapy.

References

1. Louis DN, Ohgaki H, Wiestler OD, et al. (eds). *WHO Classification of Tumours of the Central Nervous System* (4th edn). Lyon: International Agency for Research on Cancer, 2007.

2. Central Brain Tumor Registry of the United States. *2016 CBTRUS Fact Sheet*. 2016. http://www.cbtrus.org/factsheet/factsheet.html.

3. National Program of Cancer Registries [Homepage]. http://www.cdc.gov/cancer/npcr/.

4. National Program of Cancer. *Cancer Surveillance System*. http://www.cdc.gov/cancer/npcr/css.htm.

5. Surveillance, Epidemiology and End Results Program [Homepage]. http://seer.cancer.gov/.

6. Dolecek TA, Propp JM, Stroup NE, et al. CBTRUS statistical report: primary brain and central nervous system tumors diagnosed in the United States in 2005-2009. *Neuro Oncol* 2012; 14(Suppl 5):v1–49.

7. McCarthy BJ. *Descriptive Analysis of Pilocytic Astrocytomas using SEER 13 registry (1992-2002) and SEER 9 registry (1973-2002) data*. 2006. http://akidsbraintumorcure.org/6171/news/2006-jpa-statistical-data/.

8. Burkhard C, Di Patre PL, Schuler D, et al. A population-based study of the incidence and survival rates in patients with pilocytic astrocytoma. *J Neurosurg* 2003; 98(6):1170–1174.

9. United States Cancer Statistics: 1999–2011 Incidence, WONDER Online Database. United States Department of Health and Human Services, Centers for Disease Control and Prevention and National Cancer Institute. 2014. http://wonder.cdc.gov/cancer-v2011.html.

10. Claus EB, Black PM. Survival rates and patterns of care for patients diagnosed with supratentorial low-grade gliomas: data from the SEER program, 1973–2001. *Cancer* 2006; 106(6):1358–1363.

11. Okamoto Y, Di Patre PL, Burkhard C, et al. Population-based study on incidence, survival rates, and genetic alterations of low-grade diffuse astrocytomas and oligodendrogliomas. *Acta Neuropathol* 2004; 108(1):49–56.

12. Fisher MJ, Avery RA, Allen JC, et al. Functional outcome measures for NF1-associated optic pathway glioma clinical trials. *Neurology* 2013; 81(21 Suppl 1):S15–24.

13. Lee AG. Neuroophthalmological management of optic pathway gliomas. *Neurosurg Focus* 2007; 23(5):E1.

14. Fisher MJ, Loguidice M, Gutmann DH, et al. Visual outcomes in children with neurofibromatosis type 1-associated optic pathway glioma following chemotherapy: a multicenter retrospective analysis. *Neuro Oncol* 2012; 14(6):790–797.

15. Suh YL, Koo H, Kim TS, et al. Tumors of the central nervous system in Korea: a multicenter study of 3221 cases. *J Neurooncol* 2002; 56(3):251–259.

16. Katakura R, Yoshimoto T. Epidemiology and statistical analysis of gliomas. In: Suzuki J (ed) *Treatment of Glioma*. Tokyo: Springer-Verlag, 1988; 3–16.

17. Larouche V, Huang A, Bartels U, et al. Tumors of the central nervous system in the first year of life. *Pediatr Blood Cancer* 2007; 49 (7 Suppl):1074–1082.

18. Ater JL, Zhou T, Holmes E, et al. Randomized study of two chemotherapy regimens for treatment of low-grade glioma in young children: a report from the Children's Oncology Group. *J Clin Oncol* 2012; 30(21):2641–2647.

19. Parsa CF, Givrad S. Juvenile pilocytic astrocytomas do not undergo spontaneous malignant transformation: grounds for designation as hamartomas. *Br J Ophthalmol* 2008; 92(1):40–46.

20. Forsyth PA, Shaw EG, Scheithauer BW, et al. Supratentorial pilocytic astrocytomas. A clinicopathologic, prognostic, and flow cytometric study of 51 patients. *Cancer* 1993; 72(4):1335–1342.

21. Qaddoumi I, Sultan I, Gajjar A. Outcome and prognostic features in pediatric gliomas: a review of 6212 cases from the Surveillance, Epidemiology, and End Results database. *Cancer* 2009; 115(24):5761–5770.

22. Dougherty MJ, Santi M, Brose MS, et al. Activating mutations in BRAF characterize a spectrum of pediatric low-grade gliomas. *Neuro Oncol* 2010; 12(7):621–630.

23. Jeuken JW, Wesseling P. MAPK pathway activation through BRAF gene fusion in pilocytic astrocytomas; a novel oncogenic fusion gene with diagnostic, prognostic, and therapeutic potential. *J Pathol* 2010; 222(4):324–328.

24. Chen YH, Gutmann DH. The molecular and cell biology of pediatric low-grade gliomas. *Oncogene* 2014; 33(16):2019–2026.

25. Listernick R, Ferner RE, Liu GT, et al. Optic pathway gliomas in neurofibromatosis-1: controversies and recommendations. *Ann Neurol* 2007; 61(3):189–198.

26. Rodriguez FJ, Perry A, Gutmann DH, et al. Gliomas in neurofibromatosis type 1: a clinicopathologic study of 100 patients. *J Neuropathol Exp Neurol* 2008; 67(3):240–249.

27. Jentoft M, Giannini C, Cen L, et al. Phenotypic variations in NF1-associated low grade astrocytomas: possible role for increased mTOR activation in a subset. *Int J Clin Exp Pathol* 2010; 4(1):43–57.

28. Rodriguez EF, Scheithauer BW, Giannini C, et al. PI3K/AKT pathway alterations are associated with clinically aggressive and histologically anaplastic subsets of pilocytic astrocytoma. *Acta Neuropathol* 2011; 121(3):407–420.

29. Rodriguez FJ, Scheithauer BW, Burger PC, et al. Anaplasia in pilocytic astrocytoma predicts aggressive behavior. *Am J Surg Pathol* 2010; 34(2):147–160.

30. Dias-Santagata D, Lam Q, Vernovsky K, et al. BRAF V600E mutations are common in pleomorphic xanthoastrocytoma: diagnostic and therapeutic implications. *PLoS One* 2011; 6(3):e17948.

31. Schindler G, Capper D, Meyer J, et al. Analysis of BRAF V600E mutation in 1,320 nervous system tumors reveals high mutation frequencies in pleomorphic xanthoastrocytoma, ganglioglioma and extra-cerebellar pilocytic astrocytoma. *Acta Neuropathol* 2011; 121(3):397–405.

32. Giannini C, Scheithauer BW, Burger PC, et al. Pleomorphic xanthoastrocytoma: what do we really know about it? *Cancer* 1999; 85(9):2033–2045.

33. Lubansu A, Rorive S, David P, et al. Cerebral anaplastic pleomorphic xanthoastrocytoma with meningeal dissemination at first presentation. *Childs Nerv Syst* 2004; 20(2):119–122.

34. Koeller KK, Sandberg GD. From the archives of the AFIP. Cerebral intraventricular neoplasms: radiologic-pathologic correlation. *Radiographics* 2002; 22(6):1473–1505.

35. Marko NF, Weil RJ. The molecular biology of WHO grade I astrocytomas. *Neuro Oncol* 2012; 14(12):1424–1431.

36. Singhal S, Birch JM, Kerr B, et al. Neurofibromatosis type 1 and sporadic optic gliomas. *Arch Dis Child* 2002; 87(1):65–70.

37. Rodgers SD, Bassani L, Weiner HL, et al. Stereotactic endoscopic resection and surgical management of a subependymal giant cell astrocytoma: case report. *J Neurosurg Pediatr* 2012; 9(4):417–420.

38. Park KJ, Kano H, Kondziolka D, et al. Gamma Knife surgery for subependymal giant cell astrocytomas. *J Neurosurg* 2011; 114(3):808–813.

39. Franz DN, Belousova E, Sparagana S, et al. Efficacy and safety of everolimus for subependymal giant cell astrocytomas associated with tuberous sclerosis complex (EXIST-1): a multicentre, randomised, placebo-controlled phase 3 trial. *Lancet* 2013; 381(9861):125–132.

40. Krueger DA, Care MM, Agricola K, et al. Everolimus long-term safety and efficacy in subependymal giant cell astrocytoma. *Neurology* 2013; 80(6):574–80.

41. Law M, Yang S, Wang H, et al. Glioma grading: sensitivity, specificity, and predictive values of perfusion MR imaging and proton MR spectroscopic imaging compared with conventional MR imaging. *AJNR Am J Neuroradiol* 2003; 24(10):1989–1998.

42. Rachinger W, Goetz C, Popperl G, et al. Positron emission tomography with O-(2-[18F]fluoroethyl)-l-tyrosine versus magnetic resonance imaging in the diagnosis of recurrent gliomas. *Neurosurgery* 2005; 57(3):505–511.

43. Ginsberg LE, Fuller GN, Hashmi M, et al. The significance of lack of MR contrast enhancement of supratentorial brain tumors in adults: histopathological evaluation of a series. *Surg Neurol* 1998; 49(4):436–440.

44. Adriaensen ME, Schaefer-Prokop CM, Stijnen T, et al. Prevalence of subependymal giant cell tumors in patients with tuberous sclerosis and a review of the literature. *Eur J Neurol* 2009; 16(6):691–696.

45. Jenkin D, Angyalfi S, Becker L, et al. Optic glioma in children: surveillance, resection, or irradiation? *Int J Radiat Oncol Biol Phys* 1993; 25(2):215–225.

46. Wong JY, Uhl V, Wara WM, et al. Optic gliomas. A reanalysis of the University of California, San Francisco experience. *Cancer* 1987; 60(8):1847–1855.

47. Parentin F, Rabusin M, Zennaro F, et al. Chemotherapy for optic nerve glioma in a child with neurofibromatosis type-1. *Neuro-Ophthalmology* 2008; 32(3):159–162.

48. Shofty B, Ben-Sira L, Freedman S, et al. Visual outcome following chemotherapy for progressive optic pathway gliomas. *Pediatr Blood Cancer* 2011; 57(3):481–485.

49. Bouffet E, Jakacki R, Goldman S, et al. Phase II study of weekly vinblastine in recurrent or refractory pediatric low-grade glioma. *J Clin Oncol* 2012; 30(12):1358–1363.

50. Gnekow AK, Falkenstein F, von Hornstein S, et al. Long-term follow-up of the multicenter, multidisciplinary treatment study HIT-LGG-1996 for low-grade glioma in children and adolescents of the German Speaking Society of Pediatric Oncology and Hematology. *Neuro Oncol* 2012; 14(10):1265–1284.

51. Marcus KJ, Goumnerova L, Billett AL, et al. Stereotactic radiotherapy for localized low-grade gliomas in children: final results of a prospective trial. *Int J Radiat Oncol Biol Phys* 2005; 61(2):374–379.

52. Müller K, Gnekow A, Falkenstein F, et al. Radiotherapy in pediatric pilocytic astrocytomas: A subgroup analysis within the prospective multicenter study HIT-LGG 1996 by the German Society of Pediatric Oncology and Hematology (GPOH). *Strahlenther Onkol* 2013; 189(8):647–655.

53. Merchant TE, Kun LE, Wu S, et al. Phase II trial of conformal radiation therapy for pediatric low-grade glioma. *J Clin Oncol* 2009; 27(22):3598–604.

54. Debus J, Kocagoncu KO, Hoss A, et al. Fractionated stereotactic radiotherapy (FSRT) for optic glioma. *Int J Radiat Oncol Biol Phys* 1999; 44: 243–248.

55. Saran FH, Baumert BG, Khoo VS, et al. Stereotactically guided conformal radiotherapy for progressive low-grade gliomas of childhood. *Int J Radiat Oncol Biol Phys* 2002; 53(1):43–51.

56. Hug EB, Muenter MW, Archambeau JO, et al. Conformal proton radiation therapy for pediatric low-grade astrocytoma. *Strahlenther Onkol* 2002; 178:10–17.

57. Combs SE, Schulz-Ertner D, Moschos D, et al. Fractionated stereotactic radiotherapy of optic pathway gliomas: tolerance and long-term outcome. *Int J Radiat Oncol Biol Phys* 2005; 62(3):814–819.

58. Paulino AC, Mazloom A, Terashima K, et al. Intensity-modulated radiotherapy (IMRT) in pediatric low-grade glioma. *Cancer* 2013; 119(14):2654–2659.

59. Ruge MI, Simon T, Suchorska B, et al. Stereotactic brachytherapy with iodine-125 seeds for the treatment of inoperable low-grade gliomas in children: long-term outcome. *J Clin Oncol* 2011; 29(31):4151–4159.

CHAPTER 3

Astrocytic tumours: diffuse astrocytoma, anaplastic astrocytoma, glioblastoma, and gliomatosis cerebri

Michael Weller, Michael Brada, Tai-Tong Wong, and Michael A. Vogelbaum

Definition

Diffuse astrocytomas (World Health Organization (WHO) grade II) are classified by the 2007 WHO classification as fibrillary, gemistocytic, or protoplasmic and are also referred to as low-grade gliomas (1). Anaplastic astrocytoma (WHO grade III) and glioblastoma (WHO grade IV) have traditionally been collectively referred to as high-grade gliomas. The diagnosis of glioma may be suspected based on clinical history and neuroimaging findings (see later in chapter), but histological confirmation remains the diagnostic 'gold standard'. Diffuse astrocytomas are infiltrative, but slow-growing tumours without prominent angiogenesis, necrosis, or nuclear atypia. The WHO classification defines anaplastic astrocytoma as a diffusely infiltrating tumour characterized by nuclear atypia, increased cellularity, and significant proliferative activity. Vascular proliferation and necrosis are distinguishing histopathological features that allow the diagnosis of glioblastoma (WHO grade IV). The clinical significance of morphologically defined glioblastoma variants such as giant cell glioblastoma, small cell glioblastoma, glioblastoma with oligodendroglial component, or gliosarcoma remains controversial. This subclassification has no management implications at present. Gliomatosis cerebri is defined as a glial tumour confirmed by histology that affects more than two cerebral lobes as assessed by neuroimaging and is assigned the WHO grade III.

Molecular markers have not been incorporated into the 2007 WHO classification, but may be of diagnostic value: 1p/19q co-deletions detected by fluorescent in situ hybridization are common in oligodendroglial tumours, but are rare in astrocytic gliomas. Epidermal growth factor receptor (EGFR) amplification and over-expression detected by reverse transcriptase polymerase chain reaction (PCR) or immunocytochemistry are typical lesions of glioblastoma, but not anaplastic astrocytoma. O^6-methylguanine-DNA methyltransferase (MGMT) gene promoter methylation detected by methylation-specific PCR is a favourable prognostic marker in anaplastic gliomas and predicts benefit from alkylating agent chemotherapy in glioblastoma. Isocitrate dehydrogenase (IDH) mutations detected by immunohistochemistry (IDH^{R132H}) or PCR and direct sequencing for rare IDH-1 and for IDH-2 mutations are common in anaplastic astrocytoma, but rare in glioblastoma, and will have a major impact on the next revision of the WHO classification. The differential distribution of IDH gene mutations in glioblastomas versus grade II and III gliomas indicates that most glioblastomas are biologically distinct tumours that are not related to typical lower-grade precursor lesions. Thus, the detection of IDH gene mutations as a characteristic feature of grade II/III gliomas also provided a molecular post hoc rationale for separating glioblastomas into secondary glioblastoma derived from less malignant precursor lesions from the more common primary glioblastomas which present with the full histological pattern of glioblastoma at the time of first surgical intervention. Finally, IDH gene mutations are prognostically favourable across all glioma entities including gliomatosis cerebri (2), and almost never occur in elderly patients with malignant gliomas. In fact, the differential distribution of IDH mutations by age together with their favourable prognostic significance explains partially the negative prognostic impact of age in these patients (see later) (3). Altogether, these considerations justify that the upcoming revision of the WHO classification includes molecular markers, notably IDH, for diagnostic classification (4).

Epidemiology

The overall annual incidence of gliomas is in the range of 5–6 per 100,000 population. The figures for diffuse astrocytoma, anaplastic astrocytoma, and glioblastoma are 0.1, 0.4, and 3.1 per 100,000, respectively, whereas no incidence data are available for gliomatosis cerebri. Males are more often affected than females by glioblastoma (1.6:1) and anaplastic astrocytoma (1.4:1) (http://www.cbtrus.org) (Table 3.1). No large data sets are available for gliomatosis cerebri; in the Neuro-Onkologische Arbeitsgemeinschaft/German

Table 3.1 Malignant gliomas: epidemiology and outcome.

	Annual incidence per 100,000	Survival at 1 year (%)	Survival at 3 years (%)	Survival at 5 years (%)
Diffuse astrocytoma	0.1	75	56	58
Anaplastic astrocytoma	0.4	61	35	27
Glioblastoma	3.2	35	8	5

Source data from www.cbtrus.org

Neuro-Oncology Group (NOA)-05 trial, 19 of 35 patients (54%) were male (5).

There is little variation of risk across different countries and races. The natural course is rapid deterioration and death in glioblastoma, notably in the elderly within weeks, and more favourable, but still invariably lethal in anaplastic astrocytoma. In contrast, the natural course of diffuse astrocytoma and also gliomatosis cerebri is more variable, and some patients even with extensive disease remain neurologically largely asymptomatic for years.

Aetiology

The aetiology of most malignant gliomas remains unknown. Hereditary syndromes associated with an increased risk of glioma development include Li–Fraumeni syndrome and neurofibromatosis types 1 and 2 (see Chapters 15–17). Therapeutic irradiation to the skull and brain in childhood is associated with an increased risk of glioma. Since the overall incidence is low and no other major risk factors are known, and since gliomas may develop *de novo* within few weeks or months, no screening for gliomas has been implemented.

Pathogenesis

The pathogenesis of gliomas remains enigmatic. The cell of origin is likely to be a neuroglial precursor cell. It has become clear that IDH gene mutations, if present, occur early in glioma genesis. Mutant IDH proteins may promote genome-wide methylation and thereby tumour formation (6). Mutations in p53 (*TP53*) are also early events in malignant astrocytic tumours which harbour these alterations. For the IDH wild-type tumours, that is, most glioblastomas, a similar, presumably early molecular event is less clearly defined, because early glioblastomas are rarely diagnosed. Additional molecular aberrations of anaplastic astrocytomas include loss of heterozygosity (LOH) 17p (50–60%), LOH 10q (35–60%), and LOH 19q (40–50%). Glioblastomas are characterized by EGFR amplification (40–50%) which is associated with the EGFRvIII mutation in approximately half of these patients. Moreover, cell cycle control is disrupted in the majority of glioblastomas either at the level of the receptor tyrosine kinase pathway (88%), p53 signalling (87%), or the retinoblastoma pathway (78%) (7).

Clinical presentation

There are no characteristic features of clinical presentation of gliomas. A common mode of presentation is a first epileptic seizure in an individual without neurological history. Type and kinetics of evolution of focal clinical symptoms depend on the location and the growth rate of the tumour. Rapid neurological deterioration is most commonly seen in elderly patients with glioblastoma. Conversely, patients with diffuse astrocytomas and even with extensive gliomatosis cerebri can remain asymptomatic for many months and even years.

Imaging

The diagnosis of gliomas is most often made by neuroimaging in individuals suspected of harbouring an intracranial lesion because of the clinical history. Magnetic resonance imaging (MRI) is the method of choice. Computed tomography (CT) is only used when MRI is not available or not possible. Cerebral angiography is performed as deemed helpful by the surgeon and is less frequently used with the introduction of magnetic resonance angiography. Positron emission tomography (PET) using amino acid tracers is increasingly used to detect hot spots of increased metabolic activity which may indicate a higher grade of malignancy and can be used to guide surgical strategies including, but not limited to, the best site for biopsy (8).

Imaging is also the main method to assess response to therapy in gliomas. The Macdonald criteria (9) which served neuro-oncology well for almost two decades had to be revised in 2010 as a consequence of new patterns of response and progression observed with the introduction of anti-angiogenic agents (10). The four categories of complete response (CR), partial response (PR), stable disease (SD), and progressive disease (PD) were maintained, but more clearly delineated in terms of confounding factors, and the major innovation was the consideration not only of contrast-enhanced images, but also T2-weighted and fluid-attenuated inversion recovery (FLAIR) sequences. New Response Assessment in Neuro-Oncology (RANO) criteria were also proposed for patients with low-grade (non-enhancing) gliomas (11).

Pseudoprogression refers to an apparent increase in the size of the contrast-enhancing lesion that does not reflect tumour progression, but rather treatment-related reactive changes (12). It is often claimed to be related to combined modality treatment of glioblastoma, but such evolutions of CT and MRI scans can also be seen after radiotherapy alone, especially in patients with residual tumours. Its frequency and clinical significance are difficult to estimate since temozolomide is usually continued in patients with suspected pseudoprogression who are clinically stable or improved, but whose MRI scans appear to indicate progressive disease. This practice is reasonable, but precludes differentiation of pseudoprogression from delayed responses to temozolomide.

Treatment

The diagnosis, treatment, and follow-up of patients with astrocytic gliomas is an interdisciplinary challenge that is best met by specialized centres with dedicated brain tumour boards and inter-disciplinary outpatient clinics (Table 3.2). There is general agreement that surgical excision of the bulk tumour alone is insufficient treatment for patients with anaplastic astrocytoma or glioblastoma due to the diffusely infiltrative nature of the disease. In contrast, the strategies are more diverse in patients with diffuse astrocytomas. Some circumscribed lesions can be safely resected whereas others may be managed by a diagnostic biopsy alone and no further treatment initially. Similarly, young patients with gliomatosis cerebri (e.g. below the age of 40), who manifest with symptomatic epilepsy but are otherwise asymptomatic, may be managed initially by observation alone. However, the disease will inevitably progress at some point and become symptomatic. Altogether, therapy-independent factors are strong determinants of outcome specifically in patients with diffuse astrocytomas: favourable prognostic factors include age below 40, tumour diameter below 6 cm, tumour not crossing the midline, and absence of neurological deficits (13).

Adults

Surgery

All lesions suggestive of primary brain tumours require a tissue-based diagnosis before further therapeutic decisions are made. Diagnostic tissue can be obtained *via* a stereotactically guided biopsy without tumour debulking, or an open surgical resection intended to remove as much of the gross tumour as possible while minimizing the risk of a new, permanent neurological deficit. The requirement for a tissue-based diagnosis also extends to elderly patients for whom eventually no further treatment may be recommended. The rationale for histological verification in all patients relates to the risk of false diagnoses made by neuroimaging alone. Obtaining a definitive tissue diagnosis is important to reassure physicians, patients, and relatives even in situations where radiotherapy or chemotherapy are not considered viable options.

Surgery serves not only to allow pathology to establish a firm diagnosis, but there is evidence that the extent of resection (EOR) is a prognostic factor in most patients with gliomas. While there are no prospective, randomized trials of sufficient power to establish a causal link between EOR and outcome (and these trials are unlikely to be performed due to ethical concerns), there is a growing body of evidence that establishes a strong association between EOR and survival. Residual tumour is a negative prognostic factor in most studies of patients with grade II astrocytomas (14–16). Moreover, multiple studies have shown that patients with glioblastoma who have a more extensive surgery survive longer (17, 18) and this finding has been extended to patients with anaplastic gliomas treated on the NOA-04 trial (19). These studies cannot exclude the possibility that some tumours are more inherently 'resectable' than others (based upon factors such as location, size, diffuseness, or molecular profile) and that those that are more resectable are also biologically less aggressive than those that are not as resectable. Furthermore, there is evidence that surgically induced new neurological deficits are associated with a poorer outcome; hence the goal of a complete resection of bulk tumour needs to be balanced against the risk of functional loss (20).

Multiple tools have been developed to aid the surgeon in achieving the balance of maximizing EOR and minimizing risk of new neurological deficits. Surgical navigation systems are used to plan minimal access craniotomies and provide intraoperative tumour margin localization in order to aid in maximizing EOR. Intraoperative imaging with ultrasound, CT, or MRI can provide updated image data sets to these surgical navigation systems. A fluorescent tumour marker (5-aminolevulinic acid, 5-ALA) better delineates tumour tissue, in glioblastoma, under the surgical microscope and its use is associated with both an improved EOR and progression-free survival (PFS) at 6 months (21). Tools that help the surgeon to minimize the risk of new functional deficits include preoperative functional MRI, magnetoencephalography, transcranial magnetic stimulation, diffusion tensor imaging to

Table 3.2 Current treatment options for anaplastic astrocytoma and glioblastoma in adults

	Newly diagnosed	Recurrence or progression
Diffuse astrocytoma	Resection (or biopsy) and radiotherapy (or temozolomide) or both[a]	(Re-resection and) temozolomide or radiotherapy
Anaplastic astrocytoma	Resection (or biopsy) and radiotherapy or temozolomide[b,c] (or radiotherapy plus temozolomide[d])	(Re-resection and) temozolomide or radiotherapy (or re-irradiation) or bevacizumab
Glioblastoma	Resection[e] (or biopsy) and radiotherapy and chemotherapy (temozolomide)[f]	(Re-resection and) chemotherapy (dose-intense temozolomide or nitrosourea) (or re-irradiation) or bevacizumab[g]

[a] EORTC 22033-26033, RTOG 9802.

[b] NOA-04 trial (19).

[c] Temozolomide probably equieffective to nitrosoureas but better tolerated (19).

[d] Explored in the CATNON trial.

[e] 5-ALA trial (21).

[f] EORTC 26981-22981 NCIC CE.3 (38).

[g] (46, 47).

delineate important white matter tracts, and intraoperative direct cortical stimulation and motor/speech monitoring.

Approximately 20–25% of patients may be candidates for second surgery. Usually the recurrence should be circumscribed, but still exert relevant mass effect, and there should be further therapeutic options beyond the surgical intervention. In gliomatosis cerebri, the role of surgery is commonly limited to allowing a tissue-based diagnosis based on a stereotactic biopsy.

Surgical intervention may also be required for delivery of therapeutic molecules, most typically in an investigational setting. BCNU-impregnated biodegradable wafers have been shown to have a modest benefit in newly diagnosed or recurrent high-grade gliomas subjected to a complete resection of the enhancing tumour (22, 23). Many novel, investigational therapies involve the use of surgical delivery including viral-mediated gene therapy, oncolytic viruses, intracavitary radiolabelled antibodies, and conventional and experimental drugs introduced via convection-enhanced delivery.

Radiotherapy

The European Organization for Research and Treatment of Cancer (EORTC) trial 22845 carried out in the 1980s and 1990s compared early radiotherapy versus delayed radiotherapy at the time of progression in patients with WHO grade II gliomas and showed no survival benefit of early radiotherapy with longer PFS although this was in the pre-MRI era (15, 24). The conclusion from these studies is that radiotherapy achieves local control in patients with WHO grade II diffuse astrocytomas albeit temporary but is not a curative treatment. The benefit of local control needs to be weighed against the risk of neurocognitive side effects (25, 26), particularly in patients with survival measured in years. Two randomized trials compared two doses of radiotherapy in patients with low-grade gliomas. EORTC trial 22844 showed no survival difference between low-dose (45 Gy) and conventional dose (59.4 Gy) radiotherapy (14) which in itself is not surprising as even the higher dose did not result in survival benefit compared to delayed treatment. A US trial showed no survival difference between conventional/low-dose radiotherapy (50.4 Gy) and high-dose radiotherapy considered above the limits of radiation tolerance (64.8 Gy) (16) with higher toxicity in the high-dose arm. The standard policy is to manage patients with surveillance alone and consider radiotherapy either at the time of symptomatic progression or transformation. The appropriate dose for patients managed outside clinical trials should therefore be at the conventional dose range as used in high-grade gliomas.

Radiotherapy is the mainstay of treatment in anaplastic astrocytoma and glioblastoma and of proven survival benefit. The gross tumour volume commonly includes the T1-enhanced region with clinical target volume 2 cm beyond or the T2 or FLAIR abnormality; there is no universal agreement on the appropriate target definition and margins. The standard dose for radical treatment of glioblastoma is 60 Gy in thirty 2 Gy fractions; doses of 54 Gy at 1.8 Gy per fractions are used in anaplastic astrocytoma although the use of such lower doses is not evidence based and dose fractionation as used in glioblastoma is not inappropriate. A regimen of 50 Gy given in 1.8 Gy fractions was superior to best supportive care in patients aged 70 years or older (27). In general, in patients with poor prognosis defined by age and performance status, a 6-week course of radiotherapy is considered too onerous and patients may be treated with a shorter palliative regimen such as 40 Gy in 15 fractions (28, 29) without detriment to survival. Elderly patients with anaplastic astrocytoma or glioblastoma with unmethylated *MGMT* promoter (or unknown *MGMT* status) are appropriately treated with radiotherapy, while temozolomide may be the alternative for patients with methylated *MGMT* promoter (30). Altered radical fractionation schemes giving higher effective doses as accelerated hyper- or hypofractionated regimens are not associated with survival benefit. The addition of brachytherapy or radiosurgery/stereotactic radiotherapy boost also does not prolong survival (31, 32).

While re-irradiation at the time of recurrence either as high-precision localized radiotherapy (radiosurgery, fractionated stereotactic radiotherapy, or brachytherapy) or as conventional fractionated treatment has been employed, there are no reliable data showing benefit of re-irradiation in terms of survival or functional benefit, and re-irradiation is not currently the standard of care.

In gliomatosis cerebri, whole-brain radiotherapy to doses of 50 Gy or more achieves disease control in a proportion of patients but should generally be reserved for patients with progressive or symptomatic disease, or both.

Chemotherapy

Diffuse astrocytoma

Alkylating agent chemotherapy using the PCV (procarbazine, CCNU/lomustine, and vincristine) regimen initially and temozolomide more recently has assumed a firm place in the treatment of patients with low-grade gliomas, despite lack of evidence regarding clinically meaningful endpoints in randomized clinical trials. In case a decision for further treatment beyond surgery is made, chemotherapy is often preferred over radiotherapy in young patients with large, unresectable tumours because of the fear of long-term adverse effects from radiotherapy in patients possibly experiencing long-term survival. Radiological criteria to assess benefit from therapy have not been established and validated, but surrogate parameters such as decreased metabolic activity determined by PET or improved seizure control are advanced as arguments in favour of chemotherapy for patients with low-grade gliomas. EORTC 22033 compared radiotherapy with a protracted regimen of temozolomide (21 out of 28 days). While mature outcome data are not available yet, initial analyses indicate no major difference in PFS or overall survival (OS) (33). RTOG 9802 compared radiotherapy alone with radiotherapy followed by six cycles of PCV chemotherapy. While there was no difference in median survival or survival at 5 years, patients surviving for more than 2 years experienced improved survival when co-treated with radiotherapy and PCV (34). Molecular findings in this patient cohort in relation to outcome have not been reported.

Anaplastic astrocytoma

Alkylating agent chemotherapy has been used in the treatment of malignant gliomas for decades. In newly diagnosed anaplastic astrocytoma, the role of adjuvant chemotherapy in addition to radiotherapy is not firmly established. Meta-analyses suggested a gain in PFS and OS with the addition of nitrosourea-based chemotherapy to radiotherapy (35), but this was not confirmed in a British trial exploring the efficacy of a modified PCV protocol (36). Here, a median survival of 15 months with radiotherapy plus PCV versus 13 months with radiotherapy alone was reported.

Conversely, based on the more contemporary NOA-04 trial (19), temozolomide (200 mg/m^2, days 1–5, × 28 days) or PCV alone are probably equieffective alternatives to radiotherapy in patients with anaplastic astrocytoma, the safety profile favouring temozolomide. Importantly, in contrast to glioblastoma, *MGMT* promoter methylation was prognostic for longer survival irrespective of treatment in anaplastic gliomas in the NOA-04 trial (19).

Several treatment options are now available for patients with recurrent anaplastic astrocytoma. The choice depends primarily on the type of previous treatment: patients who have not been irradiated should commonly receive radiotherapy at recurrence. Patients irradiated at diagnosis should receive alkylating agent chemotherapy with temozolomide rather than nitrosoureas, considering the favourable safety and tolerability profile. Patients progressing after radiotherapy and one or two lines of alkylating agent chemotherapy may be treated with the vascular endothelial growth factor (VEGF) antibody, bevacizumab, as monotherapy (37) or another experimental treatment strategy.

Glioblastoma

Concomitant and adjuvant temozolomide chemotherapy plus radiotherapy is the standard of care for adult patients with newly diagnosed glioblastoma aged up to 70 and in good general and neurological condition (38). The benefit from temozolomide is most prominent in patients with glioblastoma with as opposed to without *MGMT* promoter methylation (39). Temozolomide is given at 75 mg/m^2 during radiotherapy and for six maintenance cycles on 5 out of 28 days at 150–200 mg/m^2 thereafter. There is no proven benefit for extending chemotherapy beyond six cycles or for increasing the dose or frequency of temozolomide administration in the setting of newly diagnosed disease (40). Since the introduction of temozolomide, the role of nitrosoureas given either systemically orally or intravenously or locally in the form of wafers has steadily declined.

The increasing population of elderly patients with glioblastoma represents a particular challenge, with surgery followed by radiotherapy as the standard of care up to 2012 (27). Data from two independent phase III now demonstrate that temozolomide alone is an alternative option to radiotherapy in elderly glioblastoma patients that is probably superior to radiotherapy alone in patients with tumours with *MGMT* promoter methylation (29, 30). Thus, *MGMT* testing should become standard practice at least in this subgroup of glioblastoma patients. Interestingly, in the growing population of elderly patients, there is no major difference in prognosis between anaplastic astrocytoma and glioblastoma (3, 30, 41).

The therapeutic options for patients with recurrent glioblastoma are steadily increasing, but standards of care are not defined and individual treatment decisions have to be based on prior treatment, age, performance score, and other factors. Beyond second surgery and re-irradiation, there are essentially three strategies of medical treatment for recurrent glioblastoma: nitrosourea-based regimens, alternative dosing regimens of temozolomide, and bevacizumab. The activity of lomustine (CCNU) has been confirmed in the control arms of randomized trials exploring the activity of the protein kinase C-β inhibitor, enzastaurin (42) or the VEGF receptor inhibitor, cediranib (43), with PFS rates at 6 months of 20%. Somewhat better control rates at 6 months have been observed in several, with the exception of the RESCUE trial, less well-conducted

explorative trials and retrospective series of using dose-dense regimens of temozolomide, for example, continuous dosing or 1 week on 1 week off or 3 weeks on 1 week off (44). Of note, a British trial in recurrent, temozolomide-naïve malignant glioma patients failed to confirm a superiority of dose-intensified temozolomide over conventionally dosed temozolomide (45), but this trial cannot be used to estimate the role of temozolomide re-challenge in a world where most glioblastoma patients receive temozolomide as part of their first-line treatment. These data suggest, however, that there is no rationale for using dose-dense temozolomide regimens in recurrent glioma patients who relapse without ever having been exposed to temozolomide before.

Bevacizumab has been approved for the treatment of recurrent glioblastoma in various countries throughout the world, but not in the European Union. The approval was based on two prospective trials that reported radiological response rates of 30% or more and promising PFS and OS times, but did not include a bevacizumab-free control arm (46, 47). The value of bevacizumab in the management of malignant gliomas in clinical practice is almost universally accepted because of transient symptom relief and steroid-sparing effects. However, many questions regarding timing and dosing schedules remain unanswered. Of note, no active combination partner for bevacizumab has been identified: all efforts at improving the results of bevacizumab in recurrent glioblastoma by combination with chemotherapy or other targeted agents have failed, including the combination with CCNU in the EORTC trial 26101 (48). Moreover, the AVAGlio and RTOG 0825 trials exploring bevacizumab versus placebo in the newly diagnosed setting prolonged PFS, but not OS (49, 50). Altogether, this series of phase III trials negative for OS allows the prediction that bevacizumab will assume no role in the standard of care of glioblastoma. Further development of the integrin antagonist, cilengitide, another candidate antiangiogenic agent, was discontinued after yet another phase III trial negative for OS (51). Tumour-treating fields are a novel treatment approach based on electrical fields that may prolong survival in newly diagnosed glioblastoma (52). To what extent this treatment will be integrated into current standards of care remains to be explored.

Gliomatosis cerebri

Alkylating agent chemotherapy is active, but the duration of tumour control is highly variable. The prospective NOA-05 trial reported a PFS rate of 50% after 8 months of intended treatment with procarbazine and CCNU alone (5). Similar tumour control rates may be obtained with temozolomide (53). Molecular profiling studies have indicated that gliomatosis cerebri is probably not a distinct entity (54).

Commentary on National Comprehensive Cancer Network and any other treatment guidelines

The treatment recommendations made here are in general consistent with those outlined in the National Comprehensive Cancer Network (NCCN) guidelines except that bevacizumab is not approved for glioblastoma in the European Union and can therefore formally not be recommended. Further, we consider temozolomide alone an appropriate treatment for glioblastoma with *MGMT* promoter methylation in the elderly (29, 30). European guidelines for WHO grade III and IV gliomas were last issued in 2014 (55).

Surveillance recommendations

In diffuse astrocytoma, anaplastic astrocytoma, and glioblastoma, MRI is commonly performed within 72 h after each resection, at 4 weeks after adjuvant radiotherapy or radiochemotherapy, and at 3-monthly intervals thereafter. These intervals may be prolonged after prolonged stable disease (e.g. after 2 years). Monitoring of disease course in gliomatosis cerebri is less standardized, but can be done accordingly. CT is reserved for patients who are not eligible for MRI monitoring. Monitoring by PET is experimental and not routinely recommended.

Children

Introduction

Astrocytic tumours are the most common primary brain and spinal cord tumours in children and constitute 25.7–52% of all childhood brain tumours (56, 57). The incidence rate for the grade I–II group (low-grade astrocytomas) was 14.1 per million and for the grade III–IV group (high-grade astrocytomas) was 4.49 (58). Low-grade astrocytoma accounts for 22.5–42.7% of all primary CNS tumours as compare to 10–13% of high-grade astrocytomas in children (58, 59). Astrocytic tumours affect children at different ages with the mean age and ranges at the diagnosis of pilocytic astrocytoma of 7 years (4.4 months to 16.4 years), astrocytoma of 7.5 years (4.4 months to 15.7 years), anaplastic astrocytoma of 8.6 years (3 days to 16.6 years) and glioblastoma of 7.0 years (2.8 months to 17.8 years) (57). Childhood astrocytic tumours may arise from any site of the brain. The common locations include cerebral hemisphere, cerebellum, brainstem, optic pathway, thalamus, and ventricle (57). Low-grade astrocytomas predominately originate in the cerebellum, cerebral hemispheres, optic pathway, lateral ventricle (subependymal giant cell astrocytoma, SEGA), brainstem (tectum, dorsal exophytic, cervicomedullary), and spinal cord. High-grade tumours locate mainly to cerebral hemispheres, thalamus, and pons. The treatment of low-grade astrocytoma aims at gross total excision. Strategies for unresectable or residual tumours may include the selection of longitudinal clinical imaging observation, chemotherapy, and radiation with either conformal radiation therapy or stereotactic radiosurgery. High-grade astrocytomas are invasive tumours with tumour spreading via subarachnoid spaces at diagnosis in some patients. The treatment of high-grade astrocytomas in children includes the integration of surgery, radiotherapy, and chemotherapy. However, the diagnosis, treatment, survival, growth and development, and quality of life follow-up should be managed by a multidisciplinary team and in an institute with prolonged experience of treating childhood brain tumours.

Surgery

As is the case with adult gliomas, as noted previously, the treatment of a childhood brain tumour starts with a tissue diagnosis via a surgical biopsy or resection. The only situation in which it is considered generally acceptable to treat with radiotherapy or chemotherapy without a tissue diagnosis is in cases of diffuse intrinsic pontine glioma in children that are radiographically typical. That said, the development of novel targeted therapies may support more widespread interest in obtaining tissue in these cases (60).

The primary treatment of low-grade astrocytoma is surgical resection. Gross total resection is the prime prognostic factor for PFS. The probability of PFS varies with the extent of surgical excision, tumour location, and histology. No visible postoperative residual, cerebellar or cerebral hemisphere tumour, and pilocytic astrocytoma have better PFS (61, 62). Correspondingly, the extent of tumour resection correlates with tumour location and histology. Circumscribed low-grade tumours in the cerebellum and cerebral hemisphere are more feasible for radical resection with minimal residual or gross total resection with no visible residual as compared with midline and chiasmatic tumours (63). Some of the deep-seated tumours may be infiltrative in nature so that extensive surgical resection is limited. Frameless stereotactic biopsy or image-guided neuroendoscopy-assisted intraparenchymal biopsy to obtain a tissue diagnosis for the reference of treatment are the preferred options in these patients (64).

Surgery for high-grade astrocytomas in children is performed to obtain a definitive histological diagnosis and achieve a radical to gross total resection of the tumours. Radical (>90%) resection of the tumour contributes to survival in non-disseminated anaplastic astrocytoma and glioblastoma; nonetheless, glioblastoma is associated with shorter PFS and OS than anaplastic astrocytoma (59, 65). In the HIT-GBM studies, gross total resection compared with biopsy of malignant gliomas in paediatric patients was associated with significantly longer PFS and OS. For the extensively resected (i.e. 'gross-totally resected') tumours, a comparison between less than 100% and less than 90% resection was associated with longer PFS, but not with improved OS. However, gross total resection was achieved in only 29.4% of all patients. Cerebral cortical tumours and cerebellar tumours more frequently underwent gross total excision as compared to tumours originating in other regions. Gross total resection of thalamic tumours was not feasible (66).

Hydrocephalus also may be present at the time of diagnosis of a primary paediatric brain or spinal tumour. The incidence of hydrocephalus varies depending upon the location of the primary tumour (67). Hydrocephalus occurs most often in association with tumours arising from midline or paramidline tumours. Among high-grade astrocytic tumours, half of deep-seated tumours and 8% of hemispheric tumours ultimately require a permanent cerebral spinal fluid shunting procedure (65). Radical resection of tumours may help to relieve obstructive hydrocephalus and thereby avoid shunting procedures, which include endoscopic third ventriculostomy or ventriculoperitoneal shunt (67). However, extensive resection may not be feasible for many midline tumours, in particular those arising from the thalamus.

The use of 5-ALA for fluorescence-guided resection with or without intraoperative MRI-guided surgery helped to increase gross total resection and to improve PFS in adult malignant gliomas (21, 68). However, the ongoing clinical trials of 5-ALA are limited to patients aged 18 years or older (NCT01128218). For recurrent tumours, careful selection of patients for second surgery is acceptable in children for relieving mass effect-related deficits.

Radiotherapy

Radiotherapy in the initial management of paediatric malignant astrocytic tumours is used in the same manner as in adults with local irradiation and margin for microscopic disease. Three-dimensional conformal radiotherapy to the MRI-defined tumour volume is the standard of care (69) with occasional use of intensity-modulated radiotherapy if specific avoidance is considered to be of clinical value. The treatment target volumes and radiotherapy doses (to 60 Gy in 1.8–2 Gy fractions) are as used for malignant glioma in adults. In extensive disease, such as gliomatosis cerebri, large-field irradiation is still needed with radiotherapy doses around 50 Gy. Concurrent and adjuvant temozolomide are used in glioblastoma as in adults (38) although a specific paediatric study to demonstrate benefit is not available.

Chemotherapy

There is no consensus regarding optimal chemotherapy regimens for paediatric patients with high-grade gliomas. There are few randomized trials compared with adult patients. In order to avoid delayed sequelae, infants and young children under 3 years of age often do not receive radiotherapy initially. Chemotherapy alone is the first-line adjuvant treatment after resection in such patients. Multi-agent chemotherapy has been considered, such as the vincristine, cisplatin, and cyclophosphamide combination (BABY POG). On the other hand, the treatment option in children old than 3 years old is radiotherapy with or without concomitant chemotherapy followed by adjuvant chemotherapy. Using the PCV regimen has suggested a survival benefit in a cohort of 58 patients (70). The 5-year event-free survival was 46% with chemotherapy plus radiotherapy and 18% with radiotherapy alone. An eight-drugs-in-1-day chemotherapeutic regimen consisting of vincristine, carmustine, procarbazine, hydroxyurea, cisplatin, cytosine arabinoside, methylprednisone, and dacarbazine was not superior to PCV in a large randomized trial (172 patients, aged between 18 months and 21 years old) conducted from 1985 to 1990 (Children's Cancer Group 945 study CCG-945) (71, 72). Temozolomide, the standard of care in adult glioblastoma (38), is also often used in many children. However, in the Children's Oncology Group Study ACNS0126, in 90 eligible patients with high-grade gliomas, concomitant chemoradiotherapy with temozolomide and following chemotherapy with temozolomide, the results showed no improvement of event-free survival and OS as comparing with the CCG-945 study (73). Intensive chemotherapy following surgery has been reported to improve survival in 97 paediatric patients with high-grade gliomas treated within the HIT-GBM-C protocol (74). Some studies suggested that high-dose myeloablative chemotherapy followed by autologous stem cell rescue might play a possible role in newly diagnosed and recurrent childhood malignant gliomas (75–78). However, it is difficult to draw conclusion from these trials. Bevacizumab has also been investigated in some phase I or II trials; however, its activity is less prominent than in adults (79).

Commentary on National Comprehensive Cancer Network and any other treatment guidelines

There are no guidelines of paediatric high-grade glioma available within the NCCN or other international guidelines.

Surveillance recommendations

Similar to adults, in anaplastic astrocytoma and glioblastoma in children, for those patients after radical resection of tumour, MRI is recommended within 72 hours after tumour resection to determine extent of resection. Follow-up MRI is performed at 4 weeks after adjuvant therapy and in 3-monthly intervals thereafter. These intervals may be increased after prolonged disease stabilization for 2 years.

Current research topics

Clinical research

The major cooperative clinical trial groups believe that future studies in patients with anaplastic gliomas should take into consideration the difficulties in subclassifying these tumours by morphology alone as well as the strong diagnostic, prognostic, and predictive impact of molecular markers. The CATNON trial (NCT00626990), in a 2×2 design, enrolled patients with anaplastic glioma *without* 1p/19q co-deletion to examine the role of concomitant or adjuvant temozolomide or both added to radiotherapy. Patients are stratified for *MGMT* gene promoter methylation in CATNON. This trial completed enrolment, and in late 2015, a scheduled preliminary analysis revealed that use of adjuvant temozolomide provided a survival benefit for these patients. Full analysis, including that of the role of concurrent temozolomide and radiotherapy, is pending maturity of the data. A companion trial for patients with anaplastic gliomas without 1p/19q co-deletions, largely oligodendroglial tumours (CODEL, NCT00887146), was placed on hold following the 2012 updates of the RTOG 9402 and EORTC 26951 trials which had indicated superiority for OS of radiotherapy plus PCV chemotherapy over radiotherapy alone (see Chapter 4). This trial has been reformulated to examine the equivalence of radiotherapy plus temozolomide to radiotherapy plus PCV in patients with WHO grade II and III gliomas with 1p/19q co-deletion in terms of prolongation of PFS.

Despite the enormous amount of information on molecular genetic aberrations in gliomas accumulated in recent years, targeted therapy is still waiting for its primetime. Instead, immuno-oncology is now the major area of clinical research for patients with gliomas, notably glioblastoma. The majority of studies focus on the study of immune checkpoint inhibitors which prevent the induction of T-cell inactivation via the target molecules, cytotoxic lymphocyte antigen 4 or programmed death 1 (80). Further, specific vaccines alone or in conjunction with autologous dendritic cells are being explored. The ACT IV phase III trial on the EGFRvIII-targeted vaccine rindopepimut was suspended for futility in March 2016. Whether immuno-oncology will meet the great expectations of neuro-oncology remains to be seen.

Laboratory research

Molecular profiling using high-throughput analyses of genomics, mRNA expression, or DNA methylation are currently used to subclassify gliomas both in adulthood and in children (7, 81–84). However, these new subtypes of gliomas have not assumed relevance for clinical decision-making yet. Laboratory science focuses on a better characterization and identification of glioma-initiating cells ('stem cells') to develop targeted therapies against the putatively most important glioma cell population within heterogeneous tumours.

References

1. Louis DN, Ohgaki H, Wiestler OD, et al. The 2007 WHO classification of tumours of the central nervous system. *Acta Neuropathol* 2007; 114:97–109.

2. Desestret V, Ciccarino P, Ducray F, et al. Prognostic stratification of gliomatosis cerebri by IDH1 R132H and INA expression. *J Neurooncol* 2011; 105:219–224.

3. Hartmann C, Hentschel B, Wick W, et al. Patients with IDH1 wild type anaplastic astrocytomas exhibit worse prognosis than IDH1-mutated glioblastomas, and IDH1 mutation status accounts for the unfavorable prognostic effect of higher age: implications for classification of gliomas. *Acta Neuropathol* 2010; 120:707–718.

4. Weller M, Stupp R, Hegi ME, et al. Personalized care in neuro-oncology coming of age: why we need MGMT and 1p/19q testing in malignant glioma patients in clinical practice. *Neuro-Oncology* 2012; 14:iv100–iv108.

5. Glas M, Bähr O, Felsberg J, et al. NOA-05 phase II trial of procarbazine and CCNU therapy in gliomatosis cerebri. *Ann Neurol* 2011; 70:445–453.

6. Turcan S, Rohle D, Goenka A, et al. IDH1 mutation is sufficient to establish the glioma hypermethylator phenotype. *Nature* 2012; 483:479–483.

7. The Cancer Genome Atlas Research Network. Comprehensive genomic characterization defines human glioblastoma genes and core pathways. *Nature* 2008; 455:1061–1068.

8. La Fougère C, Suchorska B, Bartenstein P, et al. Molecular imaging of gliomas with PET: opportunities and limitations. *Neuro-Oncology* 2011; 13:806–819.

9. Macdonald DR, Cascino TL, Schold SC, et al. Response criteria for phase II studies of supratentorial malignant glioma. *J Clin Oncol* 1990; 8:1277–1280.

10. Wen PY, Macdonald DR, Reardon DA, et al. Updated response assessment criteria for high-grade gliomas: response assessment in neuro-oncology working group. *J Clin Oncol* 2010; 28:1963–1972.

11. van den Bent MJ, Wefel JS, Schiff D, et al. Response assessment in neuro-oncology (a report of the RANO group): assessment of outcome in trials of diffuse low-grade gliomas. *Lancet Oncol* 2011; 12:583–593.

12. Brandsma D, Stalpers L, Taal W, et al. Clinical features, mechanisms, and management of pseudoprogression in malignant gliomas. *Lancet Oncol* 2008; 9:453–461.

13. Pignatti F, Van Den Bent M, Curran D, et al. Prognostic factors for survival in adult patients with cerebral low-grade glioma. *J Clin Oncol* 2002; 20:2076–2084.

14. Karim AB, Maat B, Hatlevoll R, et al. A randomized trial on dose-response in radiation therapy of low-grade cerebral glioma: European Organization for Research and Treatment of Cancer (EORTC) study 22844. *Int J Radiat Oncol Biol Phys* 1996; 36:549–556.

15. Karim AB, Afra D, Cornu P, et al. Randomized trial on the efficacy of radiotherapy for cerebral low-grade glioma in the adult: European Organization for Research and Treatment of Cancer Study 22845 with the Medical Research Council study BRO4: an interim analysis. *Int J Radiat Oncol Biol Phys* 2002; 52:316–324.

16. Shaw E, Arusell R, Scheithauer B, et al. Prospective randomized trial of low- versus high-dose radiation therapy in adults with supratentorial low-grade glioma: initial report of a North Central Cancer Treatment Group/Radiation Therapy Oncology Group/Eastern Cooperative Oncology Group study. *J Clin Oncol* 2002; 20:2267–2276.

17. Lacroix M, Abi-Said D, Fourney DR, et al. A multivariate analysis of 416 patients with glioblastoma multiforme: prognosis, extent of resection, and survival. *J Neurosurg* 2001; 95:190–198.

18. Sanai N, Polley MY, McDermott MW, et al. An extent of resection threshold for newly diagnosed glioblastomas. *J Neurosurg* 2011; 115:3–8.

19. Wick W, Hartmann C, Engel C, et al. NOA-04 randomized phase III trial of sequential radiochemotherapy of anaplastic glioma with PCV or temozolomide. *J Clin Oncol* 2009; 27:5874–5880.

20. McGirt MJ, Mukherjee D, Chaichana KL, et al. Association of surgically acquired motor and language deficits on overall survival after resection of glioblastoma multiforme. *Neurosurgery* 2009; 65:463–469.

21. Stummer W, Pichlmeier U, Meinel T, et al. Fluorescence-guided surgery with 5-aminolevulinic acid for resection of malignant glioma: a randomised controlled multicentre phase III trial. *Lancet Oncol* 2006; 7:392–401.

22. Brem H, Piantadosi S, Burger PC, et al. Placebo-controlled trial of safety and efficacy of intraoperative controlled delivery by biodegradable polymers of chemotherapy for recurrent gliomas. *Lancet* 1995; 345:1008–1012.

23. Westphal M, Hilt DC, Bortey E, et al. A phase 3 trial of local chemotherapy with biodegradable wafers (Gliadel wafers) in patients with primary malignant glioma. *Neuro-Oncology* 2003; 5:79–88.

24. Van den Bent MJ, Afra D, de Witte O, et al. Long-term efficacy of early versus delayed radiotherapy for low-grade astrocytoma and oligodendroglioma in adults: the EORTC 22845 randomised trial. *Lancet* 2005; 366:985–990.

25. Klein M, Heimans JJ, Aaronson NK, et al. Effect of radiotherapy and other treatment- related factors on mid-term to long-term cognitive sequelae in low-grade gliomas: a comparative study. *Lancet* 2002; 360:1361–1368.

26. Douw L, Klein M, Fagel SS, et al. Cognitive and radiological effects of radiotherapy in patients with low-grade glioma: long-term follow-up. *Lancet Neurol* 2009; 8:810–818.

27. Keime-Guibert F, Chinot O, Taillandier L, et al. Radiotherapy for glioblastoma in the elderly. *N Engl J Med* 2007; 356:1527–1535.

28. Roa W, Brasher PM, Bauman G, et al. Abbreviated course of radiation therapy in older patients with glioblastoma multiforme: a prospective randomized clinical trial. *J Clin Oncol* 2004; 22:1583–1588.

29. Malmström A, Grønberg BH, Marosi C, et al. Temozolomide versus standard 6-week radiotherapy versus hypofractionated radiotherapy for patients aged over 60 years with glioblastoma: the Nordic randomized phase 3 trial. *Lancet Oncol* 2012; 13(9):916–926.

30. Wick W, Platten M, Meisner C, et al. Chemotherapy *versus* radiotherapy for malignant astrocytoma in the elderly. *Lancet Oncol* 2012; 13:707–715.

31. Souhami L, Seiferheld W, Brachman D, et al. Randomized comparison of stereotactic radiosurgery followed by conventional radiotherapy with carmustine to conventional radiotherapy with carmustine for patients with glioblastoma multiforme: report of Radiation Therapy Oncology Group 93-05 protocol. *Int J Radiat Oncol Biol Phys* 2004; 60:853–860.

32. Laperriere NJ, Leung PM, McKenzie S, et al. Randomized study of brachytherapy in the initial management of patients with malignant astrocytoma. *Int J Radiat Oncol Biol Phys* 1998; 41:1005–1011.

33. Baumert BG, Mason WP, Ryan G, et al. Temozolomide chemotherapy versus radiotherapy in molecularly characterized (1p loss) low-grade glioma: a randomized phase III intergroup study by the EORTC/NCIC-CTG/TROG/MRC-CTU (EORTC 22033-26033). *J Clin Oncol* 2013; 31(Suppl):Abstract 2007.

34. Shaw EG, Wang M, Coons SW, et al. Randomized trial of radiation therapy plus procarbazine, lomustine, and vincristine chemotherapy for supratentorial adult low-grade glioma: initial results of RTOG 9802. *J Clin Oncol* 2012; 30:3065–3070.

35. Glioma Meta-analysis Trialists (GMT) Group. Chemotherapy in adult high-grade glioma: a systematic review and meta-analysis of individual patient data from 12 randomised trials. *Lancet* 2002; 359:1011–1018.

36. The Medical Research Council Brain Tumor Working Party. Randomized trial of procarbazine, lomustine, and vincristine in the adjuvant treatment of high-grade astrocytoma: a Medical Research Council trial. *J Clin Oncol* 2001; 19:509–518.

37. Chamberlain MC, Johnston S. Salvage chemotherapy with bevacizumab for recurrent alkylator-refractory anaplastic astrocytoma. *J Neurooncol* 2009; 91:359–367.

38. Stupp R, Mason WP, van den Bent MJ, et al. Radiotherapy plus concomitant and adjuvant temozolomide for patients with newly diagnosed glioblastoma. *N Engl J Med* 2005; 352:987–996.

39. Hegi ME, Diserens AC, Gorlia T, et al. MGMT gene silencing and response to temozolomide in glioblastoma. *N Engl J Med* 2005; 352:997–1003.

40. Gilbert MR, Wang M, Aldape KD, et al. Dose-dense temozolomide for newly diagnosed glioblastoma: a randomized phase III clinical trial. *J Clin Oncol* 2013; 31:4085–4091.

41. Barnholtz-Sloan JS, Williams VL, Maldonado JL, et al. Patterns of care and outcomes among elderly individuals with primary malignant astrocytoma. *J Neurosurg* 2008; 108:642–648.

42. Wick W, Puduvalli VK, Chamberlain M, et al. Enzastaurin versus lomustine in the treatment of recurrent intracranial glioblastoma: a phase III study. *J Clin Oncol* 2010; 28:1168–1174.

43. Batchelor TT, Mulholland P, Neyns B, et al. Phase III randomized trial comparing the efficacy of cediranib as monotherapy, and in combination with lomustine, with lomustine alone in patients with recurrent glioblastoma. *J Clin Oncol* 2013; 31:3212–3218.

44. Perry JR, Belanger K, Mason WP, et al. Phase II trial of continuous dose-intense temozolomide in recurrent malignant glioma: RESCUE study. *J Clin Oncol* 2010; 28:2051–2057.

45. Brada M, Stenning S, Gabe R, et al. Temozolomide versus procarbazine, lomustine, and vincristine in recurrent high-grade glioma. *J Clin Oncol* 2010; 28:4601–4608.

46. Kreisl TN, Kim L, Moore K, et al. Phase II trial of single-agent bevacizumab followed by bevacizumab plus irinotecan at tumor progression in recurrent glioblastoma. *J Clin Oncol* 2009; 27:740–745.

47. Friedman H, Prados M, Wen P, et al. Bevacizumab alone and in combination with irinotecan in recurrent glioblastoma. *J Clin Oncol* 2009; 27:4733–4740.

48. Wick W, Brandes A, Gorlia T, et al. Phase III trial exploring the combination of bevacizumab and lomustine in patients with first recurrence of a glioblastoma: the EORTC 26101 trial. *Neuro-Oncol* 2015; 17(Suppl 5):LB05.

49. Chinot O, Wick W, Mason W, et al. Bevacizumab plus radiotherapy-temozolomide for newly diagnosed glioblastoma. *N Engl J Med* 2014; 370:709–722.

50. Gilbert MR, Dignam JJ, Armstrong TS, et al. A randomized trial of bevacizumab for newly diagnosed glioblastoma. *N Engl J Med* 2014; 370:699–708.

51. Stupp R, Hegi ME, Gorlia T, et al. Cilengitide combined with standard treatment for patients with newly diagnosed glioblastoma with methylated O6-methylguanine-DNA methyltransferase (MGMT) promoter: final results of the multicentre, randomised, open-label, controlled, phase 3 CENTRIC (EORTC 26071-22072) study. *Lancet Oncol* 2014; 15:1100–1108.

52. Stupp R, Taillibert S, Kanner AA, et al. Maintenance therapy with tumor-treating fields plus temozolomide vs temozolomide alone for glioblastoma: a randomized clinical trial. *JAMA* 2015; 314:2535–2543.

53. Kaloshi G, Guillevin R, Martin-Duverneuil N, et al. Gray matter involvement predicts chemosensitivity and prognosis in gliomatosis cerebri. *Neurology* 2009; 73:445–449.

54. Herrlinger U, Jones DTW, Glas M, et al. Gliomatosis cerebri: no evidence for a separate brain tumor entity. *Acta Neuropathol* 2016; 131(2):309–319.

55. Weller M, Van den Bent M, Hopkins K, et al. EANO guideline on the diagnosis and treatment of malignant glioma. *Lancet Oncol* 2014; 15:e395–403.

56. Gurney JG, Smith MA, Bunin GR. CNS and miscellaneous intracranial and intraspinal neoplasms. In: Ries LA, Smith MA, Gurney JG, et al. (eds) *Cancer Incidence and Survival among Children and Adolescents: United States SEER Program 1975–1995*. Bethesda, MD: National Cancer Institute, SEER Program, 1999; 51–63.

57. Wong TT, Ho DM, Chang KP, et al. Primary pediatric brain tumors: statistics of Taipei VGH, Taiwan (1975–2004). *Cancer* 2005; 104:2156–2167.

58. Hjalmars U, Kulldorff M, Wahlqvist Y, et al. Increased incidences rate but no space-time clustering of childhood astrocytoma in Sweden 1973-1992. *Cancer* 1999; 85:2077–2090.

59. Campbell J, Pollack IF, Martinez AJ, et al. High-grade astrocytoma in children: radiologically complete resection is associated with an excellent long-term prognosis. *Neurosurgery* 1998; 38:258–264.

60. Grill J, Puget S, Andreiuolo F, et al. Critical oncogenic mutations in newly diagnosed pediatric diffuse intrinsic pontine glioma. *Pediatr Blood Cancer* 2012; 58:489–491.

61. Shaw EG, Wisoff JH. Prospective clinical trials of intracranial low-grade glioma in adults and children. *Neuro-oncology* 2003; 5(3):153–160.

62. Wisoff JH, Sanford RA, Sposto R, et al. Primary neurosurgery for pediatric low-grade gliomas: a prospective multi-institutional study from the children's oncology group. *Neurosurg* 2011; 68:1548–1554.

63. Pollack IF, Claassen D, al-Shboul Q, et al. Low grade gliomas of the cerebral hemispheres in children: an analysis of 71 cases. *J Neurosurg* 1995; 82:536–547.

64. Akai T, Shiraga S, Sasagawa Y, et al. Intraparenchyma tumor biopsy using neuroendoscopy with navigation. *Minim Invasive Neurosurg* 2008; 51:83–86.

65. Wisoff JH, Boyett JM, Berger MS, et al. Current neurosurgical management and the impact of the extent of resection in the treatment of malignant gliomas of childhood: a report of the Children's Cancer Group trial no. CCG-945. *J Neurosurg* 1998; 89:52–59.

66. Kramm CM, Wagner S, Van Gool S, et al. Improved survival after gross total resection of malignant gliomas in pediatric patients from the HIT-GBM studies. *Anticancer Res* 2006; 26:3773–3779.

67. Wong TT, Liang ML, Chen HH, et al. Hydrocephalus with brain tumors in children. *Childs Nerv Syst* 2011; 27:1723–1734.

68. Tsugu A, Ishizaka H, Mizokami Y, et al. Impact of the combination of 5-aminolevulinic acid-induced fluorescence with intraoperative magnetic resonance imaging-guided surgery for glioma. *World Neurosurg* 2011; 76:120–127.

69. Chan JL, Lee SW, Fraass BA, et al. Survival and failure patterns of high-grade gliomas after three dimensional conformal radiotherapy. *J Clin Oncol* 2002; 20:1635–1642.

70. Sposto R, Ertel IJ, Jenkin RD, et al. The effectiveness of chemotherapy for treatment of high grade astrocytoma in children: results of a randomized trial. A report from the Children's Cancer Study Group. *J Neurooncol* 1989; 7:165–177.

71. Finlay JL, Boyett JM, Yates AJ, et al. Randomized phase III trial in childhood high-grade astrocytoma comparing vincristine, lomustine, and prednisone with the eight-drugs-in-1-day regimen. Children's Cancer Group. *J Clin Oncol* 1995; 13:112–123.

72. Geyer JR, Finlay JL, Boyett JM, et al. Survival of infants with malignant astrocytomas. A report from the Children's Cancer Group. *Cancer* 1995; 75:1045–1050.

73. Cohen KJ, Pollack IF, Zhou T, et al. Temozolomide in the treatment of high-grade gliomas in children: a report from the Children's Oncology Group. *Neuro-Oncology* 2011; 13:317–323.

74. Wolff JE, Riever PH, Erdlenbruch B, et al. Intensive chemotherapy improves survival in pediatric high-grade glioma after gross total resection: results of the HIT-GBM-C protocol. *Cancer* 2010; 116:705–712.

75. Heideman RL, Douglass EC, Kellie SJ, et al. High-dose chemotherapy and autologous bone marrow rescue followed by interstitial and external-beam radiotherapy in newly diagnosed pediatric malignant gliomas. *J Clin Oncol* 1993; 13:1458–1465.

76. Finlay JL, Goldman S, Wong MC, et al. Pilot study of high-dose thiotepa and etoposide with autologous bone marrow rescue in children and young adults with recurrent CNS tumors. The Children's Cancer Group. *J Clin Oncol* 1996; 14:2495–2503.

77. Finlay JL, Dhall G, Boyett JM, et al. Myeloablative chemotherapy with autologous bone marrow rescue in children and adolescents with recurrent malignant astrocytoma: outcome compared with conventional chemotherapy: a report from the Children's Oncology Group. *Pediatr Blood Cancer* 2008; 51:806–11.

78. Massimino M, Gandola L, Luksch R, et al. Sequential chemotherapy, high-dose thiotepa, circulating progenitor cell rescue, and radiotherapy for childhood high-grade glioma. *Neuro-Oncology* 2005; 7:41–48.

79. Narayana A, Kunnakkat S, Chacko-Mathew J, et al. Bevacizumab in recurrent high-grade pediatric gliomas. *Neuro-Oncology* 2010; 12:985–990.

80. Preusser P, Lim M, Hafler DA, et al. Prospects of immune checkpoint modulators in the treatment of glioblastoma. *Nat Rev Neurol* 2015; 11:504–514.

81. Phillips HS, Kharbanda S, Chen R et al. Molecular subclasses of high-grade glioma predict prognosis, delineate a pattern of disease progression, and resemble stages in neurogenesis. *Cancer Cell* 2006; 9:157–173.

82. Verhaak RG, Hoadley KA, Purdom E, et al. Integrated genomic analysis identifies clinically relevant subtypes of glioblastoma characterized by abnormalities in PDGFRA, IDH1, EGFR, and NF1. *Cancer Cell* 2010; 17:98–110.

83. Noushmehr H, Weisenberger DJ, Diefes K, et al. Identification of a CpG island methylator phenotype that defines a distinct subgroup of glioma. *Cancer Cell* 2010; 17:510–522.

84. Schwartzentruber J, Korshunov A, Liu XY, et al. Driver mutations in histone H3.3 and chromatin remodelling genes in paediatric glioblastoma. *Nature* 2012; 482:226–231.

CHAPTER 4

Oligodendroglial tumours

Wolfgang Wick, Colin Watts, and Minesh P. Mehta

Definition

Oligodendroglial tumours comprise 8–12% of all gliomas. The World Health Organization (WHO) separates these into well-differentiated oligodendrogliomas (grade II) and anaplastic oligodendrogliomas (grade III) (5–6% of all gliomas). These tumours have a specific histopathological appearance. They are composed of cells with small to slightly enlarged round, dark, and compact nuclei with a small amount of eosinophilic cytoplasm. Perinuclear halos, occurring as a diagnostic fixation artefact and displaying a 'fried egg' or 'honeycomb' appearance, are commonly seen, as are calcifications and reticular (chicken wire) vessels. Occasionally, tumour cells with a small amount of strongly eosinophilic cytoplasm are encountered and these are termed 'mini-gemistocytes' (Fig. 4.1). Occasional mitoses and a Ki-67/MIB-1 labelling index up to 5% are compatible with oligodendroglioma WHO grade II. There is no immunohistochemical marker specific for oligodendrogliomas.

Some tumours show both oligodendroglial and astrocytic components (2–4%) and have been called mixed gliomas or oligoastrocytoma (WHO grade II or III) for many decades. Since a molecular classification does not allow a separation of these mixed tumours, but in contrast allows calling them either oligodendroglioma or astrocytoma, the 2016 WHO classification strongly discourages the designation oligoastrocytoma and recommends using genetic analysis for a correct diagnosis of either diffuse astrocytoma or oligodendroglioma. Application of identical diagnostic criteria poses difficulties for the separation of oligoastrocytomas from both astrocytomas and oligodendrogliomas as the diagnostic features represent a continuum from one end of the histological spectrum to the other. Because the amount of material available to the neuropathologist may be limited due to modern surgical approaches which sometimes yield very little tissue for diagnosis and also because of increased scientific interest in banking fresh tumour tissue, the diagnostic certainty is further limited (1). WHO guidelines for the diagnosis of a grade III oligodendroglial tumour include subjective criteria such as 'significant' hypercellularity and pleomorphism. In addition, the presence of low mitotic activity, vascular proliferation, and necrosis, including pseudopalisading necrosis, are insufficient by themselves to elevate the grade of these tumours. All of these factors lead to considerable interobserver diagnostic variability, which has been addressed in the most recent update of the WHO classification (2).

Although the tumour may appear to be vaguely circumscribed, it is by definition a diffusely infiltrating tumour. However, whether the grade of infiltration and growth pattern is the same in astrocytic and oligodendroglial tumours is not yet clear.

Areas of major subjectivity that are not adequately clarified by the current WHO classification include the differentiation between grade II and III gliomas, the classification of oligodendroglial tumours with necrosis, and the diagnosis of a mixed glioma, that is, an oligoastrocytoma. A set of 114 anaplastic oligodendroglial tumours from the European Organization for Research and Treatment of Cancer (EORTC) 26951 was reviewed independently by nine internationally renowned pathologists. The panel diagnosed a low-grade glioma in 1–16%, an anaplastic astrocytoma in up to 11%, and a glioblastoma in 1–27% (3). A similar exercise was performed with tissue from the Radiation Therapy Oncology Group (RTOG) 94-02 trial that had a central review to begin with. Interobserver variability was again higher than wished for, with a Cohen's kappa of 0.55 (95% confidence interval (CI) 0.44–0.65) (4). Not surprisingly, this intrinsic diagnostic variability, in addition to other confounding variables, factors at study entry, and the inherent difficulty in comparing between trials, leads to major differences in outcomes when the larger trials focusing on this entity, including EORTC 26951, RTOG 94-02, and Neuro-Oncology Working Party of the German Cancer Society (NOA)-04, are compared (5) (Table 4.1).

Epidemiology

Oligodendroglial tumours make up 4–6% of all primary central nervous system (CNS) tumours, with a male preponderance and occurrence at a lower relative proportion in children. The median age at diagnosis is 35 years. There are no known geographic or racial differences in the incidence or natural history of disease.

Data regarding the natural history after definitive diagnosis are sparse and are mainly limited to grade II gliomas with good prognostic factors, or in patients with poor underlying performance status (6, 7). Patients with prognostically favourable grade II tumours may experience clinical stability over many years without therapeutic intervention (8). Population-based observational studies are also rare. A Swiss population-based registry (9) reported median survivals of 11.6 and 3.5 years for patients with oligodendrogliomas and anaplastic oligodendrogliomas, respectively. Whether one of the later-discussed molecular markers or the oligodendroglial morphology confers a less aggressive course of disease remains unclear. Expression of N-myc downstream-regulated gene 1 (*NDRG1*), not one of the more commonly assessed molecular parameters (discussed later), has been associated with a better natural course of disease without genotoxic treatments (10).

Simple screening tests for early diagnosis are not available, and magnetic resonance imaging (MRI), can only detect macroscopic disease. Anecdotal clinical evidence indicates that glioblastomas

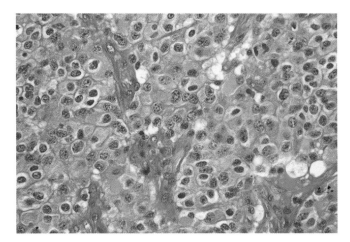

Fig. 4.1 Typical histological appearance of a grade II oligodendroglioma. These tumours are composed of cells with small to slightly enlarged round nuclei with dark, compact nuclei and a small amount of eosinophilic cytoplasm including perinuclear halos as a diagnostic fixation artefact, termed 'fried egg' or 'honeycomb' appearance, frequently containing calcifications and reticular (chicken wire) vessels. Reproduced from https://en.wikipedia.org/wiki/Oligodendroglioma#/media/File:Oligodendroglioma1_high_mag.jpg under the Creative Commons License 3.0.

may evolve within a few months, further supporting the concept that early diagnosis and screening are not feasible at a population level and should therefore be restricted, if recommended at all, to individuals at high risk for developing gliomas, such as those with neurofibromatosis types 1 and 2 or Li–Fraumeni syndrome. Whether such patients should undergo repeated neuroimaging in the absence of new neurological symptoms or signs, however, remains uncertain.

Aetiology

The only proposed risk factor for gliomas is exposure to irradiation to the brain, for example, in patients with long-term

remission from leukaemias treated with prophylactic radiotherapy to the brain (11). There is no causal relationship with head trauma, nitrosamine-containing food, or electromagnetic fields. The use of mobile phones continues to remain controversial in terms of its causal association with gliomas but increasingly, the majority of longer-term data do not demonstrate a strong association, as these have only been in major use for the past 15 years. A minority of patients with anaplastic oligodendroglial tumours have a positive family history for gliomas (7).

Pathogenesis

Among anaplastic gliomas there is high correlation between oligodendroglial morphology and the 1p/19q co-deletion, a pericentromeric unbalanced translocation. Tumours with 1p/19q co-deletion carry isocitrate dehydrogenase (*IDH*)-1/2 mutations and frequently demonstrate O^6-methylguanine DNA methyltransferase (*MGMT*) promoter methylation as well as telomerase reverse transcriptase (*TERT*) promoter mutations (12). In contrast, tumour protein p53 (*TP53*) mutation and loss of alpha-thalassemia/mental retardation syndrome X-linked (*ATRX*) expression are rare in 1p/19q co-deleted gliomas, but common in diffuse and anaplastic astrocytomas. This may help to distinguish the controversial entity of anaplastic oligoastrocytoma (13) (Fig. 4.2).

In addition to molecular markers, there are clinical prognostic factors for grade II oligodendroglial tumours including age over 40 years and the presence of preoperative neurological deficits (6, 12). Regarding neuroimaging findings, larger tumours and tumours crossing the midline correlate with shorter overall and progression-free survival (6, 14). Growth rates, based on imaging findings, are inversely correlated with survival (15). There are conflicting reports as to whether contrast enhancement is associated with a worse prognosis (16, 17). Low cerebral blood volume (CBV) on MRI (18) and a low uptake of ^{11}C-methionine (19) correlate with longer progression-free and overall survival (class III), although the value of CBV in oligodendroglial tumours is debatable (Fig. 4.3).

Table 4.1 Progression-free and overall survival of patients with anaplastic oligodendroglial tumours by trial and treatment group

Trial (reference)	Treatment group	
RTOG 94-02 (45)	RT	PCV + RT
Median PFS, months (95% CI)	20.4 (15.6–28.8)	31.2 (22.8–49.2)
Median OS, months (95% CI)	56.4 (40.8–68.4)	58.8 (39.6–86.4)
EORTC 26951 (41)	RT	RT + PCV
Median PFS, months (95% CI)	13.0 (9.2–19.4)	23.0 (17.6–43.8)
Median OS, months (95% CI)	30.6 (21.9–45.3)	40.3 (28.7–68.2)
NOA-04 (40)	RT	PCV or TMZ
Median PFS, months (95% CI)	52.1 (36.4–n.r.)	52.7 (33.9–n.r.)
Median OS, months	84+	84+

n.r., not reached; OS, overall survival; PCV, procarbazine, CCNU (lomustine), and vincristine; PFS, progression-free survival; RT, radiotherapy; TMZ, temozolomide.

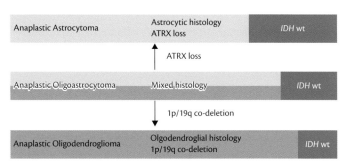

Fig. 4.2 Proposed molecular classification of anaplastic gliomas based on histology and molecular markers. Length of the green bars (right of diagram) represents the proportion of *IDH*-wild-type tumours, whereas the yellow and blue bars (top left and bottom left, respectively, of diagram) represent *IDH*-mutant tumours. Mixed anaplastic oligoastrocytomas harbouring *IDH* mutations are molecularly classified as either oligodendrogliomas (carrying 1p/19q co-deletion) or astrocytomas (carrying *ATRX* loss).
Reproduced from *Acta Neuropathol*, 126(3), Wiestler B, Capper D, Holland-Letz T, et al., ATRX loss refines the classification of anaplastic gliomas and identifies a subgroup of IDH mutant astrocytic tumors with better prognosis, pp. 443–51, Copyright (2013), with permission from Springer.

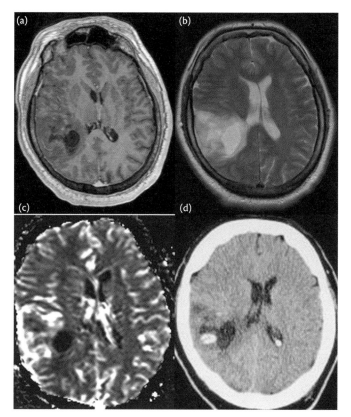

Fig. 4.3 Imaging of a grade III oligodendroglioma. (a) Typical slight, but not intense, contrast uptake and some cystic component on T1 contrast-enhanced MRI. (b) T2 gives an impression of a rather well-delineated tumour. (c) Enhanced cerebral blood flow in the solid tumour area (white signal). (d) Computed tomography gives a clear impression of intratumoural macro-calcification.
Images courtesy of Prof. Martin Bendszus, Heidelberg, Germany.

Clinical presentation

Seizures are the most common clinical presentation of grade II gliomas and may be partial or generalized. Seizures occur in 70–90% of patients and are intractable in almost 50% of patients with grade II tumours. Seizures are more frequently associated with cortically based tumours, particularly in frontal, temporal, and insular/para-insular locations and with oligodendroglial tumours (20). There is no clear association between the severity of seizures and tumour behaviour.

Another frequent presentation is headaches, which are identified in 40–50% of patients. Focal neurological deficits are unusual, developing over many years, but may present as hemiparesis or aphasia in 5–20% of patients. Raised intracranial pressure is rare in patients with supratentorial tumours and is typically seen in posterior fossa and intraventricular tumours. Intratumoural haemorrhage can occur, but is uncommon.

Imaging

Conventional MRI is useful for differential diagnosis, surgical and radiation planning, and treatment monitoring (21). Grade II oligodendroglial tumours appear as low-signal mass lesions on T1-weighted MRI and high signal on T2-weighted and fluid-attenuated inversion recovery (FLAIR) sequences. Contrast

enhancement is usually absent; when present, it may indicate a focal area of high-grade transformation, although some oligodendrogliomas have patchy enhancement, which remains stable over time (Fig. 4.3). Calcification is relatively common on computed tomography images and may appear as a low signal region on MRI. The use of advanced imaging techniques has been suggested as increasing diagnostic accuracy, but no categorical studies proving this are available (20, 22, 23). Proton magnetic resonance spectroscopy (MRS) measures the concentration and spatial distribution of metabolites like choline or N-acetylaspartate. A choline/N-acetylaspartate ratio ≥2 is believed to indicate increased cellular proliferation and reduced neuronal density and highlights metabolically more active parts of the tumour in high-grade gliomas (24). This metabolite ratio has been shown to predict survival and identify relapse location in glioblastoma, in small series (23, 25). The typical spectrum of a low-grade oligodendroglial tumour shows elevated choline, presumably reflecting increased membrane turnover, and decreased N-acetylaspartate, reflecting neuronal loss, but similar abnormal spectra may be observed in non-neoplastic lesions. Grading of gliomas is not possible by spectroscopy alone, as there is considerable overlap between low- and high-grade lesions. The presence of lactate and lipids is associated with higher proliferative activity and more aggressive behaviour (27). MRS is helpful in guiding a biopsy to an area of high-grade activity, but not in longitudinal monitoring (28). Dynamic susceptibility contrast MRI allows measurement of relative cerebral blood volume (rCBV) which correlates with vascularity at the histological level. In grade II astrocytoma, increased rCBV predicts high-grade transformation before gadolinium enhancement occurs on MR (27, 29); however, these observations have not been validated in oligodendroglioma, which per se have a high rCBV, irrespective of grade II lesion (30). Quantitative MRI in oligodendrogliomas with loss of heterozygosity of chromosome 1p/19q shows more heterogeneous T1- and T2-dependent signal, less distinct tumour margins, and higher rCBV than tumours with intact 1p/19q (29, 30) chromosomes (31, 32). Dynamic contrast-enhanced MRI, which measures the permeability of the blood–brain barrier by means of the transfer coefficient, K^{trans}, does not have a well-demonstrated role in the current diagnostic armamentarium. Apparent diffusion coefficient values, as measured by diffusion-weighted imaging, are lower and more variable in oligodendrogliomas compared to astrocytomas (33).

MRI is also the most important tool for treatment planning and monitoring response to therapy in grade III oligodendroglial tumours, which may or may not enhance after contrast administration (32). MRI criteria for treatment response are under continuous development (34). Ideally, patients should be on stable steroid doses for at least 5 days prior to imaging. When tumours are located within, or adjacent to, eloquent brain regions, functional MRI (fMRI) and white matter tractography may help to assess the feasibility of surgery and serve as a guide to planning the operation. The role of further imaging techniques including perfusion MRI, single-photon emission computed tomography, and MRS in routine clinical care still needs to be defined.

Treatment

Primary or acquired resistance to alkylating agents remains one of the major obstacles in the treatment of gliomas. Several resistance factors such as the DNA mismatch repair genes *MLH1*, *MSH2*,

MSH6, and *PMS2* (35), alkylpurine DNA *N*-glycosylase (36), DNA-(apurinic or apyrimidinic site) lyase (APEX1) (37), polynucleotide 3′-phosphatase, polynucleotide 5′-hydroxyl-kinase (PNKP), or the DNA repair protein MGMT have been identified. Of these, epigenetic silencing of the *MGMT* gene plays a critical role in mediating primary resistance to alkylating agents (38). MGMT transfers an alkyl group from the O^6 position of guanine to a cysteine residue in its active site, thereby repairing the DNA damage caused by alkylating agents, including chloroethylating (e.g. carmustine and lomustine) or methylating agents (e.g. procarbazine, streptozotocin, dacarbazine, and temozolomide), which would otherwise be cytotoxic. *MGMT* promoter hypermethylation, as assessed through methylation-specific polymerase chain reaction, is associated with greater benefit from temozolomide in glioblastoma (39). In contrast, in anaplastic gliomas the predictive value of *MGMT* promoter hypermethylation has not been established (40, 41). Retrospective subgroup analysis of the NOA-04 trial suggests that in tumours with an *IDH1* mutation, *MGMT* promoter methylation was associated with prolonged progression-free survival with combined chemoradiation or radiation alone groups, and was thus prognostic. In tumours without an *IDH1* mutation, *MGMT* promoter methylation was associated with increased progression-free survival in patients treated with chemotherapy, too, but not in those who received radiation alone as the first-line treatment, and is thus predictive of benefit from chemotherapy. Therefore, *MGMT* promoter methylation is a predictive biomarker of benefit from alkylating agents in patients with *IDH1*-wild-type, but not *IDH1*-mutant malignant gliomas of WHO grades III/IV. Combined *IDH1/MGMT* assessment may help to individualize clinical decision-making (42).

Reports from the late 1980s noted a greater chemosensitivity of many gliomas with oligodendroglial features (grade II and III oligoastrocytoma and oligodendroglioma) (43). These reports led to the establishment of the combination chemotherapy regimen of procarbazine, CCNU (lomustine), and vincristine (PCV) as a standard treatment for malignant gliomas (44). The regimen consists of four to six 6-week cycles of CCNU given at 110 mg/m² on day 1, procarbazine given at 60 mg/m² on days 7–21, and vincristine given at 1.5 mg/m² intravenously on days 8 and 29. In clinical trials (40, 41, 45), this regimen was associated with considerable toxicity, chiefly myelosuppression (CCNU and procarbazine) and neuropathy (vincristine), but is very effective either alone (40) or in combination with radiotherapy (41, 45). With the introduction of temozolomide as a novel alkylating agent in gliomas, chemotherapy options have expanded. As a single agent, temozolomide is usually given on days 1–5 of 28-day cycles at a dose of 200 mg/m². Treatment duration is typically 6–12 cycles. Although there are no formal head-to-head comparisons of PCV versus temozolomide, there are, with one exception, no major differences in terms of efficacy, based on indirect comparisons (38, 40). It is widely accepted that the tolerability of temozolomide is better than PCV. For this reason and to optimize the efficacy of temozolomide, alternative dosing schedules have been developed and implemented in clinical trials including a weekly alternating (7 days on, 7 days off) schedule at 100–150 mg/m² (46) or in a 21 days on/7 days off schedule. While in the recurrent disease setting these dosing schedules have demonstrated some activity, studies in glioblastoma have not indicated superiority over the conventional 5 days on/23 days off schedule (47). Currently used alkylating chemotherapy protocols are summarized in Table 4.2.

The greater chemosensitivity of some glial tumours could, in part, be explained by *MGMT* promoter hypermethylation, but 1p/19q co-deletion and *IDH* mutations are also potential predictive biomarkers, though the mechanisms of action remain elusive (48). It may well be that these 'predictive biomarkers' just signify a different disease biology and not a molecular alteration for sensitivity to genotoxic therapy. Furthermore, these and other molecular characteristics (49–51) may supplement the morphology-based WHO classification and thus help to resolve the discrepancy between classification and clinical outcome.

Grade II oligodendroglial tumours are usually well-differentiated, slow-growing but treatment-resistant tumours. Therefore, the question when to initiate genotoxic treatments is relevant. These tumours, although often clinically stable over a long period of time, grow linearly by a few millimetres every year (52), detectable when imaging is compared to the baseline scan rather than the immediately preceding scan. To date, no curative treatment is available, and most low-grade oligodendroglial tumours eventually transform into high-grade tumours (WHO grade III or IV) at some point during the course of the disease.

Surgery

Although earlier surgical intervention and more complete resection have never been proven in randomized studies to alter overall survival, retrospective studies suggest that more extensive resection in grade II oligodendroglial tumours improves outcome (51), also in modern series (54). Although there are no controlled data from randomized studies, it appears that the extent of resection is a major prognostic factor in patients with anaplastic oligodendroglial tumours (38, 40, 52, 53, 55, 56). Macroscopic resection also improves seizure control, particularly in patients with a long history of epilepsy and insular tumours (20). A critical point in the interpretation of data from these studies is the precise definition of total resection. For grade II gliomas that do not enhance, total resection implies removal of all the hyperintense regions on T2 or FLAIR images,

Table 4.2 Protocols with alkylating chemotherapy

Protocol	Dose and mode of administration
Temozolomide concomitant	75 mg/m² every day during the period of radiotherapy
maintenance	150–200 mg/m² days 1–5 PO × 4 weeks
ACNU, BCNU, CCNU	Different regimens, e.g. CCNU PO 110 mg/m² × 6 weeks
PCV alone or prior or parallel and after radiotherapy	Procarbazine 60 mg/m² PO days 8–21
	CCNU 110 mg/m² PO day 1
	Vincristine 1.4 mg/m² IV (maximum 2 mg) day 8 + day 29 × (6–)8 weeks

ACNU, nimustine; BCNU, carmustine; CCNU, lomustine; IV, intravenous; PCV, procarbazine, CCNU (lomustine), and vincristine; PO, per os.

Adapted from *The Lancet Oncology*, 15(9), Weller M, van den Bent M, Hopkins K, Tonn JC, Stupp R, Falini A, Cohen-Jonathan-Moyal E, Frappaz D, Henriksson R, Balana C, Chinot O, Ram Z, Reifenberger G, Soffietti R, Wick W, for the European Association for Neuro-Oncology (EANO) Task Force on Malignant Glioma, EANO Guideline on the Diagnosis and Treatment of Malignant Glioma, pp. e395–e403, Copyright (2014), with permission from Elsevier.

and thus can only be determined by comparing preoperative and postoperative tumour volumes on MRI. This has only been done in a limited number of studies, and all have shown that total/near total resection decreases the incidence of recurrence and the risk of malignant transformation, and improves progression-free and overall survival (53, 56). Nonetheless, even with intra-operative MRI-guided surgery, total resection is achieved in no more than 36% of patients (57).

In the European guidelines, the timing of surgery for oligodendroglioma is controversial in patients that are young, present with an isolated seizure (medically well controlled), and with small tumours (58). Potential surgical morbidity may compromise the otherwise intact functional status and some authors have advocated deferring surgery ('watch and wait policy') after diagnosis has been made (59, 60). The risk of deferring surgery includes managing at a later time-point a larger tumour, which may have undergone anaplastic transformation (59). Improvements in surgical techniques and imaging, together with enhanced treatment options for anaplastic oligodendrogliomas in modern practice, emphasize the importance of accurately determining a histopathological diagnosis as early as feasible.

Radiotherapy

Radiotherapy is commonly utilized in patients with symptomatic and/or progressive disease or in patients with poor prognostic factors (61, 62). However, guidance as to whether a patient with a grade II oligodendroglial tumour needs early radiotherapy or not is pivotal, as its early use at currently accepted doses (50.4 Gy in 1.8 Gy fractions of the involved part of the brain) is not associated with an overall survival benefit (63) but could possibly induce long-term sequelae (1). Although radiotherapy (54–60 Gy, 1.8–2 Gy-fractions) has been considered standard of care for anaplastic oligodendroglial tumours, their chemosensitivity to nitrosoureas and temozolomide has long been recognized, and current data suggest that combination chemoradiation significantly prolongs survival, in comparison to radiation alone for grade III oligodendroglial tumours with 1p/19q co-deletions.

Four phase III randomized trials have been performed to define the value of radiotherapy and chemoradiation in grade II gliomas (Table 4.3). The 'non-believer' EORTC 22845 trial (62, 63) investigated the role of timing of radiotherapy. Although improved progression-free survival was demonstrated for patients treated with immediate radiotherapy, this did not translate into improved overall survival. Besides prolonging the time to tumour progression, radiotherapy has several other potential benefits, such as symptom control, particularly epileptic seizures (64). Two randomized trials investigated different radiation doses. The 'believer' EORTC 22844 and North Central Cancer Treatment Group (NCCTG) studies showed no advantage for higher versus lower doses (61, 65). If higher doses are used, increased toxicity is observed, with a 2-year incidence of radiation necrosis of 2.5% (61) or lower levels of functioning and quality of life, especially for fatigue, insomnia, and emotional functioning (66). RTOG 9802 compared radiotherapy alone versus radiotherapy in combination with PCV (67). As two-thirds of the patients in the radiotherapy arm who progressed received chemotherapy at progression, this trial might be considered a trial of early chemotherapy versus chemotherapy at progression. In the first analysis of study results, progression-free survival, but not overall survival, was improved. However, beyond 2 years, the addition of PCV to radiotherapy conferred a significant overall and progression-free survival advantage, and reduced the risk of death by 48% and progression by 55%, suggesting possible delayed benefit of chemotherapy. Grades III and IV toxicities were higher among patients receiving radiotherapy plus PCV versus radiotherapy alone (67% versus 9%). However, long-term follow-up of the patients enrolled in this study demonstrated a significant improvement in overall survival for the patients who received initial radiotherapy plus PCV. Patients treated with whole-brain radiotherapy have a higher incidence of leucoencephalopathy and cognitive deficits in comparison with patients treated with focal radiotherapy (68). In studies using modern methods of radiotherapy, a more limited impact on cognition is observed (69–71), although data related to patients who had more detailed neuropsychological follow-up at a mean of 12 years and were free of tumour progression suggest that those patients treated without radiotherapy maintain their cognitive status whereas patients receiving radiotherapy fare worse on attention and executive functioning as well as information processing speed (72).

Table 4.3 Phase III trials on radiotherapy and chemotherapy for low-grade gliomas

Study (reference)	Treatment arms/patients (n)	5-year progression-free survival		5-year overall survival	
EORTC 22845	S (157)	37%		66%	
(62, 63)	S + RT (154)	44%	p = 0.02	63%	NS
EORTC 22844	S + RT 45 Gy (171)	47%		58%	
(61)	S + RT 59.4 Gy (172)	50%	NS	59%	NS
NCCTG	S + RT 50.4 Gy	55%		72%	
(65)	S + RT 64.8 Gy	52%	NS	64%	NS
RTOG 9402	S + RT (125)	46%		63%	
(67)	S + RT + PCV (126)	63%	p = 0.005	72%	NS

NS, not significant; PCV, procarbazine, CCNU (lomustine), and vincristine; S, surgery; R, radiotherapy.

Adapted from *Eur J Neurol*, 17(9), Soffietti R, Baumert B, Bello L, von Deimling A, Duffau H, Frénay M, Grisold W, Grant R, Graus F, Hoang-Xuan K, Klein M, Melin B, Rees J, Siegal T, Smits A, Stupp R, Wick W, Guidelines on management of low-grade gliomas: report of an EFNS-EANO* task force, pp. 1124–33, Copyright (2010), with permission from John Wiley and Sons.

Chemotherapy

There have been a number of pivotal chemotherapy trials in patients with anaplastic oligodendroglial tumours. The phase III RTOG trial, 9402, utilized pre-radiation PCV, whereas EORTC 26951 utilized post-radiation PCV. Initial reports in 2006 showed increased progression-free but not overall survival in patients receiving radiotherapy plus chemotherapy for both trials but at the cost of significant toxicity in those receiving PCV (41, 45).

In 2012, longer-term data for both trials demonstrated an overall survival benefit in favour of the radiotherapy plus PCV regimen, specifically for patients with 1p/19q co-deleted tumours.

EORTC 26951 randomized 368 patients with newly diagnosed anaplastic oligodendroglial tumours to radiotherapy alone versus radiotherapy followed by up to six cycles of PCV. Overall survival was 42.3 months with radiotherapy followed by PCV as opposed to 30 months with radiotherapy alone (hazard ratio (HR) = 0.75, 95% CI 0.6–0.95). In patients with 1p/19q co-deleted tumours, median overall survival was not yet reached at the time of analysis, versus 112 months in the radiotherapy followed by PCV versus radiotherapy arms, respectively (HR = 0.56, 95% CI 0.31–1.03), but only 25 versus 21 months, respectively, for non-co-deleted tumours (HR = 0.83, 95% CI 0.62–1.1). Although the addition of PCV significantly prolonged survival (HR = 0.75, 95% CI 0.60–0.95) in the full trial cohort irrespective of molecular analysis, only the patients with the 1p/19q co-deletion derived a clinically relevant overall survival benefit from the addition of PCV, especially when considering the toxicity of the combined treatment (73).

In RTOG 9402, 291 patients with newly diagnosed anaplastic oligodendroglial tumours were randomized to radiotherapy or radiotherapy preceded by up to four cycles of dose-intensified PCV. Overall survival was 4.6 years with PCV followed by radiotherapy and 4.7 years with radiotherapy alone (HR = 0.79, 95% CI 0.6–1.04). However, in the subgroup of patients with 1p/19q co-deleted tumours, the overall survival was 14.7 versus 7.3 years in the PCV followed by radiotherapy versus radiotherapy arms, respectively (HR = 0.59, 95% CI 0.37–0.95), but only 2.6 versus 2.7 years, respectively for non-co-deleted tumours (HR = 0.85, 95% CI 0.58–1.23) (74).

Despite the impressive survival benefit seen in both anaplastic oligodendroglioma trials with PCV chemotherapy and radiotherapy in 1p/19q co-deleted tumours, these results are provisional. Moreover, these trials did not specify these subgroup analyses.

Cognitive functioning and health-related quality of life (HRQOL) have been evaluated in a cohort of 32/37 Dutch and French long-term anaplastic oligodendroglioma survivors from EORTC 26951. Results were compared to healthy controls and to patients' own HRQOL 2.5 years following initial treatment. At the time of assessment, median survival for the patients was 147 months, 27 were still progression-free since initial treatment. Of these 27 progression-free patients, severe cognitive impairment was observed in 30%; 41% were employed and 81% could live independently. Patients' HRQOL was worse compared to controls as expected, but similar to quality of life status 2.5 years after initial treatment. The initial treatment (radiotherapy versus radiotherapy plus PCV) was not correlated with cognition or HRQOL. These results from a small patient cohort suggest that cognitive function could be impaired in a relevant proportion of patients treated with radiotherapy and this needs to be further evaluated in larger patient cohorts (75). The role of temozolomide has introduced further controversy. Initial results from the German NOA-04 trial, which compared radiotherapy versus temozolomide versus PCV alone (40) do not provide a conclusive answer since follow-up was too short at the time of initial publication. This phase III trial for all anaplastic gliomas was designed to study sequencing of therapies by comparing efficacy and safety of radiotherapy versus chemotherapy (temozolomide or PCV) and using an adapted cross-over design at progression. Radiotherapy and chemotherapy elicited comparable therapeutic results and the outcome of pure and mixed anaplastic oligodendroglial tumours was identical and more favourable than for astrocytoma. Only a minority of cases in this study had anaplastic oligodendrogliomas, therefore limiting definitive conclusions. The median overall survival of patients on this trial was approximately 80 months, stressing the relevance of long-term monitoring for HRQOL and toxicities, in anaplastic gliomas with good prognosis, similar to low-grade glioma (72).

Commentary on National Comprehensive Cancer Network and European Association for Neuro-Oncology guidelines

The treatment algorithms for oligodendroglial tumours adapted from the National Comprehensive Cancer Network (NCCN) and European Association for Neuro-Oncology (EANO) guidelines are summarized in Figures 4.4 and 4.5.

The NCCN guidelines in their current version and the EANO guidelines (76) support the proposed sequence for diagnosis, that is, suggestive MRI, which triggers multidisciplinary preoperative input followed by diagnostic surgery, which incorporates maximal safe resection when feasible. For a suspected grade II lesion, serial observations are an option for selected individual patients, although it is generally recommended that a histopathological diagnosis be established early in the course of the patient's management. The extent of resection remains a matter of debate and is assigned a lesser role in the EANO guidelines.

NCCN guidelines allow the intraoperative use of carmustine wafers, although this is controversial because it usually limits subsequent entry into clinical trials, is of unproven clinical benefit, specifically for oligodendroglioma, and may lead to more postoperative wound complications. An early (<72 h) postoperative MRI is recommended as a baseline, to assess potential complications and to objectively determine the extent of resection.

Postoperatively, tumour tissue is utilized to determine histopathological grade and to assess molecular or cytogenetic markers (e.g. 1p/19q chromosome status). For grade II tumours, both NCCN and EANO guidelines recommend radiotherapy or chemotherapy (with a lower evidence level) for high-risk patients or incompletely resected patients, with the option for watchful waiting in patients without symptoms. Updated results from the RTOG 9802 study will likely result in greater utilization of radiotherapy plus PCV (as in the trial) or temozolomide (because no relevant difference to PCV except lower toxicity is described in comparative trials so far) will become an option also for grade II oligodendroglial tumours with an indication for postoperative treatment (67). Grade III patients should receive adjuvant treatment with radiotherapy plus chemotherapy with PCV or temozolomide being recommended for patients with a 1p/19q co-deletion; although an option for chemotherapy alone, but not radiotherapy alone has

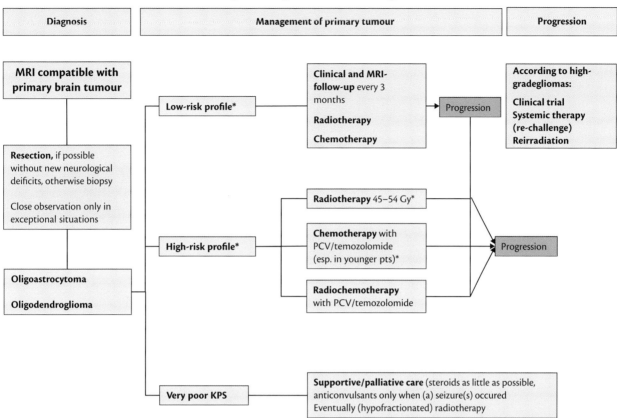

Fig. 4.4 Pragmatic approach to WHO grade II oligodendroglial tumours. Low-risk factors are age ≤40 years, Karnofsky performance score (KPS) >70, tumour diameter <6 cm, and minor or no preoperative neurological deficits. High-risk factors are essentially the converse plus crossing of the midline in the preoperative MRI, but NCCN also considers any non-radical resection a negative prognostic factor. Whether molecular parameters should be considered remains controversial (NCCN, yes and EANO, no) as is the use of increased perfusion in the MRI as a negative prognostic factor. In addition, the option for combined radiochemotherapy is a new development since the press release of RTOG 9802.
Source: data from N Engl J Med, 374(14), Buckner JC et al., Radiation plus Procarbazine, CCNU, and Vincristine in Low-Grade Glioma, pp. 1344–55, Copyright (2016), Massachusetts Medical Society.

also been proffered, this is not based on reliable data, as the randomized data to date only show the superiority of combined modality therapy over radiotherapy alone, and not that of chemotherapy alone over radiotherapy or combined modality therapy. For the 1p/19q non-co-deleted grade III patients, radiotherapy or radiotherapy plus chemotherapy are the primary options, and once again, although chemotherapy alone has been used, data supporting this option are not robust. Patients with a poor performance status may be managed with best supportive care, hypofractionated radiotherapy, or PCV/temozolomide. At recurrence, any surgical options should be discussed in a multidisciplinary setting and systemic chemotherapy, best supportive care, and re-irradiation considered within an individualized programme of care.

Follow-up recommendations

Clinical examination and MRI should be used to monitor treatment efficacy or for surveillance after completion of treatment (77). Intervals of 3 months are recommended for most patients with malignant gliomas, but longer intervals should be considered for patients with prolonged disease control, notably younger patients with 1p/19q co-deleted oligodendroglial tumours. Clinical follow-up needs to focus on tracking long-term sequelae of treatment.

Current research topics

While the WHO classification has prognostic value (40), it is prone to high interobserver variability, especially for anaplastic oligoastrocytomas (3). In recent years, large-scale genomic and epigenomic studies have greatly increased our insight into the biology of malignant gliomas, identifying key alterations and molecular subgroups (78–81) which may augment the WHO classification. The discovery of a prognostically favourable conserved point mutation in *IDH1* codon 132 (82), resulting in a neomorphic enzymatic capacity to produce 2-hydroxyglutrate from α-ketoglutarate, has considerably altered our understanding of glioma biology (83). *IDH1* (and less frequently, *IDH2*) mutations are found in the majority of secondary glioblastomas as well as diffuse oligodendroglial (WHO grade II and III) tumours. The *IDH* mutation causes epigenetic remodelling (84), resulting in a CpG island methylator phenotype (85). Indeed, gliomas across histological subtypes with an *IDH* mutation carry a very similar epigenetic profile (86). This and other studies (87) suggest that *IDH* mutant gliomas form a biologically distinct entity.

Besides *IDH*, the 1p/19q co-deletion is a strong biomarker of better prognosis (88). When two phase III trials reported their long-term follow-up, both demonstrating an overall survival benefit from combined treatment with radiotherapy and PCV chemotherapy mainly in patients with 1p/19q co-deleted

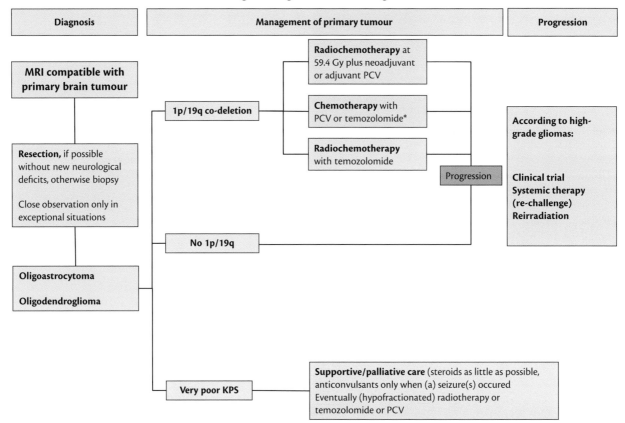

Fig. 4.5 Pragmatic approach to WHO grade III oligodendroglial tumours. A matter of debate between the NCCN and the EANO guidelines is mainly the use of carmustine wafers, which are a more realistic option in the NCCN guidelines.
* Sole chemotherapy is only an option for individual cases or trials.

tumours, the 1p/19q co-deletion gained predictive properties (88, 89). Mutations of the homolog of the *Drosophila* gene capicua (*CIC*) on chromosome 19q and far-upstream element binding protein 1 (*FUBP1*) on 1p have been identified as potential mechanisms involved in the biology of 1p/19q co-deleted gliomas (90). Gene expression clustering plus *IDH1* and 1p/19q status have revealed molecular subgroups with prognostic value among oligodendroglial tumours (91). Mutually exclusive mutations in *TERT* and *ATRX* genes have been detected in malignant gliomas (92, 93). Two point mutations in the promoter of *TERT* (C228 and C250) resulting in higher *TERT* mRNA expression

were discovered with a high frequency in oligodendrogliomas (usually co-occurring with the 1p/19q co-deletion) and primary glioblastomas. Alternative lengthening of telomeres (ALT) is another, telomerase-independent mechanism of telomere maintenance. *ATRX* gene mutations, usually leading to reduced or absent ATRX protein expression (94), have been linked to ALT (95). Consequently, loss of ATRX expression predominantly occurs in astrocytomas and mixed oligoastrocytomas without 1p/19q co-deletion (i.e. *TERT* wild-type tumours) and seems to identify a prognostically more favourable subgroup among the anaplastic astrocytoma patients (13).

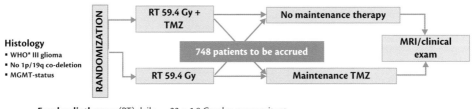

Focal radiotherapy (RT) daily — 33 × 1.8 Gy plus concomitant
Temozolomide (TMZ) 75 mg/m²/day
Temozolomide (TMZ) 150/200 mg/m² PO/day D1–5/4 weeks × 6–12

*Concurrent and **A**djuvant **T**emozolomide in **non**-deleted grade III

Fig. 4.6 EORTC CATNON trial.
MGMT, methylguanine-methyltransferase; MRI, magnetic resonance tomography; RT, radiotherapy; TMZ, temozolomide.

Unlike glioblastomas, anaplastic gliomas (89) have been (except for the gene expression array and methylation analysis on the EORTC 26951 trial (90)) less comprehensively analysed. The feasibility and prognostic value of a molecular classification of anaplastic gliomas based on epigenetic analysis is currently being investigated.

Several questions remain regarding optimal treatment of anaplastic oligodendroglial tumours: should there be concomitant, adjuvant, or combined concomitant and adjuvant temozolomide for patients with anaplastic gliomas with, or without, 1p/19q co-deletion? This is one objective of the ongoing CATNON (Concurrent and Adjuvant Temozolomide Chemotherapy in Non-1p/19q Deleted Anaplastic Glioma) trial (Fig. 4.6). Should all grade II and III (oligodendro-) gliomas with 1p/19q co-deletion be treated with radiochemotherapy? Or would chemotherapy with temozolomide (or PCV) alone be sufficient? Can PCV in the current standard radiochemotherapy for patients with 1p/19q co-deleted tumours be safely and effectively replaced by temozolomide? What novel therapeutics may prove beneficial for anaplastic oligodendroglial tumours? At present, IDH inhibitors are in early development. Apart from being a target for pharmacological intervention, mutated IDH may be an excellent target for immunotherapy. Its appearance in 100% of cells in mutated tumours, the relatively indolent course of disease, the high likelihood of immunocompetence of the respective patients, as well as a degree of spontaneous T-cell response in patients with IDH1 R132H mutated tumours, makes it a promising target for immunotherapy-based trials, some of which are underway (NCT-2013-0216, EudraCT 2014-000503-27). What is the optimal treatment at recurrence? Outside trials, these tumours can be focally irradiated or treated with standard temozolomide or other alkylating agents, especially lomustine and procarbazine. Future research will hopefully answer several of these questions and provide further insight into better classification and improved treatment options.

References

1. Soffietti R, Baumert B, Bello L, et al. Guidelines on management of low-grade gliomas: report of an EFNS-EANO task force. *Eur J Neurol* 2010; 17:1124–1233.

2. Louis DN, Perry A, Reifenberger G, et al. The 2016 World Health Organization Classification of Tumors of the Central Nervous System: a summary. *Acta Neuropathol* 2016; 131:803–820.

3. Kros JM, Gorlia T, Kouwenhoven MC, et al. Panel review of anaplastic oligodendroglioma from EORTC trial 26951: assessment of consensus in diagnosis, influence of 1p/19q loss and correlations with outcome. *J Neuropathol Exp Neurol* 2007; 66:545–551.

4. Giannini C, Burger PC, Berkey BA, et al. Anaplastic oligodendroglial tumors: refining the correlation among histopathology, 1p 19q deletion and clinical outcome in Intergroup Radiation Therapy Oncology Group Trial 9402. *Brain Pathol* 2008; 18:360–369.

5. Wick W, Weller M. Classification and management of anaplastic gliomas. *Curr Opin Neurol* 2009; 22:650–656.

6. Pignatti F, van den Bent MJ, Curran D, et al. Prognostic factors for survival in adult patients with cerebral low-grade glioma. *J Clin Oncol* 2002; 20:2076–2084.

7. Bourne TD, Schiff D. Update on molecular findings, management and outcome in low-grade gliomas. *Nat Rev Neurol* 2010; 6:695–701.

8. Weiler M, Wick W. Molecular predictors of outcome in low-grade glioma. *Curr Opin Neurol* 2012; 25:767–773.

9. Ohgaki H, Kleihues P. Population-based studies on incidence, survival rates, and genetic alterations in astrocytic and oligodendroglial gliomas. *J Neuropathol Exp Neurol* 2005; 64:479–489.

10. Blaes J, Weiler M, Sahm F, et al. NDRG1 prognosticates the natural course of disease in WHO grade II glioma. *J Neurooncol* 2014; 117:25–32.

11. Fontana M, Stanton C, Pompill A, et al. Late multifocal gliomas in adolescents previously treated for acute lymphoblastic leukemia. *Cancer* 1987; 60:1510–1518.

12. Weller M, Pfister SM, Wick W, et al. Molecular neuro-oncology entering clinical practice: a new horizon. *Lancet Oncol* 2013; 14:e370–379.

13. Wiestler B, Capper D, Holland-Letz T, et al. ATRX loss refines the classification of anaplastic gliomas and identifies a subgroup of IDH mutant astrocytic tumors with better prognosis. *Acta Neuropathol* 2013; 126:443–451.

14. Lebrun C, Fontaine D, Ramaioli A, et al. Long-term outcome of oligodendrogliomas. *Neurology* 2004; 62:1783–1787.

15. Rees J, Watt H, Jäger HR, et al. Volumes and growth rates of untreated adult low-grade gliomas indicate risk of early malignant transformation. *Eur J Radiol* 2009; 72:54–64.

16. Pallud J, Capelle L, Taillandier L, et al. Prognostic significance of imaging contrast enhancement for WHO grade II gliomas. *Neuro Oncol* 2009; 11:176–182.

17. Chaichana KL, McGirt MJ, Niranjan A. Prognostic significance of contrast-enhancing low-grade gliomas in adults and a review of the literature. *Neurol Res* 2009; 31:931–939.

18. Law M, Young RJ, Babb JS, et al. Gliomas: predicting time to progression or survival with cerebral blood volume measurements at dynamic susceptibility-weighted contrast-enhanced perfusion MR imaging. *Radiology* 2008; 247:490–498.

19. Ribom D, Eriksson A, Hartman M, et al. Positron emission tomography (11)C-methionine and survival in patients with low-grade gliomas. *Cancer* 2001; 92:1541–1549.

20. Chang EF, Potts MB, Keles GE, et al. Seizure characteristics and control following resection in 332 patients with low-grade gliomas. *J Neurosurg* 2008; 108:227–235.

21. Sanders WP, Chistoforidis GA. Imaging of low-grade primary brain tumors. In: Rock JP, Rosenblum ML, Shaw EG, et al. (eds) *The Practical Management of Low-Grade Primary Brain Tumors*. Philadelphia, PA: Lippincott Williams & Wilkins, 1999; 5–32.

22. Law M, Yang S, Wang H, et al. Glioma grading: sensitivity, specificity, and predictive values of perfusion MR imaging and proton MR spectroscopic imaging compared with conventional MR imaging. *AJNR Am J Neuroradiol* 2003; 24:1989–1998.

23. Zonari P, Baraldi P, Crisi G. Multimodal MRI in the characterization of glial neoplasms: the combined role of single-voxel MR spectroscopy, diffusion imaging and echo-planar perfusion imaging. *Neuroradiology* 2007; 49:795–803.

24. Pirzkall A, Li X, Oh J, et al. 3D MRSI for resected high-grade gliomas before RT: tumor extent according to metabolic activity in relation to MRI. *Int J Radiat Oncol Biol Phys* 2004; 59:126–137.

25. Crawford FW, Khayal IS, McGue C, et al. Relationship of pre-surgery metabolic and physiological MR imaging parameters to survival for patients with untreated GBM. *J Neurooncol* 2009; 91:337–351.

26. Laprie A, Catalaa I, Cassol E, et al. Proton magnetic resonance spectroscopic imaging in newly diagnosed glioblastoma: predictive value for the site of postradiotherapy relapse in a prospective longitudinal study. *Int J Radiat Oncol Biol Phys* 2008; 70:773–781.

27. Guillevin R, Menuel C, Duffau H, et al. Proton magnetic resonance spectroscopy predicts proliferative activity in diffuse low-grade gliomas. *J Neurooncol* 2008; 87:181–187.

28. Reijneveld JC, van der Grond J, Ramos LM, et al. Proton MRS imaging in the follow-up of patients with suspected low-grade gliomas. *Neuroradiology* 2005; 47:887–891.

29. Danchaivijitr N, Waldman AD, Tozer DJ, et al. Low-grade gliomas: do changes in rCBV measurements at longitudinal perfusion-weighted MR imaging predict malignant transformation? *Radiology* 2008; 247:170–178.

30. Cha S, Tihan T, Crawfoed C, et al. Differentiation of low-grade oligodendrogliomas from low-grade astrocytomas by using quantitative blood-volume measurements derived from dynamic susceptibility contrast-enhanced MR imaging. *AJNR Am J Neuroradiol* 2005; 26:266–273.

31. Jenkinson MD, du Plessis DG, Smith TS, et al. Histological growth patterns and genotype in oligodendroglial tumours: correlation with MRI features. *Brain* 2006; 129:1884–1891.

32. Brown R, Zlatescu M, Sijben A, et al. The use of magnetic resonance imaging to noninvasively detect genetic signatures in oligodendroglioma. *Clin Cancer Res* 2008; 14:2357–2362.

33. Khayal IS, McKnight TR, McGue C, et al. Apparent diffusion coefficient and fractional anisotropy of newly diagnosed grade II gliomas. *NMR Biomed* 2009; 22:449–455.

34. Wen PY, Macdonald DR, Reardon DA, et al. Updated response assessment criteria for high-grade gliomas: response assessment in neuro-oncology working group. *J Clin Oncol* 2010; 28:1963–1972.

35. Felsberg J, Thon N, Eigenbrod S, et al. Promoter methylation and expression of MGMT and the DNA mismatch repair genes MLH1, MSH2, MSH6 and PMS2 in paired primary and recurrent glioblastomas. *Int J Cancer* 2011; 129:659–670.

36. Silber JR, Bobola MS, Blank A, et al. The apurinic/apyrimidinic endonuclease activity of Ape1/Ref-1 contributes to human glioma cell resistance to alkylating agents and is elevated by oxidative stress. *Clin Cancer Res* 2002; 8:3008–3018.

37. Agnihotri S, Gajadhar AS, Ternamian C, et al. Alkylpurine-DNA-N-glycosylase confers resistance to temozolomide in xenograft models of glioblastoma multiforme and is associated with poor survival in patients. *J Clin Invest* 2012; 122:253–266.

38. Sarkaria JN, Kitange GJ, James CD, et al. Mechanisms of chemoresistance to alkylating agents in malignant glioma. *Clin Cancer Res* 2008; 14: 2900–2908.

39. Hegi ME, Diserens AC, Gorlia T, et al. MGMT gene silencing and benefit from TMZ in glioblastoma. *N Engl J Med* 2005; 352:997–1003.

40. Wick W, Hartmann C, Engel C, et al. NOA-04 randomized phase III trial of sequential radiochemotherapy of anaplastic glioma with PCV or temozolomide. *J Clin Oncol* 2009; 27:5874–5880.

41. Van den Bent MJ, Carpentier AF, Brandes AA, et al. Adjuvant procarbazine, lomustine, and vincristine improves progression-free

survival but not overall survival in newly diagnosed anaplastic oligodendrogliomas and oligoastrocytomas: a randomized European Organisation for Research and Treatment of Cancer. *J Clin Oncol* 2006; 24:2715–2722.

42. Wick W, Meisner C, Hentschel B, et al. IDH1 mutations determine the prognostic versus predictive value of MGMT promoter methylation in malignant gliomas. *Neurology* 2013; 81:1515–1522.

43. Cairncross JG, Macdonald DR. Successful chemotherapy for recurrent malignant oligodendroglioma. *Ann Neurol* 1988; 23:360–364.

44. Levin VA, Edwards MS, Wright DC, et al. Modified procarbazine, CCNU, and vincristine (PCV 3) combination chemotherapy in the treatment of malignant brain tumors. *Cancer Treat Rep* 1980; 64:237–244.

45. Cairncross G, Berkey B, Shaw E, et al. Phase III trial of chemotherapy plus radiotherapy compared with radiotherapy alone for pure and mixed anaplastic oligodendroglioma: Intergroup Radiation Therapy Oncology Group Trial 9402. *J Clin Oncol* 2006; 24:2707–2714.

46. Wick W, Platten M, Meisner C, et al. Chemotherapy versus radiotherapy for malignant astrocytoma in the elderly. *Lancet Oncol* 2012; 13:707–715.

47. Gilbert M, Mehta M, Aldape K, et al. Dose-dense temozolomide for newly diagnosed glioblastoma: a randomized phase III clinical trial. *J Clin Oncol* 2013; 31:4085–4091.

48. Cairncross JG, Wang M, Jenkins RB, et al. Benefit from procarbazine, lomustine, and vincristine in oligodendroglial tumors is associated with mutation of IDH. *J Clin Oncol* 2014; 32:783–790.

49. Cancer Genome Atlas Research Network. Comprehensive genomic characterization defines human glioblastoma genes and core pathways. *Nature* 2008; 455:1061–1068.

50. Noushmehr H, Weisenberger DJ, Diefes K, et al. Identification of a CpG island methylator phenotype that defines a distinct subgroup of glioma. *Cancer Cell* 2010; 17:510–522.

51. Sturm D, Witt H, Hovestadt V, et al. Hotspot mutations in H3F3A and IDH1 define distinct epigenetic and biological subgroups of glioblastoma. *Cancer Cell* 2012; 22:425–437.

52. Verhaak RGW, Hoadley KA, et al. Integrated genomic analysis identifies clinically relevant subtypes of glioblastoma characterized by abnormalities in PDGFRA, IDH1, EGFR, and NF1. *Cancer Cell* 2010; 17:98–110.

53. Mandonnet E, Delattre JY, Tanguy ML, et al. Continuous growth of mean tumor diameter in a subset of grade II gliomas. *Ann Neurol* 2003; 53:524–528.

54. Smith JS, Chang EF, Lamborn KR, et al. Role of extent of resection in the long-term outcome of low-grade hemispheric gliomas. *J Clin Oncol* 2008; 26:1338–1345.

55. Gorlia T, Delattre JY, Brandes AA, et al. New clinical, pathological and molecular prognostic models and calculators in patients with locally diagnosed anaplastic oligodendroglioma or oligoastrocytoma. A prognostic factor analysis of European Organisation for Research and Treatment of Cancer Brain Tumour Group Study 26951. *Eur J Cancer* 2013; 49:3477–3485.

56. Berger MS, Deliganis AV, Dobbins J, et al. The effect of extent of resection on recurrence in patients with low grade cerebral hemisphere gliomas. *Cancer* 1994; 74:1784–1791.

57. Claus EB, Horlacher A, Hsu L, et al. Survival rates in patients with low-grade glioma after intraoperative magnetic resonance image guidance. *Cancer* 2005; 103:1227–1233.

58. Olson JD, Riedel E, DeAngelis LM. Long-term outcome of low-grade oligodendroglioma and mixed glioma. *Neurology* 2000; 54:1442–1448.

59. Recht LD, Lew R, Smith TW. Suspected low-grade glioma: is deferring treatment safe? *Ann Neurol* 1992; 31:431–436.

60. Reijneveld JC, Sitskoorn MM, Klein M, et al. Cognitive status and quality of life in patients with suspected versus proven low-grade gliomas. *Neurology* 2001; 56:618–623.

61. Karim AB, Maat B, Hatlevoll R, et al. A randomized trial on dose-response in radiation therapy of low-grade cerebral glioma: European

Organization for Research and Treatment of Cancer (EORTC) Study 22844. *Int J Radiat Oncol Biol Phys* 1996; 36:549–556.

62. van den Bent MJ, Afra D, de Witte O, et al. Long-term efficacy of early versus delayed radiotherapy for low-grade astrocytoma and oligodendroglioma in adults: the EORTC 22845 randomised trial. *Lancet* 2005; 366:985–990.

63. Karim AB, Afra D, Cornu P, et al. Randomized trial on the efficacy of radiotherapy for cerebral low-grade glioma in the adult: European Organization for Research and Treatment of Cancer Study 22845 with the Medical Research Council study BRO4: an interim analysis. *Int J Radiat Oncol Biol Phys* 2002; 52:316–324.

64. Soffietti R, Borgognone M, Ducati A, et al. Efficacy of radiation therapy on seizures in low-grade astrocytomas. *Neuro-Oncology* 2005; 7:389.

65. Shaw E, Arusell R, Scheithauer B, et al. Prospective randomized trial of low- versus high-dose radiation therapy in adults with supratentorial low-grade glioma: initial report of a North Central Cancer Treatment Group/Radiation Therapy Oncology Group/Eastern Cooperative Oncology Group study. *J Clin Oncol* 2002; 20:2267–2276.

66. Kiebert GM, Curran D, Aaronson NK, et al. Quality of life after radiation therapy of cerebral low-grade gliomas of the adult: results of a randomised phase III trial on dose response (EORTC trial 22844). *Eur J Cancer* 1998; 34:1902–1909.

67. Shaw EG, Wang M, Coons SW, et al. Randomized trial of radiation therapy plus procarbazine, lomustine, and vincristine chemotherapy for supratentorial adult low-grade glioma: initial results of RTOG 9802. *J Clin Oncol* 2012; 30:3065–3070.

68. Surma-aho O, Niemelä M, Vilkki J, et al. Adverse long-term effects of brain radiotherapy in adult low-grade glioma patients. *Neurology* 2001; 56:1285–1290.

69. Taphoorn MJ, Schiphorst AK, Snoek FJ, et al. Cognitive functions and quality of life in patients with low-grade gliomas: the impact of radiotherapy. *Ann Neurol* 1994; 36:48–54.

70. Klein M, Heimans JJ, Aaronson NK, et al. Effect of radiotherapy and other treatment-related factors on mid-term to long-term cognitive sequelae in low-grade gliomas: a comparative study. *Lancet* 2002; 360:1361–1368.

71. Laack NN, Brown PD, Ivnik RJ, et al. North Central Cancer Treatment Group. Cognitive function after radiotherapy for supratentorial low-grade glioma: a North Central Cancer Treatment Group prospective study. *Int J Radiat Oncol Biol Phys* 2005; 63:1175–1183.

72. Douw L, Klein M, Fagel SS, et al. Cognitive and radiological effects of radiotherapy in patients with low-grade glioma: long-term follow-up. *Lancet Neurol* 2009; 8:810–818.

73. Van den Bent MJ, Brandes AA, Taphoorn MJB, et al. Adjuvant procarbazine, lomustine, and vincristine chemotherapy in newly diagnosed anaplastic oligodendroglioma: long-term follow-up of EORTC Brain Tumor Group Study 26951. *J Clin Oncol* 2013; 31:344–350.

74. Cairncross G, Wang M, Shaw E, et al. Phase III trial of chemoradiotherapy for anaplastic oligodendroglioma: long-term results of RTOG 9402. *J Clin Oncol* 2013; 31:337–343.

75. Habets EJ, Taphoorn MJ, Nederend S, et al. Health-related quality of life and cognitive functioning in long-term anaplastic oligodendroglioma and oligoastrocytoma survivors. *J Neurooncol* 2014; 116:161–168.

76. Weller M, van den Bent M, Hopkins K, et al. EANO guideline for the diagnosis and treatment of anaplastic gliomas and glioblastoma. *Lancet Oncol* 2014; 15:e395–403.

77. Wen PY, Macdonald DR, Reardon DA, et al. Updated response assessment criteria for high-grade gliomas: response assessment in neuro-oncology working group. *J Clin Oncol* 2010; 28:1963–1972.

78. Brennan CW, Verhaak RGW, McKenna A, et al. The somatic genomic landscape of glioblastoma. *Cell* 2013; 155:462–477.

79. Frattini V, Trifonov V, Chan JM, et al. The integrated landscape of driver genomic alterations in glioblastoma. *Nat Genet* 2013; 45:1141–1149.

80. Verhaak RGW, Hoadley KA, Purdom E, et al. Integrated genomic analysis identifies clinically relevant subtypes of glioblastoma characterized by abnormalities in PDGFRA, IDH1, EGFR, and NF1. *Cancer Cell* 2010; 17:98–110.

81. Sturm D, Bender S, Jones DTW, et al. Paediatric and adult glioblastoma: multiform (epi)genomic culprits emerge. *Nat Rev Cancer* 2014; 14:92–107.

82. Parsons DW, Jones S, Zhang X, et al. An integrated genomic analysis of human glioblastoma multiforme. *Science* 2008; 321:1807–1812.

83. Ward PS, Patel J, Wise DR, et al. The common feature of leukemia-associated IDH1 and IDH2 mutations is a neomorphic enzyme activity converting alpha-ketoglutarate to 2-hydroxyglutarate. *Cancer Cell* 2010; 17:225–234.

84. Turcan S, Rohle D, Goenka A, et al. IDH1 mutation is sufficient to establish the glioma hypermethylator phenotype. *Nature* 2012; 483:479–483.

85. Noushmehr H, Weisenberger DJ, Diefes K, et al. Identification of a CpG island methylator phenotype that defines a distinct subgroup of glioma. *Cancer Cell* 2010; 17:510–522.

86. Christensen BC, Smith AA, Zheng S, et al. DNA methylation, isocitrate dehydrogenase mutation, and survival in glioma. *J Natl Cancer Inst* 2011; 103:143–153.

87. Lai A, Kharbanda S, Pope WB, et al. Evidence for sequenced molecular evolution of IDH1 mutant glioblastoma from a distinct cell of origin. *J Clin Oncol* 2011; 29:4482–4490.

88. Smith JS, Perry A, Borell TJ, et al. Alterations of chromosome arms 1p and 19q as predictors of survival in oligodendrogliomas, astrocytomas, and mixed oligoastrocytomas. *J Clin Oncol* 2000; 18:636–645.

89. Van den Bent MJ, Brandes AA, Taphoorn MJB, et al. Adjuvant procarbazine, lomustine, and vincristine chemotherapy in newly diagnosed anaplastic oligodendroglioma: long-term follow-up of EORTC brain tumor group study 26951. *J Clin Oncol* 2013; 31:344–350.

90. Bettegowda C, Agrawal N, Jiao Y, et al. Mutations in CIC and FUBP1 contribute to human oligodendroglioma. *Science* 2011; 333:1453–1455.

91. Erdem-Eraslan L, Gravendeel LA, de Rooi J, et al. Intrinsic molecular subtypes of glioma are prognostic and predict benefit from adjuvant procarbazine, lomustine, and vincristine chemotherapy in combination with other prognostic factors in anaplastic oligodendroglial brain tumors: a report from EORTC stu. *J Clin Oncol* 2013; 31:328–336.

92. Killela PJ, Reitman ZJ, Jiao Y, et al. TERT promoter mutations occur frequently in gliomas and a subset of tumors derived from cells with low rates of self-renewal. *Proc Natl Acad Sci U S A* 2013; 110:6021–6026.

93. Schwartzentruber J, Korshunov A, Liu X-Y, et al. Driver mutations in histone H3.3 and chromatin remodelling genes in paediatric glioblastoma. *Nature* 2012; 482:226–231.

94. Liu X-Y, Gerges N, Korshunov A, et al. Frequent ATRX mutations and loss of expression in adult diffuse astrocytic tumors carrying IDH1/IDH2 and TP53 mutations. *Acta Neuropathol* 2012; 124:615–625.

95. Heaphy CM, de Wilde RF, Jiao Y, et al. Altered telomeres in tumors with ATRX and DAXX mutations. *Science* 2011; 333:425.

96. Buckner JC, Shaw EG, Pugh SL, et al. Radiation plus procarbazine, CCNU, and vincristine in low-grade glioma. N Engl J Med. 2016; 374(14):1344–1355.

CHAPTER 5

Ependymal tumours

Mark R. Gilbert and Roberta Rudà

Definition

Ependymomas are rare cancers of the central nervous system (CNS) that can occur at any age, although they are more prevalent in the paediatric age range and therefore account for a higher percentage of paediatric brain tumours (~8–10%) than adults where less than 4% of brain tumours are diagnosed as ependymoma (1). Ependymomas were first described by Bailey in 1924 with a report of 11 cases of a distinct tumour apparently arising from the ependymal cells lining the ventricles or spinal central canal (2). Therefore, ependymomas can occur throughout the CNS, although primary spinal cord involvement is uncommon in paediatric patients (<10%), but is the most common location in adults, estimated to be nearly 75%.

Epidemiology

Ependymomas are rare, representing approximately 3.5% of all primary CNS malignancies in all age groups (1). They constitute a higher percentage among paediatric cancers (5.2–5.7% of primary CNS cancers) than in adults where ependymomas account for 1.9% of CNS tumours, and 3.5% of primary CNS cancers. These statistics are based on compilations from tumour registries in the United States: the Surveillance, Epidemiology and End Results (SEER) programme and the Central Brain Tumor Registry of the United States (CBTRUS) statistical reports. The precise incidence of ependymoma cannot be accurately determined as these registries rely on institutional reports and there are concerns about misdiagnosis of ependymoma that has been estimated to be as high as 30%

The site of disease varies with age. Intracranial tumours are the most common location in the paediatric age group and spinal cord involvement is uncommon (3). In children, the infratentorial region is a much more common location (around two-thirds) than tumours arising supratentorially. The spinal cord is the most common location for ependymoma in adults. In contradistinction to children, intracranial tumours occur more commonly in the supratentorial region. Although ependymomas can occur at any age, there is a bimodal distribution with a peak at an early age (0–4 years) and a second peak during the fourth to fifth decade of life.

Pathogenesis

With the exception of the high-grade (anaplastic) tumours, ependymomas are typically well demarcated from the surrounding parenchyma. In fact, myxopapillary ependymomas may be encapsulated and removal without breaching this capsule may be curative. Regardless of the subtype or grade, ependymomas on gross examination may have associated haemorrhage, necrosis, and calcification.

Ependymomas are diagnosed on the basis of histological appearance. Although there may be a variety of cellular morphological characteristics, the hallmarks are perivascular pseudorosettes and ependymal rosettes. The perivascular rosettes are perivascular zones that are defined by radially arranged ependymal cell processes directed towards central blood vessels. Ependymal rosettes, unlike pseudorosettes, are composed of epithelioid cuboidal to columnar cells arranged around a central lumen. Although perivascular pseudorosettes are more commonly observed on histopathology than ependymal rosettes, the latter are more specific for ependymomas. Perivascular pseudorosettes stain for vimentin and glial fibrillary acidic protein (GFAP). Other immunohistological findings include positive staining for S100, and neural cell adhesion molecule or CD56. The absence of GFAP staining should prompt a search for another diagnosis. Epithelial membrane antigen (EMA) staining often shows a characteristic punctuate, dot type pattern. However, EMA staining is not seen in myxopapillary ependymomas.

Although the ependymal and perivascular pseudorosettes are cardinal features of ependymomas, the tumour cells can have very diverse morphological characteristics (Fig. 5.1). The cellular elements can vary from elongated fibrillary glial-type cells to an epithelioid appearance. The universally accepted histology-based grading system uses the World Health Organization (WHO) guidelines, most recently published in 2016 (4). Low-grade ependymoma typically have tumour cells with fairly uniform round to oval nuclei containing finely dispersed chromatin. In contradistinction, high-grade ependymomas show polymorphic, irregular cells, and hyperchromatic nuclei. As with other glial neoplasms, the highest grade component, even if only a small percentage of the overall tumour, dictates the grade. As is true with most primary CNS tumours, the commonly used TNM (tumour, lymph node involvement, and distant metastasis) cancer staging system does not apply to ependymomas, because these tumours only rarely spread outside the CNS or involve in adjacent lymph nodes.

Grade I ependymomas include subependymoma and myxopapillary ependymoma (Fig. 5.1c, d, respectively). Although both are slow growing and have the potential to be cured if completely removed, they have distinct characteristics including cellular morphology, localization, clinical features, and imaging findings.

Subependymomas are slow-growing lesions, are often asymptomatic, and are typically discovered as an incidental finding on brain imaging or at autopsy. Subependymomas typically attach to a

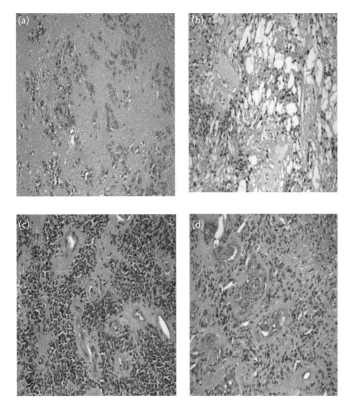

Fig. 5.1 (See colour plate section) Histology of ependymoma. (a) Ependymoma (WHO grade II). (b) Anaplastic ependymoma (WHO grade III). (c) Subependymoma (WHO grade I). (d) Myxopapillary ependymoma (WHO grade I).

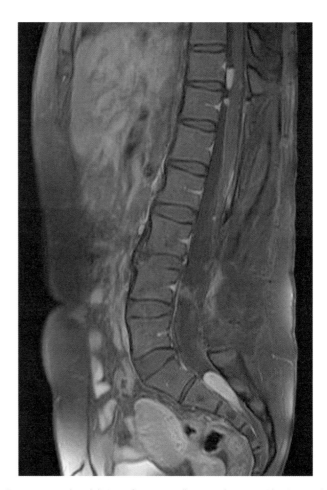

Fig. 5.2 MRI with gadolinium of a myxopapillary ependymoma with CSF spread.

ventricle wall, most commonly of the fourth ventricle or less commonly on the wall of a lateral ventricle. On magnetic resonance imaging (MRI), they typically appear as sharply demarcated nodular masses that are non-enhancing. When these tumours do present clinically, the symptoms are usually due to ventricular obstruction or haemorrhage. Although subependymomas share some histological features with ependymomas, their biology and molecular characterization has not been well elucidated. As a result, many investigators believe that subependymomas should not be grouped with ependymomas.

Myxopapillary ependymomas almost exclusively arise in the region of the conus medullaris, cauda equina, and the filum terminale of the spinal cord, although uncommon locations such as cervical thoracic spinal cord, lateral ventricle, or the brain parenchyma have been reported (5–8). Chronic back pain is typically the most common presenting symptom. On MRI, they appear to be sharply circumscribed, sausage-shaped, and enhanced by the gadolinium contrast (Fig. 5.2). As described earlier, if they remain encapsulated, complete tumour removal is often possible and may be curative. Breaching of the capsule may lead to dissemination within the spinal canal with the potential for seeding along the spinal cord and less commonly, within the brain (Fig. 5.2). Once dissemination has occurred, the prognosis is similar to patients with WHO grade II tumours.

In contrast to the typically well-circumscribed grade I tumours, ependymomas classified as grade II and III tumours tend to be infiltrative into the surrounding tissues in the brain or the spinal cord. Clinical presentation is typically dictated by the tumour location.

Grade II tumours by WHO criteria are designated by the name ependymoma, whereas grade III tumours are called anaplastic ependymoma. Although all grade II ependymomas share the histological features of perivascular pseudorosettes, and true ependymal rosettes, there are multiple histological variants including cellular, papillary, clear cell, and tanycytic ependymomas (Fig. 5.1a). To date, aside from morphological differences, there appears to be no prognostic significance to the subtyping although they may be associated with specific tumour locations and patient age. For example, clear cell ependymomas are seen predominantly in the supratentorial compartment and young adults. Histologically, they resemble oligodendrogliomas and misdiagnosis by morphology alone can usually be resolved with testing for the characteristic allelic loss of chromosomes 1p and 19q in oligodendroglioma.

Anaplastic ependymomas are designated as grade III gliomas by the WHO classification schema. Histological features include a high proliferative index using the Mib-1 staining and readily observed mitotic figures. There is typically prominent cellular pleomorphism and angiogenesis (Fig. 5.1b). The pseudorosettes and ependymal rosettes that characterize low-grade ependymoma may be distorted or lost. Transformation to glioblastoma (WHO grade IV) is rare, but has been reported (9).

Clinical outcomes for patients with ependymomas can be quite variable even within a specific WHO grade. In contradistinction to the almost binary outcomes in spinal myxopapillary ependymomas where cure is common with complete, en bloc removal, there are highly variable outcomes among patients harbouring ependymomas of comparable grade. This strongly suggests that there are differences in tumour biology that cannot be elucidated exclusively by conventional histological or pathological evaluations.

A number of studies have investigated the regional heterogeneity in ependymomas using a variety of molecular platforms. Testing for chromosomal abnormalities in spinal cord tumours revealed a high incidence of loss of heterozygosity on chromosome 22, often with neurofibromatosis type 2 (*NF2*) mutations. There is a variety of genomic losses (2q, 4q, 5q, 6q, 15q, 16q, 17p, and 19p) as well as gains (chromosome 17, 9q, 12p, 13q, 20q, and 22q) but each is relatively uncommon (10–12). There is some evidence that the changes segregate by tumour location, but the association with tumour biology is unclear. Early studies also demonstrated some characteristic changes in signalling pathways. Overexpression of *ErbB2* (*HER2*) and *ErbB4* were reported in a high percentage of paediatric tumours (13) and other studies describe increased expression of the $\alpha_v \beta_3$ integrins, annexin A1, and cyclooxygenase.

The radial glia are thought to be the stem cells that transform into ependymoma (14). Comparison of molecular profiling of these cells from the various CNS compartments demonstrates many of the molecular features of tumours from these regions. Furthermore, a cross-species study demonstrated that ependymomas from different CNS locations share the same gene expression profiles with radial glial stem cells in the corresponding region of the developing brain or spinal cord (15). Human ependymomas were evaluated using messenger RNA, microRNA, and DNA copy number alteration profiles, and it was observed that there were distinct subgroups that varied by location, demonstrating that they are truly distinct biological entities. Additionally, they demonstrated that *EPHB2*, an oncogene in human supratentorial ependymomas, transformed forebrain radial glial stem cells into ependymomas. However, *EPHB2* did not transform, in contrast, the radial glial stem cells isolated from hindbrain and spinal cord, demonstrating that this is a unique site-specific phenomenon.

A series of landmark publications have reported seminal findings based on whole-genome, whole-exome sequencing and methylation profiling of supratentorial (16), posterior fossa (17, 18), and spinal cord ependymomas (19).

An extensive genomic analysis of supratentorial ependymomas revealed relatively few abnormalities such as nucleotide insertions or deletions or copy number variations. However, the observation of genomic structural abnormalities clustered within a highly focal region on chromosome 11q12.1–q13.3 led to the discovery of inter- and intrachromosomal rearrangement, consistent with chromothripsis (16). This results in a stereotypical fusion of a poorly characterized gene, *C11orf95*, to *RELA*, a known principal effector of canonical nuclear factor kappa-light-chain-enhancer of activated B cells (NF-κB) signalling pathways. This fusion was found in approximately 70% of supratentorial ependymoma, but not in infratentorial ependymomas. Further investigation revealed that this novel RELA fusion protein drives an aberrant NF-κB transcriptional process in mouse neural stem cells and can transform stem cells to give rise to ependymomas that histologically mimic human supratentorial ependymomas. Human supratentorial RELA fusion-bearing ependymomas show marked upregulation of NF-κB target genes including *CCND1* and *L1CAM* providing additional evidence that the fusion causes activation of the NF-kB pathway. The

C11orf95-RELA translocation defines a biologically unique subset of supratentorial ependymoma and preliminary data suggest that it may negatively impact survival. However, the activation of the NF-κB pathway does represent a possible therapeutic target.

Posterior fossa (infratentorial) ependymomas occur predominantly in the paediatric population and early studies indicated that infants typically had a much worse prognosis than older children (and adults). Extensive molecular analyses from two sets of posterior fossa ependymomas determined that by transcriptional profiling there are two distinct subgroups (17). Those designated group A (PFA) predominantly occur in infants, originate more laterally in the posterior fossa, and are associated with a poor prognosis. Conversely, group B (PFB) usually occur in older children and adults, are more centrally located within the posterior fossa, and have a better prognosis. An independent study, using a separate set of posterior fossa tumours, confirmed and validated the two molecular subclasses and their respective age predilection and prognosis (20).

Although the studies described above were able to identify two distinct types of posterior fossa ependymomas, there are very few copy number and nucleotide variations to help understand the genesis of these cancers. A study of the epigenetic changes was performed to help better understand the biological basis of posterior fossa ependymomas (18). In this study, 79 ependymomas were evaluated for their DNA methylation pattern. Unsupervised consensus clustering of CpG methylation profiles demonstrated three distinct subgroups including supratentorial, posterior fossa, and a mixed spinal/posterior fossa groupings in a similar pattern as that yielded by unsupervised clustering of gene expression profiles. Importantly, the methylome patterns between PFA and PFB were distinct with a much higher degree of CpG island methylation found in PFA compared with PFB ependymomas. The investigators proposed that PFA ependymomas be referred to as PFA CPG island methylator phenotype (CIMP)-positive ependymomas, and PFB as PFB CIMP-negative ependymomas. The exact mechanism by which hypermethylation leads to tumourigenesis is not known, but the finding of H3K27 trimethylation (H3K27Me3) and H3K27Me3 target genes in PFA-CIMP-positive tumours, but not in the PFB-CIMP-negative ependymomas, suggests that tumour suppressor gene silencing by CpG hypermethylation contributes to the pathogenesis of PFA.

Spinal ependymomas are much more common in adults and are common in patients with NF2, suggesting a potential role of the *NF2* gene in ependymomas located in the spinal cord (21, 22). The spinal ependymomas in the setting of NF2 have more indolent clinical courses. A systematic analysis of 35 spinal ependymomas revealed that in addition to distinct morphological differences between grade II and myxopapillary ependymomas, there are important genomic and biological differences. Molecular analyses demonstrated that the myxopapillary ependymomas had consistent alterations in metabolic pathways such as increased expression of HIF1-alpha and other proteins indicating that myxopapillary ependymomas can be distinguished from other spinal cord ependymomas by their metabolic properties and reliance on aerobic glycolysis commonly referred to as the Warburg effect (19).

The classification of ependymoma was further refined with the use of DNA methylation profiling providing both DNA methylation information and copy number data. A cohort of 500 clinically annotated ependymoma samples from all ages and all three anatomical compartments were analysed (23). This comprehensive investigation determined that there are nine distinct subtypes of ependymoma with three definable groups within each anatomical compartment. In the supratentorial compartment there are histologically designated ependymomas (grade II and III) which either have the RELA fusion or a YAP1 fusion. The third group is histologically designated as subependymoma that has a unique phenotype and only rarely molecular abnormalities. The posterior fossa (infratentorial compartment) is comprised of three distinct groups. Histologically defined ependymomas (grade II and III) are categorized as group A with extensive DNA methylation (CIMP+) or group B without the CIMP phenotype. Subependymoma is the third posterior fossa tumour group and like the supratentorial tumour, shows few molecular abnormalities. The spinal cord is comprised of three distinct subtypes with different molecular profiles. Histological ependymomas (grade II and III) constitute one group that is molecularly and histologically distinct from the myxopapillary and (rare) subependymoma of the spinal cord.

The studies of genomic characteristics of ependymoma demonstrate that ependymomas may have different biology that is based both on location in the CNS and distinct molecular features that permit classification into biologically unique subgroups. Additionally, these seminal findings have generated important prognostic information and may provide insight into specific therapeutic targets.

Prognostic factors

The identification of prognostic factors in ependymomas is evolving. Earlier studies examining prognostic factors in ependymoma include the SEER database (1997–2005) of 2408 ependymoma cases, including 2132 grade II and 276 grade III tumours (24). This study found that younger age, male gender, higher tumour grade, intracranial location, and failure to undergo extensive surgical resection were associated with a poor clinical outcome. Although these are important findings, the use of the central registry does raise concerns regarding the accuracy of the diagnosis. In fact, review of ependymomas at a tertiary care centre revealed that approximately 20% of the cases from outside institutions were misdiagnosed as another histological type of neoplasm prior to review by a pathologist with expertise in ependymoma (25), underscoring the need for caution in using unverified cases and the need for expert verification for clinical trials.

The recent molecular findings described previously in the section on pathogenesis have defined subtypes within each anatomical compartment of the CNS so that in addition to the previously recognized prognostic factors related to age, tumour location, and extent of tumour resection, the molecular subgroup classification has proven to be a key determinant of outcome. For example, RELA-positive supratentorial tumours have a worse outcome than the YAP1-positive tumours, irrespective of age or extent of resection (16, 23). Similarly, in the posterior fossa, the group A (CIMP+) tumours are highly malignant and rarely curable, whereas the group B (CIMP−) are indolent and long-term survival is common (18). This information is critical in the management of patients with ependymoma and in the development of clinical trials. Selection criteria for molecularly targeted agents would require pre-enrolment testing and inclusive trials would need to stratify by subtype to ensure that the treatment arms of a trial are well balanced.

Grade I ependymomas (subependymomas and myxopapillary ependymoma) are distinct in their prognostic features. They are characterized by being well circumscribed and if completely removed, may be cured (26). Conversely, for myxopapillary ependymoma, if the tumour capsule ruptures and tumour cells enter the cerebrospinal fluid (CSF), tumour recurrence is common and the prognosis is similar to grade II spinal cord ependymoma (27, 28).

Treatment

Surgery

Surgery is considered the most important therapeutic intervention as extent of resection is associated with improvement of both progression-free survival (PFS) and overall survival (OS). Moreover, the surgical procedure can re-establish the normal CSF flow, and reverse hydrocephalus.

There are several studies (29–35) that support the prognostic impact of gross total resection (GTR) for ependymoma. When a complete resection has not been achieved at the first surgery and the lesion is not in an 'eloquent' area, a 'second-look' surgery is recommended (29, 32, 34, 36); however, the optimal time to perform a second surgery is still controversial.

An MRI-confirmed complete resection can be achieved in 50–75% of patients (Fig. 5.3). Some tumours are not amenable to

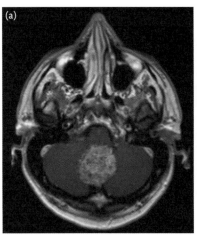
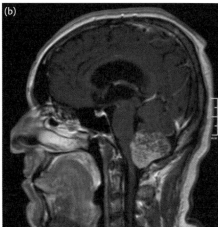
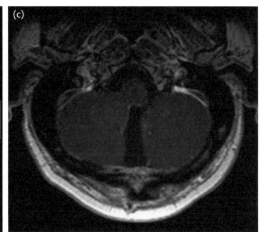

Fig. 5.3 Posterior fossa (infratentorial) grade III ependymoma. (a) MRI with gadolinium at diagnosis. (b) MRI with gadolinium at diagnosis. (c) MRI with gadolinium after gross total resection.

complete resection, as tumour location, such as intrinsic brainstem tumours, adherence to vascular structures, cranial nerves, or ventricular surface, make resection impossible. In these cases, a partial resection or a biopsy is advocated at least to provide a histological diagnosis.

As ependymomas can spread via the CSF, craniospinal MRI and CSF cytology are mandatory following surgery. The risk of dissemination varies widely in the literature, but overall it occurs in approximately 15% of patients and is more common in those with posterior fossa tumours and in those with anaplastic ependymomas (37). The occurrence of this complication at the time of presentation is less than 5% (38); however, although the incidence is relatively low, early diagnosis may impact treatment options and avoid irreversible neurological injury. Following the established paradigm for medulloblastomas, the analysis of CSF may be misleading soon after tumour resection so a minimum interval of 2 weeks from surgery is advised. Open issues are how often and how long spinal MRI and CSF examinations should be performed in the course of follow-up.

Radiotherapy

Radiotherapy is the mainstay of post-surgical treatment despite the lack of randomized clinical trials and the general opinion that ependymomas are radioresistant. There is consensus that radiation treatment is the standard of care for patients with anaplastic (grade III) ependymoma, but there are no clinical trials that demonstrate a clear dose–response relationship (39, 40). In the past, craniospinal or whole-brain radiation were employed, but many studies show that, in the absence of a CSF spread, conformal radiotherapy can be used with less toxicity. Thus, localized anaplastic ependymomas are usually treated with limited-field radiotherapy with total doses up to 60 Gy, while craniospinal irradiation is reserved in cases with CSF dissemination (41, 42).

The role of radiation treatment for grade II ependymoma is more controversial (34, 43). Most series have reported a significant advantage in survival for patients receiving adjuvant radiotherapy after incomplete resection with doses of 54–55 Gy over those treated with surgery alone (44–48). It has been suggested that for posterior fossa ependymomas, even in case of a complete resection, adjuvant radiation therapy could improve the outcome (33). These data were recently confirmed by the analysis of a large retrospective series of ependymomas collected by the Collaborative Ependymoma Research Network (28), in whom adjuvant radiotherapy was found to be beneficial in terms of a longer PFS in infratentorial tumours. Conversely, other experts advise deferral of radiotherapy to the time of tumour progression in grade II intracranial ependymomas undergoing a total resection (49, 50).

Overall, in the absence of data from randomized clinical trials, deferral of radiotherapy to the time of recurrence in patients with intracranial grade II ependymoma after complete resection is an option with a plan for careful observation with MRI.

Stereotactic radiosurgery (SRS), by increasing the dose to the tumour, could overcome the radioresistance (51–54), but the superiority over conventional techniques remains to be proven. For patients with recurrent intracranial ependymoma, SRS provides good local control and may improve survival: this is particularly true for patients with grade II tumours and small treatment volume (55). There are no studies that have evaluated the cognitive assessment after radiotherapy in ependymoma patients. The only series that focused on the quality of life in a retrospective multicentre analysis showed that local radiation therapy may have some negative impact on patients' quality of life (56).

Chemotherapy

There is no data from large, randomized trials for either intracranial or spinal ependymomas regarding the role of chemotherapy, and most information on the activity of drugs stems from small retrospective series or case reports. Thus, the role of chemotherapy as a therapeutic approach against recurrent ependymoma has remained unclear and it is only considered when local treatment options (surgery and radiotherapy) have been exhausted (38, 57, 58).

Similar to other gliomas, temozolomide has been used for the treatment of adult patients with ependymoma. Some case reports suggest that temozolomide alone or in combination is active against recurrent WHO grade II or III ependymoma (59–62). A retrospective study on 18 patients with recurrent WHO grade II and III intracranial ependymomas failing reoperation and/or re-irradiation suggested activity of temozolomide in the standard schedule both in terms of response (22% complete response + partial response) and outcome (PFS 9.69 months and OS 30.55 months) (63). Responses were observed in chemotherapy-naïve patients only, and in most cases were delayed in appearance and cumulative over time. Conversely, in another retrospective study on patients with WHO grade II intracranial ependymomas refractory to platinum-based regimens, temozolomide in the standard schedule had a more limited activity (response rate 4%, PFS 2 months) (64). A possible explanation of this difference is that all patients in the latter series were heavily pretreated, while the majority of patients of the series of Rudà et al. (63) were chemo-naïve, thus, receiving temozolomide in an earlier phase of the disease. Temozolomide has also been used in combination with lapatinib in a single-arm phase II study in patients with recurrent intracranial and spinal ependymoma. Lapatinib targets the epidermal growth factor receptor (ErbB1) and the related family member HER-2/neu (ErbB2) which is expressed on the cell surface of tumour cells. Fifty patients were enrolled in this trial and the treatment was generally well tolerated. Median PFS was 45 weeks for patients with WHO grade II, and 25.3 weeks for patients affected by WHO grade III anaplastic ependymomas (65). Responses to treatment correlated with higher *ErbB2* mRNA expression in the tumour tissue. Although speculative, the rather modest activity of temozolomide against ependymoma might be due to high levels of O^6-methylguanine-DNA-methyltransferase (MGMT) in ependymoma cells (66); however, even if is present, MGMT promoter methylation does not correlate with response to temozolomide in ependymoma (63).

There are several reports on the administration of platinum-based treatment regimens using either cisplatin or carboplatin. A retrospective series demonstrated higher response rates in patients with progressive or recurrent ependymoma treated with cisplatin compared to non-platinum agents; however, no difference in terms of PFS and OS was observed (67). Similarly, a retrospective study, including paediatric as well as adult patients, has reported a superiority of platinum-based over nitrosourea-based regimens (68). Other drugs and regimens were only used in single patients, such as tamoxifen and isotretinoin (69). The anti-angiogenic agent bevacizumab has been administered in a small series of eight patients with recurrent WHO grade II or III intracranial ependymoma with a median PFS of 6.4 and OS of 9.4 months (70).

Spinal cord ependymomas

Spinal cord ependymomas prevail in adults. There are two histological variants: the classic ependymoma is similar in morphological features to the intracranial ependymoma and occurs in the cervical spinal cord (more frequently) and in the thoracic cord. This tumour is classified as grade II by WHO criteria, although rarely an anaplastic form can be observed.

The myxopapillary ependymoma is located almost exclusively in the region of cauda equina, filum terminale, and conus medullaris. As described previously, it is classified as WHO grade I; however, recent data indicate that these tumours do not fare better in outcome compared to grade II tumours (27), suggesting that the current WHO grading system may need a further review.

The risk of CSF spread is relatively low and extraneural metastases are extremely rare. Although spinal dissemination at diagnosis is rare in adults, compared with children, many authors recommend that all patients with a biopsy-proven spinal ependymoma undergo brain and spinal MRI and CSF cytology in their initial evaluation before deciding between observation or adjuvant treatments (71).

Extent of resection is one of the key determinants of outcome (26, 71–74).

Thus, the gold standard therapy for spinal ependymomas is en bloc GTR over piecemeal subtotal resection (71, 75, 76). Overall, GTR can be achieved in up to 70% of such patients and provides a significant improvement of PFS and OS and a lower recurrence rate compared with subtotal resection. A review of the literature (74) has revealed some interesting findings: the rate of GTR is lower in grade I myxopapillary tumours (59%) compared with grade II tumours (79%), and moreover GTR plays an important role in prolonging PFS in grade II but not in grade I tumours. One hypothesis is that GTR is more difficult to obtain for grade I myxopapillary ependymomas than perceived by neurosurgeons during surgery, as microtumours may be left behind on nerve roots, cauda equina, or filum terminale. It is also possible that myxopapillary ependymomas are biologically more aggressive than the classical ependymomas. Importantly, it has been reported that there is some risk of CSF dissemination in myxopapillary ependymomas following piecemeal removal, as the opening of the tumour capsule allows a spillage of tumour cells into CSF (26). Last, functional recovery after surgery is good in the majority of patients.

Adjuvant radiotherapy generally is not prescribed after GTR of both classical and myxopapillary ependymomas. Conversely, most studies support the use of postoperative local radiotherapy for incompletely resected tumours or for the rare anaplastic variant (71, 77–81).

Some studies suggest that total radiation doses greater than 50 Gy may be superior over lower doses when given to the region of the tumour (82). The higher doses are associated with an increased risk of radiation-induced myelopathy, but it has been estimated that 55 Gy has a less than 2% risk of significant spinal cord injury (83). More extensive radiation treatment, such as complete spine or craniospinal radiation is reserved for patients with evidence of dissemination.

The management of patients with recurrent disease includes re-resection often followed by re-irradiation with either conventional external beam treatment or use of a more focused radiation technique, such as radiosurgery (84, 85). This approach may provide good local control although the risk of myelopathy from the radiation increases with repeated treatment.

Chemotherapy does not have a standard role in the treatment of patients with spinal cord ependymoma. A variety of agents have been tried, including etoposide with modest success (86). There was a minor response using imatinib in a spinal ependymoma that expressed the PDGF receptors (87).

Outcomes in patients with myxopapillary ependymomas are variable. The predominant pattern of failure is local recurrence, followed by distant spinal relapse (10%), and distant brain relapse (up to 6%) (71, 88). However, although the recurrence rates are substantial (27–37%), OS is often prolonged, even following recurrence, In a joint study from MD Anderson Cancer Center and the European Rare Cancer Network the 10-year overall survival was 92% and PFS was 61% (71).

Challenges in clinical research in ependymoma

Despite several decades of clinical and laboratory research investigating ependymomas, patient outcomes are more related to prognostic factors, underlying tumour biology, and surgical resection than to advances in tumour-specific treatments. The seminal molecular discoveries provide encouragement that in the short term, treatment decisions can be made in the context of prognosis and anticipated biological behaviour. In the long term, there is hope that these molecular discoveries can be translated into effective and tumour-specific treatments. However, given the relative rarity of ependymoma, subclassification into molecularly defined subgroups increases the challenge to accrue to target-specific clinical trials. This is a challenge faced by all rare diseases, but there is increasing interest and support for national and international collaborations such as the Collaborative Ependymoma Research Network (http://www.CERN-foundation.org) that are helping to galvanize research efforts and provide outreach to patients that can help clinical trial accrual.

References

1. Ostrom QT, Gittleman H, Liao P, et al. CBTRUS statistical report: primary brain and central nervous system tumors diagnosed in the United States in 2007-2011. *Neuro Oncol* 2014; 16(Suppl 4): iv1–63.

2. Bailey P. A study of tumors arising from ependymal cells. *Arch Neurol Psychiatry* 1924; 11:1–27.

3. Kilday JP, Rahman R, Dyer S, et al. Pediatric ependymoma: biological perspectives. *Mol Cancer Res* 2009; 7(6):765–786.

4. Louis DN, Ohgaki H, Wiestler OD, et al. *WHO Classification of Tumours of the Central Nervous System* (revised 4th edn). Lyon: International Agency for Research on Cancer, 2016.

5. Sato H, Ohmura K, Mizushima M, et al. Myxopapillary ependymoma of the lateral ventricle. A study on the mechanism of its stromal myxoid change. *Acta Pathol Jpn* 1983; 33(5):1017–1025.

6. Sonneland PR, Scheithauer, BW Onofrio BM. Myxopapillary ependymoma. A clinicopathologic and immunocytochemical study of 77 cases. *Cancer* 1985; 56(4):883–893.

7. Warnick RE, Raisanen J, Adornato BT, et al. Intracranial myxopapillary ependymoma: case report. *J Neurooncol* 1993; 15(3):251–256.

8. Lim SC, Jang SJ. Myxopapillary ependymoma of the fourth ventricle. *Clin Neurol Neurosurg* 2006; 108(2):211–214.

9. Cachia D, Wani K, Penas-Prado M, et al. C11orf95-RELA fusion present in a primary supratentorial ependymoma and recurrent sarcoma. *Brain Tumor Pathol* 2015; 32(2):105–111.

10. Scheil S, Bruderlein S, Eicker M, et al. Low frequency of chromosomal imbalances in anaplastic ependymomas as detected by comparative genomic hybridization. *Brain Pathol* 2001; 11(2):133–143.

11. Jeuken JW, Sprenger SH, Gilhuis J, et al. Correlation between localization, age, and chromosomal imbalances in ependymal tumours as detected by CGH. *J Pathol* 2002; 197(2):238–244.

12. Modena P, Lualdi E, Facchinetti F, et al. Identification of tumor-specific molecular signatures in intracranial ependymoma and association with clinical characteristics. *J Clin Oncol* 2006; 24(33):5223–5233.

13. Gilbertson RJ, Bentley L, Hernan R, et al. ERBB receptor signaling promotes ependymoma cell proliferation and represents a potential novel therapeutic target for this disease. *Clin Cancer Res* 2002; 8(10):3054–3064.

14. Taylor MD, Poppleton H, Fuller C, et al. Radial glia cells are candidate stem cells of ependymoma. *Cancer Cell* 2005; 8(4):323–335.

15. Johnson RA, Wright KD, Poppleton H, et al. Cross-species genomics matches driver mutations and cell compartments to model ependymoma. *Nature* 2010; 466(7306):632–636.

16. Parker M, Mohankumar KM, Punchihewa C, et al. C11orf95-RELA fusions drive oncogenic NF-kappaB signalling in ependymoma. *Nature* 2014; 506(7489):451–455.

17. Witt H, Mack SC, Ryzhova M, et al. Delineation of two clinically and molecularly distinct subgroups of posterior fossa ependymoma. *Cancer Cell* 2011; 20(2):143–157.

18. Mack SC, Witt H, Piro RM, et al. Epigenomic alterations define lethal CIMP-positive ependymomas of infancy. *Nature* 2014; 506(7489):445–450.

19. Mack SC, Agnihotri S, Bertrand KC, et al. Spinal myxopapillary ependymomas demonstrate a Warburg phenotype. *Clin Cancer Res* 2015; 21(16):3750–3758.

20. Wani K, Armstrong TS, Vera-Bolanos E, et al. A prognostic gene expression signature in infratentorial ependymoma. *Acta Neuropathol* 2012; 123(5):727–738.

21. Birch BD, Johnson JP, Parsa A, et al. Frequent type 2 neurofibromatosis gene transcript mutations in sporadic intramedullary spinal cord ependymomas. *Neurosurgery* 1996; 39(1):135–140.

22. Ebert C, von Haken M, Meyer-Puttlitz B, et al. Molecular genetic analysis of ependymal tumors. NF2 mutations and chromosome 22q loss occur preferentially in intramedullary spinal ependymomas. *Am J Pathol* 1999; 155(2):627–632.

23. Pajtler KW, Witt H, Sill M, et al. Molecular classification of ependymal tumors across all CNS compartments, histopathological grades, and age groups. *Cancer Cell* 2015; 27(5):728–743.

24. Rodriguez, D, Cheung MC, Housri N, et al. Outcomes of malignant CNS ependymomas: an examination of 2408 cases through the Surveillance, Epidemiology, and End Results (SEER) database (1973–2005). *J Surg Res* 2009; 156(2):340–351.

25. Armstrong TS, Vera-Bolanos E, Bekele BN, et al. Adult ependymal tumors: prognosis and the M. D. Anderson Cancer Center experience. *Neuro Oncol* 2010; 12(8):862–870.

26. Nakamura M, Ishii K, Watanabe K, et al. Long-term surgical outcomes for myxopapillary ependymomas of the cauda equina. *Spine (Phila Pa 1976)* 2009; 34(21):E756–760.

27. Tarapore PE, Modera P, Naujokas A, et al. Pathology of spinal ependymomas: an institutional experience over 25 years in 134 patients. *Neurosurgery* 2013; 73(2):247–255.

28. Vera-Bolanos E, Aldape K, Yuan Y, et al. Clinical course and progression-free survival of adult intracranial and spinal ependymoma patients. *Neuro Oncol* 2015; 17(3):440–447.

29. Healey EA, Barnes PD, Kupsky WJ, et al. The prognostic significance of postoperative residual tumor in ependymoma. *Neurosurgery* 1991; 28(5):666–671.

30. Schwartz TH, Kim S, Glick RS, et al. Supratentorial ependymomas in adult patients. *Neurosurgery* 1999; 44(4):721–731.

31. Paulino AC, Wen BC, Buatti JM, et al. Intracranial ependymomas: an analysis of prognostic factors and patterns of failure. *Am J Clin Oncol* 2002; 25(2):117–122.

32. Kawabata Y, Takahashi JA, Arakawa Y, et al. Long-term outcome in patients harboring intracranial ependymoma. *J Neurosurg* 2005; 103(1):31–37.

33. Rogers L, Pueschel J, Spetzler R, et al. Is gross-total resection sufficient treatment for posterior fossa ependymomas? *J Neurosurg* 2005; 102(4):629–636.

34. Metellus P, Barrie M, Figarella-Branger D, et al. Multicentric French study on adult intracranial ependymomas: prognostic factors analysis and therapeutic considerations from a cohort of 152 patients. *Brain* 2007; 130(Pt 5):1338–1349.

35. Metellus P, Figarella-Branger D, Guyotat J, et al. Supratentorial ependymomas: prognostic factors and outcome analysis in a retrospective series of 46 adult patients. *Cancer* 2008; 113(1):175–185.

36. van Veelen-Vincent ML, Pierre-Kahn A, Kalifa C, et al. Ependymoma in childhood: prognostic factors, extent of surgery, and adjuvant therapy. *J Neurosurg* 2002; 97(4):827–835.

37. Reni M, Gatta G, Mazza E, et al. Ependymoma. *Crit Rev Oncol Hematol* 2007; 63(1):81–89.

38. Rudà R, Gilbert M, Soffietti R. Ependymomas of the adult: molecular biology and treatment. *Curr Opin Neurol* 2008; 21(6):754–761.

39. Taylor RE. Review of radiotherapy dose and volume for intracranial ependymoma. *Pediatr Blood Cancer* 2004; 42(5):457–460.

40. Merchant TE, Fouladi M. Ependymoma: new therapeutic approaches including radiation and chemotherapy. *J Neurooncol* 2005; 75(3):287–299.

41. Merchant TE. Three-dimensional conformal radiation therapy for ependymoma. *Childs Nerv Syst* 2009; 25(10):1261–1268.

42. Merchant TE, Li C, Xiong X, et al. Conformal radiotherapy after surgery for paediatric ependymoma: a prospective study. *Lancet Oncol* 2009; 10(3):258–266.

43. Reni M, Brandes AA, Vavassori V, et al. A multicenter study of the prognosis and treatment of adult brain ependymal tumors. *Cancer* 2004; 100(6):1221–1229.

44. Mork SJ, Loken AC. Ependymoma: a follow-up study of 101 cases. *Cancer* 1977; 40(2):907–915.

45. Salazar OM, Castro-Vita H, VanHoutte P, et al. Improved survival in cases of intracranial ependymoma after radiation therapy. Late report and recommendations. *J Neurosurg* 1983; 59(4):652–659.

46. Shaw EG, Evans RG, Scheithauer BW, et al. Postoperative radiotherapy of intracranial ependymoma in pediatric and adult patients. *Int J Radiat Oncol Biol Phys* 1987; 13(10):1457–1462.

47. Vanuytsel LJ, Bessell EM, Ashley SE, et al. Intracranial ependymoma: long-term results of a policy of surgery and radiotherapy. *Int J Radiat Oncol Biol Phys* 1992; 23(2):313–319.

48. Schild SE, Nisi K, Scheithauer BW, et al. The results of radiotherapy for ependymomas: the Mayo Clinic experience. *Int J Radiat Oncol Biol Phys* 1998; 42(5):953–958.

49. Awaad YM, Allen JC, Miller DC, et al. Deferring adjuvant therapy for totally resected intracranial ependymoma. *Pediatr Neurol* 1996; 14(3):216–219.

50. Hukin J, Epstein F, Lefton D. Treatment of intracranial ependymoma by surgery alone. *Pediatr Neurosurg* 1998; 29(1):40–45.

51. Stafford SL, Pollock BE, Foote RL, et al. Stereotactic radiosurgery for recurrent ependymoma. *Cancer* 2000; 88(4):870–875.

52. Mansur DB, Drzymala RE, Rich KM, et al. The efficacy of stereotactic radiosurgery in the management of intracranial ependymoma. *J Neurooncol* 2004; 66(1–2):187–190.

53. Combs SE, Thilmann C, Debus J, et al. Local radiotherapeutic management of ependymomas with fractionated stereotactic radiotherapy (FSRT). *BMC Cancer* 2006; 6:222.

54. Lo SS, Abdulrahman R, Desrosiers PM, et al. The role of Gamma Knife radiosurgery in the management of unresectable gross disease or gross residual disease after surgery in ependymoma. *J Neurooncol* 2006; 79(1):51–56.

55. Stauder MC, Ni Laack N, Ahmed KA, et al. Stereotactic radiosurgery for patients with recurrent intracranial ependymomas. *J Neurooncol* 2012; 108(3):507–512.

56. Dutzmann S, Schatlo B, Lobrinus A, et al. A multi-center retrospective analysis of treatment effects and quality of life in adult patients with cranial ependymomas. *J Neurooncol* 2013; 114(3):319–327.

57. Gilbert MR, Rudà R, Soffietti R. Ependymomas in adults. *Curr Neurol Neurosci Rep* 2010; 10(3):240–247.

58. Iqbal MS, Lewis J. An overview of the management of adult ependymomas with emphasis on relapsed disease. *Clin Oncol (R Coll Radiol)* 2013; 25(12):726–733.

59. Rehman S, Brock C, Newlands ES. A case report of a recurrent intracranial ependymoma treated with temozolomide in remission 10 years after completing chemotherapy. *Am J Clin Oncol* 2006; 29(1):106–107.

60. Freyschlag CF, Tuettenberg J, Lohr F, et al. Response to temozolomide in supratentorial multifocal recurrence of malignant ependymoma. *Anticancer Res* 2011; 31(3):1023–1025.

61. Kim WH, Yoon SH, Kim CY, et al. Temozolomide for malignant primary spinal cord glioma: an experience of six cases and a literature review. *J Neurooncol* 2011; 101(2):247–254.

62. Khoo HM, Kishima H, Kinoshita M, et al. Radiation-induced anaplastic ependymoma with a remarkable clinical response to temozolomide: a case report. *Br J Neurosurg* 2013; 27(2):259–261.

63. Rudà R, Bosa C, Magistrello M, et al. Temozolomide as salvage treatment for recurrent intracranial ependymomas of the adult: a retrospective study. *Neuro Oncol* 2016; 18(2):261–268.

64. Chamberlain MC, Johnston SK. Temozolomide for recurrent intracranial supratentorial platinum-refractory ependymoma. *Cancer* 2009; 115(20):4775–4782.

65. Gilbert MR, Yuan Y, Wani K, et al. A phase II study of lapatinib and dose-dense temozolomide (TMZ) for adults with recurrent ependymoma: a CERN clinical trial. *Neuro Oncol* 2014; 16(Suppl 5):AT-23.

66. Buccoliero AM, Castiglione F, Rossi Degl'Innocenti D, et al. O6-Methylguanine-DNA-methyltransferase in recurring anaplastic ependymomas: PCR and immunohistochemistry. *J Chemother* 2008; 20(2):263–268.

67. Brandes AA, Cavallo G, Reni M, et al. A multicenter retrospective study of chemotherapy for recurrent intracranial ependymal tumors in adults by the Gruppo Italiano Cooperativo di Neuro-Oncologia. *Cancer* 2005; 104(1):143–148.

68. Gornet MK, Buckner JC, Marks RS, et al. Chemotherapy for advanced CNS ependymoma. *J Neurooncol* 1999; 45(1):61–67.

69. Rojas-Marcos I, Calvet D, Janoray P, et al. Response of recurrent anaplastic ependymoma to a combination of tamoxifen and isotretinoin. *Neurology* 2003; 61(7):1019–1020.

70. Green RM, Cloughesy TF, Stupp R, et al. Bevacizumab for recurrent ependymoma. *Neurology* 2009; 73(20):1677–1680.

71. Weber DC, Wang Y, Miller R, et al. Long-term outcome of patients with spinal myxopapillary ependymoma: treatment results from the MD Anderson Cancer Center and institutions from the Rare Cancer Network. *Neuro Oncol* 2015; 17(4):588–595.

72. Gomez DR, Missett BT, Wara WM, et al. High failure rate in spinal ependymomas with long-term follow-up. *Neuro Oncol* 2005; 7(3):254–259.

73. Volpp PB, Han K, Kagan AR, et al. Outcomes in treatment for intradural spinal cord ependymomas. *Int J Radiat Oncol Biol Phys* 2007; 69(4):1199–1204.

74. Oh MC, Tarapore PE, Kim JM, et al. Spinal ependymomas: benefits of extent of resection for different histological grades. *J Clin Neurosci* 2013; 20(10):1390–1397.

75. Bostrom A, von Lehe M, Hartmann W, et al. Surgery for spinal cord ependymomas: outcome and prognostic factors. *Neurosurgery* 2011; 68(2):302–308.

76. Feldman WB, Clark AJ, Safaee M, et al. Tumor control after surgery for spinal myxopapillary ependymomas: distinct outcomes in adults versus children: a systematic review. *J Neurosurg Spine* 2013; 19(4):471–476.

77. Whitaker SJ, Bessell EM, Ashley SE, et al. Postoperative radiotherapy in the management of spinal cord ependymoma. *J Neurosurg* 1991; 74(5):720–728.

78. Schwartz TH, McCormick PC. Intramedullary ependymomas: clinical presentation, surgical treatment strategies and prognosis. *J Neurooncol* 2000; 47(3):211–218.

79. Akyurek S, Chang EL, Yu TK, et al. Spinal myxopapillary ependymoma outcomes in patients treated with surgery and radiotherapy at M.D. Anderson Cancer Center. *J Neurooncol* 80(2):177–183.

80. Dickerman RD, Reynolds AS, Gilbert E, et al. The importance of early postoperative radiation in spinal myxopapillary ependymomas. *J Neurooncol* 2007; 82(3):323–325.

81. Pica A, Miller R, Villa S, et al. The results of surgery, with or without radiotherapy, for primary spinal myxopapillary ependymoma: a retrospective study from the rare cancer network. *Int J Radiat Oncol Biol Phys* 2009; 74(4):1114–1120.

82. Shaw EG, Evans RG, Scheithauer BW, et al. Radiotherapeutic management of adult intraspinal ependymomas. *Int J Radiat Oncol Biol Phys* 1986; 12(3):323–327.

83. Schultheiss TE, Stephens LC, Peters LJ. Survival in radiation myelopathy. *Int J Radiat Oncol Biol Phys* 1986; 12(10):1765–1769.

84. Kopelson G. Radiation tolerance of the spinal cord previously-damaged by tumor and operation: long term neurological improvement and time-dose-volume relationships after irradiation of intraspinal gliomas. *Int J Radiat Oncol Biol Phys* 1982; 8(5):925–929.

85. Kocak Z, Garipagaoglu M, Adli M, et al. Spinal cord ependymomas in adults: analysis of 15 cases. *J Exp Clin Cancer Res* 2004; 23(2):201–206.

86. Chamberlain MC. Recurrent intracranial ependymoma in children: salvage therapy with oral etoposide. *Pediatr Neurol* 2001; 24(2):117–121.

87. Fakhrai N, Neophytou P, Dieckmann K, et al. Recurrent spinal ependymoma showing partial remission under imatimib. *Acta Neurochir (Wien)* 2004; 146(11):1255–1258.

88. Tsai CJ, Wang, Allen PK, et al. Outcomes after surgery and radiotherapy for spinal myxopapillary ependymoma: update of the MD Anderson Cancer Center experience. *Neurosurgery* 2014; 75(3):205–214.

CHAPTER 6

Choroid plexus tumours

Maria Santos, Eric Bouffet, Carolyn Freeman,
and Mark M. Souweidane

Definition

Choroid plexus tumours (CPTs) are primary brain tumours of neuroectodermal origin derived from choroid plexus epithelium and vascularized by choroidal arteries.

The choroid plexus is composed of a superficial layer of cuboidal cell epithelium linked by tight junctions overlying a basal membrane that covers a papillary-shaped mesenchymal stromal core. The mesenchymal stroma is formed by leptomeningeal cells, fenestrated blood vessels, and connective tissue distributed in a loose pattern over an extracellular matrix. The main known function of the choroid plexus is to produce cerebrospinal fluid (CSF) and immunochemistry studies have consistently shown intense aquaporin-1 (AQP1) expression on the apical surface of the epithelial cells. However, the choroid plexus has other functions. Choroid plexus epithelial cells express major histocompatibility complex classes I and II and may play a role in autoimmune inflammation (1). In addition, they are the primary constituent of the blood–brain barrier, being connected through tight junctions (zonulae occludentes).

There are four principal locations of choroid plexus: in each lateral ventricle, in the third ventricle, and in the fourth ventricle. Regarding embryonic development of the choroid plexus, the first to form is that in the fourth ventricle followed by the lateral ventricles and finally the third ventricle.

Pathology

According to the 2007 World Health Organization (WHO) classification, CPTs are classified based on histological criteria as choroid plexus papilloma (CPP) or grade I tumour, atypical choroid plexus papilloma or grade II tumour, and choroid plexus carcinoma (CPC) or grade III tumour (2).

CPPs tend to mimic papillary choroid plexus morphology in its radiologic, macro- and microscopic 'cauliflower appearance' but have an increased number of cells, sometimes stratified and with elongated shape. They can present with areas of calcification and cystic or haemorrhagic regions but, by definition, do not invade the brain parenchyma. Oncocytic alterations, xanthogranulomatous reaction, and/or melanin pigment deposition can also be identified (3–9). By definition, they are benign and curable with surgical gross total resection.

In contrast, CPCs show mitotic figures (five or more mitoses per ten randomly selected high-power fields), nuclear atypia, increased

nuclear-to-cytoplasmic ratio, and necrosis. The papillary architecture is distorted and there is diffuse invasion of the adjacent neural tissue by the infiltrating cells on a stromal base. CPCs are considered malignant due to their potential for recurrence and dissemination.

Atypical choroid plexus papillomas are composed of cells showing any sign of atypia but confined to the ependymal lining of the ventricles. Their most distinctive feature is increased mitotic activity defined as two or more mitoses per ten randomly selected high-power fields. Grade II tumours have an increased risk of recurrence when compared to grade I tumours.

The diagnosis of CPT can usually be made on classic haematoxylin–eosin staining (10) but immunochemistry may have relevance in the differential diagnosis especially to rule out metastatic carcinomas and other central nervous system papillary tumours such as the papillary variant of ependymoma, sub-ependymoma, or papillary meningioma (11). These tumours usually have variable staining for cytokeratin (CK7, CK20, etc.), monoclonal antibodies (human epithelial antigen-125 and Ber-EP4), vimentin, glial fibrillary acidic protein, transthyretin, podoplanin, and S-100 protein and combinations of staining patterns can be used to help with the histological differential diagnosis. CPT usually stain positive for E-cadherin and laminin and negative for neural cell adhesion marker, while ependymomas express the opposite pattern of staining for these reagents. In CPC, the papillary architecture may be absent and the differential diagnosis includes supratentorial primitive neuroectodermal tumours and atypical rhabdoid/teratoid tumours. Integrase interactor 1 (INI1) is a nuclear antigen that is consistently expressed in CPCs but lost in atypical teratoid/rhabdoid tumours (12–14). Microarray techniques have revealed two markers, Kir 7.1 and stanniocalcin 1, that are sensitive and specific for CPT (15). Kir 7.1 is a potassium channel found in normal choroid plexus and stanniocalcin 1 is a glycosylated protein involved in calcium homeostasis and resistance to hypoxia. Alpha 1-antitrypsin CSF levels appear to correlate positively with progression and recurrence of CPCs (16). Ki-67/mouse intestinal bacteria 1 (MIB1) indices also appear to be measures of CPT aggressiveness.

Diffuse villous hyperplasia of the choroid plexus (DVHCP) is an extremely rare congenital, non-neoplastic entity that should be considered in the differential radiological and histological diagnosis of CPP (10, 17). The first description of this entity was made in a postmortem specimen in 1924 by Davis as diffuse and macroscopic bilateral enlargement of histologically normal choroid plexuses of the lateral ventricles (18). The increased number and macroscopic enlargement of villi are caused by normal choroid plexus cell hyperplasia and not by hypertrophy and it was shown that these cells express less *AQP1* in their membranes than CPP cells (19). DVHPC usually presents as communicating hydrocephalus as a result of CSF overproduction in neonates or infants, and magnetic resonance imaging (MRI) frequently discloses massive enlargement of the normal choroid plexus throughout the entire ventricular system and massive communicating hydrocephalus, as well as subarachnoid space enlargement (20–22). The ventriculoperitoneal shunt failure rate is high and patients usually present with ascites after being shunted or shunt track CSF accumulation (23–25). Ventriculoatrial shunt, open choroid plexus plexectomy, or endoscopic choroid plexus coagulation are usually needed to treat this condition and can eventually be used together (26–28). There is no documented progression from DVHCP to any form of CPT (26, 27).

Epidemiology

Classically described as slow-growing childhood tumours and known as uncommon, CPTs have an approximate incidence of 0.3 per 1 million population per year. Approximately 1500 cases are diagnosed worldwide annually, corresponding to 0.3–0.6% of all brain tumours, 2–4% of all paediatric intracranial tumours, and 10–23% of tumours in children younger than 1 year (29). The incidence of CPCs is higher in one region in southern Brazil due to a higher incidence of an allele (R337H) corresponding to a *TP53* gene mutation (30). The median age at diagnosis is 3.5 years with a slight preponderance in males (1.2:1) (31). There is no known race preponderance. As expected, the primary location is intraventricular, although ectopic extraventricular locations such as the suprasellar or the pineal regions have been reported (32–34). The supratentorial compartment (lateral and third ventricles) is the most common location for these tumours in children and the infratentorial compartment in adults (fourth ventricle and the cerebellopontine angle) (31, 35). In 5% of the cases, synchronous tumours are seen. Generally, 80% of CPTs are CPPs, 15% are atypical papillomas, and less than 5% are CPCs (36), the latter occurring in infants or very young children (mean age 23–32 months) in 80% of cases (11).

Although rare, progression from a benign CPP to a malignant CPC has been reported, as well as recurrence after gross total resection of a CPP (37, 38). Jeibmann et al. found a 6% recurrence rate for WHO grade I CPP but this may be overestimated as a result of a non-detailed initial classification of the tumours (39). There are only eight well-documented cases of CPP progression to CPC (38, 39). Both recurrence and progression to a higher grade seem to be correlated with mitotic activity and the Ki-67 proliferation index (monoclonal MIB1 index). Consequently, tumours that exhibit a high proliferative index should be monitored more closely (39).

Aetiology and pathogenesis

There is no identified cause for CPTs and most occur in a sporadic way although there are recognized rare syndromic associations (10). The wide range of age at diagnosis suggests different mechanisms of development. Several common chromosomal abnormalities have been identified in CPT and the chromosomal aberration pattern differs according to the grade of anaplasia. Comparative genomic hybridization has identified chromosomal imbalances (gains, losses, or duplications) in chromosomes 1, 4, 5, 7, 9, 10, 12, 14, 18, and 20 in tumoural tissue. A large study comprising 149 patients showed that gain of chromosome 9 and loss of chromosome 10 were associated with prolonged survival in patients with CPC (40).

Li–Fraumeni syndrome is an autosomal dominant cancer predisposition syndrome caused by a *TP53* germline mutation. It has an incidence of approximately 1/20,000 and is the most recognized syndrome associated with increased risk of CPC (15, 41). There are reports of CPT associated with Li–Fraumeni syndrome diagnosed *in utero*. There are also reports of coincidental diagnosis of CPC and adrenocortical carcinoma associated with *TP53* mutation. In a study of 64 patients with tumours of the choroid plexus including 42 CPC, *TP53* mutations were found in 50% of CPC. This study found both quantitative and qualitative p53 status to be predictive of survival, with patients presenting *TP53* mutations having a worse prognosis (15). Aicardi syndrome is another syndrome that is associated with CPT development (42–46).

Recently, platelet-derived growth factor receptor (PDGFR) has been implicated in CPT tumour pathogenesis. PDGFR is expressed normally in the choroid plexus. However, the beta isoform of PDGFR is highly phosphorylated in CPCs when compared to CPPs and to normal choroid plexus and seems to induce cell proliferation when bound to its ligand (47–50). It is also known that imatinib, a tyrosine kinase inhibitor, can inhibit *in vitro* CPT epithelial cell proliferation (51).

Recent evidence has associated two other genes with CPT development. *TWIST1* is a p53 suppressor and when knocked out in cellular lines, cell proliferation is reduced. *Notch 3* is an oncogene that seems to have a role in embryological development of CPP (52).

The monkey polyomavirus simian virus 40 (SV40) is a potent virus that induces tumours in laboratory animals. Polyomavirus encode viral tumour proteins that are able to deregulate the cell cycle and to induce monoclonal proliferation of cells. It is known that transgenic mice that harbour the SV40 large T-antigen gene will develop CPT. It is also known by polymerase chain reaction methods that more than 50% of human CPTs present and express SV40-like DNA sequences. This virus was a contaminant of the polio vaccines administered to adults and children between 1955 and 1963 (53–55). However, it is not possible to establish a direct correlation between the polyomavirus injection and CPT SV40 DNA sequences. Not every patient positive for SV40 DNA sequence received polio vaccines and the presence of polyomavirus DNA sequences is not consistently associated with CPT.

Clinical presentation

Hydrocephalus is by far the most common presenting symptom for most patients with CPT. The mechanism of ventricular enlargement is most commonly a combination of CSF overproduction and direct obstruction of the CSF pathways by the tumour (56). The majority of patients present with insidious intracranial hypertension symptoms such as headaches, nausea, vomiting, and double or blurred vision. On physical examination, papilloedema is the most common finding. Younger children typically present with irritability, lethargy, macrocrania, bulging fontanelles, protruding scalp veins, and diastasis of the sutures (57). Given that the disproportionate incidence of these tumours is in infants, divergent macrocephaly is universal in this population. Patients with CPTs located in the third ventricle may present with bobble-head doll syndrome due to bilateral thalamic compression (58). Seizures are a rare form of presentation. Sudden deterioration of the level of consciousness may occur as a result of intratumoural haemorrhage or decompensating hydrocephalus.

Imaging

Computed tomography scan images usually show an intraventricular tumour with a lobulated 'cauliflower-like' edge that is well demarcated from surrounding brain that shows intense and homogeneous contrast enhancement (Fig. 6.1). Cyst formation, calcification, haemorrhagic or cystic changes, and perilesional oedema are also described (59). Hydrocephalus is nearly always present, the rare exception being an incidentally diagnosed lesion.

MRI is used for preoperative evaluation to assess tumour vascularization and determine metastatic status, and postoperatively to confirm degree of resection and monitor for recurrence. Spectroscopy has been used to differentiate between high-grade and low-grade tumours and to tailor the therapeutic approach based on the preoperative data. MRI T1-weighted sequences typically show an intraventricular iso-intense mass which intensely and uniformly enhances after contrast administration, while T2-weighted sequences usually show an iso- to hyper-intense heterogeneous tumour (Fig. 6.2 and Fig. 6.3). In CPPs, spectroscopy is characterized by a single strikingly elevated myo-inositol while in CPCs there is usually a choline and lactate peak and a decrease of the *N*-acetyl aspartate level. Both express different biochemical patterns from the normal choroid plexus (60, 61). Linear or nodular leptomeningeal enhancement is a strong indication of dissemination.

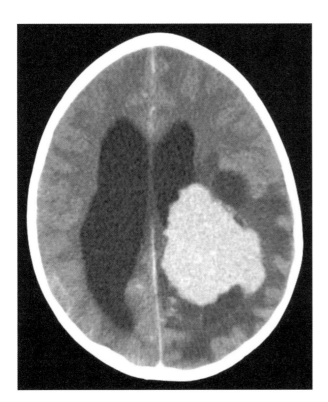

Fig. 6.1 Computed tomography with contrast showing a left intraventricular choroid plexus tumour with homogeneous contrast enhancement and intense peritumoural oedema.

Preoperative complete neuraxis MRI is recommended to rule out dissemination if there is a suspicion of a CPT on brain MRI. CPTs are highly vascularized and a considerable amount of flow voids can be identified.

Treatment

Due to the rarity of CPTs, treatment remains controversial and challenging.

CPPs are described as benign lesions and in most cases gross total resection is enough to cure the patient (57). Several series report a 5-year survival of 100% after total removal of a CPP without adjuvant therapy, with gross total resection rates as high as 96%. Even after sub-total tumour resection, the role of adjuvant therapy is controversial. Regardless, and despite the presumptive benign behaviour of CPPs, long-term clinical and radiological follow-up is needed, given reports of CPP relapses even after gross total resection sometimes many years later (31, 62–66).

CPCs are considered malignant tumours with a poor prognosis and are many times more likely to recur locally and metastasize than CPPs (11). Gross total resection is successfully achieved in less than 50% of CPCs (67, 68). The 5-year survival rate ranges from 11% to 86% after gross total resection followed by adjuvant therapy and less than 20% if no more than a partial resection is achieved (68).

The overall incidence of metastatic CPTs is 12–50% (31, 69), mainly from CPCs. The usual pattern of dissemination is spinal drop metastasis through the CSF pathways (70, 71) and every patient diagnosed with a CPT should undergo a complete neuraxis MRI to rule out dissemination (72). Shunt-related metastases are extremely rare (73).

National Comprehensive Cancer Network (NCCN) guidelines recommend testing for *TP53* mutations in any patient with a new diagnosis of CPT as this may have implication in terms of screening for associated malignancies (74).

Surgical resection

Irrespective of the histological type, gross total resection seems to play a dominant role in the treatment of CPTs, allowing symptom resolution and reducing risk of tumour recurrence, and several studies demonstrate that gross total resection is the single most important prognostic variable in CPT (56, 68, 75, 76).

Surgical resection of CPTs, and especially of CPCs, is technically demanding because they are deep seated and close to vital brain and vascular structures. Despite the great advances in diagnostic imaging techniques, neurosurgical procedures, and neuroanaesthesia, mortality rates still range up to 25% (77), the overwhelming majority of deaths being attributed to intraoperative haemorrhage due to their intense vascularization. Several case reports describe the need for abortion of the surgical procedure due to blood loss. Haemorrhage is of particular concern in very young children who have low circulating blood volumes (80 mL/kg). Solid perioperative neuroanaesthetic support is fundamental to the successful management of patients with CPTs. Patients should have adequate venous access which allows rapid and large volumes of fluid or blood transfusion and an arterial line for continuous blood pressure monitoring. Preoperative cross matching and the availability of blood, fresh frozen plasma, platelets units, and fibrinogen are

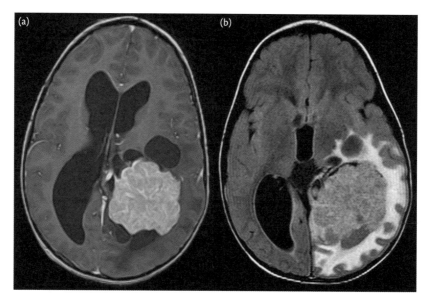

Fig. 6.2 (a) Axial T1-weighted MRI with contrast showing a left intraventricular choroid plexus tumour, intensely enhancing with associated peripheral cysts. (b) Axial T2-weighted MRI demonstrating the same lesion and emphasizing the peritumoural oedema.

mandatory. Using a microneurosurgery technique, it is critical to find the vascular pedicle of the tumour as early as possible (78–80). Generous coagulation of the tumour surface prior to sharp dissection or debulking can minimize risk of haemorrhage. Because of the recognized risk of massive bleeding during CPC resection, some teams have advocated a two-stage approach, with an initial biopsy followed by neoadjuvant chemotherapy and second-look surgery (69, 81). Following resection of CPT, subdural collections are common (82).

Neuroendoscopy, although not a mainstay, might have a role in the management of select CPTs because most of them are purely intraventricular. Endoscopic approaches have the well-recognized advantages of any endoscopic surgery, namely minimal parenchyma disruption, improved visualization, and improved cosmetic results. In the case of CPTs, endoscopic approaches allow not only tumour resection but also the treatment of hydrocephalus and possibly avoidance of ventriculoperitoneal shunt placement (83).

However, the use of endoscopic surgery in CPTs has been limited due to the lack of equipment for endoscopic dissection and the limited endoscopic visual field in the context of their exceptional vascularization and typically voluminous size. The discrepancy between the tumour and the endoscopic working channel can be overcome by a piecemeal dissection of the tumour. Endoscopic removal is feasible for small third ventricular tumors with a dominant vascular pedicle.

Interventional neuroradiology

Interventional neuroradiology has both diagnostic and therapeutic roles in the management of CPT. CPTs are vascularized by hypertrophied choroid vessels that can arise from anterior or posterior circulation, can be single or multiple, and dominant or not (80). Angiography is helpful for diagnosis and also helps in defining therapeutic options and the feasibility of preoperative embolization.

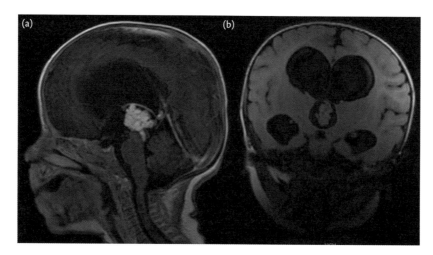

Fig. 6.3 (a) Sagittal T1-weighted MRI with contrast showing a solid choroid plexus papilloma of the third ventricle. (b) Coronal T2-FLAIR-weighted MRI showing the same tumour. There is a concomitant associated obstructive hydrocephalus. The patient was an infant and had a purely endoscopic gross total tumour resection.

Due to their characteristic high vascularization and predominance in children, CPTs are ideally suited for embolization. However, the reported success rates in performing meaningful embolization are low (84–86). Embolization is technically difficult because of elongated, tortuous, and narrow feeding vessels and the lack of adequate collateral supply to the optic pathways and internal capsule (77, 88). The relative low weight of these young children also limits the volume of contrast and amount of diagnostic radiation that can be used. Nevertheless, interventional neuroradiology is in constant technological evolution and there are progressive advances in the development of angiographic microcatheters, microguidewires, and embolization materials that reduce the risk of morbidity of interventional procedures in young children.

In addition, embolization may have a therapeutic role (87). Wind et al. reported endovascular embolization of a third-ventricle CPT in a 3-month-old patient that resulted in steady regression of the tumour with no visible lesion on an MRI performed 7 months after the procedure (88).

Radiation therapy

The role of radiotherapy in CPTs remains unclear. In a review of the literature that included data on 524 patients with a diagnosis of CPT, the 5-year projected survival rate was 68% for patients with CPCs that had undergone gross total resection followed by radiotherapy, compared to 16% for those that had not received radiotherapy (89). The clinical relevance of this finding is unknown, however, since, as in any retrospective review, multiple biases are possible. Despite this, a relative consensus exists that postoperative radiotherapy may increase the survival rate of patients who have undergone gross or partial resection of a CPC. However, there is evidence that some completely resected CPC patients can be successfully treated without radiation and future studies should aim to identify those patients who could avoid adjuvant radiation treatment. Radiotherapy is more routinely considered after incomplete resection of a CPC. However, the outlook for CPC patients with incomplete resection is dismal regardless as to whether they receive radiation or not (31).

The choice of radiotherapy target volume (neuraxis, whole brain, or involved-field) is also controversial. Given the propensity for dissemination, craniospinal irradiation (CSI) has been the standard for CPC and a recent literature review on this topic suggests that CSI improves progression-free and overall survival when compared to involved-field irradiation (90). However, this review pointed out the large diversity of radiation approaches, particularly for the treatment of younger children. As an illustration, doses to the primary site ranged from 10 to 78 Gy and doses to the neuraxis from 18 to 46 Gy. In general, CSI will now be used only in older patients with CPC and those with metastatic disease.

Chemotherapy

Due the rarity of CPCs and the lack of large prospective trials, the role of chemotherapy for CPCs also remains unclear. Retrospective data suggest that chemotherapy may decrease the risk of recurrence and increase the survival rate after gross total surgical resection (81). In infants and younger children, it may allow deferment or avoidance of postoperative radiotherapy. There is also evidence that neoadjuvant chemotherapy (prior to tumour resection) can facilitate second-look surgery and in particular reduce the risk of intraoperative bleeding (91). In some studies, a combination of etoposide and platinum compounds was considered the most effective chemotherapeutic regimen (69).

There is no reliable information regarding treatment of CPC at relapse apart from isolated clinical reports or small series. At the time of relapse, 50% of cases show distant patterns of failure and the mortality rate is near 100%. High-dose chemotherapy with autologous stem cell transplant is a therapeutic option that has demonstrated anecdotal success (80).

CPT-SIOP-2000 is a multicentre, prospective, and randomized controlled trial that was started in 2000 to test adjuvant chemotherapeutic agents in order to identify optimal treatment for localized and disseminated CPCs and incompletely resected atypical plexus papillomas. For children older than 3 years old, the study included radiation therapy. The first analysis of a group of atypical plexus papilloma patients showed a favourable response to chemotherapy (92). The current CPT-SIOP-2009 study compares four different chemotherapeutic protocols.

Treatment of choroid plexus tumour-associated hydrocephalus

CPTs present with hydrocephalus in 30–70% of cases as the result of a combination of a communicating and an obstructive mechanism. Shunt placement prior to tumour resection is often needed despite the risk of ascites and congestive cardiac failure that has been reported as a consequence of large volumes of CSF production (up to 900 mL/day) (56, 93). The literature reports rates of permanent shunting between 26% and 50%. Embolization may reduce the rate of CSF production by the tumour (84). Total removal of the CPT can itself be curative of hydrocephalus (93, 95). The persistence of microinflammatory changes of the ependyma (arachnoiditis), intraventricular tumour debris, or haemorrhage, however, commonly contributes to the persistence to both intraventricular and extraventricular obstruction of CSF pathways. Endoscopic third ventriculostomy has not gained widespread appeal in CPT-associated hydrocephalus owing to the typical tumour location and CSF overproduction.

Next steps

CPTs are challenging tumours that require a multidisciplinary approach. Progress in the management of CPCs in particular has been slow due to the rarity of these tumours. Improvement will only be possible through international collaborations that include cooperative molecular biology and genomic studies with the final objective of identifying new therapies for this still poor-prognosis disease.

References

1. Wolburg H, Paulus W. Choroid plexus: biology and pathology. *Acta Neuropathol* 2010; 119(1):75–88.
2. Louis DN, Oghaki H, Wiestler OD, et al. The 2007 WHO classification of tumors of central nervous system. *Acta Neuropathol* 2001; 114(2):97–109.
3. Aquilina K, Nanra JS, Allcut DA, et al. Choroid plexus adenoma: case report and review of the literature. *Childs Nerv Syst* 2005; 21(5):410–415.
4. Bucoliero AM, Bacci M, Mennonna P, et al. Pathologic quiz case: infratentorial tumor in a middle aged woman. Oncocytic variant of choroid plexus papilloma. *Arch Pathol Lab Med* 2004; 128(12):1448–1450.
5. Corcoran GM, Frazier SR, Prayson RA. Choroid plexus papilloma with osseous and adipose metaplasia. *Ann Diagn Pathol* 2001; 5(1):43–47.
6. Gaudio RM, Tacconi L, Rossi ML. Pathology of choroid plexus papillomas: a review. *Clin Neurol Neurosurg* 1998; 100 (3):165–186.
7. Ikota H, Tanaka Y, Yokoo H, et al. Clinicopathological and immunohistochemical study of 20 choroid plexus tumors: their histological diversity and the expression of markers useful for differentiation from metastatic cancer. *Brain Tumor Pathol* 2011; 28(3):215–221.
8. Tena-Suck ML, Lopez-Gomez M, Salinas-Lara C, et al. Psammomatous choroid plexus papilloma: three cases with atypical characteristics. *Surg Neurol* 2006; 65 (6):604–610.
9. Watanabe K, Ando Y, Iwanaga H, et al. Choroid plexus papilloma containing melanin pigment. *Clin Neuropathol* 1995; 14(3):159–161.
10. Gupta N. Choroid plexus tumors in children. *Neurosurg Clin N Am* 2003; 4:621–631.
11. Gopal P, Parker JR, Debski R, et al. Choroid plexus carcinoma. *Arch Pathol Lab Med* 2008; 132(8):1350–1354.
12. Ang LC, Taylor AR, Bergin D, et al. An immunohistochemical study of papillary tumors in the central nervous system. *Cancer* 1990; 65(12):2712–2719.
13. Kepes JJ, Collins J. Choroid plexus epithelium (normal and neoplastic) expresses synaptophysin. A potential useful aid in differentiating carcinoma of the plexus from metastatic papillary carcinomas. *J Neuropathol Exp Neurol* 1999; 58(4):398–401.
14. Paulus W, Janisch W. Clinicopathologic correlations in epithelial choroid plexus neoplasms: a study of 52 cases. *Acta Neuropathol* 1990; 80(6):635–641.
15. Tabori U, Shilen A, baskin B, et al. TP53 alterations determine clinical subgroups and survival of patients with choroid plexus tumors. *J Clin Oncol* 2010; 28(12):1995–2001.
16. Qualman SJ, Shannon BT, Boesel CP, et al. Ploidy analysis and cerebrospinal fluid nephelometry as measures of clinical outcome in childhood choroid plexus neoplasia. *Pathol Annu* 1992; 27(Pt1):305–320.
17. Barreto AS, Vassalo J, Queiroz L de S. Papillomas and carcinomas of the choroid plexus: histological and immunohistochemical studies and comparison with normal fetal choroid plexus. *Arq Neuropsiquiatr* 2004; 62:600–607.
18. Davis L. A physio-pathologic study of the choroid plexus with the report of a case of villous hypertrophy. *J Med Res* 1924; 44:521–534.
19. Smith Z, Moftakhar P, Malkasian D, et al. Choroid plexus hyperplasia: surgical treatment and immunohistochemical results. Case report. *J Neurosurg* 2007; 107:255–262.
20. Asai A, Hoffmann HJ, Matsutani M, et al. Choroid plexus tumors in infancy. *No Shinkei Geka* 1991; 19:21–26.
21. Ceddia A, Di Rocco C, Carlucci A. Hypersecretive congenital hydrocephalus due to choroid plexus villous hypertrophy associated with contralateral papilloma. *Minerva Pediatr* 1993; 45:363–367.
22. Chow E, Reardon DA, Shah AB, et al. Pediatric choroid plexus neoplasms. *Int J Radiat Oncol Biol Phys* 1999; 44:249–254.
23. Britz GW, kim DK, Loeser JD. Hydrocephalus secondary to diffuse vollous hyperplasia of the choroid plexus. Case report and review of the literature. *J Neuro*surg 1996; 85:689–691.
24. Casey KF, Vries JK. Cerebral fluid overproduction in the absence of tumor or villous hypertrophy of the choroid plexus. *Childs Nerv Syst* 1989; 5:332–334.
25. Iplikcoglu AC, Bek S, Gokduman CA, et al. Diffuse villous hyperplasia of choroid plexus. *Acta Neurochir (Wien)* 2006; 148:691–694.
26. Bucholz RD, Pittman T. Endoscopic coagulation of the choroid plexus using the ND:YAG laser: initial experience and proposal for management. *Neurosurgery* 1991; 28:421–427.
27. Philips MF, Shanno G, Duhaime AC. Treatment of villous hypertrophy of the choroid plexus by endoscopic contact coagulation. Technical case report. *Pediatr Neurosurg* 1998; 28:252–256.
28. Welch K, Strand R, Bresnan M, et al. Congenital hydrocephalus due to villous hypertrophy of the telencephalic choroid plexuses. Case report. *J Neurosurg* 1983; 59:172–175.
29. Koh EJ, Wang KC, Phi JH, et al. Clinical outcome of pediatric choroid plexus tumors; retrospective analysis from a single institute. *Childs Nerv Syst* 2014; 30(2):217–25.
30. Custodio G, Taques GR, Figueiredo BC, et al. Increased incidence of choroid plexus carcinoma due to the germline TP53 R337H mutation in southern Brazil. *PloS One* 2011; 6(3):e18015.
31. Wolff JE, Sajedi M, Brant R, et al. Choroid plexus tumors. *Br J Cancer* 2002; 87:1086–1191.
32. Carter A, Price D, Tucci K, et al. Choroid plexus carcinoma presenting as an intraparenchymal mass. *J Neurosurg* 2001; 95:1040–1044.
33. Kimura M, Takayasu M, Suzuki Y, et al. Primary choroid plexus papilloma located in the suprasellar region: case report. *Neurosurgery* 1992; 31:563–566.
34. Rickert CH, Paulus W. Tumors of the choroid plexus. *Microsc Res Tech* 2001; 52:104–111.
35. McGirr SJ, Ebersold MJ, Scheithauer BW, et al. Choroid plexus papillomas: long term follow-up results in a surgically treated series. *J Neurosurg* 1988; 69:843–849.
36. Koeller KK, Sandberg GD. From the archives of the AFIP. Cerebral intraventricular neoplasms: radiologic-pathologic. *Radiographics* 2002:22:1473–505.
37. Dhillon RS, Wang YY, McKelvie PA, et al. Progression of choroid plexus papilloma. *J Clin Neurosci* 2013; 20(12):1775–1778.
38. Niikawa S, Ito T, Murakawa T, et al. Recurrence of choroid plexus papilloma with malignant transformation-case report and lectin histochemistry study. *Neurol Med Chir (Tokyo)* 1993; 33:32–35.
39. Jeibmann A, Wrede B, Peters O, et al. Malignant progression in choroid plexus papillomas. *J Neurosurg* 2007; 107:199–202.
40. Rickert CH, Wiestler OD, Paulus W. Chromosomal imbalances in choroid plexus tumors. *Am J Pathol* 2002; 160:1105–1113.
41. Krutilkova V, Trkova M, Fleitz J. Identification of five new families strengthens the link between childhood choroid plexus carcinoma and germline TP53 mutations. *Eur J Cancer* 2005; 41:1597–1603.
42. Aicardi J. Aicardi syndrome. *Brain Dev* 2005; 27(3):164–171.
43. Muchardt C, Sardet C, Bourachot B, et al. A human protein with homology to Saccharomyces cerevisae SNF5 interacts with the potential helicase hbrm. *Nucleic Acids Res* 1995; 23(7):1127–1132.
44. Sevenet N, Sheridan E, Amran D, et al. Constitutional mutations of the hSNF5/INI1 gene predispose to a variety of cancers. *Am J Hum Genet* 1999; 65(5):1342–1348.
45. Versteege I, Sevenet N, Lange J, et al. Truncating mutations of hSNF5/INI1 in aggressive pediatric cancers. *Nature* 1998; 394(6689):203–206.
46. Wade PA, Wolffe P. Transcriptional regulation: SWItching circuitry. *Curr Biol* 1999; 9(6):R221–R224.
47. Andrae J, Gallini R, Betsholtz C. Role of platelet-derived growth factors in physiology and medicine. *Genes Dev* 2008; 22(10):1276–1312.
48. Enge M, Wilhelmsson U, Abramsson A, et al. Neuron-specific ablation of PDGF-B is compatible with normal central nervous system development and astroglial response to injury. *Neurochem Res* 2003; 28(2):271–279.
49. Hellstrom M, Kalen M, Lindahl P, et al. Role of PDGF-B and PDGFR-beta in recruitment of vascular smooth muscle cells and pericytes

during embryonic blood vessel formation in the mouse. *Development* 1999; 126(14):3047–3055.

50. Kaminski WE, Lindahl P, Lin NL, et al. Basis of hematopoietic defects in platelet-derived growth factor (PDGF)-B and PDGF beta-receptor null mice. *Blood* 2001; 97(7):1990–1998.

51. Koos B, Paulsson J, Jarvius M, et al. Platelet-derived growth factor receptor expression and activation in choroid plexus tumors. *Am J Pathol* 2009; 175(4):1631–1637.

52. Safaee M, Oh MC, Bloch O, et al. Choroid plexus papillomas: advances in molecular biology and understanding of tumorigenesis. *Neuro Oncol* 2013; 15(3):255–267.

53. Bergsagel DJ, Finegold MJ, Butel JS, et al. DNA Sequences similar to those of simian virus 40 in ependymomas and choroid plexus tumors of childhood. *N Engl J Med* 1992; 326:988–993.

54. Engels EA, Katki HA, Nielsen NM, et al. Cancer incidence in Denmark following exposure to poliovirus vaccine contaminated with simian virus 40. *J Natl Cancer Inst* 2003; 95(7):532–539.

55. Hosoya K, Hori S, Ohtsuki S, et al. A new in vitro model for blood-cerebrospinal fluid barrier transport studies: an immortalized choroid plexus epithelial cell line derived from the tsA58 SV40 large T-antigen gene transgenic rat. *Adv Drug Deliv Rev* 2004; 56(12):1875–1885.

56. Eisenberg HM, McComb JG, Lorenzo AV. Cerebrospinal fluid overproduction and hydrocephalus associated with choroid plexus papilloma. *J Neurosurg* 1974; 40:381–5.

57. Ellenbogen RG, Winston KR, Kuspsky WJ. Tumors of the choroid plexus in children. *Neurosurgery* 1989; 25:327–35.

58. Keating RF, Goodrich JT, Packer RJ. *Tumors of the Pediatric Central Nervous System*. New York: Thieme; 2001.

59. Hopper KD, Foley LC, Nieves NL, Smirniotopoulos JG. The intraventricular extension of choroid plexus papillomas. *AJNR Am J Neuroradiol* 1987; 8:469–472.

60. Horská A, Ulug AM, Melhem ER, et al. Proton magnetic resonance spectroscopy of choroid plexus tumors in children. *J Magn Reson Imaging* 2001; 14(1):78–82.

61. Krieger MD, Panigrahy A, McComb JG, et al. Differentiation of choroid plexus tumors by advanced magnetic resonance spectroscopy. *Neurosurg Focus* 2005; 18(6A):E4.

62. Bettegowda C, Adogwa O, Metha V, et al. Treatment of choroid plexus tumors: a 20-year single institutional experience. *J Neurosurg Pediatr* 2012; 10(5):398–405.

63. Due Tonnessen C, Heseth E, Shullerud K, et al. Choroid plexus tumors in children and young adults: report of 16 consecutive cases. *Child Nerv Syst* 2001; 17(4-5):252–256.

64. Krishnan S, Brown PD, Scheithauer BW, et al. Choroid plexus papillomas: a single institutional experience. *J Neurooncol* 2004; 68(1):49–55.

65. Lafay-Cousin, Keene D, Carret AS, et al. Choroid plexus tumors in children less than 36 months: the Canadian Pediatric Brain Tumor Consortium (CPBTC) experience. *Childs Nerv Syst* 2011; 27(2):259–264.

66. McEvoy AW, Harding BN, Phipps KP, et al. Management of choroid plexus in children: 20 years experience at a single neurosurgical centre. *Pediatr Neurosurg* 2000; 32(4):192–199.

67. Packer RJ, Perilongo G, Johnson D, et al. Choroid plexus carcinoma of childhood. *Cancer* 1992; 69(2):580–585.

68. Pierga JY, Kalifa C, Terrir-Lacombe MJ, et al. Carcinoma of the choroid plexus: a pediatric experience. *Med Pediatr Oncol* 1993; 21:480–487.

69. Berger C, Thiesse P, Lellouch-Tubiana A, et al. Choroid plexus carcinomas in childhood: clinical features and prognostic factors. *Neurosurgery* 1998; 42(3):470–475.

70. McCall T, Binning M, Blumenthal DT, et al. Variations of disseminated choroid plexus papilloma: 2 case reports and a review of the literature. *Surg Neurol* 2006; 66(1):62–67.

71. Yoshida K, Sato K, Kitai R, et al. Coincident choroid plexus carcinoma and adrenocortical tumor in an infant. *Brain Tumor Pathol* 2013; 30(2):104–8.

72. Ahn SS, Cho YD. Spinal drop metastasis from a posterior fossa choroid plexus papilloma. *J Korean Neurosurg Soc* 2007; 42(6):475–477.

73. Donovan DJ, Prauner RD. Shunt related abdominal metastases in a child with choroid plexus carcinoma; case report. *Neurosurg* 2005; 56(2):e412.

74. Daly MB, Pilarski R, Axilbund JE, et al. NCCN Clinical Practice Guidelines in Oncology: genetic/familial high risk assessment: breast and ovarian, version 1.2014. *J Natl Compr Canc Netw* 2014; 12(9):1326–1338.

75. Dohrmann GJ, Collias JC. Choroid plexus carcinoma. Case report. *J Neurosurg* 1975; 43:225–232.

76. Sharma R, Rout D, Gupta AK, et al. Choroid plexus papillomas. *Br J Neurosurg* 1994; 8:169–177.

77. Pencalet P, Sainte-Rose C, Lellouch-Tubiana A, et al. Papillomas and carcinomas of the choroid plexus in children. *J Neurosurg* 1998; 88(3):521–528.

78. Hawkins JC III. Treatment of choroid plexus papillomas in children: a brief analysis of twenty years' experience. *Neurosurgery* 1980; 6:380–384.

79. Matson DD, Crofton FDL. Papilloma of the choroid plexus in childhood. *J Neurosurg* 1960; 17:1002–1027.

80. Raimondi AJ, Gutierrez FA. Diagnosis and surgical treatment of choroid plexus papillomas. *Childs Brain* 1975; 1:81–115.

81. Lafay-Cousin L, Mabbot DJ, Halliday W, et al. Use of ifosfamide, carboplatin, and etoposide chemotherapy in choroid plexus carcinoma. *J Neurosurg Pediatr* 2010; 5(6):615–621.

82. Kumar R, Singh S. Childhood choroid plexus papillomas: operative complications. *Childs Nerv Syst* 2005; 21(2):138–143.

83. Reddy D, Gunnarsson T, Scheinemann K, et al. Combined staged endoscopic and microsurgical approach of a third ventricular choroid plexus papilloma in an infant. *Minim Invasive Neurosurg* 2011; 54(5–6):264–267.

84. Haliasos N, Brew S, Robertson F, et al. Pre-operative embolisation of choroid plexus tumours in children. Part II. Observations on the effects on CSF production. *Childs Nerv Syst* 2013; 29(1):71–76.

85. Otten ML, Riina HA, Gobin YP, et al. Preoperative embolization in the treatment of choroid plexus papilloma in an infant. Case report. *J Neurosurg* 2006; 104(6 Suppl):419–421.

86. Trivelato FP, Manzato LB, Rezende MT, et al. Preoperative embolization of choroid plexus papilloma with Onyx via the anterior choroidal artery: technical note. *Childs Nerv Syst* 2012; 28(11):1955–1958.

87. Hoffman C, Riina HA, Stieg P, et al. Associated aneurysms in pediatric arteriovenous malformations and the implications for treatment. *Neurosurgery* 2011; 69(2):315–322.

88. Wind JJ, Bell RS, Bank WO, et al. Treatment of third ventricular choroid plexus papilloma in an infant with embolization alone. *J Neurosurg Pediatr* 2010; 6(6):579–582.

89. Wolff JE, Sajedi M, Coppes MJ, et al. Radiation therapy and survival in choroid plexus carcinoma. *Lancet* 1999; 353:2126.

90. Mazloom A, Wolff JE, Paulino AC. The impact of radiotherapy fields in the treatment of patients with choroid plexus carcinoma. *Int J Radiat Oncol Biol Phys* 2010; 78(1):79–84.

91. Souweidane MM, Johnson JH Jr, Lis E. Volumetric reduction of a choroid plexus carcinoma using preoperative chemotherapy. *J Neurooncol* 1999; 43(2):167–171.

92. Wrede B, Hasselblatt M, Peters O, et al. Atypical choroid plexus papilloma: clinical experience in the CPT-SIOP-2000 study. *J Neurooncol* 2009; 95(3):383–392.

93. Ghatak NR, McWhorter JM. Ultrastructural evidence for CSF production by a choroid plexus papilloma. *J Neurosurg* 1976; 45:409–415.

94. Husag L, Costabile G, Probst C. Persistent hydrocephalus following removal of choroid plexus papilloma of the lateral ventricle. *Neurochirurgia* 1984; 27:82–85.

95. McDonald JV. Persistent hydrocephalus following the removal of papillomas of the choroid plexus of the lateral ventricles. Report of two cases. *J Neurosurg* 1969; 30:736–740.

CHAPTER 7

Other neuroepithelial tumours: astroblastoma, angiocentric glioma, and chordoid glioma

Martin J. van den Bent, Frederic Dhermain, and Walter Stummer

Astroblastoma

Definition (histology)

Astroblastoma is a rare tumour, originally described by Bailey and Cushing, which is still a controversial entity (1). Nonetheless, it continues to be part of the 2016 World Health Organization (WHO) classification and its histological features are described as: 'A glial neoplasm characterized by a typical perivascular pattern of GFAP positive astrocytic cells with broad, non-tapering processes radiating towards a central blood vessel' (2). Perivascular pseudorosettes and prominent perivascular hyalinization are typical features. Tumours are strongly positive for S-100, glial fibrillary acid protein (GFAP), and vimentin. A distinction is made between low-grade and high-grade astroblastomas based on the presence of nuclear atypia, degree of cellularity, and the frequency of mitotic figures (3). Necrosis has been reported regardless of histological type. The clinical significance of the grading of these tumours is not completely clear, but in several larger series anaplastic histology was found to be a poor prognostic feature with more frequent recurrences (3–5). Unexpected rapid recurrences in low-grade astroblastoma have been described however (6). These tumours must be distinguished in particular from ependymomas, astrocytomas, and certain non-neuroepithelial tumours. Recurrent lesions often show increasing anaplasia, and have been diagnosed as glioblastoma or gliosarcoma.

Epidemiology

The incidence is low, but reliable estimates are lacking. It is reasonable to estimate the incidence below 1% of primary brain tumours. In almost all case series, females are more frequently affected than males; in a large review, 70 females to 30 males were found (7). It is predominantly a tumour of childhood and young adults (3, 5, 7).

Aetiology

There are no known aetiological factors. Hereditary cases have not been reported.

Pathogenesis

In view of the anecdotal nature of reports, no systematic accounts of pathogenesis of these lesions exist. One report described chromosomal abnormalities in seven cases as assessed by classical comparative genomic hybridization (5). The most frequent alterations were gains of chromosome arm 20q (four out of seven) and 19 (three out of seven). In two cases, gain of 9p was noted. Another case report observed loss of heterozygosity of chromosome 9 (8).

Clinical presentation

The clinical presentation of astroblastoma is not specific, depending on growth rate and localization. Many patients present with non-localizing signs and symptoms, suggestive of an increased intracranial pressure. Others present with focal deficits or seizures.

Imaging

In several papers, detailed neuroimaging features have been described (9, 10). The available data suggest these tumours are often diagnosed once they are quite large (in 50%, >5 cm diameter, suggestive of a low growth rate) (7). The classical appearance is one of a peripheral or even extra-axial located, supratentorial, and lobulated mass often with multiple cysts. The tumours usually appear well demarcated from normal brain parenchyma. On computed tomography (CT) imaging, calcified foci are frequent. On T1-weighted magnetic resonance imaging (MRI), the lesion is often hypo- or isointense compared to normal white matter. The multiple cysts in combination with the heterogeneous enhancement of the solid component on T1-weighted images after contrast administration may give the tumour a 'bubbly' appearance. Frequently a striking enhancing rim around the cysts is present

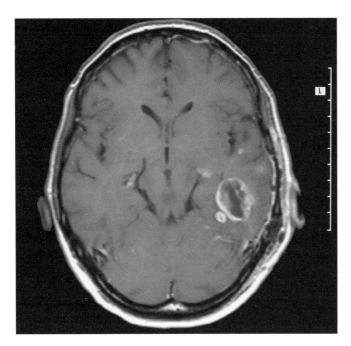

Fig. 7.1 Magnetic resonance imaging of an astroblastoma (T1-weighted image after contrast administration).

(Fig. 7.1). On T2-weighted images, the solid component frequently has a decreased signal intensity, and despite the size of the lesion there is often very little oedema around the tumour.

Treatment

All outcome reports are based on retrospective case series of limited size, with some larger series and one detailed review report available (3, 7, 11). In these series, childhood cases are mixed with adult cases. There are at present no data to suggest that childhood tumours should be treated differently than adult cases.

Surgery

Radical resection is the treatment of choice of these usually non-infiltrative growing, well-demarcated, and peripherally located lesions. Because of these features, most of these tumours are candidates for a gross complete tumour resection, even when very large. Five-year progression-free survival after gross total resection was 83%, versus 55% after subtotal resection in one large review (7). With the clear clinical benefit of gross total tumour removal, it seems reasonable to re-resect incompletely resected patients if a complete removal appears feasible (but data on this approach are not available).

Radiotherapy

With the clear role of complete resection, the question is what the role of adjuvant treatments and in particular of radiotherapy is, especially after complete resection in low-grade lesions. With most data from retrospective case reports, this remains a difficult question. Even many long-surviving, completely resected low-grade astroblastoma patients received postoperative radiotherapy as part of initial management (3, 11). However, in some series, long-term survival was reported after complete resection of low-grade lesions without radiotherapy (3, 4). There are several indications that astroblastoma may indeed be radiosensitive. Good responses and

long-term survival have been described after radiotherapy alone or in incompletely resected recurrences (3, 6). One case of gamma knife-based radiosurgery of a recurrent astroblastoma resulted in good local control for at least 17 months (12). A reasonable approach is to consider adjuvant postsurgical radiotherapy in anaplastic astroblastoma, except for very young children so as to avoid severe radiotherapy-induced toxicities. Radiotherapy should also be considered in incompletely resected low-grade cases. The role of radiotherapy in completely resected low-grade cases is unclear.

Chemotherapy

There are no clear data on chemotherapy and astroblastoma. Some anaplastic astroblastomas have been treated with chemotherapy as part of initial treatment. As this was mainly administrated to anaplastic lesions which tend to have worse survival, it is unclear whether this has contributed to survival. Data on chemotherapy outcome in recurrent lesions are very scattered, but complete remissions have been described (13).

Commentary on National Comprehensive Cancer Network and any other treatment guidelines

There are no evidence-based guidelines available for the follow-up of these lesions. It seems reasonable to follow patients with high-grade lesions more closely. Completely resected low-grade astroblastomas have a good outcome, especially after radiotherapy. In case no radiotherapy has been given, a more stringent follow-up should be considered.

Current research topics

These lesions are typical tumours that should be part of a prospective rare tumour registry.

Angiocentric glioma

This recently described entity continues to be present in the 2016 WHO classification and is characterized by a perivascular pattern of growth, and although tumour cells show diffuse infiltration, they tend to cluster around vessels in a manner resembling the pseudorosettes of ependymoma and astroblastoma (14). In 2005, two different groups described ten cases and eight cases of a particular unifocal, supratentorial brain tumour, infiltrating the cortex and subcortical white matter of children and young adults, showing both astrocytic and ependymal differentiation with a marked angiocentric growth pattern. Lellouch-Tubiana et al. designated this stable or slowly growing neoplasm as an 'angiocentric neuroepithelial tumor' (ANET) (15) whereas Wang et al. described a 'monomorphous angiocentric glioma' (AG) (16). In 2007, eight new cases were reported with comparable clinicopathological findings (17). The tumours are characterized by an angiocentric growth pattern of bipolar spindle cells with slender nuclei that radiate from a central vessel to form pseudorosettes (14–22). Mostly composed of a focal solid part with areas of nested clear epithelioid-like cells, a locally infiltrative border is visible with a subpial aggregation of streaming spindled cells, possibly associated with microcalcifications (20–24). When sufficient adjacent non-tumour tissue is resected, often a focal cortical dysplasia is described, suggesting a developmental basis (20, 22). This entity is considered as grade I glioma in the last 2007 WHO classification of brain tumours, due to its benign clinical behaviour and the possibility of curative surgery (19). Ki-67 labelling indices usually range from less than 1% to 5%, but at least three cases of angiocentric glioma with a mitotic index as high as 10% have been reported (14–16, 21, 25–27). One patient suffered from an early recurrence and finally died, but the benign clinical behaviour of the other two was confirmed.

Epidemiology

This is a very rare tumour. In 2012, fewer than 45 cases had been reported and AG represented only 2.3% of a selected series of 129 children with chronic epilepsy encountered over a 20-year period (28). There is no sex predilection.

Aetiology

There are no known factors.

Pathogenesis

Lellouch-Tubiana et al. hypothesized a dysembryoplastic process from a radial glial cell or neuronal origin, while Wang et al. suggested an astrocytic or ependymal origin (15, 16). Characteristic 'dot-like' epithelial membrane antigen (EMA) staining of microlumens within these tumours suggests an ependymomatous differentiation of lesion cells. The neoplasm is variably immunoreactive for GFAP (14–22, 29). No isocitrate dehydrogenase-1 mutation was found in a recent series of three new cases (30).

Clinical presentation

The patients present mostly during childhood or early adulthood. Median age at surgery is around 12 years (range 2–70 years), with most patients presenting initial symptoms many years before (14, 20, 21, 29). Adult cases have been reported with mesial temporal lobe locations, without clear prognostic implications (21, 25). Typically, patients present with epilepsy of many years' duration. A few patients present with headaches or motor deficits.

Imaging

The typical image is that of a non-enhancing cortico-subcortical glioma, mainly located in the frontotemporal lobes. On MRI, T2/ FLAIR-weighted images show a hyperintense lesion often extending to the nearest lateral ventricle with an intrinsic rim-like hyperintensity on T1 images, without enhancement after gadolinium injection (Fig. 7.2) (14–22, 29). These tumours are centred in the cortical grey matter and extend into the underlying white matter for a short distance, in the frontoparietal and temporal lobes as well as in the hippocampal region (14, 16, 20–22, 29, 31). Based on imaging characteristics, other benign tumours should be considered: pilomyxoid variant of astrocytoma (32, 33), cortical ependymomas (20, 34, 35), gangliogliomas, and dysembryoplastic neuroepithelial tumours (22, 28, 29). Importantly, all of these other slowly growing lesions are usually strongly enhancing after gadolinium administration.

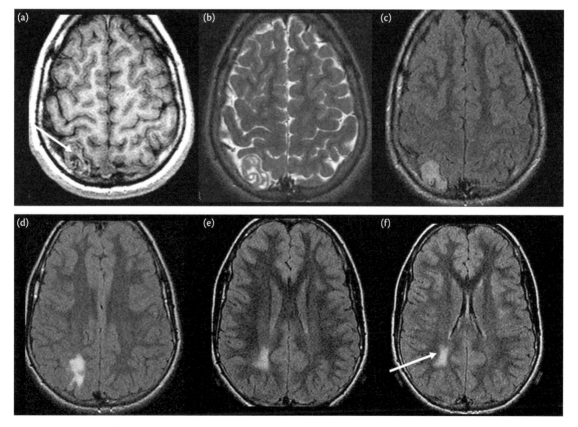

Fig. 7.2 Magnetic resonance imaging of an angiocentric glioma. Intrinsic cortical rim of hyperintensity on T1 SE-weighted sequences (a, see arrow) and clear cortico-subcortical hyperintensity on T2-weighted sequences (b) and FLAIR-weighted sequences (c) are observed. Different level on axial FLAIR slices showed that the white matter hyperintensity extends to the nearest lateral ventricle (d, e, f; see arrow).

Treatment

Surgery

Gross total resection alone has proved to be curative in most cases with a follow-up range of 1–10 years. In addition, in most patients this results in complete cessation of epileptic symptoms, although some patients continue to suffer from usually non-disabling simple partial seizures, especially after incomplete resections (22, 29). Importantly, obtaining a surgical margin of several millimetres (when possible) in the surrounding macroscopically 'uninvolved' cerebral tissue may encompass most of the microscopic infiltration, resulting in potentially better tumour control. As long-term video-electroencephalography monitoring recording disclosed epileptic activities extending beyond the margin of the radiological lesion, extended cortical resection might also result in better control of seizures (20, 36).

Radiotherapy

For non-resectable tumours located in highly eloquent areas, radiotherapy can be considered, with good local control in three published cases (17, 20, 21).

Chemotherapy

No reports are available regarding chemotherapy for angiocentric gliomas.

Commentary on National Comprehensive Cancer Network and any other treatment guidelines

There are no evidence-based guidelines available for the follow-up of these lesions.

Current research topics

These lesions are typical tumours that should be part of a prospective rare tumour registry.

Chordoid glioma

Introduction

Chordoid glioma, the name of which was derived from its glial and chordoid characteristics, is a rare tumour with features suggesting it to be low grade in nature. The 2016 WHO classification has retained this diagnosis. Histologically, the tumour consists of clusters and cords of ovoid and polygonal epithelioid cells embedded within a mucinous matrix (37–39). This tumour was first defined as a distinct neuropathological entity in 1998 but was probably already described 3 years earlier as a 'third ventricular meningioma' with a 'peculiar' expression of GFAP (38, 40). Chordoid glioma was included in the 2000 WHO classification of tumours of the central nervous system as a 'neuroepithelial tumour of uncertain origin' and provisionally defined as a grade II tumour (41). The 2016 version of the WHO classification maintains the chordoid glioma as a grade II (9444/1) tumour (42).

Epidemiology

To date, fewer than 80 cases of chordoid glioma have been reported in the literature (42). Most cases are found in adults with a median age of 45 years (43). Only three tumours have been reported in children (44). There is a distinct female preponderance (1:2), although oestrogen or progesterone receptor reactivity could not be found *in vitro* (42, 43, 45).

Aetiology

Data on the aetiology of these tumours are not available.

Pathogenesis

An ependymal histogenesis has been suggested for these tumours due to some cases showing tumour cells arranged in papillary structures (46–48). With electron microscopy, features have been observed that support the ependymal origin of many chordoid gliomas, such as microvilli, intermediate filaments, intercellular lumina, hemidesmosomes, and a basal lamina (43, 44, 47, 49–51). The expression of D2-40 has also been observed in chordoid gliomas, which is assumed to be a useful marker for ependymal tumours, especially in combination with epithelial membrane antigen (EMA) (42, 52). Since papillary structures have been observed in tumours of the ependymal layer, this would explain the intraventricular location of chordoid gliomas (46). A strong CD34 expression in conjunction with GFAP and vimentin co-expression was found to be a pattern unique for differentiating chordoid glioma of the third ventricle from other tumours. Since CD34-positive cells have been assumed to represent dysplastic or undifferentiated neural precursors, this suggests chordoid glioma to have a neural differentiation (42, 53, 54). In one series, array comparative genomic hybridization showed losses at several loci, and fluorescence *in situ* hybridization confirmed consistent genetic alterations at 9p21 and 11q13 (55). Others, however, failed to demonstrate chromosomal imbalances (39).

Histopathology

Chordoid gliomas are usually reactive for GFAP, vimentin, and slightly and focally immunoreactive for EMA, cytokeratin, and S-100 protein immunostaining (37, 39, 42, 45, 49).

On the other hand, a small fraction of chordoid gliomas reported in the literature appear to stain for neurofilament protein but the majority do not (37, 39, 43, 56). Overall, tumour cells have a low proliferative rate, with a Ki-67 of 2–5% (39, 42, 50).

Imaging

Most cases are located in the anterior part of the third ventricle or suprasellar region with an association with the hypothalamus (42, 43, 49, 57, 58). The tumour may cause hydrocephalus through obstruction of the third ventricle (Fig. 7.3) (42). However, lesions distant to this region have been described, for example, being located extraventricularly in the temporoparietal brain, in the corona radiata and thalamus in a juxtaventricular location, and in the thalamus (44, 59, 60).

Radiologically, these tumours are rather consistent. The mass is hyperdense on CT, hypointense to isointense on T1, and shows homogeneous contrast enhancement (Fig. 7.2) (42, 44, 58, 61). The shape is usually ovoid. The tumours are mostly located above or anterior to the infundibulum, displacing the chiasm caudally. The largest diameter is usually from inferior to superior (39, 43, 45, 47, 49–51, 55). Based on imaging alone, possible differential diagnosis are pilocytic astrocytoma, meningioma, craniopharyngioma, germ cell tumour, or pituitary adenoma.

Clinical presentation

Symptoms of chordoid gliomas are related to their usual location in the third ventricle, causing compression of the hypothalamus

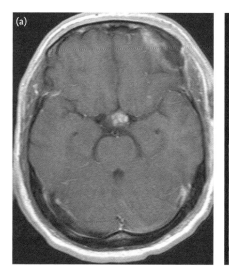 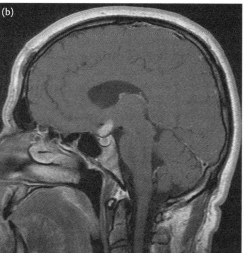 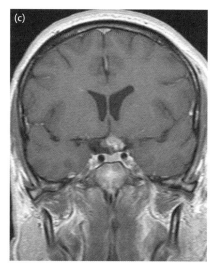

Fig. 7.3 (a–c) Sagittal, axial, and coronal T1-weighted magnetic resonance images after contrast administration of a chordoid glioma. The tumour is located in the recessus infundibularis of the third ventricle above the chiasm.

and the fornices, as well as hydrocephalus. Thus, typical symptoms for these tumours are headache, dizziness, decline in visual acuity, hypothalamic dysfunction (amenorrhoea) with endocrine disturbances, and memory deficits (42, 45, 62).

Treatment

Among approximately 50 patients from the literature in whom follow-up data are available, one patient survived 72 months and died of trauma, whereas two patients died of recurrence at 36 months and at 4 months (47, 49, 63). The latter observation suggests that aggressive subtypes may exist. The relationship to the hypothalamus might render outcome poor (64). Together, confident conclusions regarding optimal therapy are difficult to draw due to the low number of patients and the diversity of treatments.

Surgery

Surgery is usually attempted for these low-grade, well-defined, and moderately vascularized masses with the aim of gross total removal (46). Surgical routes to be considered are translamina terminalis (62), transcallosal transventricular (58, 61), or transcortical transventricular (45). While gross total resection may be associated with long-term recurrence-free survival, the immediate postoperative mortality has been observed to be higher with maximal tumour removal, with almost half of patients dying from pulmonary embolism, than after subtotal resection (46, 65). This finding may in part be explained by hypothalamic dysfunction and associated

dehydration. Thus, while it appears that gross total removal may be oncologically beneficial or even curative, attempts at gross total removal must be weighed against risks involved by surgery in the delicate region of the hypothalamus (46).

To minimize morbidity, some groups have argued strongly in favour of a translamina terminalis approach due to the putative origin of these tumours at the lamina terminalis (62). Mortality and morbidity using this approach have been found to be lowest (37, 38, 46, 66, 67).

Radiotherapy

Radiotherapy and radiosurgery have been proposed; however, the efficacy of these approaches is as yet unclear (37, 46, 64, 68).

Chemotherapy

No reports are available regarding chemotherapy for chordoid gliomas.

Commentary on National Comprehensive Cancer Network and any other treatment guidelines

There are no evidence-based guidelines available for the follow-up of these lesions.

Current research topics

These lesions are typical tumours that should be part of a prospective rare tumour registry.

References

1. Bailey P, Cushing H. *Classification of the Tumors of the Glioma Group.* Philadelphia, PA: Lippincott, 1926.

2. Louis DN, Ohgaki H, Wiestler OD, et al. *WHO Classification of Tumours of the Central Nervous System.* Lyon: International Agency for Research on Cancer, 2007.

3. Bonnin JM, Rubinstein LJ. Astroblastomas: a pathological study of 23 tumors, with a postoperative follow-up in 13 patients. *Neurosurgery* 1989; 25:6–13.

4. Thiessen B, Finlay J, Kulkarni R, et al. Astroblastoma: does histology predict biologic behavior? *J Neurooncol* 1998; 40:59–65.

5. Brat DJ, Hirose Y, Cohen KJ, et al. Astroblastoma: clinicopathologic features and chromosomal abnormalities defined by comparative genomic hybridization. *Brain Pathol* 2000; 10:342–352.

6. Lau PP, Thomas TM, Lui PC, et al. 'Low-grade' astroblastoma with rapid recurrence: a case report. *Pathology* 2006; 38:78–80.

7. Sughrue ME, Choi J, Rutkowski MJ, et al. Clinical features and post-surgical outcome of patients with astroblastoma. *J Clin Neurosci* 2011; 18:750–754.

8. Hata N, Shono T, Yoshimoto K, et al. An astroblastoma case associated with loss of heterozygosity on chromosome 9p. *J Neurooncol* 2006; 80:69–73.

9. Port JD, Brat DJ, Burger PC, et al. Astroblastoma: radiologic-pathologic correlation and distinction from ependymoma. *AJNR Am J Neuroradiol* 2002; 23:243–247.

10. Bell JW, Osborn AG, Salzman KL, et al. Neuroradiologic characteristics of astroblastoma. *Neuroradiology* 2007; 49:203–209.

11. Salvati M, D'Elia A, Brogna C, et al. Cerebral astroblastoma: analysis of six cases and critical review of treatment options. *J Neurooncol* 2009; 93:369–378.

12. Weintraub D, Monteith SJ, Yen CP, et al. Recurrent astroblastoma treated with gamma knife radiosurgery. *J Neurooncol* 2011; 103:751–754.

13. Bergkasa M, Sundstrom S, Gulati S, et al. Astroblastoma—a case report of a rare neuroepithelial tumor with complete remission after chemotherapy. *Clin Neuropathol* 2011; 30:301–306.

14. Shakur SF, McGirt MJ, Johnson MW, et al. Angiocentric glioma: a case series. *J Neurosurg Pediatr* 2009; 3:197–202.

15. Lellouch-Tubiana A, Boddaert N, Bourgeois M, et al. Angiocentric neuroepithelial tumor (ANET): a new epilepsy-related clinicopathological entity with distinctive MRI. *Brain Pathol* 2005; 15:281–286.

16. Wang M, Tihan T, Rojiani AM, et al. Monomorphous angiocentric glioma: a distinctive epileptogenic neoplasm with features of infiltrating astrocytoma and ependymoma. *J Neuropathol Exp Neurol* 2005; 64:875–881.

17. Preusser M, Hoischen A, Novak K, et al. Angiocentric glioma: report of clinico-pathologic and genetic findings in 8 cases. *Am J Surg Pathol* 2007; 31:1709–1718.

18. Chakravarti A, Seiferheld W, Tu X, et al. Immunohistochemically determined total epidermal growth factor receptor levels not of prognostic value in newly diagnosed glioblastoma multiforme: report from the Radiation Therapy Oncology Group. *Int J Radiat Oncol Biol Phys* 2005; 62:318–327.

19. Louis DN, Ohgaki H, Wiestler OD, et al. The 2007 WHO classification of tumours of the central nervous system. *Acta Neuropathol* 2007; 114:97–109.

20. Lehman NL. Patterns of brain infiltration and secondary structure formation in supratentorial ependymal tumors. *J Neuropathol Exp Neurol* 2008; 67:900–910.

21. Mott RT, Ellis TL, Geisinger KR. Angiocentric glioma: a case report and review of the literature. *Diagn Cytopathol* 2010; 38:452–456.

22. Marburger T, Prayson R. Angiocentric glioma: a clinicopathologic review of 5 tumors with identification of associated cortical dysplasia. *Arch Pathol Lab Med* 2011; 135:1037–1041.

23. Varikatt W, Dexter M, Mahajan H, et al. Usefulness of smears in intra-operative diagnosis of newly described entities of CNS. *Neuropathology* 2009; 29:641–648.

24. Rho GJ, Kim H, Kim HI, et al. A case of angiocentric glioma with unusual clinical and radiological features. *J Korean Neurosurg Soc* 2011; 49:367–369.

25. Ma X, Ge J, Wang L, et al. A 25-year-old woman with a mass in the hippocampus. *Brain Pathol* 2010; 20:503–506.

26. Li JY, Langford LA, Adesina A, et al. The high mitotic count detected by phospho-histone H3 immunostain does not alter the benign behavior of angiocentric glioma. *Brain Tumor Pathol* 2012; 29:68–72.

27. Pokharel S, Parker JR, Parker JC, Jr., et al. Angiocentric glioma with high proliferative index: case report and review of the literature. *Ann Clin Lab Sci* 2011; 41:257–261.

28. Prayson RA. Tumours arising in the setting of paediatric chronic epilepsy. *Pathology* 2010; 42:426–431.

29. Koral K, Koral KM, Sklar F. Angiocentric glioma in a 4-year-old boy: imaging characteristics and review of the literature. *Clin Imaging* 2012; 36:61–64.

30. Raghunathan A, Olar A, Vogel H, et al. Isocitrate dehydrogenase 1 R132H mutation is not detected in angiocentric glioma. *Ann Diagn Pathol* 2012; 16:255–259.

31. Miyata H, Ryufuku M, Kubota Y, et al. Adult-onset angiocentric glioma of epithelioid cell-predominant type of the mesial temporal lobe suggestive of a rare but distinct clinicopathological subset within a spectrum of angiocentric cortical ependymal tumors. *Neuropathology* 2012; 32(5):479–491.

32. Darwish B, Koleda C, Lau H, et al. Juvenile pilocytic astrocytoma 'pilomyxoid variant' with spinal metastases. *J Clin Neurosci* 2004; 11:640–642.

33. Nagaishi M, Yokoo H, Hirato J, et al. Clinico-pathological feature of pilomyxoid astrocytomas: three case reports. *Neuropathology* 2011; 31:152–157.

34. Lum DJ, Halliday W, Watson M, et al. Cortical ependymoma or monomorphous angiocentric glioma? *Neuropathology* 2008; 28:81–86.

35. Van Gompel JJ, Koeller KK, Meyer FB, et al. Cortical ependymoma: an unusual epileptogenic lesion. *J Neurosurg* 2011; 114:1187–1194.

36. Takada S, Iwasaki M, Suzuki H, et al. Angiocentric glioma and surrounding cortical dysplasia manifesting as intractable frontal lobe epilepsy—case report. *Neurol Med Chir (Tokyo)* 2011; 51:522–526.

37. Nakajima M, Nakasu S, Hatsuda N, et al. Third ventricular chordoid glioma: case report and review of the literature. *Surg Neurol* 2003; 59:424–428.

38. Pomper MG, Passe TJ, Burger PC, et al. Chordoid glioma: a neoplasm unique to the hypothalamus and anterior third ventricle. *AJNR Am J Neuroradiol* 2001; 22:464–469.

39. Reifenberger G, Weber T, Weber RG, et al. Chordoid glioma of the third ventricle: immunohistochemical and molecular genetic characterization of a novel tumor entity. *Brain Pathol* 1999; 9:617–626.

40. Wanschitz J, Schmidbauer M, Maier H, et al. Suprasellar meningioma with expression of glial fibrillary acidic protein: a peculiar variant. *Acta Neuropathol* 1995; 90:539–544.

41. Kleihues P, Cavenee WK. *World Health Classification of Tumours: Pathology and Genetics of Tumours of the Nervous System.* Lyon: International Agency for Research on Cancer, 2000.

42. Louis DN, Perry A, Reifenberger G, et al. The 2016 World Health Organization classification of tumors of the central nervous system: a summary. *Acta Neuropathol* 2016; 131:803–820.

42. Ni HC, Piao YS, Lu DH, et al. Chordoid glioma of the third ventricle: four cases including one case with papillary features. *Neuropathology* 2013; 33:134–139.

43. Pasquier B, Peoc'h M, Morrison AL, et al. Chordoid glioma of the third ventricle: a report of two new cases, with further evidence supporting an ependymal differentiation, and review of the literature. *Am J Surg Pathol* 2002; 26:1330–1342.

44. Jain D, Sharma MC, Sarkar C, et al. Chordoid glioma: report of two rare examples with unusual features. *Acta Neurochir (Wien)* 2008; 150:295–300.

45. Liu WP, Cheng JX, Yi XC, et al. Chordoid glioma: a case report and literature review. *Neurologist* 2011; 17:52–56.

46. Raizer JJ, Shetty T, Gutin PH, et al. Chordoid glioma: report of a case with unusual histologic features, ultrastructural study and review of the literature. *J Neurooncol* 2003; 63:39–47.

47. Kawasaki K, Kohno M, Inenaga C, et al. Chordoid glioma of the third ventricle: a report of two cases, one with ultrastructural findings. *Neuropathology* 2009; 29:85–90.

48. Lehman NL. Central nervous system tumors with ependymal features: a broadened spectrum of primarily ependymal differentiation? *J Neuropathol Exp Neurol* 2008; 67:177–188.

49. Brat DJ, Scheithauer BW, Staugaitis SM, et al. Third ventricular chordoid glioma: a distinct clinicopathologic entity. *J Neuropathol Exp Neurol* 1998; 57:283–290.

50. Sato K, Kubota T, Ishida M, et al. Immunohistochemical and ultrastructural study of chordoid glioma of the third ventricle: its tanycytic differentiation. *Acta Neuropathol* 2003; 106:176–180.

51. Cenacchi G, Roncaroli F, Cerasoli S, et al. Chordoid glioma of the third ventricle: an ultrastructural study of three cases with a histogenetic hypothesis. *Am J Surg Pathol* 2001; 25:401–405.

52. Ishizawa K, Komori T, Shimada S, et al. Podoplanin is a potential marker for the diagnosis of ependymoma: a comparative study with epithelial membrane antigen (EMA). *Clin Neuropathol* 2009; 28:373–378.

53. Lin G, Finger E, Gutierrez-Ramos JC. Expression of CD34 in endothelial cells, hematopoietic progenitors and nervous cells in fetal and adult mouse tissues. *Eur J Immunol* 1995; 25:1508–1516.

54. Deb P, Sharma MC, Tripathi M, et al. Expression of CD34 as a novel marker for glioneuronal lesions associated with chronic intractable epilepsy. *Neuropathol Appl Neurobiol* 2006; 32:461–468.

55. Horbinski C, Dacic S, McLendon RE, et al. Chordoid glioma: a case report and molecular characterization of five cases. *Brain Pathol* 2009; 19:439–448.

56. Iwami K, Arima T, Oooka F, et al. Chordoid glioma with calcification and neurofilament expression: case report and review of the literature. *Surg Neurol* 2009; 71:115–120.

57. Vajtai I, Varga Z, Scheithauer BW, et al. Chordoid glioma of the third ventricle: confirmatory report of a new entity. *Hum Pathol* 1999; 30:723–726.

58. Sugita Y, Ohshima K, Shigemori M, et al. The tumor of the third ventricle. *Neuropathology* 2010; 30:97–100.

59. Kim JW, Kim JH, Choe G, et al. Chordoid glioma: a case report of unusual location and neuroradiological characteristics. *J Korean Neurosurg Soc* 2010; 48:62–65.

60. Goyal R, Vashishta RK, Singhi S, et al. Extraventricular unusual glioma in a child with extensive myxoid change resembling chordoid glioma. *J Clin Pathol* 2007; 60:1294–1295.

61. Tu A, Yeo T, Steinke D, et al. Chordoid glioma: imaging pearls of a unique third ventricular tumor. *Can J Neurol Sci* 2010; 37:677–680.

62. Carrasco R, Pascual JM, Reina T, et al. Chordoid glioma of the third ventricle attached to the optic chiasm. Successful removal through a trans-lamina terminalis approach. *Clin Neurol Neurosurg* 2008; 110:828–833.

63. Jung TY, Jung S. Third ventricular chordoid glioma with unusual aggressive behavior. *Neurol Med Chir (Tokyo)* 2006; 46:605–608.

64. Kurian KM, Summers DM, Statham PF, et al. Third ventricular chordoid glioma: clinicopathological study of two cases with evidence for a poor clinical outcome despite low grade histological features. *Neuropathol Appl Neurobiol* 2005; 31:354–361.

65. Vanhauwaert DJ, Clement F, Van DJ, et al. Chordoid glioma of the third ventricle. *Acta Neurochir (Wien)* 2008; 150:1183–1191.

66. Ricoy JR, Lobato RD, Baez B, et al. Suprasellar chordoid glioma. *Acta Neuropathol* 2000; 99:699–703.

67. Taraszewska A, Bogucki J, Andrychowski J, et al. Clinicopathological and ultrastructural study in two cases of chordoid glioma. *Folia Neuropathol* 2003; 41:175–182.

68. Tonami H, Kamehiro M, Oguchi M, et al. Chordoid glioma of the third ventricle: CT and MR findings. *J Comput Assist Tomogr* 2000; 24:336–338.

CHAPTER 8

Neuronal and mixed neuronal–glial tumours

Riccardo Soffietti, Hugues Duffau,
Glenn Bauman, and David Walker

Introduction

Neuronal and mixed neuronal-glial tumours are rare tumours of the central nervous system (CNS) that are composed of either a pure population of neoplastic neuronal cells, or neuronal tumour cells admixed with one or more subpopulations of neoplastic glial cells. Anaplastic transformation may occur. Overall, they represent between 1% and 6.5% of primary brain tumours in adults, and up to 10% of brain tumours in children. Despite their generally benign course, most tumours have been increasingly implicated in causing medically intractable seizures: in this regard they have been denominated 'long-term epilepsy-associated tumours' (LEATs) (1). The World Health Organization (WHO) classification (2) distinguishes nine histological variants.

Dysplastic gangliocytoma of the cerebellum/Lhermitte–Duclos disease

Definition

Dysplastic gangliocytomas of the cerebellum/Lhermitte–Duclos disease (LDD) are cerebellar lesions composed of dysplastic ganglion cells. It is not clear whether these lesions are neoplastic (grade I WHO) or hamartomatous (3). A case of LDD with focal areas of nodular dysembryoplastic neuroepithelial tumour (DNET) differentiation has been reported (4).

Epidemiology

These tumours are very rare (>100 patients have been described so far). Most cases occur in adults between the third and fourth decades; however, they have been reported in younger children and in the elderly.

Aetiology

The occurrence of LDD can be linked to Cowden disease, an autosomal dominant developmental syndrome, that is caused, at least in some families, by germline mutation or loss of the phosphatase and tensin homologue (*PTEN*) suppressor gene; some authors feel that the two diseases represent a single phacomatosis, with variable clinical manifestations (5–7).

Pathogenesis

A *PTEN* mutation has been identified in virtually all adult-onset LDD but not in childhood-onset cases (8), suggesting that the biology of the two forms is different.

Clinical presentation

The symptoms are usually chronic and present for 3–4 years before the diagnosis is made, and comprise cerebellar symptoms and symptoms related to raised intracranial pressure secondary to hydrocephalus. Macrocephaly, mental retardation, and seizures can be present.

Imaging

The appearance on neuroimaging is suggestive (9, 10). T2-weighted and fluid-attenuated inversion recovery (FLAIR) images demonstrate a homogenous and hyperintense lesion, with a striated or 'corduroy' pattern, that does not enhance after contrast administration. The lesion usually involves one hemisphere and may extend into the vermis.

Treatment of adults and children

Surgery

The optimal treatment consists of complete resection (3). In case of recurrence, a reoperation should be attempted.

Radiotherapy

Radiotherapy should be considered only for patients with persistent recurrent disease.

Chemotherapy

No data are available in the literature.

Commentary on National Comprehensive Cancer Network and any other treatment guidelines

There are no guidelines available in the National Comprehensive Cancer Network (NCCN) guidelines or other international guidelines.

Surveillance recommendations

Monitoring with magnetic resonance imaging (MRI) is recommended, more closely in case of incomplete resection.

As cerebellar lesions may develop before the appearance of other features of the Cowden disease, patients with LDD should be monitored for the development of additional tumours, such as breast, endometrial, and non-medullary thyroid carcinomas.

Current research topics

There are no ongoing clinical trials.

Desmoplastic infantile astrocytoma and ganglioglioma

Definition

Desmoplastic infantile astrocytoma (DIA) and desmoplastic infantile ganglioglioma (DIG) are tumours that involve the cerebral cortex and leptomeninges, and are often attached to dura (11, 12). Histologically, they are composed of a prominent desmoplastic stroma with a neoplastic population either restricted to astrocytes (DIA) or characterized by astrocytes together with a variable neuronal component (DIG). In addition, poorly differentiated neuroepithelial cells are present: because of this immature component, tumours may be misdiagnosed as malignant cerebral tumours, such as neuroblastomas, malignant gliomas or malignant meningiomas. Both tumours have been assigned WHO grade I.

Epidemiology

In the original report, DIA represented 1.25% of 483 intracranial tumours in children (11), while DIG accounted for only 0.4% in a series of more than 6500 CNS tumours from all ages (13). When studies have been limited to brain tumours in infancy, DIA/DIG accounted for 16% of intracranial tumours (14). Lönnrot et al. (15) reported five cases of DIG resulting in an incidence of 0.03 new cases per 10,000 people annually in Finland. Most cases present during the first year of life (16, 17) with a male:female ratio of 1.5:1. Some non-infantile cases (ages between 5 and 25 years) have been reported, with a strong male predominance (18–20). At surgery, the tumours may appear plaque-like, attached to the dura and surface of the brain, and commonly involve more than one lobe (frontal, parietal, or temporal in decreasing order). The tumours are large (3–13 cm), and a deeply located cystic component is common. A case presenting with multiple intracranial localizations has been described (21).

Aetiology

There are no data available in the literature.

Pathogenesis

Molecular studies of DIA revealed no *TP53* mutations or loss of heterozygosity on chromosomes 10 or 17: overall, the lack of genetic alterations typical of diffuse astrocytomas suggests that they are not related to these neoplasms (13, 22). The cellular origin of DIA/DIG has not been established. As the primitive neuroepithelial cells express both glial and neuronal markers, DIA/DIG could be embryonal neoplasms programmed to progressive maturation.

Clinical presentation

Symptoms are of short duration, and include progressive megalocephaly, tense and bulging fontanelles, and lethargy. Rarely, patients present with seizures, focal motor signs, or skull bossing over the tumour.

Imaging

On MRI, DIA/DIG (23) appear as large cystic lesions, hypointense on T1- and hyperintense on T2-weighted images, that are deeply located, and associated with a superficial solid portion that enhances with gadolinium. Oedema is usually absent or moderate.

Treatment of adults and children

Surgery

Surgery is the treatment of choice, and no adjuvant treatment is needed in cases of complete tumour resection (13, 24–29). Long-term tumour control can be achieved by total resection despite the presence of primitive neuroepithelial cells, mitotic activity, and foci of necrosis.

Radiotherapy

Radiotherapy is indicated in incompletely resected tumours that are deeply located or when anaplastic features are present, as they can be associated with tumour relapse and unfavourable outcome (30–36).

Chemotherapy

There are no data available in the literature.

Commentary on NCCN and any other treatment guidelines

There are no guidelines available in the NCCN guidelines or other international guidelines

Surveillance recommendations

Monitoring with MRI is recommended, more closely in case of incomplete resection.

Current research topics

There are no ongoing clinical trials.

Dysembryoplastic neuroepithelial tumour

Definition

Dysembryoplastic neuroepithelial tumour (DNET) is a tumour entity defined by cortical topography and a 'specific glioneuronal element' (37–39). This 'specific glioneuronal element' is characterized by columns orientated perpendicularly to the cortical surface and formed by bundles of axons lined by small oligodendrocytic-like cells. Between these columns neurons are floating in a paleeosinophilic matrix, with scattered stellate astrocytes. Several histological variants of DNET have been described (38, 40–43). The simple form consists of unique glioneuronal elements, while in the complex form they are associated with glial nodules conferring a typical multinodular architecture. The non-specific or diffuse forms include a spectrum of tumours that cannot be easily distinguished from ordinary gliomas or oligodendrogliomas, especially when limited material is available (44). In association with the tumour, a dysplastic organization of the cortex is observed in up to 80% of cases, and sometimes ectopic neurons are found in the adjacent white matter. Both in the tumour and foci of cortical dysplasia, mature neurons show cytological abnormalities; however, DNET does not contain atypical neurons resembling dysplastic ganglion cells as in gangliogliomas. Some multinodular tumours with associated ganglioglioma and DNET features (45) and an unusual case with combined histological features of DNET and rosette-forming glioneuronal tumour (46) have been described. Characteristically,

DNET lesions are devoid of anaplastic features, and correspond to WHO grade I.

Epidemiology

DNET is an important fraction of all the lesions encountered in surgical resections for intractable epilepsy: their incidence in these specimens ranges from 6% to 25%. In about 90% of cases the first seizure occurs before 20 years of age. At diagnosis, the patients are often in the second or third decade of life, but detection of DNET by imaging in children or young adults with recent-onset seizures has become more common (47–49). Males are more frequently affected. DNET may be located in any part of the supratentorial cortex, but they show a predilection for the temporal lobe, in particular the mesial structures. In agreement with their chronicity, associated bone deformities may be present.

Aetiology

No data are available in the literature.

Pathogenesis

The pathogenesis of DNET remains unsolved: no deletion on 1p, 17p, or 19q and no *TP53* gene mutations have been detected (50–52).

Clinical presentation

Patients who harbour supratentorial DNET typically present with drug-resistant partial seizures, with or without secondary generalization, and absence of neurological deficits (53).

Imaging

Magnetic resonance imaging typically shows cortically-based lesions, without peritumoural oedema and mass effect. These lesions appear hyperintense on T2-weighted or FLAIR images and hypointense or, less often, isointense on T1-weighted images, and may have a pseudocystic or multicystic appearance (47, 54) (Fig. 8.1). Calcifications are frequently seen on computed tomography (CT). About one-third of DNET enhance on CT or MRI: more often the enhancement appears as multiple rings rather than homogeneous. The simple and complex histological forms correspond to a highly characteristic, well-delineated tumour with cystic or polycystic appearance on MRI (55–57). Conversely, the non-specific histological forms have a more heterogeneous MRI structure and are less clearly delineated (58).

Treatment of adults and children

Surgery

The outcome of DNET after surgical resection is excellent (54). Long-term clinical follow-up usually demonstrates no evidence of

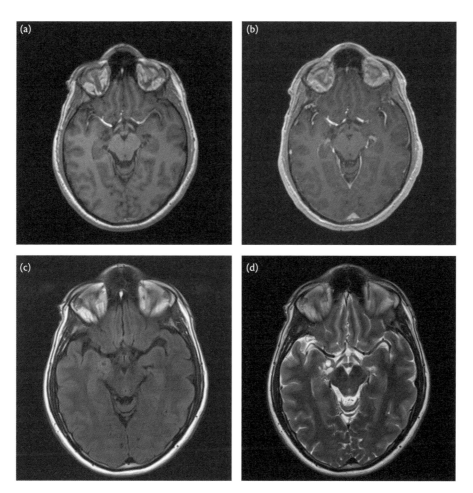

Fig. 8.1 (a–d) Typical right temporal DNET (T1 without and with GD, FLAIR, T2).

recurrence, even after incomplete resection. On imaging follow-up, ring enhancement may develop in a previously non-enhancing tumour, and increased size, with or without peritumoural oedema, may also be observed, but these changes can be due to ischaemic and/or haemorrhagic changes (54, 59). However, some reports have described an aggressive behaviour, requiring reoperation (60). Complete tumour resection yields a long-term epilepsy control (58, 61–66): seizure-free patients range between 70% and 90% (67). It is easier to achieve a complete tumour removal in simple and complex histological forms as they are circumscribed on MRI and the epileptic zone co-localizes with the tumour, while in non-specific forms a more extensive resection, including the perilesional cortex, is necessary as they are poorly delineated on MRI, and the epileptic zone frequently extends beyond the tumour (68). Risk factors for recurrent/resistant seizures are older age, long preoperative history of seizures, and the association with a cortical dysplasia.

Radiotherapy

Radiotherapy can be useful in cases of aggressive behaviour.

Chemotherapy

There are no data available in the literature.

Commentary on NCCN and any other treatment guidelines

There are no guidelines available in the NCCN guidelines or other international guidelines.

Surveillance recommendations

Monitoring with MRI is recommended in case of incomplete resection.

Current research topics

There are no ongoing clinical trials.

Gangliocytoma and ganglioglioma

Definition

Gangliocytoma (GC) is a neuroepithelial tumour composed of a pure population of neoplastic mature ganglion cells. The neoplastic cells may have dysplastic features and multiple nuclei. They stain for neuronal markers (synaptophysin, neurofilament epitopes), and frequently for the oncofetal CD34 antigen. Ganglioglioma (GG) is a neuroepithelial tumour composed of a combination of neoplastic, mature ganglion cells with neoplastic glial cells that sometimes may resemble fibrillary astrocytoma, oligodendroglioma, or pilocytic astrocytoma. Staining for glial fibrillary acidic protein (GFAP) confirms the astrocytic component. GC and most GG correspond to WHO grade I. A GG with anaplastic features in the glial component (prominent nuclear atypia, hypercellularity, high proliferative Ki-67 labelling index, frequent mitoses, vascular proliferations, and necrosis) is considered WHO grade III, and can be associated with unfavourable outcome (69). Cortical dysplasia, neuronal heterotopias, and other migration disorders frequently occur in the neighbourhood of GGs.

Epidemiology

Gangliocytoma has an estimated incidence of 0.1–0.5%, while GG is more frequent with an incidence ranging from 0.5% to 6.25% of all primary brain tumours and up to 10% of CNS tumours in children (70–71). The age range varies from very young children to elderly adults, but the majority of cases present in the second and third decades of life. Some series suggest a slight male predilection. GC and GG can arise anywhere in the CNS (cerebrum, hypothalamus, brain stem, upper spinal cord), and the most common location is the temporal lobe (72).

Aetiology

No data are available in the literature.

Pathogenesis

Gain of chromosome 7 and partial loss of chromosome 9p are the most frequent genetic alterations, while *TP53* mutation is generally absent. A *BRAF* V600E mutation has been reported in 18–57 % of cases with GG both in the glial and neuronal component (73–75), and *KIAA1549–BRAF* fusions have been found in some low-grade glioneuronal/neuroepithelial tumours (76). The possibility of using drugs targeting the *BRAF* V600E mutation has recently been shown to be effective in malignant melanoma (77). The histogenesis of these tumours is still unknown: an origin from a dysplastic malformative glioneuronal precursor lesion with neoplastic transformation of the glial element has been hypothesized.

Clinical presentation

Seizures are the most common presenting symptom, affecting between 65% and 85% of patients (78–80). Generally seizures are of the partial complex type, and are drug resistant: this explains why GC is the tumour most frequently resected for treatment of chronic epilepsy (81). The duration of seizures prior to diagnosis can be in fact quite long (>15 years), with a median of approximately 4 years.

Imaging

On CT the tumours can present either as a solid or as a cystic isodense or hypodense mass with a mural nodule, and calcifications in approximately 50% of cases. Oedema and mass effect are uncommon while enhancement is absent to mild (82). Scalloping of the calvarium may be seen adjacent to superficially located tumours. On MRI, T2-weighted and FLAIR images the tumour appears as a well circumscribed hyperintense mass that may be solid or cystic. T1-weighted images consistently show the mass to be hypointense in comparison to surrounding brain. After gadolinium, the degree of enhancement is variable. Anaplastic GG is often more infiltrative on MRI, and demonstrates a higher degree of enhancement and peritumoural oedema.

Treatment of adults and children

Surgery

Similar to other neuronal CNS tumours, surgical resection is the first therapeutic option to consider. Because the tumours are usually non-infiltrative and well demarcated from the normal tissue, gross total resection is often feasible. In the SEER series, 92% of patients had surgery with 68% achieving a gross total resection (72). Gross total resection is the best predictor of prolonged overall and progression-free survival (83). In a large series patients who received a complete resection had a significantly higher 7.5 year recurrence-free survival rate than those who received a partial resection (99% versus 92%) (80). Patients with a subtotal resection may have a good prognosis as well (84). Patients who have tumours in the midline, brain stem and spinal cord, that more often undergo a limited resection or biopsy, have a greater risk of recurrence and death (78). In case of relapse GGs may undergo malignant transformation with a rate ranging between 2% and 5% (85): this anaplastic transformation occurs usually in the glial component, but there are some reports of malignant changes within the neuronal component (86, 87). Patients with recurrent tumours should be reoperated on to optimize the extent of resection as well as to obtain a second pathological diagnosis. Interestingly, in a study on 58 anaplastic gangliogliomas from the Surveillance, Epidemiology and End Results (SEER) database, the median overall survival was only 28.5 months, and univariate and multivariate analysis identified surgical resection, in addition to unifocal disease, as a significant predictor of survival (88). This scenario is exemplified in Fig. 8.2.

Patients with classic grade I glioneuronal tumours often survive many years (89), making seizure freedom a critical factor in optimizing quality of life. A review of the timing of resection for GGs across the literature has demonstrated the role of early intervention in achieving seizure control (90, 91). Other series have shown that the strongest predictors of seizure freedom after surgery were duration of epilepsy for 1 year or less and gross total lesionectomy, with extended surgical resection (including hippocampectomy and/or corticectomy) conferring additional benefit in temporal lobe tumours, particularly when there was evidence of dual pathology (e.g. hippocampal sclerosis) existed on neuroimaging (92, 93). In a study by Englot et al. (94) seizure outcome did not differ significantly between adults and children or between patients with medically controlled and refractory seizures. Interestingly, they also observed similar rates of seizure freedom among tumours that were removed with or without intraoperative Electrocorticography (ECoG) to guide the extent of resection, suggesting that its use is not associated with improved seizure outcome. Maximal resection can be challenging for tumours that are deeply located or for tumours involving eloquent areas, with an increased risk of postoperative neurological deficits. With the aim of maximizing extent of resection while preserving quality of life, intrasurgical mapping and monitoring may be beneficial—as already demonstrated in diffuse low-grade and high-grade gliomas (95). Moreover, new methodologies, such as neuronavigation and intraoperative MRI diffusion tensor imaging, have also been suggested to reduce the postsurgical morbidity.

Radiotherapy

Conformal radiotherapy is generally reserved for patients with anaplastic or grade I incompletely resected tumours (96). However, in the latter case, it is not clear whether adjuvant radiotherapy provides a significant advantage over careful surveillance with treatment delayed at time of recurrence/progression. Rades et al. (97), in summarizing the literature for GG, noted a local control advantage but not an overall survival advantage at 10 years for those patients treated with adjuvant radiotherapy for subtotally resected tumours. Radiotherapy is indicated for persistent recurrent low-grade tumours (98). In the SEER series, radiotherapy use was reported in only 3.5% of patients, lower than older case series, suggesting a decline in the use of this modality, perhaps because of improvements in surgical technique and concerns regarding late toxicity of radiotherapy (88). In cases where radiation therapy is required, treatment doses and volumes are typically selected by analogy to low-grade glial neoplasms with conformal radiation delivery of doses in the range of 45–54 Gy in 1.8–2.0 Gy/day fractions given

the absence of evidence to suggest dose response above 54 Gy for low-grade lesions.

Recommendations for atypical or anaplastic lesions include treatment to higher doses (54–60 Gy) but the dose response of these lesions remains poorly defined given their rarity. Given the typically indolent behaviour and expected long-term survival of individuals with these tumours, careful radiation planning and delivery is necessary to minimize the chance of long term neurocognitive sequelae and focal deficits such as optic pathway injury. The principles of stereotactic radiotherapy should be applied with reproducible non-invasive immobilization with mask or bite block-based systems, careful target delineation using fusion of planning CT and MRI, conservative target volumes (typically 0.5–1.0 cm expansion on the imaging evident tumour with an additional 0.3–0.5 cm expansion for setup variation for a total 'safety margin' (planning target volume) of 1.0–1.5cm), and focused delivery using three-dimensional conformal or intensity-modulated radiotherapy techniques (99) (Fig. 8.3).

Chemotherapy

Chemotherapy should be considered for patients with persistent recurrent low- and high-grade tumours not amenable to re-resection or re-irradiation (100). Both in children and adults responses have been reported after nitrosoureas, temozolomide, etoposide, carboplatin, and cyclophosphamide. Recently, a case of a patient with a brainstem ganglioglioma successfully treated with vemurafenib (inhibitor of *BRAF* V600E mutation) and vinblastine has been described (101).

Commentary on NCCN and any other treatment guidelines

There are no guidelines available in the NCCN guidelines or other International guidelines.

Surveillance recommendations

Monitoring with MRI every 12 months is recommended in case of incomplete resection of grade I and II tumours. Monitoring with MRI every 4–6 months is recommended in case of anaplastic tumours.

Current research topics

Ongoing studies will define the role of *BRAF* V600E mutation inhibitors in these rare forms of the gliomas.

Central neurocytoma and extraventricular neurocytoma

Definition

Neurocytomas are neuroepithelial tumours composed of uniform round cells with neuronal differentiation, located within the lateral ventricles with frequent attachment to the septum pellucidum near the foramen of Monro (central neurocytoma, CN) or within the brain parenchyma (extraventricular neurocytoma, EVN). CN has been recognized as a separate clinicopathological entity only since 1982 (102). The neuronal phenotype of the tumour is consistent with the immunohistochemical profile, characterized by a diffuse positivity for synaptophysin and negativity for neurofilament and chromogranin. Despite their superficial resemblance to oligodendrogliomas, they rarely express glial markers and do not present *IDH-1* R132H mutations. CN corresponds histologically to WHO grade II. Atypical neurocytomas are defined as a

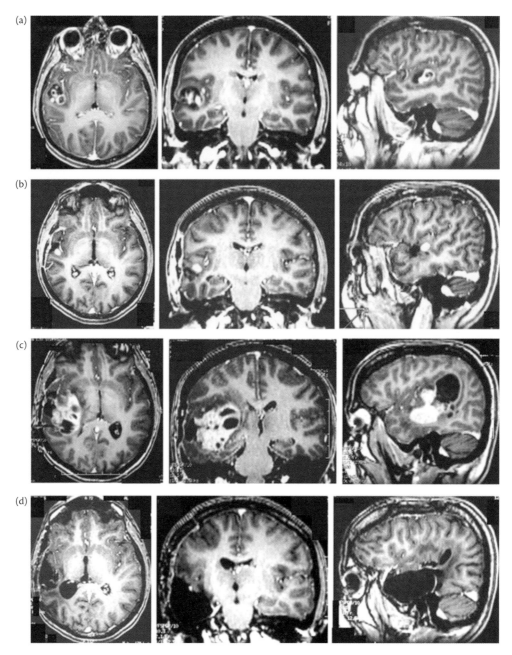

Fig. 8.2 (a) Axial (left), coronal (middle), and sagittal (right) enhanced T1-weighted MRI before the first operation, showing a grade I ganglioglioma within the right superior temporal gyrus. (b) Axial (left), coronal (middle), and sagittal (right) enhanced T1-weighted MRI following the first operation, showing the tumour removal, with a small residue which remained stable for 1.5 years (no adjuvant therapy). (c) Axial (left), coronal (middle), and sagittal (right) enhanced T1-weighted MRI before the second operation, demonstrating a huge and malignant recurrence of the ganglioglioma 2 years after the first resection. (d) Axial (left), coronal (middle), and sagittal (right) enhanced T1-weighted MRI 10 years after the second operation (which consisted of an extensive right temporal lobectomy performed using intraoperative electrical subcortical motor mapping) followed by radiotherapy.

Reproduced from *Acta Neurochir*, 150(6), Benzagmout M, Chaoui Mel F, Duffau H, Reversible deficit affecting the perception of tone of a human voice after tumour resection from the right auditory cortex, pp. 589–93, Copyright (2008), with permission from Springer.

subgroup of tumours variably exhibiting vascular proliferation, necrosis, nuclear atypia, high mitotic index, or high Ki-67 proliferation index (>2–3%). This atypical group may have a higher risk of relapse and/or a worse prognosis (103–107). However, the individual histological factors do not seem to predict the outcome (108): some CNs with anaplastic features have an indolent course, while others with a benign appearance are associated with leptomeningeal dissemination and poor outcome (109–111). Overall,

the tendency to recur of CNs is in the range of 18–23%, and is more commonly late. EVNs share key histological features with the more common CNs, but exhibit a wider morphological spectrum (112). Compared to CN, EVN presents a higher degree of gangliomic differentiation, more frequent glial differentiation, and one-third of tumours tend to recur within a relatively short period of follow-up (113). Cases of EVNs with spinal dissemination have been reported (114). Typical EVNs have a significantly

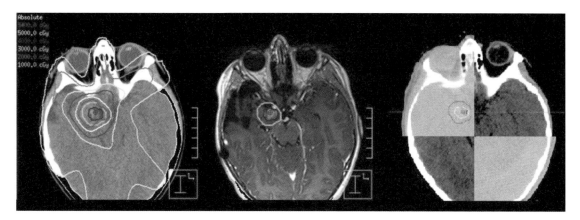

Fig. 8.3 (See colour plate section) Radiation plan for a 12-year-old boy with recurrent ganglioglioma, prescription dose was 5400 cGy in 30 fractions (left panel). Fusion of the diagnostic MRI (middle panel) allows the delineation of the gross tumour volume (GTV, blue line) and planning target volume (PTV, green line) that incorporates a safety margin for tumour infiltration and daily setup variation. CT acquisition on the linear accelerator (right panel) allows co-registration and comparison of the 'CT of the day' (light grey checker) with the planning CT (dark grey checker) to detect and correct positioning variation with millimetre accuracy.

better prognosis than atypical ones (5-year recurrence rate of 36% compared to 68%) (115).

Epidemiology

The incidence of neurocytomas is between 0.1% and 0.5% (116–118). They do not have a gender predilection. The tumours usually present between the third and fourth decades, but the range spans from 8 to 69 years (119): older age seems to be a poor prognostic factor. EVNs can be found in the cerebral hemispheres (frontal and temporal lobe), thalamus, cerebellum, spinal cord, and retina (120).

Aetiology

There are no available data in the literature.

Pathogenesis

Chromosomal gains (on chromosome 7, 2p, 10q, 18q, and 13q) have been reported in up to 20% of cases. A 1p/19q co-deletion is generally absent, while 1p deletion is more common (107, 121): these data confirm that CNs are genetically distinct from oligodendrogliomas. Moreover, p53 mutation and *EGFR* amplification are absent. As for the histogenesis, neurocytomas could derive from a precursor cell, with a predominant neuronal commitment, originating from the subependymal plate of the lateral ventricles (122).

Clinical presentation

Central neurocytoma is typically discovered because of symptoms of raised intracranial pressure secondary to obstructive hydrocephalus. Visual or memory problems, and hormonal dysfunctions have been reported as well. The clinical manifestations of EVNs vary according to the location of the tumour and include partial complex seizures, headache, cranial nerve paralysis, precious puberty, and rarely haemorrhage.

Imaging

Neuroimaging of CNs is quite typical (119, 123–125). In 50–60% of cases CT shows a heterogeneous, multicystic, hyperdense mass with calcifications, that are usually nodular and scattered; contrast enhancement is heterogeneous and mild to moderate. On MRI the

tumour margins are clearly demarcated from surrounding brain; the solid parts of the tumour are hypo-to-isointense in T1-weighted and isointense to grey matter on T2-weighted images. Clusters of cysts give the tumour a 'Swiss cheese/soap bubble' homogeneous hyperintense appearance on T2-weighted and FLAIR images. A moderate inhomogeneous contrast enhancement is present (Fig. 8.4).

The differential diagnosis for CN includes many tumours, such as choroid plexus papilloma, ependymoma, subependymoma, and intraventricular meningioma. Neuroimaging of EVN can show differences in comparison with CN: some cases are characterized by a cyst with mural nodule or are non-enhancing, and the 'soap bubble' appearance is less common (126–128). The peritumoural oedema is mild or absent. Magnetic resonance spectroscopy has

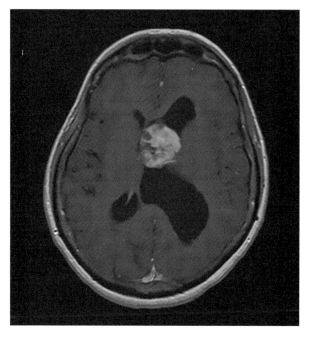

Fig. 8.4 Typical central neurocytoma with inhomogeneous contrast enhancement.

been employed in few cases: both CN and EVN show a choline peak, while in some cases of CN there is an increase of glycine. Moreover, in the EVN there is a strong decrease or even absence of N-acetylaspartate peak.

Treatment of adults and children

Surgery

The mainstay of treatment for CN is total surgical removal that seems to be associated with longer progression-free survival (106, 107, 119, 129, 130). However, in more than 50% of patients the tumour cannot be completely resected due to the risk of postoperative neurological deficits (non-communicating hydrocephalus, decreased memory, seizures) (119, 129, 131, 132). Even following total resection, the 10-year local control rate was only 61% in a large series (106): nonetheless, most authors recommend observation with MRI without adjuvant treatment after total resection. Gross total resection is superior to subtotal resection for typical EVNs.

Radiotherapy

After incomplete resection and/or in case of atypical lesions, conformal radiotherapy (45–54 Gy in conventional fractionation) yields improved local control rates and survival (133, 134). Patients with atypical lesions may benefit from higher doses (54–60 Gy) (103). A potential limiting factor for fractionated radiotherapy is represented by the risk of long-term complications: Paek et al. (135) reported radiation-induced complications (cognitive deterioration due to the white matter injury) in three out of six patients with CN who were treated with conventional radiotherapy with a median dose of 54 Gy. Radiosurgery may result in a high rate of tumour control and a lower complication rate (asymptomatic hydrocephalus), making it an attractive alternative to fractionated radiotherapy for smaller tumours (136, 137). A systematic review of the radiotherapy literature suggested a somewhat lower risk of local recurrence (7% vs 12%, hazard ratio 0.57) in patients treated with radiosurgery compared to fractioned radiotherapy (138). Overall, the long-term clinical outcome of CN after multimodal treatment is excellent: a recent retrospective evaluation of CN over 30 years in a single institution (132) showed an overall survival rate of 91% at 5 years and 88% at 10 years. In case of recurrence after initial surgery, radiotherapy or radiosurgery may be indicated, alone or following reoperation (Fig. 8.5).

Regarding typical EVNs, Kane et al. (139) have investigated the prognosis and management of 85 cases and there was a trend for adjuvant radiotherapy being beneficial for patients with subtotal resection. Adjuvant radiotherapy is generally recommended in atypical EVNs.

Chemotherapy

Chemotherapy has yielded some responses with various regimens (BCNU, PCV, platinum compounds, etoposide) in case of recurrence (140).

Commentary on NCCN and any other treatment guidelines

There are no guidelines available in the NCCN guidelines or other international guidelines.

Surveillance recommendations

Monitoring with MRI is recommended in case of incomplete resection.

Current research topics

There are no ongoing clinical trials.

Cerebellar liponeurocytoma

Definition

Cerebellar liponeurocytoma is a rare tumour of the cerebellum, consisting of isomorphic small neuronal cells with the cytology of neurocytes and focal lipomatous-differentiation, characterized by lipidized cells resembling mature adipose tissue (141, 142). The small uniform cells are similar to the 'small blue' cells of medulloblastoma, but can also resemble neoplastic oligodendroglial cells or cells of the clear cell ependymoma. Anaplastic features, such as mitoses, microvascular hyperplasia, and areas of necrosis, are rare or absent. The tumour has a low proliferative potential (Ki-67/MIB-1 labelling index 1–3%). Both small and lipidic cells are positive for neuronal markers, such as synaptophysin, neuron-specific enolase (NSE), and MAP2, and this indicates that the adipose cells represent the product of an aberrant differentiation of tumour cells.

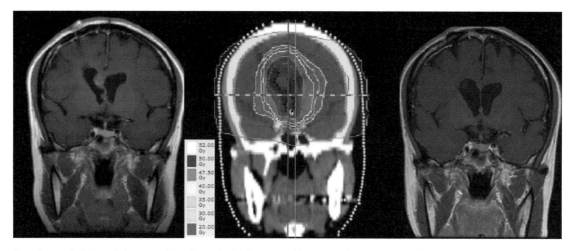

Fig. 8.5 (See colour plate section) Pre-radiation coronal T1-enhanced MRI of a 38-year-old woman with recurrent central neurocytoma (left panel) treated with image-guided conformal radiotherapy (middle panel) and with a near total radiographic response to treatment and subsequently stable disease 5 years post radiation (right panel).

Focal GFAP expression, indicating astrocytic differentiation, is seen in the majority of cases (143). The current WHO classification assigns the cerebellar liponeurocytoma to WHO grade II.

Epidemiology

The mean age is 50 (range 24–77 years): this is in contrast with the age distribution of cerebellar medulloblastoma, more than 70% of which occur in children. No gender predilection has been noted so far.

Aetiology

There are no data available in the literature.

Pathogenesis

The genetic profile has been analysed by an International Consortium that collected tumour samples from 20 patients (144). *TP53* missense mutations were found in 20% of cases, while there was no case with *PTCH, APC,* or beta-catenin mutations (all characterizing the different subsets of medulloblastomas). Isochromosome 17q, a hallmark of classic medulloblastoma, was absent. Cluster analysis of the DNA expression profile revealed similarity of cerebellar liponeurocytomas to neurocytomas: however, the presence of *TP53* mutations, which are absent in CNs, suggests that they develop through different genetic pathways. Two novel molecular markers (NEUROG1 and fatty acid binding protein 4, FABP4) have been recently identified (145).

Clinical presentation

Headache and other symptoms of raised intracranial pressure are the most common presenting symptoms.

Imaging

The MRI appearance is variable (146, 147). On T1-weighted images, the tumour is generally hypointense, relatively well demarcated, and presents numerous scattered foci of high signal intensity consistent with lipids. Enhancement after gadolinium administration is typically patchy and mild.

Treatment of adults and children

Surgery

Maximal surgical resection is the treatment of choice. However, despite the lack of anaplastic features, recurrence with a latency ranging from 1 to 12 years occurs in at least 50% of cases, and the 5-year survival rate is 48%.

Radiotherapy

Radiotherapy is to be considered for recurrent or progressive tumours (148).

Chemotherapy

There are no reports on the use of chemotherapy.

Commentary on NCCN and any other treatment guidelines

There are no guidelines available in the NCCN guidelines or other international guidelines.

Surveillance recommendations

Monitoring with MRI is recommended in case of incomplete resection.

Current research topics

There are no ongoing clinical trials.

Papillary glioneuronal tumour

Definition

Papillary glioneuronal tumours (GNTs), reported first in 1997, are rare tumours characterized by a prominent pseudopapillary architecture in which hyalinized blood vessels are surrounded by small cuboidal GFAP-positive glial cells, and interpapillary spaces are occupied by neurocytes, or ganglion cells that stain positively for synaptophysin and NSE (149, 150). The MIB-1 labelling index is typically low, and features and anaplasia, such as endothelial proliferation and necrosis, are uncommon. Papillary GNT corresponds to WHO grade I. Rare cases exhibiting more aggressive behaviour, including dissemination and local spread of disease, have been reported (151–152).

Epidemiology

Papillary GNTs are rare tumours: only several dozen have been reported. They occur over a wide range of ages (4–75 years), without a gender predilection, and preferentially involve the cerebral hemispheres (in particular the temporal lobe).

Aetiology

There are no data available in the literature.

Pathogenesis

The underlying histogenesis is uncertain, although a common progenitor cell origin (capable of glial and neuronal differentiation) from the subependymal matrix or the secondary germinal layer has been postulated (153, 154). Genetic studies in a limited number of cases have recently shown the absence of a 1p/19q deletion and *EGFR* amplification. Recently Bridge et al. (155) have identified in three cases a translocation, t(9;17) (q31;q24) resulting in an in-frame fusion of *SLC44A1* and *PKCA* genes. Thus, it has been suggested that the demonstration of this translocation may be useful for the differential diagnosis toward other mixed neuronal-glial tumours.

Clinical presentation

Headache and seizures are the main symptoms at onset.

Imaging

Magnetic resonance and CT imaging frequently show a cystic lesion with a mural nodule or a solid to cystic mass, contrast-enhancing with little mass effect (156).

Treatment of adults and children

Surgery

In most cases, gross total resection results in long-term survival (157–159).

Radiotherapy

While the use of adjuvant radiotherapy has been reported, the benefit is unclear (160).

Chemotherapy

There are no data available in the literature regarding chemotherapy.

Commentary on NCCN and any other treatment guidelines

There are no guidelines available in the NCCN guidelines or other international guidelines.

Surveillance recommendations

Monitoring with MRI is recommended in case of incomplete resection.

Current research topics

There are no ongoing clinical trials.

Rosette forming glioneuronal tumour of the fourth ventricle

Definition

Rosette-forming glioneuronal tumour (RGNT) of the fourth ventricle was first described as a novel type of glioneuronal tumour (161). It is composed of two distinct cellular components, one with uniform neurocytes forming rosette and/or perivascular pseudorosettes, the other being astrocytic and resembling pilocytic astrocytoma. Mitoses and necrosis are absent, and Ki-67 labelling index is less than 3%. RGNT of the fourth ventricle corresponds to WHO grade I.

Epidemiology

Recent reviews of the English literature have reported between 41 and 63 cases (162–164). These tumours mainly affect young adults with an average age at the time of diagnosis of 32 years (range 8–70 years) and have a high prevalence in females (61%). While initially these tumours were described in the fourth ventricle, they may be found in a larger variety of locations, although the vast majority are infratentorial. There are reports in the optic chiasm, third and lateral ventricle, thalamus, pineal region, and spinal cord.

Aetiology

There are no data available in the literature.

Pathogenesis

Genetic analysis of RGHT has revealed a mutation in the *PIK3CA* gene (165), wild-type *IDH1* and *IDH2* (166), intact *NF1* gene (167), and no 1p/19q loss (168, 169). *KIAA1549–BRAF* fusions have not been detected (170). Recent immunohistochemical studies have reported a co-expression of neuronal markers (synaptophysin), glial markers (GFAP, OLIG2, cyclin D1and PDGFRα) and stem cell markers (CD133) (171–173), thus confirming the hypothesis of a biphenotypic differentiation from a pluripotential progenitor cell in the subependymal plateau (174).

Clinical presentation

Headache and ataxia are the most common presenting symptoms, and the duration of symptoms before diagnosis ranges from 1 day to 15 years with a median of 10 months. About 12% of cases are asymptomatic or incidentally discovered.

Imaging

On MRI, most RGNT are visualized as midline lesions arising from the floor of the fourth ventricle, and can invade dorsally into the vermis or ventrally into the brain stem; additionally, they may extend superiorly into cerebral aqueduct. Conversely, RGNT of the fourth ventricle almost never extend into foramina of Magendie and Luschka, which normally occurs in other tumour types located in the fourth ventricle, such as ependymomas. RGNT can display solid, cystic, or mixed features, and calcifications on CT are present in about 20% of cases. Focal enhancement is frequently seen, but non-enhancing lesions are not uncommon: these findings can be useful in the differential diagnosis toward medulloblastomas and ependymomas that tend to enhance homogeneously.

Treatment of adults and children

Surgery

The treatment of choice is surgical resection. Gross total resection can be achieved in fewer than half of patients due to the high propensity of the tumour for adherence to the ventricular wall and/or infiltration into surrounding structures. Overall, after resection postoperative neurological deficits are around 47% of patients. The rate and time to recurrence seem similar with gross total and subtotal resection.

Radiotherapy

Radiotherapy has been employed in few cases after partial resection/biopsy and/or ventricular spreading (160, 165).

Chemotherapy

Chemotherapy (temozolomide and cis-retinoic acid) have been associated with radiotherapy in few cases after partial resection/biopsy and/or ventricular spreading.

Commentary on NCCN and any other treatment guidelines

There are no guidelines available in the NCCN guidelines or other international guidelines.

Surveillance recommendations

Owing to the lack of lengthy follow-up of patients after treatments, monitoring with MRI is recommended both after complete and incomplete surgical resection.

Current research topics

There are no ongoing clinical trials.

Spinal paraganglioma

Definition

Paraganglioma is a neuroectodermal tumour commonly found in the adrenal medulla. Paraganglioma of the CNS is very rare, and occurs almost exclusively in the cauda equine region as a solid, highly vascularized and well encapsulated tumour. Lerman et al (175) first reported this tumour in 1972. Histologically, paragangliomas resemble normal paraganglia, and are composed of chief cells disposed in nests or lobules ('Zellballen pattern'), separated by vascular channels, and subtentacular cells (176). Chief cells are round and oval in shape with abundant eosinophilic granular cytoplasm, while subtentacular cells are spindle-shaped. Immunohistochemistry permits the characterization of cells (177): chief cells are positive for synaptophysin and chromogranin, while subtentacular cells are reactive for S-100 protein, and often for GFAP. Expression of serotonin and various neuropeptides has been reported. Paraganglioma of the filum terminale correspond histologically to WHO grade I.

Epidemiology

Cauda equina paragangliomas comprise 3–4% of all tumours affecting this region. Other spinal levels are far less often involved. Rare examples of intracranial localization have been described. Cauda equina paragangliomas generally affect adults with a peak incidence in the fourth through the sixth decades. There is a slight predominance in males.

Aetiology

Several autosomal dominant inherited syndromes predispose to paraganglioma, such as von Hippel–Lindau disease or NF1, but most spinal paragangliomas are non-familial.

Pathogenesis

Among 22 spinal paragangliomas a germline mutation in the gene encoding the subunit D of the succinate dehydrogenase (*SDHD*) gene in one patient with recurrent tumour and cerebellar metastasis has been reported (178).

Clinical presentation

The most frequent clinical presentation is low-back pain and sciatica, while sensory, motor, and sphincter disturbances are infrequent (179). Rarely (until now only five cases in the literature), paraganglioma can exhibit a secreting function, causing paroxysmal hypertension, even during surgical manipulation, due to release into the systemic circulation of vasoactive substances, probably catecholamines (180). Some spinal paragangliomas presenting with symptoms of raised intracranial pressure have been reported (181).

Imaging

On MRI, findings are non-specific, as the tumour is usually hypo- or isointense on T1 sequences, hyperintense on T2 sequences, with uniform contrast enhancement (182–184). Some findings could be helpful in differentiating paraganglioma from myxopapillary ependymoma or schwannoma: an hypointense margin on T2-weighted images, with a 'salt and pepper' appearance, and serpiginous defects around the tumour suggesting serpentine vessels (185).

Treatment of adults and children

Surgery

Complete resection is the treatment of choice. Although they are benign, paragangliomas recur in about 10–12% of patients (176).

Radiotherapy

Adjuvant radiotherapy may be reserved for incompletely excised lesions, although its effectiveness has not been established. CSF seeding of spinal paragangliomas has been occasionally documented (186).

Chemotherapy

There are no data available in the literature.

Commentary on NCCN and any other treatment guidelines

There are no guidelines available in the NCCN guidelines or other international guidelines.

Surveillance recommendations

Monitoring with MRI is recommended in case of incomplete resection.

Current research topics

There are no ongoing clinical trials.

Conclusion

Due to the rarity of glioneuronal tumours, the level of evidence supporting therapeutic interventions described is low, but some management concepts seem well established from a clinical point of view. Early surgery with complete resection may significantly improve the likelihood of postoperative epilepsy freedom. This could reduce the need for a long-term antiepileptic medication in a long surviving young population. After surgery, especially if incomplete, careful surveillance with MRI is suggested (commonly every 6 or 12 months in the first years). It is not clear how long to maintain the surveillance as late recurrences are described. Conformal radiotherapy can be considered in case of patients with incompletely resected symptomatic tumours, atypical or high-grade tumours, or in the case of multiple recurrences despite resections. The role of chemotherapy in these lesions remains poorly defined. Further progress into the molecular biology of these tumours will help us to understand why some grade I tumours behave aggressively despite a 'benign' histological appearance, and will identify common molecular alterations across different histologies that can inform more targeted medical therapies.

References

1. Luyken C, Blümcke I, Fimmers R, et al. The spectrum of long-term epilepsy-associated tumors: long-term seizure and tumor outcome and neurosurgical aspects. *Epilepsia* 2003; 44:822–830.

2. Louis DN, Ohgaki H, Wiestler OD, et al. The 2007 WHO classification of tumours of the central nervous system. *Acta Neuropathol* 2007; 114(2):97–109.

3. Nowak DA, Trost HA. Lhermitte-Duclos disease (dysplastic cerebellar gangliocytoma): a malformation, hamartoma or neoplasm? *Acta Neurol Scand* 2002; 105(3):137–145.

4. Nair P, Pal L, Jaiswal AK, et al. Lhermitte-Duclos disease associated with dysembryoplastic neuroepithelial tumor differentiation with characteristic magnetic resonance appearance of 'tiger striping'. *World Neurosurg* 2011; 75(5–6):699–703.

5. Padberg GW, Schot JD, Vielvoye GJ, et al. Lhermitte-Duclos disease and Cowden disease: a single phakomatosis. *Ann Neurol* 1991; 29(5):517–523.

6. Derrey S, Proust F, Debono B, et al. Association between Cowden syndrome and Lhermitte-Duclos disease: report of two cases and review of the literature. *Surg Neurol* 2004; 61(5):447–454.

7. Robinson S, Cohen AR. Cowden disease and Lhermitte-Duclos disease: characterization of a new phakomatosis. *Neurosurgery* 2000; 46(2):371–383.

8. Zhou XP, Marsh DJ, Morrison CD, et al. Germline inactivation of PTEN and dysregulation of the phosphoinositol-3-kinase/Akt pathway cause human Lhermitte-Duclos disease in adults. *Am J Hum Genet* 2003; 73(5):1191–1198.

9. Kulkantrakorn K, Awwad EE, Levy B, et al. MRI in Lhermitte-Duclos disease. *Neurology* 1997; 48(3):725–731.

10. Raizer JJ and Naidich MJ. Neuronal tumors. In: Newton HB, Jolesz FA (eds) *Handbook of Neuro-Oncology.* Amsterdam: Elsevier/Academic Press, 2007; 435–448.

11. Taratuto AL, Monges J, Lylyk P, Leiguarda R. Superficial cerebral astrocytoma attached to dura. Report of six cases in infants. *Cancer* 1984; 54(11):2505–2512.

12. VandenBerg SR, May EE, Rubinstein LJ, et al. Desmoplastic supratentorial neuroepithelial tumors of infancy with divergent differentiation potential ('desmoplastic infantile gangliogliomas'). Report on 11 cases of a distinctive embryonal tumor with favorable prognosis. *J Neurosurg* 1987; 66(1):58–71.

13. VandenBerg SR. Desmoplastic infantile ganglioglioma and desmoplastic cerebral astrocytoma of infancy. *Brain Pathol* 1993; 3(3):275–281.

14. Zuccaro G, Taratuto AL, Monges J. Intracranial neoplasms during the first year of life. *Surg Neurol* 1986; 26(1):29–36.

15. Lönnrot K, Terho M, Kähärä V, et al. Desmoplastic infantile ganglioglioma: novel aspects in clinical presentation and genetics. *Surg Neurol* 2007; 68(3):304–308.

16. Ávila de Espìndola A, Matsushita H, et al. Brain tumors in the first three years of life: a review of twenty cases. *Arq Neuropsiquiatr* 2007; 65(4A):960–964.

17. Alexiou GA, Stefanaki K, Sfakianos G, et al. Desmoplastic infantile ganglioglioma: a report of 2 cases and a review of the literature. *Pediatr Neurosurg* 2008; 44(5):422–425.

18. Ganesan K, Desai S, Udwadia-Hegde A. Non-infantile variant of desmoplastic ganglioglioma: a report of 2 cases. *Pediatr Radiol* 2006; 36(6):541–545.

19. Pommepuy I, Delage-Corre M, Moreau JJ, et al. A report of a desmoplastic ganglioglioma in a 12-year-old girl with review of the literature. *J Neurooncol* 2006; 76(3):271–275.

20. Khubchandani SR, Chitale AR, Doshi PK. Desmoplastic non-infantile ganglioglioma: a low-grade tumor, report of two patients. *Neurol India* 2009; 57(6):796–799.

21. Uro-Coste E, Ssi-Yan-Kai G, Guilbeau-Frugier C, et al. Desmoplastic infantile astrocytoma with benign histological phenotype and multiple intracranial localizations at presentation. *J Neurooncol* 2010; 98(1):143–149.

22. Tamburrini G, Colosimo C Jr, Giangaspero F, et al. Desmoplastic infantile ganglioglioma. *Childs Nerv Syst* 2003; 19(5–6):292–297.

23. Trehan G, Bruge H, Vinchon M, et al. MR imaging in the diagnosis of desmoplastic infantile tumor: retrospective study of six cases. *AJNR Am J Neuroradiol* 2004; 25(6):1028–1033.

24. Duffner PK, Burger PC, Cohen ME, et al. Desmoplastic infantile gangliogliomas: an approach to therapy. *Neurosurgery* 1994; 34:583–589.

25. Taratuto AL, Sevlever G, Schultz M, et al. Desmoplastic cerebral astrocytoma of infancy (DCAI). Survival data of the original series and report of two additional cases, DNA, kinetic an molecular genetic studies. *Brain Pathol* 1994; 4:423.

26. Sugiyama K, Arita K, Shima T, et al. Good clinical course in infants with desmoplastic cerebral neuroepithelial tumor treated by surgery alone. *J Neurooncol* 2002; 59(1):63–69.

27. Bächli H, Avoledo P, Gratzl O, et al. Therapeutic strategies and management of desmoplastic infantile ganglioglioma: two case reports and literature overview. *Childs Nerv Syst* 2003; 19(5–6):359–366.

28. Nanassis K, Tsitsopoulos PP, Marinopoulos D, et al. Long-term follow-up of a non-infantile desmoplastic ganglioglioma. *Cent Eur Neurosurg* 2010; 71(1):50–53.

29. Gelabert-Gonzalez M, Serramito-García R, Arcos-Algaba A. Desmoplastic infantile and non-infantile ganglioglioma. Review of the literature. *Neurosurg Rev* 2010; 34(2):151–158.

30. Parisi JE, Scheithauer BW, Priest JR, et al. Desmoplastic infantile ganglioglioma (DIG): a form of gangliogliomatosis? *J Neuropathol Exp Neurol* 1992; 51:365.

31. Komori T, Scheithauer BW, Parisi JE, et al. Mixed conventional and desmoplastic infantile ganglioglioma: an autopsied case with 6-year follow-up. *Mod Pathol* 2001; 14:720–726.

32. De Munnynck K, Van Gool S, Van Calenbergh F, et al. Desmoplastic infantile ganglioglioma: a potentially malignant tumor? *Am J Surg Pathol* 2002; 26(11):1515–1522.

33. Darwish B, Arbuckle S, Kellie S, et al. Desmoplastic infantile ganglioglioma/astrocytoma with cerebrospinal metastasis. *J Clin Neurosci* 2007; 14(5):498–501.

34. Hoving EW, Kros JM, Groninger E, et al. Desmoplastic infantile ganglioglioma with a malignant course. *J Neurosurg Pediatr* 2008; 1(1):95–98.

35. Phi JH, Koh EJ, Kim SK, et al. Desmoplastic infantile astrocytoma: recurrence with malignant transformation into glioblastoma: a case report. *Childs Nerv Syst* 2011; 27(12):2177–2181.

36. Al-Kharazi K, Gillis C, Steinbok P, et al. Malignant desmoplastic infantile astrocytoma? A case report and review of the literature. *Clin Neuropathol* 2013; 32(2):100–106.

37. Daumas-Duport C, Scheithauer BW, Chodkiewicz JP, et al. Dysembryoplastic neuroepithelial tumor: a surgically curable tumor of young patients with intractable partial seizures. Report of thirty-nine cases. *Neurosurgery* 1988; 23:545–556.

38. Daumas-Duport C, Varlet P, Bacha S, et al. Dysembryoplastic neuroepithelial tumors: nonspecific histological forms—a study of 40 cases. *J Neurooncol* 1999; 41:267–280.

39. Prayson RA, Estes ML. Dysembryoplastic neuroepithelial tumor. *Am J Clin Pathol* 1992; 97:398–401.

40. Honovar M and Janota I. 73 cases of dysembrioplastic neuroepithelial tumor: the range of histological appearance. *Brain Pathol* 1994; 4:428–435.

41. Pasquier B, Péoc'H M, Fabre-Bocquentin B, et al. Surgical pathology of drug-resistant partial epilepsy. A 10-year-experience with a series of 327 consecutive resections. *Epileptic Disord* 2002; 4(2):99–119.

42. Thom M, Toma A, An S, et al. One hundred and one dysembryoplastic neuroepithelial tumors: an adult epilepsy series with immunohistochemical, molecular genetic, and clinical correlations and a review of the literature. *J Neuropathol Exp Neurol* 2011; 70(10):859–878.

43. Bodi I, Selway R, Bannister P, et al. Diffuse form of dysembryoplastic neuroepithelial tumour: the histological and immunohistochemical

features of a distinct entity showing transition to dysembryoplastic neuroepithelial tumour and ganglioglioma. *Neuropathol Appl Neurobiol* 2012; 38(5):411–425.

44. Prayson RA. Diagnostic challenges in the evaluation of chronic epilepsy-related surgical neuropathology. *Am J Surg Pathol* 2010; 34(5):e1–13.

45. Prayson RA, Napekoski KM. Composite ganglioglioma/ dysembryoplastic neuroepithelial tumor: a clinicopathologic study of 8 cases. *Hum Pathol* 2012; 43(7):1113–1118.

46. Xiong J, Ding L, Chen H, et al. Mixed glioneuronal tumor: a dysembryoplastic neuroepithelial tumor with rosette-forming glioneuronal tumor component. *Neuropathology* 2013; 33(4):431–435.

47. Fernandez C, Girard N, Paz Paredes A, Bouvier-Labit C, Lena G, Figarella-Branger D (2003). The usefulness of MR imaging in the diagnosis of dysembryoplastic neuroepithelial tumor in children: a study of 14 cases. *AJNR Am J Neuroradiol* 24(5):829–834.

48. Nolan MA, Sakuta R, Chuang N, et al (2004). Dysembryoplastic neuroepithelial tumors in childhood: long-term outcome and prognostic features. *Neurology* 62(12):2270–2276.

49. Giulioni M, Galassi E, Zucchelli M, et al. Seizure outcome of lesionectomy in glioneuronal tumors associated with epilepsy in children. *J Neurosurg* 2005; 102(3 Suppl):288–293.

50. Fujisawa H, Marukawa K, Hasegawa M, et al. Genetic differences between neurocytoma and dysembryoplastic neuroepithelial tumor and oligodendroglial tumors. *J Neurosurg* 2002; 97(6):1350–1355.

51. Prayson RA, Castilla EA, Hartke M, et al. Chromosome 1p allelic loss by fluorescence in situ hybridization is not observed in dysembryoplastic neuroepithelial tumors. *Am J Clin Pathol* 2002; 118(4):512–517.

52. Johnson MD, Vnencak-Jones CL, Toms SA, et al. Allelic losses in oligodendroglial and oligodendroglioma-like neoplasms: analysis using microsatellite repeats and polymerase chain reaction. *Arch Pathol Lab Med* 2003; 127(12):1573–1579.

53. Rudà R, Bello L, Duffau H, et al. Seizures in low-grade gliomas: natural history, pathogenesis, and outcome after treatments. *Neuro Oncol* 2012; 14(Suppl 4):iv55–64.

54. Stanescu CR, Varlet P, Beuvon F, et al. Dysembrioblastic neuroepithelial tumors: CT, MR findings and imaging follow-up: a study of 53 cases. *J Neuroradiol* 2001; 28:230–240.

55. Lee DY, Chung CK, Hwang YS, et al. Dysembryoplastic neuroepithelial tumor: radiological findings (including PET, SPECT, and MRS) and surgical strategy. *J Neurooncol* 2000; 47(2):167–174.

56. Campos AR, Clusmann H, von Lehe M, et al. Simple and complex dysembryoplastic neuroepithelial tumors (DNT) variants: clinical profile, MRI, and histopathology. *Neuroradiology* 2009; 51(7):433–443.

57. Sharma MC, Jain D, Gupta A, et al. Dysembryoplastic neuroepithelial tumor: a clinicopathological study of 32 cases. *Neurosurg Rev* 2009; 32(2):161–170.

58. Chassoux F, Rodrigo S, Mellerio C, et al. Dysembryoplastic neuroepithelial tumors: an MRI-based scheme for epilepsy surgery. *Neurology* 2012; 79(16):1699–1707.

59. Jensen, Caamano E, Jensen EM, et al. Development of contrast enhancement after long-term observation of a dysembryoplastic neuroepithelial tumor. *J Neurooncol* 2006; 78(1):59–62.

60. Mano Y, Kumabe T, Shibahara I, et al. Dynamic changes in magnetic resonance imaging appearance of dysembryoplastic neuroepithelial tumor with or without malignant transformation. *J Neurosurg Pediatr* 2013; 11(5):518–525.

61. Raymond AA, Halpin SF, Alsanjari N, et al. Dysembryoplastic neuroepithelial tumor. Features in 16 patients. *Brain* 994; 117 (Pt 3):461–475.

62. Hennessy MJ, Elwes RD, Honavar M, et al. Predictors of outcome and pathological considerations in the surgical treatment of intractable epilepsy associated with temporal lobe lesions. *J Neurol Neurosurg Psychiatry* 2001; 70(4):450–458.

63. Burneo JG, Burneo JG, Tellez-Zenteno J, et al. Adult-onset epilepsy associated with dysembryoplastic neuroepithelial tumors. *Seizure* 2008; 17(6):498–504.

64. Bilginer B, Yalnizoglu D, Soylemezoglu F, et al. Surgery for epilepsy in children with dysembryoplastic neuroepithelial tumor: clinical spectrum, seizure outcome, neuroradiology, and pathology. *Childs Nerv Syst* 2009; 25(4):485–491.

65. Chang EF, Christie C, Sullivan JE, et al. Seizure control outcomes after resection of dysembryoplastic neuroepithelial tumor in 50 patients. *J Neurosurg Pediatr* 2010; 5(1):123–130.

66. Ozlen F, Gunduz A, Asan Z. Dysembryoplastic neuroepithelial tumors and gangliogliomas: clinical results of 52 patients. *Acta Neurochir* 2010; 152(10):1661–1671.

67. Bonney PA, Boettcher LB, Conner AK, et al. Review of seizure after surgical resection of dysembryoplastic neuroepithelial tumors. *J Neurooncol* 2016; 126:1–10.

68. Chassoux F, Landré E, Mellerio C, et al. Dysembryoplastic neuroepithelial tumors: Epileptogenicity related to histologic subtypes. *Clin Neurophysiol* 2013; 124(6):1068–1078.

69. Hakim R, Loeffler JS, Anthony DC, et al. Gangliogliomas in adults. *Cancer* 1997; 79(1):127–131.

70. Prayson RA, Khajavi K, Comair YG. Cortical architectural abnormalities and MIB1 immunoreactivity in gangliogliomas: a study of 60 patients with intracranial tumors. *J Neuropathol Exp Neurol* 1995; 54(4):513–520.

71. Krouwer HG, Davis RL, McDermott MW, et al. Gangliogliomas: a clinicopathological study of 25 cases and review of the literature. *J Neurooncol* 1993; 17(2):139–154.

72. Dudley RWR, Torok MR, Gallegos DR, et al. Pediatric low grade Ganglioglioma/gangliocytoma: epidemiology, treatments, and outcome analysis on 348 children from the SEER database. *Neurosurgery* 2015; 76(3):313–320.

73. Schindler G, Capper D, Meyer J, et al. Analysis of BRAF V600E mutation in 1,320 nervous system tumors reveals high mutation frequencies in pleomorphic xanthoastrocytoma, ganglioglioma and extra-cerebellar pilocytic astrocytoma. *Acta Neuropathol* 2011; 121(3):397–405.

74. Dougherty MJ, Santi M, Brose MS, et al. Activating mutations in BRAF characterize a spectrum of pediatric low-grade gliomas. *Neuro Oncol* 2010; 12(7):621–630.

75. Koelsche C, Wöhrer A, Jeibmann A, et al. Mutant BRAF V600E protein in ganglioglioma is predominantly expressed by neuronal tumor cells. *Acta Neuropathol* 2013; 125(6):891–900.

76. Lin A, Rodriguez FJ, Karajannis MA, et al. BRAF alterations in primary glial and glioneuronal neoplasms of the central nervous system with identification of 2 novel KIAA1549:BRAF fusion variants. *J Neuropathol Exp Neurol* 2012; 71(1):66–72.

77. Chapman PB, Hauschild, A, Robert C. Improved survival with vemurafenib in melanoma with BRAF V600E Mutation for the BRIM-3 Study Group. *N Engl J Med* 2011; 364:2507–2516.

78. Lang FF, Epstein FJ, Ransohoff J, et al. Central nervous system gangliogliomas. Part 2: clinical outcome. *J Neurosurg* 1993; 79(6): 867–873.

79. Blümcke I, Wiestler OD. Gangliogliomas: an intriguing tumor entity associated with focal epilepsies. *J Neuropathol Exp Neurol* 2002; 61(7):575–584.

80. Luyken C, Blümcke I, Fimmers R, et al. Supratentorial gangliogliomas: histopathologic grading and tumor recurrence in 184 patients with a median follow-up of 8 years. *Cancer* 2004; 101(1):146–155.

81. Wolf HK, Wiestler OD. Surgical pathology of chronic epileptic seizure disorders. *Brain Pathol* 1995; 3(4):371–380.

82. Im SH, Chung CK, Cho BK, et al. Intracranial ganglioglioma: preoperative characteristics and oncologic outcome after surgery. *J Neurooncol* 2002; 59(2):173–183.

83. Zentner J, Wolf HK, Ostertun B, et al. Gangliogliomas: clinical, radiological, and histopathological findings in 51 patients. *J Neurol Neurosurg Psychiatry* 1994; 57(12):1497–1502.

84. Celli P, Scarpinati M, Nardacci B, et al. Gangliogliomas of the cerebral hemispheres. Report of 14 cases with long-term follow-up and review of the literature. *Acta Neurochir (Wien)* 1993; 125(1–4):52–57.

85. Majores M, von Lehe M, Fassunke J, et al. Tumor recurrence and malignant progression of gangliogliomas. *Cancer* 2008; 113(12):3355–3363.

86. Tarnaris A, O'Brien C, Redfern RM. Ganglioglioma with anaplastic recurrence of the neuronal element following radiotherapy. *Clin Neurol Neurosurg* 2006; 108(8):761–776.

87. Mittelbronn M, Schittenhelm J, Lemke D, et al. Low grade ganglioglioma rapidly progressing to a WHO grade IV tumor showing malignant transformation in both astroglial and neuronal cell components. *Neuropathology* 2007; 27(5):463–467.

88. Selvanathan SK, Hammouche S, Salminen HJ, et al. Outcome and prognostic features in anaplastic ganglioglioma: analysis of cases from the SEER database. *J Neurooncol* 2011; 105(3):539–545.

89. Phi JH, Kim SK, Cho BK, et al. Long-term surgical outcomes of temporal lobe epilepsy associated with low-grade brain tumors. *Cancer* 2009; 115(24):5771–5779.

90. Yang I, Chang EF, Han SJ, et al. Early surgical intervention in adult patients with ganglioglioma is associated with improved clinical seizure outcomes. *J Clin Neurosci* 2011; 18(1):29–33.

91. Radhakrishnan A, Abraham M, Vilanilam G, et al. Surgery for 'Long-term epilepsy associated tumors (LEATs)': seizure outcome and its predictors. *Clin Neurol Neurosurg* 2016; 141:98–105.

92. Giulioni M, Rubboli G, Marucci G, et al. Seizure outcome of epilepsy surgery in focal epilepsies associated with temporomesial glioneuronal tumors: lesionectomy compared with tailored resection. *J Neurosurg* 2009; 111(6):1275–1282.

93. Zaghloul KA, Schramm J. Surgical management of glioneuronal tumors with drug-resistant epilepsy. *Acta Neurochir* 2011; 153(8):1551–1559.

94. Englot DJ, Berger MS, Barbaro NM, et al. Factors associated with seizure freedom in the surgical resection of glioneuronal tumors. *Epilepsia* 2012; 53(1):51–57.

95. De Witt Hamer PC, Robles SG, Zwinderman AH, et al. Impact of intraoperative stimulation brain mapping on glioma surgery outcome: a meta-analysis. *J Clin Oncol* 2012; 30(20):2559–2565.

96. Mehta MP. Neuro-oncology: gangliogliomas--what is the appropriate management strategy? *Nat Rev Neurol* 2010; 6(4):190–191.

97. Rades D, Zwick L, Leppert J, et al. The role of postoperative radiotherapy for the treatment of gangliogliomas. *Cancer* 2010; 116(2):432–442.

98. Liauw SL, Byer JE, Yachnis AT, et al. Radiotherapy after subtotally resected or recurrent ganglioglioma. *Int J Radiat Oncol Biol Phys* 2007; 67(1):244–247.

99. Bauman G, Wong E, McDermott M. Fractionated radiotherapy techniques. *Neurosurg Clin N Am* 2006; 17(2):99–110.

100. Mohile N, Raizer JJ. Chemotherapy for glioneuronal tumors. In: Newton HB (ed) *Handbook of Brain Tumor Chemotherapy*. Amsterdam: Elsevier/Academic Press, 2006; 432–438.

101. Chamberlain MC. Recurrent ganglioglioma in adults treated with BRAF inhibitors. *CNS Oncol* 2016; 5(1):27–29.

102. Hassoun J, Gambarelli D, Grisoli F, et al. Central neurocytoma. An electron-microscopic study of two cases. *Acta Neuropathol* 1982; 56(2):151–156.

103. Söylemezoglu F, Scheithauer BW, Esteve J, et al. Atypical central neurocytoma. *J Neuropathol Exp Neurol* 1997; 56(5):551–556.

104. Rades D, Schild SE, Fehlauer F. Prognostic value of the MIB-1 labeling index for central neurocytomas. *Neurology* 2004; 62(6):987–989.

105. Rades D, Schild SE. Treatment recommendations for the various subgroups of neurocytomas. *J Neurooncol* 2006; 77(3):305–309.

106. Leenstra JL, Rodriguez FJ, Frechette CM, et al. Central neurocytoma: management recommendations based on a 35-year experience. *Int J Radiat Oncol Biol Phys* 2007; 67(4):1145–1154.

107. Hallock A, Hamilton B, Ang LC, et al. Neurocytomas: long-term experience of a single institution. *Neuro Oncol* 2011; 13(9):943–949.

108. Vasiljevic A, François P, Loundou A, et al. Prognostic factors in central neurocytomas: a multicenter study of 71 cases. *Am J Surg Pathol* 2012; 36(2):220–227.

109. Eng DY, DeMonte F, Ginsberg L, et al. Craniospinal dissemination of central neurocytoma. Report of two cases. *J Neurosurg* 1997; 86(3):547–552.

110. Tomura N, Hirano H, Watanabe O, et al. Central neurocytoma with clinically malignant behavior. *AJNR Am J Neuroradiol* 1997; 18(6):1175–1178.

111. Takao H, Nakagawa K, Ohtomo K. Central neurocytoma with craniospinal dissemination. *J Neurooncol* 2003; 61(3):255–259.

112. Giangaspero F, Cenacchi G, Losi L, et al. Extraventricular neoplasms with neurocytoma features. A clinicopathological study of 11 cases. *Am J Surg Pathol* 1997; 21(2):206–212.

113. Brat DJ, Scheithauer BW, Eberhart CG, et al. Extraventricular neurocytomas: pathologic features and clinical outcome. *Am J Surg Pathol* 2001; 25(10):1252–1260.

114. Kawaji H, Saito O, Amano S, et al. Extraventricular neurocytoma of the sellar region with spinal dissemination. *Brain Tumor Pathol* 2014; 31(1):51–56.

115. Kane AJ, Sughrue ME, Rutkowski MJ, et al. The molecular pathology of central neurocytomas. *J Clin Neurosci* 2011; 18(1):1–6.

116. Kim DG, Chi JG, Park SH, et al. Intraventricular neurocytoma: clinicopathological analysis of seven cases. *J Neurosurg* 1992; 76(5):759–765.

117. Hassoun J, Söylemezoglu F, Gambarelli D, et al. Central neurocytoma: a synopsis of clinical and histological features. *Brain Pathol* 1993; 3(3):297–306.

118. Schild SE, Scheithauer BW, Haddock MG, et al. Central neurocytomas. *Cancer* 1997; 79(4):790–795.

119. Schmidt MH, Gottfried ON, von Koch CS, et al. Central neurocytoma: a review. *J Neurooncol* 2004; 66(3):377–384.

120. Ahmad F, Rosenblum MK, Chamyan G, et al. Infiltrative brainstem and cerebellar neurocytoma. *J Neurosurg Pediatr* 2012; 10(5):418–422.

121. Tong CY, Ng HK, Pang JC, et al. Central neurocytomas are genetically distinct from oligodendrogliomas and neuroblastomas. *Histopathology* 2000; 37(2):160–165.

122. von Deimling A, Kleihues P, Saremaslani P, et al. Histogenesis and differentiation potential of central neurocytomas. *Lab Invest* 1991; 64(4):585–591.

123. Zhang B, Luo B, Zhang Z, et al. Central neurocytoma: a clinicopathological and neuroradiological study. *Neuroradiology* 2004; 46(11):888–895.

124. Niiro T, Tokimura H, Hanaya R, et al. MRI findings in patients with central neurocytomas with special reference to differential diagnosis from other ventricular tumours near the foramen of Monro. *J Clin Neurosci* 2012; 19(5):681–686.

125. Ramsahye H, He H, Feng X, et al. Central neurocytoma: radiological and clinico-pathological findings in 18 patients and one additional MRS case. *J Neuroradiol* 2013; 40(2):101–111.

126. Yi KS, Sohn CH, Yun TJ, et al. MR imaging findings of extraventricular neurocytoma: a series of ten patients confirmed by immunohistochemistry of IDH1 gene mutation. *Acta Neurochir (Wien)* 2012; 154(11):1973–1979.

127. Huang WY, Zhang BY, Geng DY, et al. Computed tomography and magnetic resonance features of extraventricular neurocytoma: A study of eight cases. *Clin Radiol* 2013; 68(4):e206–e212.

128. Liu K, Wen G, Lv XF, et al. MR imaging of cerebral extraventricular neurocytoma: a report of 9 cases. *AJNR Am J Neuroradiol* 2013; 34(3):541–546.

129. Choudhari KA, Kaliaperumal C, Jain A, et al. Central neurocytoma: a multi-disciplinary review. *Br J Neurosurg* 2009; 23(6):585–595.

130. Kim DG, Park CK. Central neurocytoma: establishment of the disease entity. *Neurosurg Clin N Am* 2015; 26(1):1–4.

131. Qian H, Lin S, Zhang M, Cao Y. Surgical management of intraventricular central neurocytoma: 92 cases. *Acta Neurochir (Wien)* 2012; 154(11):1951–1960.

132. Kim JW, Kim DG, Kim IK, et al. Central neurocytoma: long-term outcomes of multimodal treatments and management strategies based on 30 years' experience in a single institute. *Neurosurgery* 2013; 72(3):407–414.

133. Imber BS, Braunstein SE, Wu FY, et al. Clinical outcome and prognostic factors for central neurocytoma: twenty year institutional experience. *J Neurooncol* 2016; 126(1):193–200.

134. Chen YD, Li WB, Feng J, et al. Long-term outcomes of adjuvant radiotherapy after surgical resection of central neurocytoma. *Radiat Oncol* 2014; 9:242.

135. Paek SH, Han JH, Kim JW, et al. Long-term outcome of conventional radiation therapy for central neurocytoma. *J Neurooncol* 2008; 90(1):25–30.

136. Chen MC, Pan DH, Chung WY, et al. Gamma knife radiosurgery for central neurocytoma: retrospective analysis of fourteen cases with a median follow-up period of sixty-five months. *Stereotact Funct Neurosurg* 2011; 89(3):185–193.

137. Karlsson B, Guo WY, Kejia T, et al. Gamma Knife surgery for central neurocytomas. *J Neurosurg* 2012; 117(Suppl):96–101.

138. Garcia RM, Ivan ME, Oh T, et al. Intraventricular neurocytomas: a systematic review of stereotactic radiosurgery and fractionated conventional radiotherapy for residual or recurrent tumors. *Clin Neurol Neurosurg* 2014; 117:55–64.

139. Kane AJ, Sughrue ME, Rutkowski MJ, et al. Atypia predicting prognosis for intracranial extraventricular neurocytomas. *J Neurosurg* 2012; 116(2):349–354.

140. Newton HB, Rudà R, Soffietti R. Neuronal and mixed neuronal-glial tumors. In: Grisold W, Soffietti R (eds) *Handbook of Clinical Neurology, Neuro-Oncology*. Amsterdam: Elsevier/Academic Press, 2012; 551–567.

141. Budka H, Chimelli L. Lipomatous medulloblastoma in adults: a new tumor type with possible favorable prognosis. *Hum Pathol* 1994; 25(7):730–731.

142. Nishimoto T, Kaya B. Cerebellar liponeurocytoma. *Arch Pathol Lab Med* 2012; 136(8):965–969.

143. Söylemezoglu F, Soffer D, Onol B, et al. Lipomatous medulloblastoma in adults. A distinct clinicopathological entity. *Am J Surg Pathol* 1996; 20(4):413–418.

144. Horstmann S, Perry A, Reifenberger G, et al. Genetic and expression profiles of cerebellar liponeurocytomas. *Brain Pathol* 2004; 14(3):281–289.

145. Anghileri E, Eoli M, Paterra R, et al. FABP4 is a candidate marker of cerebellar liponeurocytomas. *J Neurooncol* 2012; 108(3):513–519.

146. Alkadhi H, Keller M, Brandner S, et al. Neuroimaging of cerebellar liponeurocytoma. Case report. *J Neurosurg* 2001; 95(2):324–331.

147. Akhaddar A, Zrara I, Gazzaz M, et al. Cerebellar liponeurocytoma (lipomatous medulloblastoma). *J Neuroradiol* 2003; 30(2):121–126.

148. Oudrhiri MY, Raouzi N, El Kacemi I. Understanding cerebellar liponeurocytomas: case report and literature review. *Case Rep Neurol Med* 2014; 2014:186826.

149. Komori T, Scheithauer BW, Anthony DC, et al. Papillary glioneuronal tumor: a new variant of mixed neuronal-glial neoplasm. *Am J Surg Pathol* 1998; 22(10):1171–1183.

150. Vajtai I, Kappeler A, Lukes A, et al. Papillary glioneuronal tumor. *Pathol Res Pract* 2006; 202(2):107–112.

151. Newton HB, Dalton J, Ray-Chaudhury A, et al. Aggressive papillary glioneuronal tumor: case report and literature review. *Clin Neuropathol* 2008; 27(5):317–324.

152. Javahery RJ, Davidson L, Fangusaro J, et al. Aggressive variant of a papillary glioneuronal tumor. Report of 2 cases. *J Neurosurg Pediatr* 2009; 3(1):46–52.

153. Myung JK, Byeon SJ, Kim B, et al. Papillary glioneuronal tumors: a review of clinicopathologic and molecular genetic studies. *Am J Surg Pathol* 2011; 35(12):1794–1805.

154. Gelpi E, Preusser M, Czech T, et al. Papillary glioneuronal tumor. *Neuropathology* 2007; 27(5):468–473.

155. Bridge JA, Liu XQ, Sumegi J, et al. Identification of a novel, recurrent SLC44A1-PRKCA fusion in papillary glioneuronal tumor. *Brain Pathol* 2013; 23(2):121–128.

156. Xiao H, Ma L, Lou X, et al. Papillary glioneuronal tumor: radiological evidence of a newly established tumor entity. *J Neuroimaging* 2011; 21(3):297–302.

157. Pimentel J, Barroso C, Miguéns J, et al. Papillary glioneuronal tumor--prognostic value of the extension of surgical resection. *Clin Neuropathol* 2009; 28(4):287–294.

158. Demetriades AK, Al Hyassat S, Al-Sarraj S, et al. Papillary glioneuronal tumour: a review of the literature with two illustrative cases. *Br J Neurosurg* 2012; 27(3):401–404.

159. Zhao RJ, Zhang XL, Chu SG, et al. Clinicopathologic and neuroradiologic studies of papillary glioneuronal tumors. *Acta Neurochir (Wien)* 2016; 158(4):695–702.

160. Schlamann A, von Bueren AO, Hagel C, et al. An individual patient data meta-analysis on characteristics and outcome of patients with papillary glioneuronal tumor, rosette glioneuronal tumor with neuropil-like islands and rosette forming glioneuronal tumor of the fourth ventricle. *PLoS One* 2014; 9(7):e101211.

161. Komori T, Scheithauer BW, Hirose T. A rosette-forming glioneuronal tumor of the fourth ventricle: infratentorial form of dysembryoplastic neuroepithelial tumor? *Am J Surg Pathol* 2002; 26(5):582–591.

162. Hsu C, Kwan G, Lau Q, et al. Rosette-forming glioneuronal tumour: imaging features, histopathological correlation and a comprehensive review of literature. *Br J Neurosurg* 2012; 26(5):668–673.

163. Thurston B, Gunny R, Anderson G, et al. Fourth ventricle rosette-forming glioneuronal tumour in children: an unusual presentation in an 8-year-old patient, discussion and review of the literature. *Childs Nerv Syst* 2013; 29(5):839–847.

164. Zhang J, Babu R, McLendon RE, et al. A comprehensive analysis of 41 patients with rosette-forming glioneuronal tumors of the fourth ventricle. *J Clin Neurosci* 2013; 20(3):335–341.

165. Ellezam B, Theeler BJ, Luthra R, et al. Recurrent PIK3CA mutations in rosette-forming glioneuronal tumor. *Acta Neuropathol* 2012; 123(2):285–287.

166. Solis OE, Mehta RI, Lai A, et al. Rosette-forming glioneuronal tumor: a pineal region case with IDH1 and IDH2 mutation analyses and literature review of 43 cases. *J Neurooncol* 2011; 102(3):477–484.

167. Kinno M, Ishizawa K, Shimada S, et al. Cytology is a useful tool for the diagnosis of rosette-forming glioneuronal tumour of the fourth ventricle: a report of two cases. *Cytopathology* 2010; 21(3):194–197.

168. Wang Y, Xiong J, Chu SG, et al. Rosette-forming glioneuronal tumor: report of an unusual case with intraventricular dissemination. *Acta Neuropathol* 2009; 118(6):813–819.

169. Xiong J, Liu Y, Chu SG, et al. Rosette-forming glioneuronal tumor of the septum pellucidum with extension to the supratentorial ventricles: rare case with genetic analysis. *Neuropathology* 2012; 32(3):301–305.

170. Gessi M, Lambert SR, Lauriola L, et al. Absence of KIAA1549-BRAF fusion in rosette-forming glioneuronal tumors of the fourth ventricle (RGNT). *J Neurooncol* 2012; 110(1):21–25.

171. Chakraborti S, Mahadevan A, Govindan A, et al. Rosette-forming glioneuronal tumor—evidence of stem cell origin with biphenotypic differentiation. *Virchows Arch* 2012; 461(5):581–588.

172. Matsumura N, Yokoo H, Mao Y, et al. Olig2-positive cells in glioneuronal tumors show both glial and neuronal characters: The implication of a common progenitor cell? *Neuropathology* 2012; 1440–1789.

173. Matsumura N, Wang Y, Nakazato Y. Coexpression of glial and neuronal markers in the neurocytic rosettes of rosette-forming glioneuronal tumors. *Brain Tumor Pathol* 2013; 31(1):17–22.

174. Marhold F, Preusser M, Dietrich W, et al. Clinicoradiological features of rosette-forming glioneuronal tumor (RGNT) of the fourth ventricle: report of four cases and literature review. *J Neurooncol* 2008; 90(3):301–308.

175. Lerman RI, Kaplan ES, Daman L. Ganglioneuroma-paraganglioma of the intradural filum terminale. Case report. *J Neurosurg* 1972; 36(5):652–658.

176. Sonneland PR, Scheithauer BW, LeChago J, et al. Paraganglioma of the cauda equina region. Clinicopathologic study of 31 cases with special reference to immunocytology and ultrastructure. *Cancer* 1986; 58(8):1720–1735.

177. Moran CA, Rush W, Mena H. Primary spinal paragangliomas: a clinicopathological and immunohistochemical study of 30 cases. *Histopathology* 1997; 31(2):167–173.

178. Masuoka J, Brandner S, Paulus W, et al. Germline SDHD mutation in paraganglioma of the spinal cord. *Oncogene* 2001; 20(36):5084–5086.

179. Hong JY, Hur CY, Modi HN, et al. Paraganglioma in the cauda equina. A case report. *Acta Orthop Belg* 2012; 78(3):418–423.

180. Agrawal V, Rahul M, Khan S, et al. Functional paraganglioma: a rare conus-cauda lesion. *J Surg Tech Case Rep* 2012; 4(1):46–49.

181. Haslbeck KM, Eberhardt KE, Nissen U, et al. Intracranial hypertension as a clinical manifestation of cauda equina paraganglioma. *Neurology* 1999; 52(6):1297–1298.

182. Olsen WL, Dillon WP, Kelly WM, et al. MR imaging of paragangliomas. *AJR Am J Roentgenol* 1987; 148(1):201–204.

183. Levy RA. Paraganglioma of the filum terminale: MR findings. *AJR Am J Roentgenol* 1993; 160(4):851–852.

184. Boncoeur-Martel MP, Lesort A, Moreau JJ, et al. MRI of paraganglioma of the filum terminale. *J Comput Assist Tomogr* 1996; 20(1):162–165.

185. Araki Y, Ishida T, Ootani M, et al. MRI of paraganglioma of the cauda equina. *Neuroradiology* 1993; 35(3):232–233.

186. Thines L, Lejeune JP, Ruchoux MM, et al. Management of delayed intracranial and intraspinal metastases of intradural spinal paragangliomas. *Acta Neurochir (Wien)* 2006; 148(1):63–66.

CHAPTER 9

Embryonal and pineal tumours

Roger E. Taylor, Barry L. Pizer, Nancy J. Tarbell,
Alba A. Brandes, and Stephen Lowis

Introduction

Embryonal tumours account for approximately 20% of paediatric central nervous system (CNS) tumours. They arise from transformation of undifferentiated and immature neuroepithelial cells with the capacity for divergent differentiation. They include medulloblastoma (MB), atypical teratoid/rhabdoid tumour (AT/RT), and pineoblastoma. Embryonal tumours also include a group of neoplasms that were until recently referred to as central nervous system primitive neuro-ectodermal tumours (CNS-PNETs) but have recently been reclassified both histologically and molecularly as other entities.

Medulloblastoma in childhood

Introduction

Medulloblastoma (MB) accounts for between 15% and 20% of paediatric CNS tumours and arises in the cerebellum. The median age at presentation is approximately 6 years. Pathologically MB tends to exhibit predominantly neuronal differentiation. Classical MB is comprised of densely packed cells with round to oval hyperchromatic nuclei and scanty cytoplasm. Round cells with condensed chromatin are frequently intermingled. Neuroblastic rosettes are seen in approximately 40% of cases.

Histological subtypes

The following subtypes are recognized. This list reflects the most recent revision of the World Health Organization (WHO) update of the pathological classification of tumours of the CNS (1). This new classification reflects both our traditional understanding of the pathology of MB but also recent advances in the molecular characterisation of this tumour The currently accepted genetic characterisation is as follows:

(i)   Medulloblastoma, WNT-activated.

(ii) Medulloblastoma, SHH-activated, TP53-mutant.

(iii) Medulloblastoma, SHH-activated, TP53-wildtype.

(iv) Medulloblastoma, non-WNT/non-SHH, Group 3.

(v)   Medulloblastoma, non-WNT/non-SHH, Group 4.

With respect to histology, the WHO classification is as follows:

(i)   Medulloblastoma, classic

(ii) Medulloblastoma, desmoplastic/nodular

(iii) Medulloblastoma with extensive nodularity

(iv) Medulloblastoma, large cell/anaplastic

(v)   Medulloblastoma, NOS

Desmoplastic MB is associated with a better prognosis, particularly in very young children. Large cell/anaplastic MBs (LC/A MBs) appear to carry an adverse prognosis..

MB generally arises in the cerebellar vermis and projects into the fourth ventricle. Patients typically present with the symptoms and signs of obstructive hydrocephalus such as headache and vomiting. Approximately 35% of patients present with leptomeningeal metastases within the supratentorial or spinal meninges. MB is one of the few CNS tumours that can spread outside the CNS. This is rarely seen at initial presentation, but sometimes seen at relapse. Staging studies such as a bone scan or bone marrow aspiration or biopsy are justified only if suggested by symptoms.

On computed tomography (CT) or magnetic resonance imaging (MRI), MBs appear as solid masses that are generally contrast enhancing, either uniformly or patchily (Fig. 9.1).

Initial staging investigations include gadolinium-enhanced MRI of the craniospinal axis and cerebrospinal fluid (CSF) cytology. Spinal MRI should ideally be performed preoperatively. A postoperative MRI to detect the degree of residual tumour should be performed within 24–48 hours following surgical resection. Lumbar puncture for CSF cytology should be performed at least 15 days following surgery. Chang staging is described in Table 9.1 (2).

Risk status

For the purposes of stratification of therapy, patients with MB are categorized as having standard-risk or high-risk disease, based on evaluation of the impact of prognostic factors on outcome in a series of multi-institutional studies. Factors that correlate with outcome include age at diagnosis, the presence or absence of leptomeningeal spread at diagnosis, and the completeness of the surgical resection.

Standard risk: patients at least 3 years of age who have undergone complete or subtotal resection with less than 1.5 cm^2 of residual tumour on postoperative MRI and no evidence of CSF dissemination (M0) are considered to have standard-risk disease.

High risk: patients who have larger volume residual tumour and/or those with evidence of CSF dissemination (Chang stage M1–3) at diagnosis.

Overall, approximately two-thirds of patients will be standard risk and one-third will be high risk.

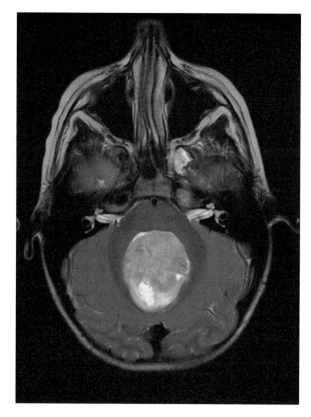

Fig. 9.1 Magnetic resonance imaging T2 sequence, demonstrating medulloblastoma within the fourth ventricle.

Influence of biological factors

Classification of histological subtypes of MB have traditionally been based on morphology, and included the variants classical MB, desmoplastic/nodular MB, MBEN (MB with extensive nodularity), large cell, and anaplastic MB. As a consequence of the ability to monitor transcription across the genome, various research groups have applied a classification of MB into subgroups on the basis of differences in the transcriptome. The four principal subgroups of MB are referred to as WNT, SHH (TP53 mutated and wildtype), Group 3, and Group 4 (3–5). This is reflected in the updated WHO classification.

The WNT subgroup is characterized by very good prognosis compared with the other subgroups with long-term survival in excess of 90%. The majority of WNT subgroup MBs have classic

Table 9.1 Chang staging

M0	No metastases
M1	Unequivocal MB cells in lumbar CSF. No evidence of metastases on craniospinal MRI
M2	Supratentorial leptomeningeal metastases on MRI
M3	Spinal leptomeningeal metastases (alone or together with supratentorial metastases) on MRI
M4	Metastases beyond the CNS

Source data from *Radiology*, 93(6), Chang CH, Housepian EM, Herbert C, Jr., An operative staging system and a megavoltage radiotherapeutic technique for cerebellar medulloblastomas, pp. 1351–9, Copyright (1969), Radiological Society of North America.

histology with these tumours demonstrating beta-catenin nucleo-positivity (6), *CTNNB1* gene mutations, and monosomy 6. Rarely the WNT subgroup may include large cell/anaplastic cases. WNT MB can occur at all ages, but is infrequent in infants. Although overall MB is more common in males, the male-to-female (M:F) ratio for the WNT subgroup is approximately 1:1. Germline mutations of the WNT pathway inhibitor APC predispose to Turcot syndrome, which includes a predisposition to MB. A minority of cases with large cell/anaplastic histology have also been reported to be WNT positive. However, these are associated with the same good prognosis as other histological subtypes of MB within this subgroup (see Fig. 9.2).

The SHH MB subgroups include *TP53*-mutant and *TP53*-wildtype subgroups. They are named after the sonic hedgehog signalling pathway, which is considered to drive tumour initiation in the majority of cases. The frequency of SHH subgroups of MB is bimodal, and is frequent in both infants aged less than 3 years and adults. The M:F ratio is approximately 1:1. The majority of nodular/desmoplastic MBs are included within the SHH subgroup. However around 50% of SHH subgroup MB have other histological subtypes, including classical, large cell/anaplastic, and MBEN varieties. The prognosis for SHH *TP53*-wildtype appears to be similar to Group 4 (see below) and intermediate between WNT and Group 3. SHH *TP53*-mutant tumours that arise in the context of constitutional TP53 mutation (Li-Fraumeni syndrome) carry an extremely poor prognosis. Individuals with germline mutations of the SHH receptor PTCH have Gorlin's syndrome, which for several decades has been recognized as carrying a predisposition to the development of MB. MBs in the SHH subgroup are identified predominantly by transcriptional profiling, but alternative approaches such as immunohistochemical staining for SFRP1 or GAB1 have also been employed. Deletion of chromosome 9q appears to be limited to SHH MB. Preliminary clinical trials are being designed to target the SHH pathway to improve outcome for this subgroup.

Group 3 MB represents the subgroup of MB with the worst prognosis. The majority of MBs in Group 3 are classical MB and include the majority of large-cell/anaplastic tumours. They occur more commonly in males than females, and arise in infants and older children, but only rarely in adults. They frequently present with metastases. Group 3 MB is typically characterized by high-level amplification of the *MYC* proto-oncogene, and almost all cases exhibit aberrant *MYC* expression. The Group 3 MB genome exhibits high levels of genomic instability and often harbours gains of chromosomes 1q, 7, and 17q, and deletions of 10q, 11, 16q, and 17p.

Patients with Group 4 MB have an intermediate to good prognosis similar to patients with SHH tumours. They include classical and large cell/anaplastic histologies. Group 4 tumours account for approximately 30–40% of MB cases. This subgroup represents the archetypal MB, for example, a 7-year-old boy with a classical histology MB who has an isochromosome 17q. The M:F ratio is approximately 3:1. As the molecular pathogenesis of Group 4 MB is not currently clear, the generic name 'Group 4' has been allocated pending further insight into molecular characteristics.

Improvements in the understanding of the molecular mechanisms of MB tumourigenesis are emerging as important factors in clinical trial design leading to a tailored approach for different histological and molecular biological subtypes. Collaborative clinical trial groups are developing studies that will investigate prospectively the stratification of therapy according to pathological,

WNT subgroup	SHH subgroup	Group 3	Group 4
CTNNB1 mutations, monosomy 6	Identified predominantly by transcriptional profiling, or IHC staining for SFRP1 or GAB1, deletion of chromosome 9q	Typically characterized by high-level amplification of MYC proto-oncogene, and aberrant MYC expression, high levels of genomic instability and often harbours gains of chromosomes 1q, 7, and 17q, and deletions of 10q, 11, 16q, and 17p	Molecular pathogenesis of Group 4 not currently clear, pending further insight into molecular characteristics, isochromosome 17q
Very good prognosis Long-term survival >90%	Prognosis similar to Group 4, intermediate between WNT and Group 3	Subgroup with worst prognosis	Intermediate prognosis similar to SHH
Majority have classical histology	Includes majority of nodular/desmoplastic MBs. 50% have other histological subtypes	Majority classical histology, include majority of large cell anaplastic tumours	30–40% of MB cases 'Archetypal MB', e.g. a 7-year-old boy with a classical histology medulloblastoma
Beta-catenin nucleo-positivity	Frequency bimodal, frequent in both infants and adults	Arise in infants and older children, rarely adults, more common in males than females	M:F ratio 3:1
Occur at all ages, but infrequent in infants	M:F ratio 1:1	Frequently present with metastases	
M:F ratio 1:1			

Fig. 9.2 Molecular subtypes of medulloblastoma.

biological, as well as the more traditional clinical parameters. In particular, clinical studies are beginning to involve a cautious lowering of the treatment intensity for patients with WNT MB and maintaining intensity for those in Group 3. This approach requires a timely and well-coordinated approach to tumour sample collection and analysis of biological parameters prior to treatment decisions (5).

Initial surgical treatment

Patients who present with obstructive hydrocephalus frequently require emergency management with either third ventriculostomy or ventricular drain. The first definitive treatment is complete, or near complete, surgical resection of the primary tumour. Following radical resection, approximately 25% of patients experience post-operative cerebellar mutism, a symptom complex characterized by decreased or absent speech and irritability that may also be associated with hypotonia, ataxia, and the inability to coordinate voluntary movements(posterior fossa syndrome). This requires additional rehabilitation, sometimes over several months, and can be problematic in that this can make preparations for radiotherapy more difficult, or occasionally the child may require anaesthesia for radiotherapy at an age where this is usually not required.

Post-surgical adjuvant treatment

Standard-risk disease

In view of the propensity of MB for metastasis via the CSF, cranio-spinal radiotherapy (CSRT) is an important component of treatment. Until the 1990s, the international standard of care was CSRT to a dose of 35–36 Gy followed by a whole posterior fossa boost to a total dose of 54–55.8 Gy. In multi-institutional studies, such treatment resulted in long-term event-free survival (EFS) in 60–65% of patients (7). However, sequelae of treatment include hormonal deficits, impaired bone growth, and neurocognitive deficits that correlate with a number of factors but particularly the age of the child and the craniospinal radiation dose (8). Other factors include the direct and indirect effects of the tumour and surgery, including hydrocephalus. Since the 1990s, an important aim of North American and European collaborative group studies has been to reduce the dose of CSRT in order to try to minimize late sequelae.

The Children's Cancer Group (CCG) 9892 study (9) was a limited, multi-institutional, non-randomized trial which employed a reduced dose of CSRT, 23.4 Gy in 13 fractions followed by a posterior fossa dose to a total dose of 55.8 Gy in 1.8 Gy fractions, together with weekly vincristine. This was followed by eight cycles of chemotherapy with cisplatin, CCNU, and vincristine. Five-year progression-free survival (PFS) was 79%. This study established the lower dose of CSRT as standard of care for patients with standard-risk disease. The Children's Oncology Group (COG) A9961 study continued with the principle of lower-dose CSRT and compared two different post-radiotherapy chemotherapy regimens, namely cisplatin with vincristine and either CCNU or cyclophosphamide. EFS at 4 years was approximately 85% in both arms (9). Such an approach continues to be the standard of care for children with standard-risk MB in North America, namely reduced-dose CSRT followed by chemotherapy (10).

During the 1990s, in North America and Europe there had been an increasing use of chemotherapy as an additional treatment modality. The benefit of chemotherapy combined with radiotherapy compared with radiotherapy alone was confirmed in the

International Society of Paediatric Oncology/United Kingdom Children's Cancer Study Group (SIOP/UKCCSG) PNET-3 trial (7) which recruited patients between 1992 and 2000, and demonstrated a significant improvement in EFS of 78.5% versus 64.8% with the use of pre-radiotherapy chemotherapy with carboplatin, cyclophosphamide, etoposide, and vincristine.

Studies of radiotherapy dose and fractionation for standard-risk medulloblastoma

Several treatment strategies designed to reduce the morbidity associated with the use of radiotherapy have been tested. The French Cooperative Group (SFOP) reduced the radiotherapy target volume to avoid supratentorial radiation together with chemotherapy but this resulted in a very high risk of recurrence (11). The use of reduced-dose CSRT (23.4 Gy) alone (without chemotherapy) in the North American intergroup study (CCG 923/POG 8631) resulted in a significantly increased risk of isolated neuraxis failure compared with 36.0 Gy and an EFS at 5 and 8 years of only 52% (12).

In Europe, the role of hyperfractionated radiotherapy (HFRT) has been investigated. A SFOP (French Pediatric Oncology Society) pilot study tested HFRT 36 Gy to CSRT in 1 Gy b.i.d. fractions without chemotherapy and demonstrated that early toxicity was reduced and PFS at 3 years was very good at 81% (13). Subsequently, HFRT was tested in the European SIOP PNET-4 randomized trial in which patients were randomized to HFRT or conventional radiotherapy. All patients received post-radiotherapy adjuvant chemotherapy with cisplatin, CCNU, and vincristine. This trial demonstrated no advantage for HFRT in terms of disease control, but provided further confirmation of acceptable survival for reduced-dose CSRT when combined with adjuvant chemotherapy (14). In an analysis of health status of long-term survivors, long-term quality of survival and growth in the two arms of the PNET-4 study were compared (15). Participants and their parents or caregivers completed standardized questionnaires on executive functioning, health status, behaviour, health-related quality of life, as well as employment, educational, and social information. Compared with standard radiation therapy, HFRT was associated with better scores for executive functioning, but health status, behavioural issues, and health-related quality of life were similar in the two treatment arms. HFRT was associated with greater decrement in height (15).

Traditionally, CSRT is followed by a boost to the posterior fossa to a total dose of 54–55.8 Gy. With a combination of careful contouring and conformal treatment techniques it is possible to reduce the dose to the inner ear, with the aim of minimizing hearing loss in children who will also be receiving chemotherapy with cisplatin. Better sparing of the cochlea, pituitary, hypothalamus, and the temporal lobes can be achieved with a reduced target volume for the boost, limited to the tumour/surgical bed with a margin rather than the whole posterior fossa. In a series of 114 patients, Fukunaga-Johnson et al. found a low risk of isolated failure outside the tumour bed in the posterior fossa (16). In addition, the SFOP pilot study referred to earlier also reported good outcomes following a boost limited to the tumour and surgical bed plus a margin (13). The recently reported COG randomized study compared a boost to the whole posterior fossa with a tumour/surgical bed plus margin boost. This study also tested the efficacy of an even lower dose of CSRT (18 Gy) in children aged 3–8 years. Preliminary results have recently been reported (17). There was no significant difference in EFS for patients treated with a tumour/surgical bed plus margin boost compared with those treated with a whole posterior fossa boost. However patients treated with 18 Gy CSRT had a reduced 5-year EFS of 71.4% compared with 82.1% for those treated with 23.4 Gy (17).

Current management of standard-risk medulloblastoma

Currently the standard of care for children with standard-risk MB is with CSRT 23.4 Gy with a tumour boost to a total dose of 54.0 Gy, followed by eight cycles of chemotherapy with vincristine, CCNU, and cisplatin. With this approach, a 5-year EFS of 83% has been achieved (18). The initial results of the recent COG trial suggest equivalence in survival between tumour bed and whole posterior fossa boosts and this, together with other data has led to a tumour bed boost becoming a standard of care.

Management of standard-risk medulloblastoma in infants

Medulloblastoma accounts for approximately 20–40% of all CNS tumours in 'infants' (defined as aged <3 years). Approximately half of infants have more favourable histological types (desmoplastic/nodular or MBEN). However, the prognosis overall is worse than in older children. In addition to the impact of biological factors, the frequency of metastatic disease is higher, approximately 50%, and the rate of complete tumour resection is lower in this age group. Furthermore, because of the concern about late effects in this age group, most patients receive low doses of CSRT or no radiotherapy at all. Infants with M0 disease who have undergone total resection may do well with chemotherapy alone, with a 5-year overall survival (OS) of 69% in the first POG infant study and a variable outcome in the German study with survival of around 90 % for infants with desmoplastic tumours (19), although treatment in the latter included intraventricular methotrexate. In other studies, results were less satisfactory. In some, the need for aggressive salvage regimens was associated with significant long-term sequelae. In fact, with the possible exception of very young children with desmoplastic/nodular MB without residual disease, evidence suggests that radiotherapy is an important component of treatment. The recently reported North American P9934 study employed early focal radiotherapy to a limited treatment volume consisting of the tumour bed plus an anatomically confined margin for patients without leptomeningeal seeding (20). Four-year EFS and OS were 50% and 69% respectively with better outcomes for those with completely resected disease and desmoplastic histology. The German study also highlighted the importance of the impact of desmoplastic histological subtype on outcome with infants with M0 disease treated with chemotherapy alone (19). The 'Headstart' chemotherapy-alone protocol delivered to M0 patients has reported 5-year EFS of 52% for all patients and 64% for those with less than gross total resection (40). However, this approach is very intensive, incorporating induction chemotherapy with cisplatin, cyclophosphamide, etoposide, and vincristine, and myeloablative therapy with high-dose carboplatin, etoposide, and thiotepa supported by autologous stem cell rescue.

Management of high-risk medulloblastoma

Clinicopathological factors indicating high-risk disease

Metastatic disease at presentation, as diagnosed by the presence of meningeal enhancement on MRI of the brain (stage M2) or spine (stage M3) clearly confers a poor prognosis (1, 2, 21, 22). A careful metastatic evaluation is critical to the success of the current radiation therapy dose reduction strategy in MB. A review of patients registered in the recent North American COG A9961 trial has demonstrated an unacceptable failure rate in patients with overlooked M2 or M3 disease in a central radiology review (10). The prognostic significance of Chang stage M1 disease, in which tumour cells are found within the CSF without radiological evidence of metastasis, is now accepted by both the COG and the European SIOP Europe PNET Group as an adverse prognostic factor, with now clear evidence that patients with M1 disease have a poorer prognosis than those without evidence of such tumour spread (21, 23).

Residual disease

Both the COG and SIOP groups accept the prognostic importance of achieving a gross total or near gross total surgical excision, as shown in the CCG-921 study (24). More recently, the HIT-SIOP PNET-4 trial also showed that the presence of residual disease, defined by at least 1.5 cm^2 (maximum cross-sectional area) of residual tumour after surgery, conferred a poorer prognosis (14). The latest analysis of this trial noted 30 patients (9.7%) out of 308 trial patients with residual disease greater than or equal to 1.5 cm^2. Five-year EFS was 64% ± 9% for those with residual disease as compared to 81% ± 3% for those with a postoperative tumour volume of less than 1.5 cm^2. More recent evidence which takes into account molecular classification and its impact on outcome, has suggested that the impact of extent of resection is attenuated after taking into account molecular characterization (25). Maximum safe surgical resection remains the standard of care. However, attempted surgical removal of minimal residual disease is not recommended if the risk of subsequent morbidity is high, as there is no definitive benefit from gross total resection compared with near-total resection.

Histology: anaplasia

Previous reports suggested that anaplasia was associated with a poorer prognosis than that for classic, desmoplastic/nodular, and MBEN (26–28). The situation is, however, complicated by a number of factors:

- Variability in the criteria adopted by groups and individual institutions for the diagnosis of the anaplastic phenotype.
- Overlap with the large cell MB phenotype and the confounding impact of tumour biology (e.g. *MYC* amplification).

The incidence of anaplastic MB is unclear. In the COG 9961 study, anaplastic cases were reported as comprising around 15% of the total trial population. It is likely that the proportion of cases with anaplasia as defined by the WHO (2007) classification of CNS tumours, where anaplasia is both diffuse and severe, will be less than this. For example, in the HIT-SIOP PNET-4 trial, there were only 14 large cell/anaplastic cases (4.5%) out of 313 analysed at central review. At the SIOP PNET Group meeting in Hamburg 2009, it was agreed that patients with large cell/anaplastic MB be regarded as high-risk patients.

Large cell/anaplastic medulloblastoma

Large cell/anaplastic MB is a rare and phenotypically distinct MB subtype that accounts for less than 5% of cases. Traditionally, large cell/anaplastic MB was regarded as being associated with a worse outlook (26–28). However, this concept has now been superseded by combined histological and molecular biological classification.

Biology of high-risk disease

MYC and *MYCN* represent the most commonly amplified genetic loci in MB, each affecting about 5% of cases, and have been associated with large cell/anaplastic MB, although can be observed in other MB phenotypes, which a mostly included in Group 3.

Amplification of *MYC* or *MYCN* is associated with a poor outcome and is accepted as an adverse prognostic factor (high-risk disease) by international collaborative groups, particularly when metastatic (29, 27).

Other biological factors that have been shown to be associated with an adverse outcome in some studies include defects of chromosome 17 (9), expression of the *ERBB-2* receptor tyrosine kinase (10), expression of the *c-MYC* oncogene or the absence of expression of the *TRKC* neurotrophin receptor. The evidence base for the prognostic importance of these factors is less strong than that for *MYC* or *MYCN* amplification. At present, the only biological factor that has been accepted as conferring high-risk status for MB is amplification of *MYC* or *MYCN*.

SIOP Europe Embryonal Group definition of high-risk medulloblastoma

- Metastatic disease (Chang stage M1, M2, M3, M4).
- Residual disease greater than 1.5 cm^2 (maximum cross-sectional area).
- Large cell/anaplastic MB.
- Amplification of *MYC* or *MYCN*.

As opposed to standard/average-risk disease, metastatic MB must be considered a poor-prognosis tumour. Previous treatments consisted of surgical excision of the primary tumour followed by conventional radiotherapy with doses of radiotherapy of 35–36 Gy to the craniospinal axis together with a boost of 18 Gy to the posterior fossa. In addition, further boosts to sites of metastatic disease are frequently administered.

Chemotherapy is accepted as having an important role in treatment of metastatic MB, although the optimal chemotherapy regimen has yet to be defined. Various large multicentre studies including the CCG-921, HIT-91, and PNET-3 have reported survival figures of between 30% and 40% for patients with M2/M3 status at diagnosis (21, 30, 31). Indeed for M2/M3 disease, no reasonably sized North American or European study has shown survival in excess of 50% where treatment consists of 35–36 Gy with addition of conventional chemotherapy.

A number of more recent trials have shown more encouraging results in the treatment of high-risk MB, with a survival rate for M2/3 patients of greater than 50%, including studies using higher-dose CSRT as well as standard-dose CSRT with concurrent chemotherapy. The POG group studied CSRT to greater than 36 Gy in study 9031. Patients with high-risk MB were randomized to pre-irradiation chemotherapy with cisplatin and etoposide or to immediate radiotherapy followed by the same chemotherapy. Both arms then received identical chemotherapy with vincristine and cyclophosphamide. For all patients the 5-year EFS was 66.0% in the early chemotherapy arm and 70.0% in the early radiotherapy arm (32). Five-year OS was 73.1% and 76.1%, respectively. Of note, the POG-9031 study used a higher CSRT dose of 39.6 Gy for patients with metastatic disease with boosts of up to 45 Gy to sites of macroscopic spread (32).

In the St Jude Medulloblastoma-96 study, children with high-risk MB received four cycles of cyclophosphamide-based, dose-intensive chemotherapy following radiotherapy (18). Although the survival for M2/M3 patients was not reported in the paper, Dr Gajjar has reported 65% 5-year EFS for the 33 patients with M2/M3 disease. For these high-risk patients, a CSRT dose of 39 Gy was used.

The result from both of these studies may indicate a dose–response effect for radiotherapy doses above 35–36 Gy, although there must be concern with regard to late neuropsychological sequelae at such high CSRT doses.

For high-risk patients, COG has completed a dose escalation trial of carboplatin used as a radiosensitizer given concomitantly with daily CSRT for patients with high-risk MB and ST-PNET (CCG-99701) (33). All patients underwent surgical debulking followed by 36 Gy CSRT with boosts to the posterior fossa and sites of bulk disease. During CSRT, patients received weekly vincristine as well as carboplatin doses ranging from 30 mg/m^2/dose × 15 to 45 mg/m^2/dose × 30 given 1–4 hours prior to each radiotherapy fraction, using a phase I design. Six weeks after completing chemoradiotherapy, patients received six courses of monthly cyclophosphamide (2 g/m^2) and vincristine.

Myelosuppression was dose limiting and 35 mg/m^2/dose × 30 was selected as the maximum tolerated carboplatin dose. Median follow-up for surviving patients was 4.5 years. Four-year OS and EFS for the entire group was 81% ± 5% and 66% ± 6% respectively. The established phase I dose of carboplatin from this study now forms the basis of a current phase III randomized trial that formally tests the benefit of carboplatin concomitant with radiotherapy as well as testing the addition of 13-cis-retinoic acid along with maintenance chemotherapy.

Studies using hyperfractionated radiotherapy

Altered radiotherapy fractionation schedules, such as HFRT, can theoretically increase the dose to tumour without an increase in the dose to normal nervous tissue. Hyperfractionated accelerated radiotherapy (HART) aims to exploit the therapeutic advantage of twice-daily radiotherapy but in addition uses a higher dose per fraction and thus a shorter overall treatment time. This approach theoretically may improve tumour control by reducing tumour cell repopulation between fractions. Encouraging results were published from the Milan group, who use a programme of high-dose sequential chemotherapy followed by HART (34).

Between 1998 and 2007, 33 consecutive patients received postoperative methotrexate (8 g/m^2), etoposide (2.4 g/m^2), cyclophosphamide (4 g/m^2), and carboplatin (0.8 g/m^2) in a 2-month schedule, then HART with a maximal dose to the neuroaxis of 39 Gy (1.3 Gy b.i.d.) and a posterior fossa boost (1.5 Gy b.i.d.) up to 60 Gy. After radiotherapy, patients received maintenance chemotherapy with six courses of lomustine and vincristine. Patients with persistent disseminated disease before HART were consolidated with two myeloablative courses of thiotepa (900 mg/m^2 per course) which replaced maintenance chemotherapy in these patients. Seven patients younger than 10 years old who achieved complete response after chemotherapy received a lower dose to the neuroaxis (31.2 Gy). The 5-year EFS, PFS, and OS rates were 70%, 72%, and 73%, respectively. However, more recently, with more widespread use of this regimen, cases of unexpected toxicity have emerged, assumed to be an interaction between the high-dose chemotherapy and HART radiotherapy regimens. There has been discussion around identifying factors which may have given rise to unexpected toxicity and how this should be avoided (35).

CCLG HART protocol

The CCLG was also interested in the potential of HART, which formed the basis of CCLG CNS 2001 06, to evaluate the feasibility and toxicity of a regimen comprising HART (1.24 Gy b.i.d.) with chemotherapy for M1–3 MB. The CSRT dose was 39.68 Gy in 32 fractions, followed by a boost to the whole posterior fossa of 22.32 Gy in 18 fractions. Where appropriate, boosts to metastases of 9.92 Gy in eight fractions were given. Chemotherapy was given after radiotherapy and comprised eight planned courses of vincristine, lomustine, and cisplatin (36). Between 2002 and 2008, 34 patients were entered into the study. At a median follow-up of 14 months, 2-year EFS was 68.1% (95% confidence interval (CI) 40.9–84.9%) and 3-year EFS = 53.0% (95% CI 26.0–74.1%). There was no unexpected toxicity.

MET-HIT 2000-AB4

The HIT Group's most recent study for metastatic MB is included in the HIT 2000 series of studies. This study recruited patients aged between 4 and 21 years at diagnosis with metastatic MB. Children received two cycles of HIT-SKK chemotherapy consisting of systemic multi-agent chemotherapy (cisplatin/vincristine, methotrexate/vincristine, carboplatin/etoposide) and intraventricular methotrexate. Patients then received HFRT (1 Gy b.i.d. to a total CSRT dose of 40 Gy) with 60 Gy to the posterior fossa, 68 Gy to the tumour bed, and 50–60 Gy boost to metastatic deposits. Following radiotherapy, patients received four cycles of lomustine, vincristine, and cisplatin chemotherapy. There was an option for patients who had a very good response to systemic chemotherapy to receive additional high-dose chemotherapy with stem cell rescue, although only a very small number of patients actually received high-dose chemotherapy.

Preliminary results from MET-HIT 2000-AB4 were presented in 2009 for patients that did not receive the high-dose chemotherapy arm. One hundred and forty patients with a median of age of 7.8 years were registered between 2001 and 2007. There were 90 patients eligible for analysis that did not receive high-dose chemotherapy, with a median follow-up of 3.7 years. Three-year EFS was 67 ± 5% and OS was 81 ± 4%. Three-year survival rates were not different between the 25 patients with M1 disease and those with M2/3 disease. There were no significant differences in survival rates of 73 children with classic, 13 with desmoplastic, and 4 large cell/anaplastic MB. There were no major unexpected toxicities and no treatment-related deaths. The preliminary outcome from the HIT 2000 study is thus encouraging and appears better for this cohort of patients who received HFRT as opposed to those entered into the HIT 91 study who received conventional radiotherapy. However, there is concern about using these high doses of radiotherapy particularly when conventionally fractionated, with respect to the long-term neuropsychological outcome.

A pre-radiotherapy chemotherapy approach may have the advantage of allowing therapy to commence immediately and to reduce the burden of disease at the time of the radiotherapy. In the HIT 91 study there appeared to be a survival advantage for those patients with metastatic MB receiving sandwich chemotherapy as opposed to those receiving immediate radiotherapy. On the other hand, data from POG 9031 study showed no difference in survival between those patients receiving immediate or delayed radiotherapy.

Management of high-risk PNET/ medulloblastoma in infants

The outcomes following treatment of infants with metastatic MB are generally poor compared with older children with metastatic MB and infants without metastases at presentation.

The results of a recent international meta-analysis of children from Europe and the United States were published in 2010 (37). In this analysis, which included children up to the age of 5 and with a median age of 1.89 years, there were in total 260 children, of whom 75 had metastatic disease at presentation. Fifty-five of the 75 had M2 or M3 disease. The 8-year survival rate was 27%.

In a UK series of children under the age of 3 with brain tumours treated between 1992 and 2003 and reported in 2010 (38), 31 had MB, of whom 15 had metastases at presentation. Although the aim was to try and avoid radiotherapy, the majority (72%) ended up receiving it. At follow-up, 5 of the 15 were alive, with a 5-year OS of 33% for those with the classical histological variety of MB.

Outcomes for young children treated in Germany have been similar (39). In the HIT SKK92 German protocol, an intensive chemotherapy regimen that included intraventricular methotrexate was used in 45 patients. For infants without metastases at presentation, 77% of those with complete resection, (particularly those with the desmoplastic histological variety), and 42% of those without complete resection, were free of relapse at 4 years. However, for children with metastases at presentation, only 27% were free of recurrence at 4 years.

The Headstart protocols have been developed with the aim of delivering very intensive chemotherapy in order to try to delay or even possibly avoid radiotherapy in young children (with both high-risk and standard-risk MB) (40). This series of protocols was developed in the United States but in recent years has become more widely used in Europe.

There are no data available on the longer-term outcomes of treatment for infants with high-risk PNET, and achieving long-term tumour control with acceptable morbidity is a major challenge.

Pineal tumours

Definition

About 20% of tumours in this location are pineal parenchymal tumours (PPTs). They are classified as PC (grade I), pineoblastomas (grade IV), as well as PPT of intermediate differentiation (PPTID). There is also the rare papillary tumour of the pineal region. Their biological behaviour is variable.

Pineocytomas are generally well circumscribed and do not spread through the CNS. PPTs are classified as grade II–III according to the WHO classification.

Epidemiology

The incidence of pineal region tumours is low, accounting for less than 1% of brain tumours. Pineal region tumours are much more common among paediatric brain tumours than among adults with brain tumours. The most common type of tumour found is germ cell tumours which represent at least 50% of all paediatric pineal region tumours. Germ cell tumours are discussed separately in Chapter 14. PPTs have been reported to occur with no gender predilection and at a median age of 12 years (41).

Clinical presentation of pineal tumours

The most common presenting symptoms from tumours in the pineal region are those symptoms resulting from hydrocephalus (headache, nausea, vomiting). In addition, Parinaud syndrome is a relatively common presenting finding.

Imaging

Most pineal tumours demonstrate heterogeneous enhancement on MRI studies. There are no clear diagnostic differences on imaging to the type of pineal tumour (see Fig. 9.3) (42).

The prognosis follows the disease extent and histology. Thus, treatment is guided by histological subtype. Surgery is required in pineocytoma while pineoblastomas will be discussed in greater detail in later sections. A biopsy is required in most pineal tumours to establish the diagnosis and guide treatment. For patients with PPTs, we recommend surgical resection if possible.

Radiotherapy techniques for medulloblastoma

The clinical target volume (CTV) for CSRT includes the meninges surrounding the whole brain and spinal cord and extending to the lower limit of the thecal sac. Conventionally the lower borders of lateral whole-brain fields are carefully matched to the superior border of one or more posterior spinal fields, usually with a moving junction between the brain and spine fields to minimize the risk of underdose or overdose in the region of the field junction in cervical spinal cord.

Treatment planning and delivery

CSRT is one of the most complex techniques employed in most radiotherapy departments. Modern tools for treatment planning and delivery should be employed leading to a more streamlined technique and can substantially reduce planning and delivery times. One such technique is shown in Fig. 9.4. Quality control of radiotherapy planning and delivery has been shown to improve outcomes for treating patients with MB. In the SFOP M-7 protocol, 50% of relapses could be correlated with targeting deviations. In the MSFOP-93 and MSFOP-98 studies the relapse rate was 17% in patients who had inadequate coverage of one component of the CTV (e.g. the cribriform plate), 28% for patients who had inadequate coverage at two sites, and 67% for patients who had inadequate coverage at three or more sites (13, 43, 44).

With regard to planning the posterior fossa boost, careful attention to detail is also necessary. The optimal CTV for a reduced-volume posterior fossa boost remains to be defined although an anatomically confined expansion of 1.5 cm around any macroscopic residual tumour and the surgical bed seems to be reasonable and this was the volume under investigation in the recently completed COG study for standard-risk disease.

CSRT should commence in a timely manner. Delay has been associated with poorer outcomes and CSRT should ideally start within 30 days following surgery (45).

New treatment modalities for craniospinal irradiation

Protons provide a dose distribution for craniospinal irradiation that cannot be achieved by even the most sophisticated photon beam treatment planning, with significant reduction in low-dose

Age at time of scan is 13 years old

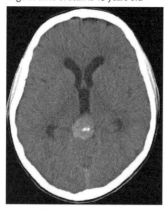

CT non-contrast shows
mineralization in lesion

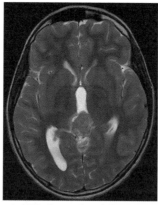

Axial T2 shows relatively low signal

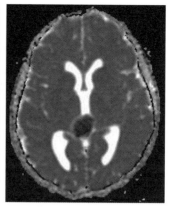

Axial ADC shows low signal
consistent with more cellular lesion

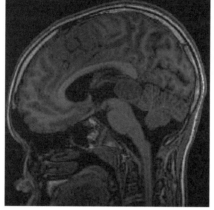

Non-contrast sagittal T1 BRAVO volumetric
type T1 sequence

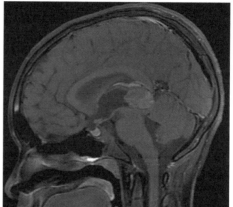

Fat-saturated sagittal T1
shows lesion enhancement

Fig. 9.3 Pineoblastoma.

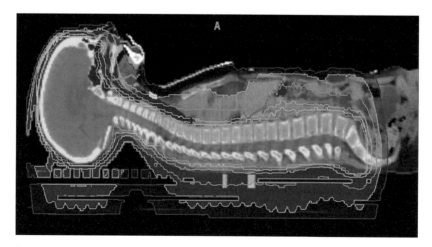

Fig. 9.4 (See colour plate section) Tomotherapy plan for craniospinal radiotherapy.

Reproduced from Hoskin P, *Radiotherapy in Practice - External Beam Therapy*, Second Edition, Copyright (2012), with permission from Oxford University Press.

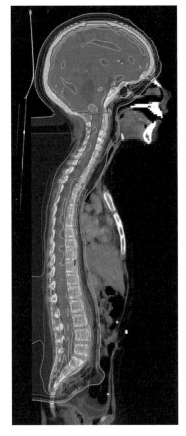
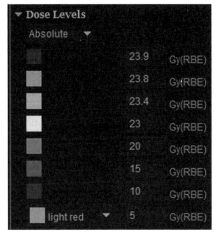

Fig. 9.5 (See colour plate section) Pencil beam scanning dose distribution for craniospinal irradiation in a child with medulloblastoma.

exposure to organs anterior to the spine in the exit region of the spinal field. This should achieve equivalent tumour control but with reduced long-term morbidity (46–48) including the risk of radiation-induced second cancer (47–50). Planning studies predict a significant reduction in the risk of second malignancy from the use of protons for CSRT due to reduced irradiation of organs anterior to the spine (see Fig. 9.5) (50).

Long-term effects of radiotherapy for medulloblastoma

The quality of survival of children with brain tumours including MB and other embryonal tumours may be compromised by long-term sequelae. There may be direct and indirect effects on musculoskeletal development, predominantly impaired spinal growth as a consequence of the effect of the spinal component of CSRT on spinal growth. Osteopenia is possible, particularly in those with residual neurological deficits.

Recently the neurocognitive sequelae of radiotherapy have become much better characterized. It is now realized that functional maturation and myelination of the CNS continue until well into adolescence and even into the young adult age range. Through its effect on the microvasculature and on the oligodendrocyte precursor cells that produce myelin, radiotherapy results in impaired neurogenesis and cortical atrophy. Patients fail to acquire new knowledge and skills at an age-appropriate rate and show a progressive decline in IQ over time (62). The magnitude of the deficit depends on age at treatment with younger children worst affected,

but other factors which apply include constitutional/genetic (e.g. *NF1*), tumour (e.g. location, presence or absence of hydrocephalus), treatment factors (e.g. radiotherapy (51, 52)), and use of chemotherapy (53). Furthermore, for children treated for MB, hearing impairment due to cisplatin may have a compounding effect on educational activities. As a consequence, many children exhibit impaired school and social performance which tends to deteriorate over several years. There is increasing evidence that intervention providing additional targeted support with schooling or using cognitive or behavioural therapy or pharmacotherapy may be useful, and that this should commence as soon after treatment as feasible for optimum benefits (50, 54, 55).

Endocrine deficits are very common after radiotherapy (56). Even though a substantial proportion of patients may have had deficits prior to radiotherapy due to the tumour or to surgery, and even though there may be modulating factors such as chemotherapy that affect the frequency of deficits, radiotherapy is primarily responsible for the growth hormone deficiency that correlates with the dose of radiotherapy to the hypothalamic–pituitary axis and the primary hypothyroidism seen after CSRT (55).

Medulloblastoma/PNET in adults

Epidemiology

The European annual incidence of CNS embryonal tumours is approximately 0.2/100,000, 0.1/100,000 and less than 0.1/100,000 per year in patients 20–39 years, 40–59 years, and older than

60 years of age, respectively (57). The survival analysis in the population-based cancer registries of around 20 European countries in the EUROCARE study (58) covered 867 adults diagnosed with PNETs of the brain during the period 1995–2002. In these patients, the survival was 78% at 1 year, 61% at 3 years, and 52% at 5 years. The 5-year relative survival decreased with age: from 56% in the younger (15–44 years) age group to 9% in the older group (45 years and over).

In the paediatric population it is now evident from molecular analysis that most tumours previously diagnosed as supratentorial PNET should now be reclassified as other entities. It is necessary for the equivalent analyses to be undertaken in the adult population.

Clinical outcomes and genetic alterations

The tendency for metastatic spread is somewhat lower in adults than in children (59, 60). However, late relapses are more common, since the 5-year relapse rate, 62%, decreases to approximately 40% at 10 years (59, 61). Metastatic spread outside the CNS is rare. Bone is the most common site of metastasis in adults, accounting for 80% of metastases found outside the CNS (62).

During recent years, genetic and molecular alterations have been claimed to explain morphological and survival differences. In particular, amplification and overexpression of *MYC* and *MYCN* occur in 5–10% of MB, being increased levels of *MYC* expression significant predictors of worse outcome (63, 64). Other frequent genetic abnormalities in MB are chromosomal alterations, in particular on chromosome 17, that occur in up to 40–50% of primary tumours. Several authors have observed that chromosome 17p deletion as shown in PNET-4 is correlated with a worse prognosis (65, 66). Ray et al. (67) showed that protein expression of MYC, p53, PDGFR-alpha, ERBB2, MIB-1, and TrkC combined with clinical characteristics could accurately predict relapse risk in paediatric MB patients.

Pomeroy et al. studied the gene expression profile in paediatric MB using oligonucleotide microarrays and demonstrated that the expression profile of eight genes helped to predict outcomes. Patients with a good prognosis pattern had a 5-year OS of 80% compared with 17% for those with a poor prognosis pattern (68).

During the past few years, array-based transcriptional profiling has uncovered the existence of distinct molecular subgroups and substantial differences have been identified between paediatric and adult MB patients (3, 69, 70), overall identifying four molecular subtypes: sonic hedgehog (SHH—about 30% of patients), WNT (10%), Group 3 (25%), and Group 4 (35%).

A recent meta-analysis of seven studies, where adults (defined as >16 years) represented 12% of the analysed population (71), identified that SHH tumours were most prominent in adults and infants, but not in older children, while Group 3 tumours were almost absent in adults. Group 4 was mainly represented in childhood, and patients in this group have an intermediate prognosis similar to the SHH subgroup, but adults with Group 4 MBs may do significantly worse (69, 71). At the time of recurrence, MBs maintain their subgroup affiliation and that the anatomical pattern of recurrence is highly subgroup specific. SHH MBs almost always recur locally, while almost all recurrences of Group 3 and Group 4 MB are metastatic, with recurrence in the posterior fossa in radiated patients being very rare (72).

Preliminary analysis of the mutational spectra of adult MB suggests that adults harbour significantly more somatic single nucleotide variations which are somatic, non-silent mutations, than subgroup-matched paediatric counterparts (73).

Prognosis

Risk factors

The Chang staging system is the same as is used in children (2). Patients with M0–1 and T1–2 disease fared best, claiming for a risk stratification.

The definitions of 'low-risk' (or 'standard-risk', 'average-risk') and high-risk (or 'poor-risk') groups, respectively, have been shown to be of controversial clinical utility. Some authors consider that patients with residual tumour of less than 1.5 cm^2 in size and no metastatic disease are at average risk (74, 75) whereas others also incorporate T stage in the risk assessment, and include patients T1–T2 and T3a tumours in the average-risk group (76).

However, despite risk definitions, it is generally agreed that patients without metastases have a lower risk for recurrence.

Metastatic disease

While in paediatric MB, M stage has been consistently associated with prognosis, its importance in adult disease is not as clear. Preliminary data reported in the prospective series of Brandes et al. suggest that patients without metastases have a significantly better outcome than those with metastatic spread (75% PFS at 5 years, compared to 45%, respectively) (76). Updated data on the same population, after a median follow-up of 7.6 years, showed that the difference was not maintained. PFS at 5 years was 61% and 78% in metastatic and non-metastatic patients, respectively, which did not achieve statistical significance (77). These data were consistent with what was obtained by other groups (78). However, it is not clear if, as in the paediatric counterpart (79), no significant difference could be found between M0 and M1.

T status

T staging may retain a prognostic role in adult MB, as suggested in a prospective trial, and in a large retrospective series of 253 patients where brainstem and fourth ventricle involvement was a negative prognostic factor on multivariate analysis (77, 78).

Residual disease

In the paediatric population, it is a generally accepted criterion that residual tumour of greater than 1.5 cm^2 in size predicts for a poorer prognosis (80). On the contrary, in adults, the largest studies were not able to find a significant impact on the 5-year PFS difference (77).

Treatment

In the past, it was assumed that MBs in adults had equivalent clinical features and responses to therapy to those in children. Adult patients therefore were frequently treated with paediatric protocols, with simple variations in drug dosages and schedules. There is a paucity of prospective controlled trials in adults, and current experience is based mainly on small retrospective studies investigating a variety of different treatments.

Surgery

Findings from several recent studies confirm the prognostic importance of achieving a total or near total surgical excision for adults and children (23).

Radiation therapy

Surgery alone is associated with a high recurrence rate, thus calling for adjuvant radiotherapy (81, 82). Postoperative radiotherapy consists of craniospinal irradiation followed by a boost to the posterior fossa as outlined earlier. Over the past 40 years, treatment outcomes have progressively improved, and the current long-term survival rate for adults is approximately 70%. The dose–response relationships for treatment of tumours within the posterior fossa have been clearly documented in paediatric patients as well as in adults (83, 87). In adults, a dose of 54 Gy provides a 5-year disease control of about 70–90%, compared to 40% with doses of less than 50 Gy (86, 87). Dose reductions in the adjacent areas of the neuraxis appear to be of critical importance. If combined with chemotherapy, however, these dose reductions appear to be feasible (9), as in paediatric patients, but the only study available in adults, by Bloom and Bessell, reports an increase in the recurrence rate after dose reductions (32–35 Gy reduced to 15–25 Gy) (85).

Chemotherapy

Standard-risk medulloblastoma

The role of chemotherapy in adults is far from clear, since despite MB remaining a chemosensitive disease also in adults, chemotherapy tolerance, especially after craniospinal irradiation is a limiting factor. Large retrospective series suggested that in the average-risk subgroup of patients, there was no overall survival difference between patients treated with axial doses of greater than 34 Gy and those treated with craniospinal doses of less than 34 Gy plus chemotherapy (76). Of note, since the updated data with long-term follow-up, reported by Brandes et al., demonstrated that the risk of recurrence increased markedly after 7 years of follow-up in average-risk patients, it raised the issue of a role for chemotherapy in average-risk patients (77). Data from the HIT 2000 trial showed that the delivery of maintenance chemotherapy for non-metastatic (mainly standard-risk) patients aged 21 years and over is feasible, but after the relatively short follow-up of 3.7 years, did not significantly improve 4-year PFS and OS (88).

Thus, the recommendation for average-risk patients is surgery followed by postoperative radiotherapy (craniospinal followed by a boost to the entire posterior fossa) using conventional doses (without dose reductions). In contrast to the paediatric counterpart, adult patients have fewer growth and hormonal issues after radiotherapy. To date, adjuvant chemotherapy is still controversial, since its effect and possible toxicity when administered for this disease are less well studied.

High-risk medulloblastoma

The efficacy of adjuvant chemotherapy in adults appears to be similar to that in children. However, because of the heterogeneity of patients and protocols, one regimen cannot be considered preferable to another (77).

Historical data showed that treatment with radiotherapy alone is insufficient for high-risk patients, while the use of chemotherapy is associated with a 5-year PFS rate of 40–45% (61, 76).

For high-risk patients, it is impossible to establish detailed treatment recommendations. Data from the prospective trial conducted by Brandes et al. suggest that upfront chemotherapy followed by radiotherapy is feasible, and provides long-term outcomes similar to those obtained with radiotherapy alone in standard-risk patients (76, 84).

Recurrent disease

As in children, there is currently no standard therapy after relapse and the prognosis is generally very poor for those patients that relapsed after having previously received radiotherapy.. Thus, new strategies are under investigation in this setting. Novel subgroup-specific therapies are being explored in clinical trials, particularly for the SHH subgroup.

The HH pathway can be activated by mutations in PTCH1 or SUFU (loss of function), or SMO (gain of function) that lead to ligand-independent, constitutive signalling. Such mutations have been identified in approximately 20–30% of MBs. Thus, it is expected that oral HH-pathway inhibitors, would most likely provide clinical benefit only in patients with HH-pathway activated (HH+) tumours, and are currently under active investigation. Despite showing a pronounced initial response to treatment with anti-SMO small molecule (i.e. vismodegib, LDE225), both humans and mice acquired resistance to this drug and relapsed (89). However, the outcome of adult and paediatric MB after anti-SMO treatment is yet to be defined. Moreover, novel SHH targets identified here are excellent candidates for combinatorial therapy with SMO inhibitors, to avoid the resistance encountered in both humans and mice (89–91).

Atypical teratoid/rhabdoid tumours

Atypical teratoid rhabdoid tumours (AT/RTs) are rare embryonal tumours, arising most commonly in infancy. There is an association of renal rhabdoid tumours with other CNS embryonal tumours, such as PNET, and in addition, areas within AT/RTs may show differentiation towards PNET, sarcoma, or carcinoma (92, 93). Most tumours show an abnormality of chromosome 22, and this led to the identification of mutations in the gene *hSNF5/INI1* in almost all cases (94). Familial cases have been reported, and a rhabdoid predisposition syndrome is now increasingly recognized.

Tumours arise in all parts of the CNS, more commonly in the infratentorial compartment, and spread contiguously or by dissemination: one-third are metastatic at diagnosis. These are highly malignant tumours, and can spread through dense fibrous structures such as tentorium.

Epidemiology

Most tumours present in early childhood, median age 20 months, and show a preponderance of males (M >F 1.6:1). Most arise within the posterior fossa or cerebral hemisphere, but may arise in the spinal cord or be multifocal.

Presentation

As for all tumours, the presentation of AT/RT depends on where the tumour arises and the age of the child. These tumours tend to grow rapidly, and may be extremely invasive. Symptoms and signs of raised intracranial pressure are expected. Radiological features are not characteristic, but such tumours appear as large, hyperdense lesions, which enhance strongly, reflecting a highly vascular structure. There may be haemorrhage or calcification, and occasionally, signs of leptomeningeal spread.

Molecular genetics

Loss of the gene *SMARCB1* (also known as *INI1, hSNF5*, and *BAF47*) is the main event leading to AT/RT development. SMARCB1 is a component of the hSWI/SNF nucleosome-remodelling complex, which is present in prokaryotes and eukaryotes. hSWI/SNF consists of 8–11 proteins, and SMARCB1 is a core member, present in all variants of the complex. The complex has elements which disrupt DNA binding to histones, enhancing transcription.

Loss of function of SMARCB1 is seen in the large majority of AT/RTs (95–97), and is the only mutation necessary in these. Loss of immunohistochemical staining for the gene product allows rapid identification of these tumours.

Although originally identified to be important in rhabdoid tumours, mutations of SMARCB1 are found in up to 20% of all cancers. Loss-of-function mutations of SMARCB1 are important factors in the oncogenesis in a subset of highly aggressive cancers in young children (94). However, loss of *only* SMARCB1 is seen in AT/RT, whilst many other mutations are typically seen in other malignancies. In the series of patients with AT/RT reported by Hasselblatt, using high-resolution genome-wide analysis with a molecular inversion probe single-nucleotide polymorphism (MIP SNP) assay, alterations at this locus were identified in 15/16 cases, but not in any other cancer-relevant genes (98). AT/RT is most unusual in carrying such limited diversity of mutation.

Approximately 5% of AT/RTs lack a *SMARCB1* gene deletion. It is likely that another member of the chromatin remodelling complex, *SMARCA4*, is lost in some of these cases, although the general importance of this gene is not clear (99).

Although the downstream molecular actions are not clear, it is known that the complex regulates the cell cycle and cooperates with p53 to prevent oncogenic transformation (100, 101). INI1/hSNF5 appears to cause transcriptional repression of the cyclin D1 gene, through histone deacetylase (102, 103).

Familial rhabdoid tumours

Ten to fifteen per cent of children with rhabdoid tumours have synchronous or metachronous brain tumours, and many of these are second primary malignant rhabdoid tumours. Germline mutations of *SMARCB1* are common, particularly in younger children, and these are associated both with familial predisposition, and multiple tumours. In the series of von Hoff et al., a germline mutation was identified in 35% of patients, and in these, younger, patients, an adverse outcome was seen. A high frequency of germline mutation in younger patients and a more aggressive clinical course has been reported in these (104–106). The identification of a familial rhabdoid tumour without *INI1* mutation indicated a second locus for this tumour, being *SMARCA4* (99) (107).

Familial schwannomatosis

In recent years, the association of the *SMARCB1* gene with familial schwannomatosis has presented an interesting additional question (106, 108–110). Although normally associated with neurofibromatosis type 2 (NF2), loss of the *NF2* locus is not seen in familial cases of Schwannoma without vestibular Schwannoma (111). The candidate gene most likely to be responsible is *SMARCB1*: the gene is located centromeric to *NF2*, very close to a linkage marker for familial schwannomatosis (108). Why loss of expression might lead to differing tumours is not fully understood, although the loss of exon 1 is associated with schwannomata, whereas most mutations in rhabdoid tumours involve exons 2, 4, 5, 6, 7, and 9 (112, 113).

Treatment and prognosis for AT/RT

The prognosis for AT/RT had, until relatively recently, been extremely poor. In the series originally reported by Rorke et al., median time to progression was 4.5 months, and median OS was 6 months (93). The Cleveland AT/RT registry included 42 patients, of whom 20 received radiotherapy (114). Median survival was 48 months (range 10–96 months). An analysis of patients with AT/RT from 1988 to 2004, in the German HIT database showed a median survival of 1.0 (range 0.1–3.1) year (115). EFS and OS at three years were 13% ± 5% and 22% ± 6%.

More recently, the development of more systematic strategies has led to significant improvement, and the identification of important prognostic factors. Most strategies have included radiotherapy, although there is no study comparing radiotherapy with other approaches such as high-dose chemotherapy.

The first prospective series of patients treated with a consistent approach was reported by Chi et al. (116). Twenty-five patients, aged 2.4 months to 19.5 years, were enrolled, and treated with aggressive multimodality therapy including craniospinal radiation, intrathecal chemotherapy, and intensive systemic chemotherapy. Toxicity was severe, with one treatment-related death and a further patient developing spinal radiation recall and transverse myelitis. However the 2-year OS and EFS reported of 70% ± 10% and 53% ± 13% were encouraging. Patients who achieved complete remission (CR) during therapy did well, whilst those with residual (progressive) disease almost all died. In this series, 15/25 patients received radiotherapy, but the importance of radiotherapy cannot be inferred from the data.

The role of surgery in AT/RT

There is a clear benefit for patients who achieve surgical CR in most reported cases. In the report by Hilden et al. (114), 10/21 patients remained alive having achieved a surgical complete clearance, compared to 4/21 who did not. Comparable data were found for the patients identified in the UK review (6/13 alive after surgical CR compared to 4/20 where this was not achieved and 0/14 where information was not available).

Further support for surgical resection being of prognostic value comes from the recent DFCI study (see below).

The role of radiotherapy in AT/RT

Radiotherapy has been used for the majority of patients treated successfully for AT/RT, and it is an important component of current strategies. There is some confounding of data, however, since patients who have not received radiotherapy are likely to be those who show early progression, poor clinical state, or are very young. Radiotherapy is often part of a systematic approach to treatment, and there may be a beneficial effect from this alone.

The data reported by Hilden et al. (114) showed some benefit associated with radiotherapy (8/13 patients alive after radiotherapy compared to 6/29 alive who had not received radiotherapy). Tekautz et al. reported 22 patients treated under the age of 3 years were treated according to the SJMB96 protocol without radiotherapy, of whom only one patient survived (117). Two patients received radiation therapy in addition to chemotherapy, and both were alive at the time of publication.

Chen et al. reported survival of only three of seventeen patients who underwent complete surgical resection and craniospinal radiation therapy. In this setting, radiotherapy appeared to be ineffective (118).

It seems reasonable to conclude that radiation therapy is associated with a higher rate of local control in patients who also receive chemotherapy, and may improve long-term survival. CSRT does not seem to be associated with a higher OS. The concern for young children is are the severe neuropsychological sequelae produced by radiotherapy to the brain, and efforts continue to attempt to avoid this.

Intrathecal therapy

Intrathecal (IT) therapy in the presence of bulky disease does not affect outcome. Reports by Chou and Anderson (119) as well as Weinblatt and Kochen (120) showed no benefit in patients with significant disease after surgical resection.

The role of IT therapy with minimal residual (microscopic) disease is unclear, and again, no systematic study has been done. IT therapy was used with the earliest successful regimens (121), and anecdotal evidence is available elsewhere. Hilden et al. reported four patients who received intrathecal thiotepa following subtotal tumour resection, chemotherapy, and high-dose chemotherapy (114).

Zimmerman et al. reported four patients who received chemotherapy, triple intrathecal therapy (MTX, ara-C, hydrocortisone), and two with radiotherapy (123). All were alive without evidence of disease at the time of publication.

Data are still limited to support the role of IT therapy in AT/RT. Many of the patients who have been successfully treated have undergone treatment in a systematic manner where all available therapies have been administered. Again, the value or otherwise is unlikely to be addressed until consistent reports of improved survival are seen.

High-dose chemotherapy

High-dose therapy has been used most often in infants, which is a selected group for whom a higher likelihood of germline mutation is expected. Most data are anecdotal, but indicate a possible role in some patients (114, 122, 124–129).

Dallorso et al. reviewed the role of high-dose chemotherapy in a series of 29 AT/RT patients included into the AIEOP trial (130). Thirteen patients received myeloablative chemotherapy. The EFS at 5 years did not differ between patients who received conventional chemotherapy and those who received high-dose chemotherapy. Thus, the authors concluded that the role of high-dose chemotherapy has to be judged as questionable.

A recent report by Lafay-Cousin et al. is informative (131). Forty patients (median age 16.7 months) were treated with surgery, chemotherapy and radiotherapy, or high-dose chemotherapy. Surgical CR was associated with significantly better survival (2-year OS 60% vs 21.7%, $P = 0.03$). Eighteen patients received high-dose therapy, and OS for these patients at 2 years was 47.9% ± 12.1% compared to 27.3% ± 9.5% for the group who underwent conventional chemotherapy. Radiotherapy was not associated with any significant improvement in survival compared to those who did not receive it (median survival 17.8 months vs 14 months, $P = 0.64$). Six of the twelve survivors received no radiotherapy.

It would seem that there may be a useful role for high-dose therapy in AT/RT, and its purpose may be to avoid the need for, or allow a reduced dose of, radiotherapy in those patients where this would be unduly hazardous. There is now a need for a multi-national study to compare these options.

Pineoblastoma

Until recently, pineoblastoma was considered a type of CNS-PNET, a disease group now no longer considered a diagnostic entity (see below). Cytogenetic and subsequently genomic and epigenetic-based techniques clearly showed that pineal and non-pineal CNS-PNET differed not only in their site of origin but also in their genetic identities. In the current WHO classification of CNS tumours, pineoblastoma is now clearly defined as a distinct tumour (132).

Pineoblastomas are very rare, with around one or two cases per year in the United Kingdom. As with other tumours previously diagnosed as PNET, treatment has been given with protocols principally designed for high-risk MB. Thus patients over the age of 3–5 years have been treatment with surgical excision, radiotherapy with a dose of 35–36 Gy to the craniospinal axis, and various chemotherapy regimens.

It is clear from a number of series (133–136) that pineoblastomas have a superior outcome to other non-MB embryonal tumours with 3–5-year EFS/PFS in the order of 60–75%. These reasonably good outcomes may, however, just apply to older non-metastatic patients, as noted for the PNET-3 series where the prognosis for those with metastatic disease was very poor (137) as is the outcome for infants not treated with radiotherapy.

The St Jude study of PNETs suggested that so-called average-risk patients (completely resected and non-metastatic) with these tumours, including pineoblastomas may have good survival with reduced dose CSRT (i.e. 23.4 Gy), although this needs to be conformed in larger series (136).

Other embryonal tumours

As with other CNS tumour groups, there has been an explosion in our knowledge and understanding of embryonal tumours. Until recently, the majority of embryonal tumours not diagnosed as either MB or AT/RT were included in the diagnostic category of CNS-PNET. In turn, the concept of PNETs was originally proposed by Hart and Earle in recognition of the similar histological characteristics of cerebellar PNETs (MB) and supratentorial PNETs (StPNETs) (138). Although this was accepted for many years, there appeared clear evidence of differences between the molecular biology and the cells of origin of MB and StPNETs (139). The term CNS-PNET was then used in preference to StPNET in recognition of the fact that non-MB PNET may rarely arise in the posterior fossa as well as the supratentorial region.

As a group, embryonal tumours previously diagnosed as CNS-PNET are rare, around 2–3% of CNS tumours in childhood, with a mean age of presentation of 5.5 years (137, 140). Most are cortical tumours but until recently the spectrum of CNS-PNET included pineoblastoma.

In 2000, Eberhart et al. described a variant of StPNET, the 'embryonal tumour with abundant neuropil and true rosettes (ETANTR)' as a tumour exhibiting prominent ependymoblastic rosettes, neuronal differentiation, and a neuropil background (141). This tumour was predominantly reported in young children and was accepted as having a very poor prognosis. The Heidelberg group subsequently described a novel genomic amplification targeting the microRNA cluster at 19q13.42 in ETANTRs (142). More recently, in 2014, the same team reported that a group that appears to clearly separate from other embryonal tumours are the now termed embryonal tumours with multilayer rosettes (ETMRs). ETMR is now recognized as containing the three histological variants ETANTR, ependymoblastoma, and medulloepithelioma (143). Although histologically these three tumour types may appear different, they are genetically indistinguishable. Almost all of them harbour the C19MC amplicon and are highly positive for LIN28A, although LIN28A is not totally specific for ETMRs, for example, some expression in AT/RTs and in germ cell tumours. Similar findings were reported by Spence et al. (144).

Of particular importance has been the observation from genomics and especially epigenetic studies appear to clearly show that the tumour group that was understood as CNS-PNET is a very heterogeneous group of tumours of which many are often misdiagnosed.

The Newcastle group in the United Kingdom, in collaboration with others, has demonstrated the utility of DNA methylation profiling for the discovery and distinction of clinical and molecular subclasses of brain tumour types (145). Using DNA methylation profiling, they assessed a series of 29 institutionally diagnosed archival CNS-PNET alongside assessment of clinical and molecular characteristics. CNS-PNET did not form a single discrete group; indeed, CNS-PNET clustered into six different tumour groups, showing closer similarities to other clinically and molecularly defined paediatric brain tumour groups investigated in parallel. For example, around 30% clustered with high-grade glioma. This work showed that despite a defining histological homogeneity using accepted diagnostic criteria, tumours diagnosed as CNS-PNET displayed highly heterogeneous DNA methylation patterns that are more commonly related to other paediatric brain tumour types than to each other.

The Heidelberg group in Germany has also used DNA methylation together with gene expression arrays to compare the data generated from a large number of institutionally diagnosed 'CNS-PNET' to a very large cohort of other brain tumours. They also noted that the majority of these tumours can be reclassified into known entities like ETMR, AT/RT, glioblastoma, or ependymoma (146).

These studies and others based on new genomic and epigenetic information have completely altered understanding and indeed nosology of embryonal tumours other than MB and AT/RT. This together with a re-evaluation of the histological aspects of embryonal tumours has resulted in the term CNS-PNET being removed from the 2016 WHO classification of CNS tumours (132). Instead, the classification refers to the following diagnoses within the overarching embryonal group: ETMR C19MC-altered, ETMR NOS, medulloepithelioma, CNS neuroblastoma, CNS ganglioneuroblastoma, CNS embryonal tumour NOS.

Alongside the histological reclassification of embryonal tumours, further work has proposed new molecular classifications of this heterogenous tumour group. In 2016, Sturm et al. from the Heidelburg group proposed four new CNS tumour entities, each associated with a recurrent genetic alteration and distinct histopathological and clinical features. These new molecular entities were designated: 'CNS neuroblastoma with FOXR2 activation (CNS NB-FOXR2)', 'CNS Ewing sarcoma family tumour with CIC alteration (CNS EFT-CIC)', 'CNS high-grade neuroepithelial tumour with MN1 alteration (CNS HGNET-MN1)', and 'CNS high-grade neuroepithelial tumour with BCOR alteration (CNS HGNET-BCOR)' (143).

In conclusion, these and other data confirm that the group of embryonal tumours previously recognized as CNS-PNETs are a heterogeneous group of tumours and a significant proportion may represent a subgroup of recognized tumour types including high-grade glioma as well as new histological and molecularly defined groups now entering the lexicon of CNS tumour classification.

Management

Embryonal tumours previous referred to as CNS-PNETs have generally been treated with protocols designed for children with high-risk MB with many historical trials and series including both tumour groups. Thus the accepted standard therapy is to remove the tumour as completely as possible. Historically, for children aged at least 3 years of age, CSRT is delivered with a dose of 35–36 Gy with a boost to the primary tumour of approximately 18 Gy. Conventional intensity chemotherapy is generally administered according to combinations of drugs used in high-risk MB protocols, although some protocols have also included myeloablative chemotherapy with stem cell rescue.

Examples of older series of embryonal tumours classified as CNS-PNET come from the SIOP PNET-3 (135), HIT 88/89 and 91 (134), and CCG-921 (146) studies. More recently, the COG reported the outcome and prognostic factors for children with 'ST PNETs' treated with carboplatin during radiotherapy in accordance to the phase II trial for high-risk MB (147).

Prognosis for these and other series reported survivals for 'non-pineal CNS-PNETs' of around 30–45%. It is of note, however, that these series may contain patients with other tumour types including high-grade glioma and do not take into account the new histological and molecular classification of embryonal tumours.

The observation that embryonal tumours other than MB, AT/RT, and pineoblastoma consist of a number of entities requires further study to fully classify these tumours and to develop focused therapeutic protocols. It also suggests that such tumours should be subject to molecular characterization as well as central pathological review, at least to enable the diagnosis of ETMR and to rule out well-defined entities such as high-grade glioma which, for example, may not require CSRT. Further translational and clinical research is needed to fully classify these tumours and to develop focused therapeutic protocols and because of the rarity of these tumours, global collaboration is clearly required.

References

1. Louis DN, Perry A, Reifenberger G, et al. The 2016 World Health Organization Classification of Tumors of the Central Nervous System: a summary. *Acta Neuropathol* 2016; 131:803–820.

2. Chang CH, Housepian EM, Herbert C, Jr. An operative staging system and a megavoltage radiotherapeutic technique for cerebellar medulloblastomas. *Radiology* 1969; 93:1351–1359.

3. Taylor MD, Northcott PA, Korshunov A, et al. Molecular subgroups of medulloblastoma: the current consensus. *Acta Neuropathol* 2012; 123:465–472.

4. Northcott PA, Jones DTW, Kool M, et al. Medulloblastomics: the end of the beginning. *Nat Rev Cancer* 2012; 12:818–834.

5. Pizer BL, Clifford SC. The potential impact of tumor biology on improved clinical practice for medulloblastoma: progress towards biologically driven clinical trials. *Br J Neurosurg* 2009; 23:364–375.

6. Ellison DW, Onilude OE, Lindsey JC, et al. beta-Catenin status predicts a favorable outcome in childhood medulloblastoma: the United Kingdom Children's Cancer Study Group Brain Tumour Committee. *J Clin Oncol* 2005; 23(31):7951–7957.

7. Taylor RE, Bailey CC, Robinson K, et al. Results of a randomized study of preradiation chemotherapy versus radiotherapy alone for nonmetastatic medulloblastoma: The International Society of Paediatric Oncology/United Kingdom Children's Cancer Study Group PNET-3 Study. *J Clin Oncol* 2003; 21:1581–1591.

8. Mulhern RK, Kepner JL, Thomas PR, et al. Neuropsychologic functioning of survivors of childhood medulloblastoma randomized to receive conventional or reduced-dose craniospinal irradiation: a Pediatric Oncology Group study. *J Clin Oncol* 1998; 16:1723–1728.

9. Packer RJ, Goldwein J, Nicholson HS, et al. Treatment of children with medulloblastomas with reduced-dose craniospinal radiation therapy and adjuvant chemotherapy: a Children's Cancer Group Study. *J Clin Oncol* 1999; 17:2127–2136.

10. Packer RJ, Gajjar A, Vezina G, et al. Phase III study of craniospinal radiation therapy followed by adjuvant chemotherapy for newly diagnosed average-risk medulloblastoma. *J Clin Oncol* 2006; 24:4202–4208.

11. Bouffet E, Bernard JL, Frappaz D, et al. M4 protocol for cerebellar medulloblastoma: supratentorial radiotherapy may not be avoided. *Int J Radiat Oncol Biol Phys* 1992; 24:79–85.

12. Thomas PR, Deutsch M, Kepner JL, et al. Low-stage medulloblastoma: final analysis of trial comparing standard-dose with reduced-dose neuraxis irradiation. *J Clin Oncol* 2000; 18:3004–3011.

13. Carrie C, Muracciole X, Gomez F, et al. Conformal radiotherapy, reduced boost volume, hyperfractionated radiotherapy, and online quality control in standard-risk medulloblastoma without chemotherapy: results of the French M-SFOP 98 protocol. *Int J Radiat Oncol Biol Phys* 2005; 63:711–716.

14. Lannering B, Rutkowski S, Doz F, et al. Hyperfractionated vs conventional radiotherapy followed by chemotherapy in standard-risk medulloblastoma: Results from the randomized multicenter study HIT-SIOP PNET 4. *J Clin Oncol* 2012; 30:3187–3193.

15. Kennedy C, Bull K, Chevignard M, et al. Quality of survival and growth in children and young adults in the PNET4 European controlled trial of hyperfractionated versus conventional radiation therapy for standard-risk medulloblastoma. *Int J Radiat Oncol Biol Phys* 2014; 88:292–300.

16. Fukunaga-Johnson N, Lee JH, Sandler HM, et al. Patterns of failure following treatment for medulloblastoma: is it necessary to treat the entire posterior fossa? *Int J Radiat Oncol Biol Phys* 1998; 42:143–146.

17. Michalski J, Vezina G, Burger P, et al. Preliminary results of COG ACNS 0331: a phase III trial of involved field radiotherapy (IFRT) and low dose craniospinal irradiation (LD-CSI) with chemotherapy in average risk medulloblastoma: a report from the children's oncology group. *Neuro-Oncology* 2016; 18:iii97–iii122.

18. Gajjar A, Chintagumpala M, Ashley D, et al. Risk-adapted craniospinal radiotherapy followed by high-dose chemotherapy and stem-cell rescue in children with newly diagnosed medulloblastoma (St Jude Medulloblastoma-96): long-term results from a prospective, multi centre trial. *Lancet Oncol* 2006; 7:813–820.

19. Rutkowski S, Gerber NU, von Hoff K, et al. Treatment of early childhood medulloblastoma by postoperative chemotherapy and deferred radiotherapy. *Neuro Oncol* 2009; 11:201–210.

20. Ashley DM, Merchant TE, Strother D, et al. Induction chemotherapy and conformal radiation therapy for very young children with nonmetastatic medulloblastoma: Children's Oncology Group study P9934. *J Clin Oncol* 2012; 30:3181–3186.

21. Zeltzer PM, Boyett JM, Finlay JL, et al. Metastasis stage, adjuvant treatment, and residual tumor are prognostic factors for medulloblastoma in children: conclusions from the Children's Cancer Group 921 randomized phase III study. *J Clin Oncol* 1999; 17:832–845.

22. Bailey CC, Gnekow A, Wellek S, et al. Prospective randomised trial of chemotherapy given before radiotherapy in childhood medulloblastoma. International Society of Paediatric Oncology (SIOP) and the (German) Society of Paediatric Oncology (GPO): SIOP II. *Med Pediatr Oncol* 1995; 25:166–178.

23. Dufour C, Beaugrand A, Pizer B, et al. Metastatic medulloblastoma in childhood: Chang's classification revisited. *Int J Surg Oncol* 2012; 2012:245385.

24. Albright AL, Wisoff JH, Zeltzer PM, et al. Effects of medulloblastoma resections on outcome in children: a report from the Children's Cancer Group. *Neurosurgery* 1996; 38:265–271.

25. Thompson EM, Hielscher T, Bouffet E, et al. Prognostic value of medulloblastoma extent of resection after accounting for molecular subgroup: a retrospective integrated clinical and molecular analysis. *Lancet Oncol* 2016; 17:484–495.

26. Ellison DW. Classifying the medulloblastoma: insights from morphology and molecular genetics. *Neuropathol Appl Neurobiol* 2002; 28:257–282.

27. Eberhart CG, Burger PC. Anaplasia and grading in medulloblastomas. *Brain Pathol* 2003; 13:376–385.

28. McManamy CS, Lamont JM, Taylor RE, et al. Morphophenotypic variation predicts clinical behaviour in childhood non-desmoplastic medulloblastomas. *J Neuropath Exp Neurol* 2003; 62:627–632.

29. Lamont JM, MacManamy CS, Taylor RE, et al. Molecular pathological stratification of disease risk in medulloblastoma. *Clin Cancer Res* 2004; 10:5482–5493.

30. Kortmann RD, Kuhl J, Timmermann B, et al. Postoperative neoadjuvant chemotherapy before radiotherapy as compared to immediate radiotherapy followed by maintenance chemotherapy in the treatment of medulloblastoma in childhood: results of the German prospective randomized trial HIT '91. *Int J Radiat Oncol Biol Phys* 2000; 46:269–279.

31. Taylor RE, Bailey CC, Robinson KJ, et al. Outcome for patients with metastatic (M2-3) medulloblastoma treated with SIOP/UKCCSG PNET-3 chemotherapy. *Eur J Cancer* 2005; 41:727–734.

32. Tarbell NJ, Friedman H, Polkinghorn WR, et al. High-risk medulloblastoma: a pediatric oncology group randomized trial of chemotherapy before or after radiation therapy (POG 9031). *J Clin Oncol* 2013; 31:2936–2941.

33. Jakacki RI, Burger PC, Zhou T, et al. Outcome of children with metastatic medulloblastoma treated with carboplatin during craniospinal radiotherapy: a Children's Oncology Group Phase I/II study. *J Clin Oncol.* 2012; 30:2648–2653.

34. Gandola L, Massimino M, Cefalo G, et al. Hyperfractionated accelerated radiotherapy in the Milan strategy for metastatic medulloblastoma. *J Clin Oncol* 2009; 27:566–571.

35. Gandola L, Horan G, Meroni S, et al. Intensive treatment of high-risk medulloblastoma (HR-MB): how to learn from toxicities in an European setting of radiotherapists and physicists of the SIOP Brain Tumor Working Group. *Neuro-Oncology* 2016 18:iii97–iii122.

36. Taylor RE, Howman, AJ, Wheatley K, et al. Hyperfractionated accelerated radiotherapy (HART) with maintenance chemotherapy for metastatic (M1-3) Medulloblastoma—a safety feasibility study. *Radiother Oncol* 2014; 111:41–46

37. Rutkowski S, von Hoff K, Emser A, et al. Survival and prognostic factors of early childhood medulloblastoma: an international meta-analysis. *J Clin Oncol* 2010; 28:4961–4968.

38. Grundy RG, Wilne SH, Robinson KJ, et al. Primary postoperative chemotherapy without radiotherapy for treatment of brain tumors other than ependymoma in children under 3 years: results of the first UKCCSG/SIOP CNS 9204 trial. Children's Cancer and Leukaemia Group (formerly UKCCSG) Brain Tumour Committee. *Eur J Cancer* 2010; 46:120–133.

39. von Bueren AO, von Hoff K, Pietsch T, et al. Treatment of young children with localized medulloblastoma by chemotherapy alone: results of the prospective, multicenter trial HIT 2000 confirming the prognostic impact of histology. *Neuro-Oncology* 2011; 13:669–679.

40. Dhall G, Grodman H, Ji L, et al. Outcome of children less than three years old at diagnosis with non-metastatic medulloblastoma treated with chemotherapy on the "Head Start" I and II protocols. *Pediatr Blood Cancer* 2008; 50:1169–1175.

41. Mandera M, Marcol W, Kotulska K, et al. Childhood pineal parenchymal tumors: clinical and therapeutic aspects. *Neurosurg Rev* 2010; 34(2):191–196.

42. Dumrongpisutikul N, Intrapiromkul J, Yousem DM. Distinguishing between germinomas and pineal cell tumors on MR imaging. *AJNR Am J Neuroradiol* 2012; 33(3):550–555.

43. Carrie C, Alapetite C, Mere P, et al. Quality control of radiotherapeutic treatment of medulloblastoma in a multicentric study: the contribution of radiotherapy technique to tumor relapse. The French Medulloblastoma Group. *Radiother. Oncol* 1992; 24:77–81.

44. Carrie C, Hoffstetter S, Gomez F, et al. Impact of targeting deviations on outcome in medulloblastoma: study of the French Society of Pediatric Oncology (SFOP). *Int J Radiat Oncol Biol Phys* 1999; 45:435–439.

45. Taylor RE, Lucraft H, Bailey CC, et al. Impact of radiotherapy parameters on outcome in the International Society of Paediatric Oncology (SIOP)/United Kingdom Children's Cancer Study Group (UKCCSG) PNET-3 study of pre-radiotherapy chemotherapy for M0-1. *Int J Radiat Oncol Biol Phys* 2004; 58:1184–1193.

46. Chung, CS, Yock TI, Nelson K, et al. Incidence of second malignancies among patients treated with proton versus photon radiation. *Int J Radiat Oncol Biol Phys* 2013; 87(1):46–52.

47. St. Clair WH, Adams JA, Bues M, et al. Advantage of protons compared to conventional X-ray or IMRT in the treatment of a pediatric patient with medulloblastoma. *Int J Radiat Oncol Biol Phys* 2004; 58(3):727–734.

48. Eaton BR, MacDonald SM, Yock TI, et al. Secondary malignancy risk following proton radiation therapy. *Front Oncol* 2015; 5:261.

49. Zhang R, Howell RM, Giebeler A, et al. Comparison of risk of radiogenic second cancer following photon and proton craniospinal irradiation for a pediatric medulloblastoma patient. *Phys Med Biol* 2013; 58:807–823.

50. Mulhern RK, Merchant TE, Gajjar A, et al. Late neurocognitive sequelae in survivors of brain tumors in childhood. *Lancet Oncol* 2004; 5:399–408.

51. Miralbell R, Lomax A, Bortfeld T, et al. Potential role of proton therapy in the treatment of pediatric medulloblastoma/primitive neuroectodermal tumors: reduction of the supratentorial target volume. *Int J Radiat Oncol Biol Phys* 1997; 38:477–484.

52. Yock TI, Yeap BY, Ebb DH, et al. Long-term toxic effects of proton radiotherapy for paediatric medulloblastoma: a phase 2 single-arm study. *Lancet Oncol* 2016; 17(3):287–298.

53. Ris MD, Packer R, Goldwein J, et al. Intellectual outcome after reduced-dose radiation therapy plus adjuvant chemotherapy for medulloblastoma: a Children's Cancer Group study. *J Clin Oncol* 2001; 19:3470–3476.

54. Butler RW, Mulhern RK. Neurocognitive interventions for children and adolescents surviving cancer. *J Pediatr Psychol* 2005; 30:65–78.

55. Mabbott DJ, Spiegler BJ, Greenberg ML, et al. Serial evaluation of academic and behavioral outcome after treatment with cranial radiation in childhood. *J Clin Oncol* 2005; 23:2256–2263.

56. Eaton BR, Esiashvili N, Kim S, et al. Endocrine outcomes with proton and photon radiotherapy for standard risk medulloblastoma. *Neuro-Oncology* 2016; 18(6):881–887.

57. Merchant TE, Williams T, Smith JM, et al. Preirradiation endocrinopathies in pediatric brain tumor patients determined by dynamic tests of endocrine function. *Int J Radiat Oncol Biol Phys* 2002; 54:45–50.

58. Gurney JG, Kadan-Lottick NS, Packer RJ, et al. Endocrine and cardiovascular late effects among adult survivors of childhood brain tumors: Childhood Cancer Survivor Study. *Cancer* 2003; 97:663–673.

59. Crocetti E, Trama A, Stiller C, et al. Epidemiology of glial and non-glial brain tumors in Europe. *Eur J Cancer* 2012; 48:1532–1542.

60. Verdecchia A, Francisci S, Brenner H, et al. Recent cancer survival in Europe: a 2000-02 period analysis of EUROCARE-4 data. *Lancet Oncol* 2007; 8:784–796.

61. Chan AW, Tarbell NJ, Black PM, et al. Adult medulloblastoma: prognostic factors and patterns of relapse. *Neurosurgery* 2000; 47:623–631.

62. Rochkind S, Blatt I, Sadeh M, et al. Extracranial metastases of medulloblastoma in adults: literature review. *J Neurol Neurosurg Psychiatry* 1991; 54:80–86.

63. Herms J, Neidt I, Luscher B, et al. C-MYC expression in medulloblastoma and its prognostic value. *Int J Cancer* 2000; 89:395–402.

64. Grotzer MA, Hogarty MD, Janss AJ, et al. MYC messenger RNA expression predicts survival outcome in childhood primitive neuroectodermal tumor/medulloblastoma. *Clin Cancer Res* 2001; 7:2425–2433.

65. Biegel JA, Janss AJ, Raffel C, et al. Prognostic significance of chromosome 17p deletions in childhood primitive neuroectodermal tumors (medulloblastomas) of the central nervous system. *Clin Cancer Res* 1997; 3:473–478.

66. Batra SK, McLendon RE, Koo JS, et al. Prognostic implications of chromosome 17p deletions in human medulloblastomas. *J Neurooncol* 1995; 24:39–45.

67. Ray A, Ho M, Ma J, et al. A clinicobiological model predicting survival in medulloblastoma. *Clin Cancer Res* 2004; 10:7613–7620.

68. Pomeroy SL, Tamayo P, Gaasenbeek M, et al. Prediction of central nervous system embryonal tumor outcome based on gene expression. *Nature* 2002; 415:436–442.

69. Remke M, Hielscher T, Northcott PA, et al. Adult medulloblastoma comprises three major molecular variants. *J Clin Oncol* 2011; 29:2717–2723.

70. Northcott PA, Korshunov A, Witt H, et al. Medulloblastoma comprises four distinct molecular variants. *J Clin Oncol* 2011; 29:1408–1414.

71. Kool M, Korshunov A, Remke M, et al. Molecular subgroups of medulloblastoma: an international meta-analysis of transcriptome, genetic aberrations, and clinical data of WNT, SHH, Group 3, and Group 4 medulloblastomas. *Acta Neuropathol* 2012; 123:473–484.

72. Ramaswamy V, Remke M, Bouffet E, et al. Recurrence patterns across medulloblastoma subgroups: an integrated clinical and molecular analysis. *Lancet Oncol* 2013; 14:1200–1207.

73. Northcott PA, Korshunov A, Pfister SM, et al. The clinical implications of medulloblastoma subgroups. *Nat Rev Neurol* 2012; 8:340–351.

74. Packer RJ, Rood BR, MacDonald TJ. Medulloblastoma: present concepts of stratification into risk groups. *Pediatr Neurosurg* 2003; 39:60–67.

75. Tabori U, Sung L, Hukin J, et al. Distinctive clinical course and pattern of relapse in adolescents with medulloblastoma. *Int J Radiat Oncol Biol Phys* 2006; 64:402–407.

76. Brandes AA, Ermani M, Amista P, et al. The treatment of adults with medulloblastoma: a prospective study. *Int J Radiat Oncol Biol Phys* 2003; 57:755–761.

77. Brandes AA, Franceschi E, Tosoni A, et al. Long-term results of a prospective study on the treatment of medulloblastoma in adults. *Cancer* 2007; 110:2035–2041.

78. Padovani L, Sunyach MP, Perol D, et al. Common strategy for adult and pediatric medulloblastoma: a multicenter series of 253 adults. *Int J Radiat Oncol Biol Phys* 2007; 68:433–440.

79. Kortmann RD, Kuhl J, Timmermann B, et al. Postoperative neoadjuvant chemotherapy before radiotherapy as compared to immediate radiotherapy followed by maintenance chemotherapy in the treatment of medulloblastoma in childhood: results of the German prospective randomized trial HIT '91. *Int J Radiat Oncol Biol Phys* 2000; 46:269–279.

80. Shonka N, Brandes A, De Groot JF. Adult medulloblastoma, from spongioblastoma cerebelli to the present day: a review of treatment and the integration of molecular markers. *Oncology (Williston Park)* 2012; 26:1083–1091.

81. Hubbard JL, Scheithauer BW, Kispert DB, et al. Adult cerebellar medulloblastomas: the pathological, radiographic, and clinical disease spectrum. *J Neurosurg* 1989; 70:536–544.

82. Ferrante L, Mastronardi L, Celli P, et al. Medulloblastoma in adulthood. *J Neurosurg Sci* 1991; 35:23–30.

83. Kortmann RD, Kuhl J, Timmermann B, et al. [Current and future strategies in interdisciplinary treatment of medulloblastomas, supratentorial PNET (primitive neuroectodermal tumors) and intracranial germ cell tumors in childhood]. *Strahlenther Onkol* 2001; 177:447–461.

84. Berry MP, Jenkin RD, Keen CW, et al. Radiation treatment for medulloblastoma. A 21-year review. *J Neurosurg* 1981; 55:43–51.

85. Bloom HJ, Bessell EM. Medulloblastoma in adults: a review of 47 patients treated between 1952 and 1981. *Int J Radiat Oncol Biol Phys* 1990; 18:763–772.

86. Hazuka MB, DeBiose DA, Henderson RH, et al. Survival results in adult patients treated for medulloblastoma. *Cancer* 1992; 69:2143–2148

87. Abacioglu U, Uzel O, Sengoz M, et al. Medulloblastoma in adults: treatment results and prognostic factors. *Int J Radiat Oncol Biol Phys* 2002; 54:855–860.

88. Friedrich C, von Bueren AO, von Hoff K, et al. Treatment of adult nonmetastatic medulloblastoma patients according to the paediatric HIT 2000 protocol: a prospective observational multicentre study. *Eur J Cancer* 2013; 49:893–903.

89. Rudin CM, Hann CL, Laterra J, et al. Treatment of medulloblastoma with hedgehog pathway inhibitor GDC-0449. *N Engl J Med* 2009; 361:1173–1178.

90. Yauch RL, Dijkgraaf GJ, Alicke B, et al. Smoothened mutation confers resistance to a hedgehog pathway inhibitor in medulloblastoma. *Science* 2009; 326:572–574.

91. Buonamici S, Williams J, Morrissey M, et al. Interfering with resistance to smoothened antagonists by inhibition of the PI3K pathway in medulloblastoma. *Sci Transl Med* 2010; 2:51ra70.

92. Rorke LB, Packer R, Biegel J. Central nervous system atypical teratoid/rhabdoid tumors of infancy and childhood. *J Neurooncol* 1995; 24:21–28.

93. Rorke LB, Packer RJ, Biegel JA. Central nervous system atypical teratoid/rhabdoid tumors of infancy and childhood: definition of an entity. *J Neurosurg* 1996; 85:56–65.

94. Sevenet N, Sheridan E, Amram D, et al. Constitutional mutations of the hSNF5/INI1 gene predispose to a variety of cancers. *Am J Hum Genet* 1999; 65:1342–1348.

95. Versteege I, Sevenet N, Lange J, et al. Truncating mutations of hSNF5/INI1 in aggressive paediatric cancer. *Nature* 1998; 394:203–206.

96. Biegel JA, Zhou JY, Rorke LB, et al. Germ-line and acquired mutations of INI1 in atypical teratoid and rhabdoid tumors. *Cancer Res* 1999; 59:74–79.

97. Sigauke E, Rakheja D, Maddox DL, et al. Absence of expression of SMARCB1/INI1 in malignant rhabdoid tumors of the central nervous system, kidneys and soft tissue: an immunohistochemical study with implications for diagnosis. *Mod Pathol* 2006; 19:717–725.

98. Hasselblatt M, Isken S, Linge A, et al. High-resolution genomic analysis suggests the absence of recurrent genomic alterations other than SMARCB1 aberrations in atypical teratoid/rhabdoid tumors. *Genes Chromosomes Cancer* 2013; 52:185–190.

99. Schneppenheim R, Fruhwald MC, Gesk S, et al. Germline nonsense mutation and somatic inactivation of SMARCA4/BRG1 in a family with rhabdoid tumor predisposition syndrome. *Am J Hum Genet* 2010; 86:279–284.

100. Isakoff MS, Sansam CG, Tamayo P, et al. Inactivation of the Snf5 tumor suppressor stimulates cell cycle progression and cooperates with p53 loss in oncogenic transformation. *Proc Natl Acad Sci U S A* 2005; 102:17745–17750.

101. Sansam CG, Roberts CW. Epigenetics and cancer: altered chromatin remodeling via Snf5 loss leads to aberrant cell cycle regulation. *Cell Cycle* 2006; 5:621–24.

102. Fujisawa H, Misaki K, Takabatake Y, et al. Cyclin D1 is overexpressed in atypical teratoid/rhabdoid tumor with hSNF5/INI1 gene inactivation. *J Neurooncol* 2005; 73:117–124.

103. Zhang ZK, Davies KP, Allen J, et al. Cell cycle arrest and repression of cyclin D1 transcription by INI1/hSNF5. *Mol Cell Biol* 2002; 22:5975–5988.

104. Kordes U, Gesk S, Fruhwald MC et al. Clinical and molecular features in patients with atypical teratoid rhabdoid tumor or malignant rhabdoid tumor. *Genes Chromosomes Cancer* 2010; 49:176–181.

105. Bourdeaut F, Dufour C, Delattre O. [Rhabdoid tumors: hSNF/INI1 deficient cancers of early childhood with aggressive behaviour]. *Bull Cancer* 2010; 97:37–45.

106. Eaton KW, Tooke LS, Wainwright LM, et al. Spectrum of SMARCB1/INI1 mutations in familial and sporadic rhabdoid tumors. *Pediatr Blood Cancer* 2011; 56:7–15.

107. Fruhwald MC, Hasselblatt M, Wirth S, et al. Non-linkage of familial rhabdoid tumors to SMARCB1 implies a second locus for the rhabdoid tumor predisposition syndrome. *Pediatr Blood Cancer* 2006; 47:273–278.

108. Hulsebos TJ, Plomp AS, Wolterman RA, et al. Germline mutation of INI1/SMARCB1 in familial schwannomatosis. *Am J Hum Genet* 2007; 80:805–810.

109. Hulsebos TJ, Kenter SB, Jakobs ME, et al. SMARCB1/INI1 maternal germ line mosaicism in schwannomatosis. *Clin Genet* 2010; 77:86–91.

110. Brennan PM, Barlow A, Geraghty A, et al. Multiple schwannomatosis caused by the recently described INI1 gene – molecular pathology, and implications for prognosis. *Br J Neurosurg* 2011; 25:330–332.

111. MacCollin M, Willett C, Heinrich B et al. Familial schwannomatosis: exclusion of the NF2 locus as the germline event. *Neurology* 2003; 60:1968–1974.

112. Janson K, Nedzi LA, David O, et al. Predisposition to atypical teratoid/rhabdoid tumor due to an inherited INI1 mutation. *Pediatr Blood Cancer* 2006; 47:279–284.

113. Biegel JA, Tan L, Zhang F, et al. Alterations of the hSNF5/INI1 gene in central nervous system atypical teratoid/rhabdoid tumors and renal and extrarenal rhabdoid tumors. *Clin Cancer Res* 2002; 8:3461–3467.

114. Hilden JM, Meerbaum S, Burger P, et al. Central nervous system atypical teratoid/rhabdoid tumor: results of therapy in children enrolled in a registry. *J Clin Oncol* 2004; 22:2877–2884.

115. von Hoff K, Hinkes B, Dannenmann-Stern E, et al. Frequency, risk-factors and survival of children with atypical teratoid rhabdoid tumors (AT/RT) of the CNS diagnosed between 1988 and 2004, and registered to the German HIT database. *Pediatr Blood Cancer* 2011; 57:978–985.

116. Chi SN, Zimmerman MA, Yao X, et al. Intensive multimodality treatment for children with newly diagnosed CNS atypical teratoid rhabdoid tumor. *J Clin Oncol* 2009; 27:385–389.

117. Tekautz TM, Fuller CE, Blaney S, et al. Atypical teratoid/rhabdoid tumors (ATRT): improved survival in children 3 years of age and older with radiation therapy and high-dose alkylator-based chemotherapy. *J Clin Oncol* 2005; 23:1491–1499.

118. Chen YW, Wong TT, Ho DM, et al. Impact of radiotherapy for pediatric CNS atypical teratoid/rhabdoid tumor (single institute experience). *Int J Radiat Oncol Biol Phys* 2006; 64:1038–1043.

119. Chou SM, Anderson JS. Primary CNS malignant rhabdoid tumor (MRT): report of two cases and review of literature. *Clin Neuropathol* 1990; 10:1–10.

120. Weinblatt M, Kochen J. Rhabdoid tumor of the central nervous system. *Med Pediatr Oncol* 1992; 20:258.

121. Olson TA, Bayar E, Kosnik E, et al. Successful treatment of disseminated central nervous system malignant rhabdoid tumor. *J Pediatr Hematol Oncol* 1995; 17:71–75.

122. Ronghe MD, Moss TH, Lowis SP. Treatment of CNS malignant rhabdoid tumors. *Pediatr Blood Cancer* 2004; 42:254–260.

123. Zimmerman MA, Goumnerova LC, Proctor M, et al. Continuous remission of newly diagnosed and relapsed central nervous system atypical teratoid/rhabdoid tumor. *J Neurooncol* 2005; 72:77–84.

124. Katzenstein HM, Kletzel M, Reynolds M, et al. Metastatic malignant rhabdoid tumor of the liver treated with tandem high-dose therapy and autologous peripheral blood stem cell rescue. *Med Pediatr Oncol* 2003; 40:199–201.

125. Sahdev I, James-Herry A, Scimeca P, et al. Concordant rhabdoid tumor of the kidney in a set of identical twins with discordant outcomes. *J Pediatr Hematol Oncol* 2003; 25:491–494.

126. Fujita M, Sato M, Nakamura M, et al. Multicentric atypical teratoid/rhabdoid tumors occurring in the eye and fourth ventricle of an infant: case report. *J Neurosurg* 2005; 102:299–302.

127. Watanabe H, Watanabe T, Kaneko M, et al. Treatment of unresectable malignant rhabdoid tumor of the orbit with tandem high-dose chemotherapy and gamma-knife radiosurgery. *Pediatr Blood Cancer* 2006; 47:846–850.

128. Beschorner R, Mittelbronn M, Koerbel A, et al. Atypical teratoid-rhabdoid tumor spreading along the trigeminal nerve. *Pediatr Neurosurg* 2006; 42:258–263.

129. Madigan CE, Armenian SH, Malogolowkin MH, ET AL. Extracranial malignant rhabdoid tumors in childhood. *Cancer* 2007; 110:2061–2066.

130. Dallorso S, Dini G, Ladenstein R, et al. Evolving role of myeloablative chemotherapy in the treatment of childhood brain tumors. *Bone Marrow Transplant* 2005; 35:S31–S34.

131. Lafay-Cousin L, Hawkins C, Carret AS, et al. Central nervous system atypical teratoid rhabdoid tumors: the Canadian Paediatric Brain Tumour Consortium experience. *Eur J Cancer* 2012; 48:353–359.

132. Louis DN, Ohgaki H, Wiestler OD, et al. The 2016 World Health Organization Classification of Tumors of the Central Nervous System. *Acta Neuropathol* 2016; 131(6):803–820.

133. Cohen, BH, Packer RJ. Chemotherapy for medulloblastomas and primitive neuroectodermal tumors. *J Neurooncol* 1996; 29:55–68.

134. Timmermann B, Kortmann RD, Kuhl J, et al. Role of radiotherapy in the treatment of supratentorial primitive neuroectodermal tumors in childhood: results of the prospective German brain tumor trials HIT 88/89 and 91. 2002 *J Clin Oncol* 20:842–849.

135. Pizer BL, Weston CL, Robinson KJ, et al. Analysis of patients with supratentorial primitive neuro-ectodermal tumours entered into the SIOP/UKCCSG PNET 3 study. *Eur J Cancer* 2006; 42:1120–1128.

136. Chintagumpala M, Hassall Palmer S, et al. A pilot study of risk-adapted radiotherapy and chemotherapy in patients with supratentorial PNET. *Neuro Oncol* 2009; 11:33–40.

137. Pizer B, Hayden J. Supratentorial PNETs: treatment. In: Hayat MA (ed) *Pediatric Cancer: Diagnosis, Therapy, and Prognosis* (Vol 4). Dordrecht: Springer, 2013.

138. Hart MN, Earle KM. Primitive neuroectodermal tumors of the brain in children. *Cancer* 1973; 32:890–897.

139. Pomeroy SL, Tamayo P, Gaasenbeek M, et al. Prediction of central nervous system embryonal tumour outcome based on gene expression. *Nature* 2002; 415(6870):436–442.

140. Dai AI, Backstrom JW, Burger PC, et al. Supratentorial primitive neuroectodermal tumors of infancy: clinical and radiologic findings. *Pediatr Neurol* 2003; 29:430–434.

141. Eberhart CG, Brat DJ, Cohen KJ, et al. Pediatric neuroblastic brain tumors containing abundant neuropil and true rosettes. *Pediatr Dev Pathol* 2000; 3:346–352.

142. Pfister S, Remke M, Castoldi M, et al. Novel genomic amplification targeting the microRNA cluster at 19q13.42 in a pediatric embryonal tumor with abundant neuropil and true rosettes. *Acta Neuropathol* 2009; 117:457–464.

143. Sturm D, Orr BA, Toprak UH, et al. New brain tumor entities emerge from molecular classification of CNS-PNETs. *Cell* 2016; 164(5):1060–1072.

144. Spence T, Sin-Chan P, Picard D, et al. CNS-PNETs with C19MC amplification and/or LIN28 expression comprise a distinct histogenetic diagnostic and therapeutic entity. *Acta Neuropathol* 2014; 128(2):291–303.

145. Schwalbe EC, Hayden JT, Rogers HA, et al. Histologically defined central nervous system primitive neuro-ectodermal tumours (CNS-PNETs) display heterogeneous DNA methylation profiles and show relationships to other paediatric brain tumour types *Acta Neuropathol* 2013; 126(6):943–946.

146. Cohen BH, Zeltzer PM, Boyett JM, et al. Prognostic factors and treatment results for supratentorial primitive neuroectodermal tumors in children using radiation and chemotherapy: a Children's Cancer Group randomized trial. *J Clin Oncol* 1995; 13(7):1687–1696.

147. Jakacki RI, Burger PC, Kocak M, et al. Outcome and prognostic factors for children with supratentorial primitive neuroectodermal tumors treated with carboplatin during radiotherapy: a report from the Children's Oncology Group. *Pediatr Blood Cancer* 2015; 62(5):776–783.

CHAPTER 10

Tumours of the cranial nerves

Joerg-Christian Tonn and Douglas Kondziolka

Definition

Most tumours of the cranial nerves are schwannomas (formerly neuromas), which develop from the Schwann cells. The olfactory nerve very rarely develops a so-called ectopic paediatric olfactory schwannoma. The optic nerve has no Schwann cells and therefore does not give rise to any schwannoma.

The second, less frequent, tumour type of cranial nerve tumours, is the optic nerve sheath meningioma (ONSM). Since the optic nerve is the only cranial nerve with its own arachnoidal cell layer, nerve sheath meningiomas are restricted to only this location.

Epidemiology

The most frequent tumours of the cranial nerves are schwannomas, which account for 8% of all intracranial tumours. The most common tumour is the schwannoma of the vestibular nerve (formerly, often misleadingly, termed 'acoustic neuroma') with an incidence of 1.3 per 100,000 population per year (1). In patients with neurofibromatosis type 2 (NF2), the incidence is much higher (see Chapter 15).

Optic nerve sheath meningiomas are very rare, accounting for only 1% of all meningiomas (2). Another rare, primary tumour of the cranial nerves is the optic nerve glioma, which can extend to the optic pathway and is much more common in children with NF1, compared to non-NF1 patients and adults. The incidence is 1:10,000 (3).

The esthesioneuroblastoma (also termed olfactory neuroblastoma) is a very rare, malignant tumour of the olfactory nerve and the olfactory bulb. Approximately one thousand cases of this clinically malignant tumour have been described so far (4).

Malignant peripheral nerve sheath tumours (MPNST) are extremely rare in cranial nerves with a preponderance of the trigeminal nerve and the vestibulocochlear nerve (5).

Clinical symptoms

Usually the first clinical symptom of a tumour arising from a cranial nerve is directly related to its impaired function.

For the most frequent tumours of the cranial nerves (vestibular schwannoma), vertigo, progressive hearing loss, and tinnitus are the first symptoms. Since they are rather unspecific and usually slowly progressive, they can precede the diagnosis sometimes by years. Although vestibular schwannomas have a very close anatomical relation to the facial nerve, facial nerve symptoms occur rather infrequently in this type of tumour, and if—mostly incomplete—facial nerve palsy occurs, it is rather more likely due to a tumour primarily arising from the facial nerve. These very rare primary facial nerve schwannomas in most instances involve the ganglion geniculi. Very large tumours arising from the nerves of the cerebellopontine angle can affect the trigeminal nerve at a later stage, resulting in facial hypaesthesia or facial pain syndromes such as trigeminal neuropathy or trigeminal neuralgia. Schwannomas of the caudal cranial nerves or the jugular foramen can cause a hoarse voice, swallowing difficulties, or a sensation of having a lump in the throat. Very large tumours can cause ataxia or, due to obstruction of the cranial spinal fluid pathways, the symptoms of obstructive hydrocephalus (6).

Optic nerve sheath meningiomas and optic gliomas typically lead to a slowly progressive impairment of vision, bulbar protrusion, or both. Bulbar protrusion is more common in large optic gliomas in childhood. ONSMs in particular lead to very slow progression of symptoms. Any unilateral progressive loss of vision must draw the ophthalmologist's attention towards this potential differential diagnosis.

The very rare malignant esthesioneuroblastoma causes a slow, progressive loss of olfactory function; however, this is rarely realized by the patient. Hence, epistaxis due to larger and already aggressively destructive tumours are the leading symptoms.

Diagnosis

Once the clinical symptoms are suspicious of a tumour of the cranial nerves, imaging with high-resolution magnetic resonance imaging (MRI) is warranted. Usually these tumours have very typical features in MRI conducted with and without administration of gadolinium-DTPA as a contrast medium. Schwannomas of the cranial nerves in particular usually do not raise many diagnostic difficulties due to the tumour extension into the foramen of the skull base (Fig. 10.1). The most frequent differential diagnosis is a meningioma growing in close vicinity to the nerve. Typically the lack of a broad contact area to the dura of the skull base and a missing 'dural tail', a contrast enhancement of adjacent infiltrated dura, indicates the schwannoma (7).

For ONSMs, an enhancement of the outer sleeve of the optical nerve without contrast enhancement of the nerve itself leads to the characteristic 'railroad sign' on axial contrast-enhanced T1 planes. On coronal sections, a contrast-enhancing ring around the optic nerve is typical.

In contrast, the optic nerve glioma is characterized by intrinsic growth of the tumour with gross enlargement of the diameter of the optic nerve with a high T2 signal intensity and the absence of the features typical for meningiomas (8). However, cavernous haemangiomas of the orbit, granulomatous disease, sarcoidosis, and other

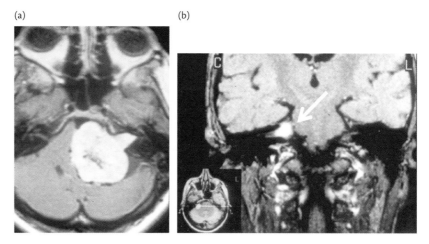

Fig. 10.1 Large vestibular schwannoma with brainstem compression (a) and small intra/extracanalicular vestibular schwannoma without contact with the brainstem (b).

inflammatory lesions might appear rather similar. Even intraorbital schwannomas, although very rare, have to be considered.

Tumours involving the bony structure of the skull base (e.g. vestibular schwannomas with growth inside the internal meatus, trigeminal schwannomas growing in Meckel's cave) require additional high-resolution CT scans of the skull base. These benign lesions usually cause a well-delineated bony defect, typical for long-lasting, slow, expansive growth. This is also a very good diagnostic tool for the differentiation against the destructive growth of skull base metastases (9).

Another differential diagnosis for lesions closely related to the jugular foramen is tumours of the glomus jugulare (also referred to as paraganglioma) with a characteristic extension into the middle ear and below the skull base. Typically, they show an excessive enhancement after the application of contrast media. Angiography, either as magnetic resonance angiography or digital subtraction angiography, reveals a highly vascularized tumour thus leading to the correct diagnosis (9, 10).

Destructive lesions of the skull base (e.g. chordoma or chondrosarcoma) can be very well differentiated from schwannomas. The epidermoid tumour of the cerebellopontine angle has also a completely different growth pattern and can be easily diagnosed via diffusion-weighted MRI (10).

Grading and classification

Clinical course and prognosis are reflected by the grading system of the World Health Organization (WHO).

Schwannomas are graded as WHO I. Very rare malignant peripheral nerve sheath tumours are assigned to WHO III or IV (11).

The ONSM corresponds to WHO I (11).

Usually gliomas of the optic nerve are classified as pilocytic astrocytoma WHO I. However, even the more malignant spectrum like anaplastic gliomas grade III and glioblastomas grade IV can be found, although very seldomly (12).

Esthesioneuroblastoma is always classified as malignant being WHO IV due to its aggressive growth, the poor prognosis, and the capability to metastasize (13).

Tumour classification systems have been proposed for schwannomas, and are referred to in Tables 10.1–10.3 (14–18). For

Table 10.1 Classification of vestibular schwannomas

Size(Tos)	Grade (Koos)	Class (Samii)	Definition of tumour size
	Grade I	T1	Purely intracanalicular lesion
	Grade II	T2	Vestibular schwannoma protruding into the cerebellopontine angle without brainstem contact
<1 cm	IIA	T2	Tumour diameter <1 cm
1–1.8 cm	IIB	T2	Tumour diameter 1–1.8 cm
	Grade III	T3a	Filling cerebellopontine angle cistern
		T3b	Reaching the brainstem
	Grade IV	T4a	Brainstem compression
		T4b	Severely dislocating the brainstem and compressing the fourth ventricle

Source data from Tos M, Thomsen J, Proposal of classification of tumor size in acoustic neuroma surgery. In: Tos M, Thomsen J (eds.), *Acoustic Neuroma: Proceedings of the First International Conference on Acoustic Neuroma*, pp. 133–137, Copyright (1991), Kugler Publications; *J Neurosurg*, 88(3), Koos W T, Day J D, Matula C, Levy D I, Neurotopographic considerations in the microsurgical treatment of small acoustic neurinomas, pp. 506–512, Copyright (1998), American Association of Neurological Surgeons; *Neurosurgery*, 40(1), Samii, M, Matthies, C, Management of 1000 vestibular schwannomas (acoustic neuromas): surgical management and results with an emphasis on complications and how to avoid them, pp. 11–21, Copyright (1997), Wolters Kluwer Health, Inc.

Table 10.2 Surgical classification of trigeminal schwannomas

Type	Definition of tumour extension
A	Intracranial predominantly in the middle fossa
B	Intracranial predominantly in the posterior fossa
C	Intracranial dumbbell-shaped in the middle and posterior fossa
D	Extracranial with intracranial extension

Source data from *J Neurosurg*, 82(5), Samii M, Migliori MM, Tatagiba M, Babu R, Surgical treatment of trigeminal schwannomas, pp. 711–718, Copyright (1995), American Association of Neurological Surgeons.

Table 10.4 Staging of esthesioneuroblastomas

Group	Definition
A	The tumour is limited to the nasal cavity
B	The tumour is localized to the nasal cavity and paranasal sinuses
C	The tumour extends beyond the nasal cavity and paranasal sinuses

Source data from *Cancer*, 37(3), Kadish S, Goodman M, Wang CC, Olfactory neuroblastoma. A clinical analysis of 17 cases, pp. 1571–1576, Copyright (1976), John Wiley and Sons.

esthesioneuroblastomas, a grading system into three groups has been proposed reflecting location and, thereby, invasive and distant growth (Table 10.4) (19).

Treatment

Due to the widespread availability of high-resolution MRI, tumours of the cranial nerves are nowadays diagnosed at a rather early stage in disease, with tumours being smaller and with function, although impaired, often still present. Accordingly, preservation of function is nowadays considered to be equally important to tumour control in those lesions which are histologically and clinically benign. Whereas the (very rare) malignant tumours of the cranial nerves such as esthesioneuroblastoma and malignant peripheral nerve sheath tumours require a most radical resection with adjuvant radio- and chemotherapy, the therapeutic concept for benign tumours of the cranial nerves is different. Microsurgial resection, radiosurgery, radiotherapy, and watchful waiting are options. They have to be selected either alone or in combination, on an individual basis according to the principles of 'personalized therapy' (20, 21).

Optic nerve sheath meningiomas

Optic nerve sheath meningiomas grow circumferentially around the optic nerve being adherent to the nerve itself and its vascular supply which is typically located on the surface of the nerve. Hence, surgical resection has an extremely high risk of complete loss of function leaving the patient blind in the respective eye. Therefore, surgical resection is not a valid option for ONSMs with the exception of tumour growth towards the optic chiasm and the respective

Table 10.3 Surgical classification of jugular foramen schwannomas (CNS)

Type	Definition of tumour extension
A	Primarily at the cerebellopontine angle with minimal enlargement of the FJ
B	Tumours primarily in the FJ with intracranial extension
C	Primarily extracranial tumour with extension into the FJ
D	Dumbbell-shaped tumours with both intra- and extracranial components

FJ, foramen jugulare.

Source data from *J Neurosurg*, 82(6), Samii M, Babu R P, Tatagiba M, Sepehrnia A, Surgical treatment of jugular foramen schwannomas, pp. 924–932, Copyright (1995) American Association of Neurological Surgeons.

eye already being blind. In all other cases, fractionated radiotherapy provides the best results of growth control and maintenance of visual acuity (22–25). In contrast to small meningiomas in other locations, radiosurgical procedures are usually not recommended in ONSM, unless vision is already lost or the tumour is small and eccentric to the nerve. Favourable results have been published using different concepts of conformal and stereotactic fractionated radiotherapy. However, these treatments should only be administered in case of symptomatic, especially progressive ONSM. In case of an asymptomatic tumour, a watchful wait-and-scan strategy can be applied since these tumours might stay biologically and clinically stable for longer periods (2). In rare cases, where compression of the optic nerve within the optic canal is likely to be the reason for functional decompensation, a microsurgical unroofing of the canal by drilling away the bone *without* removal of the meningioma itself might be warranted. In ONSM restricted to the intraorbital space, such a decompression is not necessary (26, 27).

Optic nerve glioma

The vast majority of optic nerve gliomas occur in childhood and young adolescence. In the very young (up to the age of 10–14 years), a close monitoring with watchful waiting and ophthalmological check-up every 3 months and bi-annual MRI are advocated since a rather large proportion of the lesions tend to stop growing at the beginning of adolescence. In case of any doubt concerning the proper diagnosis based on high-resolution MRI, a biopsy is warranted to obtain a histology. However, any therapeutic intervention in optic nerve gliomas bears a very high risk of functional deterioration. Whenever radiological and/or clinical progression is proven, fractionated stereotactic radiotherapy is the treatment modality of first choice (28, 29). There have even been reports of improved vision thereafter. In case of exophytic tumours and whenever progression with growth towards the chiasm is documented, surgical resection should be considered (30). In these cases, the resection plane should be some millimetres away from the chiasm in order not to destroy Meyer's loop, which would result in visual field deficits on the contralateral side. Therefore, these tumours should be resected before they have reached the chiasm. Since resection of intrinsic optic nerve gliomas nearly always result in blindness of that eye, the indication has to be very strict. In exophytic lesions, high-resolution MRI may help to visualize a resection plane allowing the removal of the tumour without severe impairment of visual function. In selected, very well-delineated and circumscribed lesions, stereotactic brachytherapy with implantation of radioactive ^{125}I-seeds have been shown to be effective with low treatment-related permanent morbidity (31).

In the very rare cases of adult malignant optic nerve glioma, a combination of radio/chemotherapy remains the only treatment option due to a lack of alternatives, although they mostly progress rapidly (12).

Schwannomas

Preservation of function is key in schwannomas, especially with regard to the biologically benign nature of the lesion. Microsurgical resection, radiosurgery, and fractionated stereotactic radiotherapy are the treatment options. For the growing number of incidental findings, a watchful waiting/wait-and-scan policy may be acceptable as long as the tumour remains asymptomatic and shows no growth on MRI. However, recent natural history studies show a tumour doubling time between 1.5 and 4.5 years (20, 32–34).

For most cases, especially the very small lesions, stereotactic radiosurgery and microsurgical removal are the best alternatives. Generally, the imaging obtained by high-resolution MRI is typical, especially any tumour extending out of the auditory canal into the cerebellopontine angle. However, in case of any doubt, a proper histology obtained before microsurgery is mandatory. The risk of microsurgical removal compared to radiosurgery has to be calculated against the potential benefit of a lower recurrence rate after tumour removal. Whenever the tumour has exceeded an extracanalicular diameter of 30 mm, radiosurgical options are less effective at rapidly improving symptoms and microsurgery is the treatment of choice (20). Patients with disabling ataxia, trigeminal neuralgia, hydrocephalus, intractable headache, or an unclear diagnosis should consider resection first. In case of microsurgical tumour removal, online functional neuromonitoring is mandatory. By means of modern techniques, several nerves can be monitored via electromyography. These techniques include the facial nerve, cranial nerves XII, XI, IX and the motor part of cranial nerve V. In specialized centres cranial nerves III, IV, and VI can be monitored as well (35–38).

In large tumours, which at surgery turn out to be not completely resectable without a considerable risk of a severe functional deficit, it can be wise to perform an incomplete resection with a very small remnant being left in order not to compromise function (Fig. 10.2). These small remnants may undergo planned radiosurgery several months later once they progress. If there is a stable enhancement without progression, only residual linear enhancement that may not be tumour, close imaging follow-up is warranted. This combined concept has greatly improved the functional results (39, 40).

Vestibular schwannoma stereotactic radiosurgery using the Gamma Knife® has been practised for more than 40 years. Long-term outcome results have established stereotactic radiosurgery as an important minimally invasive alternative to resection. Advanced dose planning software, intraoperative high-resolution MRI, dose optimization, and robotic delivery reflect the evolution of this technology. To reduce risk, various image-guided linear accelerator devices (Trilogy®, Synergy S®, Novalis®, and CyberKnife®) might require fractionation of the radiation delivery in 5–30 sessions. Proton beam technology is also used to deliver fractionated radiation therapy. The goals of vestibular schwannoma radiosurgery include prevention of further tumour growth and preservation of existing neurological function. Stereotaxy, dose planning, and dose delivery are three critical components of successful radiosurgery. Complete volumetric conformal and selective tumour radiosurgery improves the rates of facial, cochlear, and trigeminal nerve preservation. Reduction of dose delivered to the brainstem is especially relevant during treatment of larger tumours.

Commonly, a radiosurgery dose of 11–13 Gy is typically prescribed to the 50% (or other) isodose line that conforms to the three-dimensional tumour margin. These marginal doses are associated with a low complication rate and yet maintain a high rate of tumour control (41–43). Long relaxation time (T2), 1 mm axial plane volumetric MRI is necessary to identify the cochlea for dose planning. A mean cochlear dose less than 4.2 Gy may be important for hearing preservation. The stereotactic radiosurgery technology must also be able to restrict dose to adjacent structures by having a very sharp dose gradient at the tumour edge. While many radiosurgical centres have evolved towards similar dose-selection parameters, the doses and regimens chosen for fractionated radiotherapy continue to vary.

Fractionated radiosurgery or fractionated stereotactic radiotherapy can also be used for vestibular schwannomas. In 2009, Andrews et al. published the Thomas Jefferson University experience using stereotactic radiotherapy at total dose of 50.4 or 46.8 Gy (44). In patients with class I or II hearing, the median follow-up was 65 weeks. Although no patient had later tumour growth, the hearing preservation rates were better at the lower dose. At 3 years, the hearing preservation rate was 55–60%, and no patient with class II

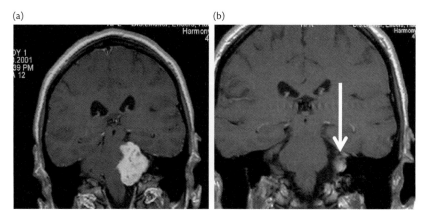

(a)   (b)

Fig. 10.2 Large vestibular schwannoma with brainstem compression (a) and small intracanalicular remnant at the facial nerve—being stable in size 10 years after surgery (b).

hearing maintained hearing if they received the 50 Gy dose (44). Based on these findings, the group reported the use of even lower doses to try to improve hearing outcomes. Recently, they updated their experience at the 46.8 Gy dose in 154 patients at median follow-up of 35 months. Overall, hearing preservation was 66% and 54% at 3 and 5 years, respectively. However, for patients with class II hearing, it was only 45% at 3 years and 29% at 5 years (45).

Rasmussen et al. concluded that fractionated radiotherapy at a dose of 54 Gy (higher than used in the Thomas Jefferson University report) appeared to accelerate hearing loss (46). Kapoor et al. published outcomes after fractionated stereotactic radiotherapy from Johns Hopkins Hospital in 496 patients of whom 385 had follow-up (47). Radiation was administered in five 5-Gy fractions or ten 3-Gy fractions. Resection was later performed in 3%. Attempted hearing preservation is often given as reason why some centres choose to use fractionated radiotherapy, but hearing results were not provided.

During recent years, anti-angiogenic therapy with bevacizumab (Avastin®) has been proposed as medical therapy in patients with vestibular or acoustic schwannomas, mostly in NF2 (48), and partial regression of the tumour and improvement of hearing function have been reported (see Chapter 15 for more details).

Esthesioneuroblastoma

In esthesioneuroblastoma, a most radical resection with tumour-free margins is the treatment of choice with significant improvement of the patient's prognosis. To achieve this goal, combined craniofacial procedures have to be chosen. In tumours limited to the nasal cavity (Kadish stage A), surgery alone is appropriate; in Kadish group B (tumour is localized in the nasal cavity and paranasal sinuses), additional radiotherapy with up to 60 Gy is necessary. In Kadish group C (tumour extends beyond the nasal cavity and the paranasal sinuses), additional chemotherapy either prior to surgery or after irradiation is advocated. Concerning metastases, local excision of metastases should be performed with subsequent radiotherapy and, in case of distant and multifocal metastases, chemotherapy; 5-year survival rates of approximately 55% can be achieved. Due to a sometimes very late appearance of metastatic spread, long-term follow-up is necessary. Radiosurgery can be effective for locally recurrent disease (19, 49–55).

Current research topics

In terms of optic nerve gliomas, research focusing on glioma biology and individualized treatment based on the molecular signature of tumours is warranted.

In cranial nerve schwannomas, the concept of anti-angiogenic treatment with bevacizumab is emerging (47). However, many questions remain to be resolved, including: (i) up to now this therapy has mainly been tested in patients with NF2—whether this seems to be effective in non-NF2 patients still remains unclear; and (ii) there is a debate on whether bevacizumab has to be given lifelong. It remains to be elucidated whether 'drug holidays' might increase the risk of a relapse. Since bevacizumab may impair fertility in women with child-bearing potential, this aspect of therapy has to be investigated more thoroughly since patients with neurofibromatosis usually are younger (see Chapter 15).

References

1. Tos M, Stangerup SE, Caye-Thomasen P, et al. What is the real incidence of vestibular schwannoma? *Arch Otolaryngol Head Neck Surg* 2004; 130:216–220.

2. Saeed P, Rootman J, Nugent RA, et al. Optic nerve sheath meningiomas. *Ophthalmology* 2003; 110(10):2019–2030.

3. Astrup J. Natural history and clinical management of optic pathway glioma. *Br J Neurosurg* 2003; 17:327–335.

4. Bockmuhl U, You X, Pacyna-Gengelbach M, et al. CGH pattern of esthesioneuroblastoma and their metastases. *Brain Pathol* 2004; 14:158–163.

5. Baehring JM, Betensky RA, Batchelor TT. Malignant peripheral nerve sheath tumor: the clinical spectrum and outcome of treatment. *Neurology* 2003; 61:696–698.

6. Roser F, Honegger J, Schuhmann MU, et al. Meningiomas, nerve sheath tumors, and pituitary tumors: diagnosis and treatment. *Hematol Oncol Clin North Am* 2012; 26(4):855–879.

7. Choudhri AF, Parmar HA, Morales RE, et al. Lesions of the skull base: imaging for diagnosis and treatment. *Otolaryngol Clin North Am* 2012; 45(6):1385–1404.

8. Hintschich C, Rose G. Orbital tumors. In: Tonn JC, Westphal M, Rutka JT (eds) *Oncology of CNS Tumors* (2nd edn). Heidelberg: Springer, 2010; 309–330.

9. Choudhri AF, Parmar HA, Morales RE, et al. Lesions of the skull base: imaging for diagnosis and treatment. *Otolaryngol Clin North Am* 2012; 45(6):1385–1404.

10. Bonneville F, Savatovsky J, Chiras J. Imaging of cerebellopontine angle lesions: an update. Part 1: enhancing extra-axial lesions. *Eur Radiol* 2007; 17(10):2472–2482.

11. Louis DN, Ohgaki H, Wiestler OD, et al. The 2007 WHO classification of tumours of the central nervous system. *Acta Neuropathol* 2007; 114(2):97–109.

12. Wabbels B, Demmler A, Seitz J, et al. Unilateral adult malignant optic nerve glioma. *Graefes Arch Clin Exp Ophthalmol* 2004; 242(9):741–748.

13. Kleihues P, Cavenee WK. *Pathology and Genetics of Tumours of the Nervous System.* Lyon: International Agency for Research on Cancer, 2000.

14. Tos M, Thomsen J. Proposal of classification of tumor size in acoustic neuroma surgery. In: Tos M, Thomsen J (eds) *Proceedings of the First International Conference on Acoustic Neuroma Copenhagen, Denmark, August 25–29, 1991.* Amsterdam: Kugler Publications, 1992; 133–137.

15. Koos WT, Day JD, Matula C, et al. Neurotopographic considerations in the microsurgical treatment of small acoustic neurinomas. *J Neurosurg* 1998; 88:506–512.

16. Samii M, Matthies C. Management of 1000 vestibular schwannomas (acoustic neuromas): surgical management and results with an emphasis on complications and how to avoid them. *Neurosurgery* 1997; 40:11–21.

17. Samii M, Migliori MM, Tatagiba M, et al. Surgical treatment of trigeminal schwannomas. *J Neurosurg* 1995; 82:711–718.

18. Samii M, Babu RP, Tatagiba M, et al. Surgical treatment of jugular foramen schwannomas. *J Neurosurg* 1995; 82:924–932.

19. Kadish S, Goodman M, Wang CC. Olfactory neuroblastoma. A clinical analysis of 17 cases. *Cancer* 1976; 37:1571–1576.

20. Sarmiento JM, Patel S, Mukherjee D, et al. Improving outcomes in patients with vestibular schwannomas: microsurgery versus radiosurgery. *J Neurosurg Sci* 2013; 57(1):23–44.

21. Maniakas A, Saliba I. Microsurgery versus stereotactic radiation for small vestibular schwannomas: a meta-analysis of patients with more than 5 years' follow-up. *Otol Neurotol* 2012; 33(9):1611–1620.

22. Turbin RE, Thompson CR, Kennerdell JS, et al. A long-term visual outcome comparison in patients with optic nerve sheath meningioma managed with observation, surgery, radiotherapy, or surgery and radiotherapy. *Ophthalmology* 2002; 109:890–899.

23. Pitz S, Becker G, Schiefer U, et al. Stereotactic fractionated irradiation of optic nerve sheath meningioma: a new treatment alternative. *Br J Ophthalmol* 2002; 86:1265–1268.

24. Narayan S, Cornblath WT, Sandler HM, et al. Preliminary visual outcomes after three-dimensional conformal radiation therapy for optic nerve sheath meningioma. *Int J Radiat Oncol Biol Phys* 2003; 56:537–543.

25. Subramanian PS, Bressler NM, Miller NR. Radiation retinopathy after fractionated stereotactic radiotherapy for optic nerve sheath meningioma. *Ophthalmology* 2004; 111:565–567.

26. Shimano H, Nagasawa S, Kawabata S, et al. Surgical strategy for meningioma extension into the optic canal. *Neurol Med Chir (Tokyo)* 2000; 40:447–451.

27. Shapey J, Sabin HI, Danesh-Meyer HV, et al. Diagnosis and management of optic nerve sheath meningiomas. *J Clin Neurosci* 2013; 20(8):1045–1056.

28. Binning MJ, Liu JK, Kestle JR, et al. Optic pathway gliomas: a review. *Neurosurg Focus* 2007; 23(5):E2.

29. Walker D. Recent advances in optic nerve glioma with a focus on the young patient. *Curr Opin Neurol* 2003; 16:657–664.

30. Bessero AC, Fraser C, Acheson J, et al. Management options for visual pathway compression from optic gliomas. *Postgrad Med J* 2013; 89(1047):47–51.

31. Schwarz SB, Thon N, Nikolajek K, et al. Iodine-125 brachytherapy for brain tumours – a review. *Radiat Oncol* 2012; 7:30.

32. Kondziolka D, Mousavi SH, Kano H, et al. The newly diagnosed vestibular schwannoma: radiosurgery, resection, or observation? *Neurosurg Focus* 2012; 33(3):E8.

33. Fong B, Barkhoudarian G, Pezeshkian P, et al. The molecular biology and novel treatments of vestibular schwannomas. *J Neurosurg* 2011; 115(5):906–914.

34. Charabi S, Tos M, Thomsen J. Vestibular schwannoma growth – long-term results. *Acta Otolaryngol Suppl* 2000; 543:7–10.

35. Matthies C, Samii M. Management of vestibular schwannomas (acoustic neuromas): the value of neurophysiology for intraoperative monitoring of auditory function in 200 cases. *Neurosurgery* 1997; 40:459–466.

36. Matthies C, Samii M. Direct brainstem recording of auditory evoked potentials during vestibular schwannoma resection: nuclear BAEP recording. Technical note and preliminary results. *J Neurosurg* 1997; 86:1057–1062.

37. Tonn JC, Schlake HP, Goldbrunner R, et al. Acoustic neuroma surgery as an interdisciplinary approach: a neurosurgical series of 508 patients. *J Neurol Neurosurg Psychiatry* 2000; 69:161–166.

38. Matthies C, Samii M. Management of 1000 vestibular schwannomas (acoustic neuromas): clinical presentation. *Neurosurgery* 1997; 40:1–9.

39. Theodosopoulos PV, Pensak ML. Contemporary management of acoustic neuromas. *Laryngoscope* 2011; 121(6):1133–1137.

40. Gurgel RK, Theodosopoulos PV, Jackler RK. Subtotal/near-total treatment of vestibular schwannomas. *Curr Opin Otolaryngol Head Neck Surg* 2012; 20(5):380–384.

41. Flickinger JC, Kondziolka D, Niranjan A, et al. Acoustic neuroma radiosurgery with marginal tumor doses of 12 to 13 Gy. *Int J Radiat Oncol Biol Phys* 2003; 57:S325.

42. Hempel JM, Hempel E, Wowra B, et al. Functional outcome after gamma knife treatment in vestibular schwannoma. *Eur Arch Otorhinolaryngol* 2006; 263:714–718.

43. Pollock BE, Driscoll CL, Foote RL, et al. Patient outcomes after vestibular schwannoma management: a prospective comparison of microsurgical resection and stereotactic radiosurgery. *Neurosurgery* 2006; 59:77–85.

44. Andrews D, Werner-Wasik M, Den R, et al. Toward dose optimization for fractionated stereotactic radiotherapy for acoustic neuromas: comparison of two dose cohorts. *Int J Radiat Oncol Biol Phys* 2009; 74:419–426.

45. Champ CE, Shen X, Shi W, et al. Reduced-dose fractionated stereotactic radiotherapy for acoustic neuromas: maintenance of tumor control with improved hearing preservation. *Neurosurgery* 2013; 73:489–496.

46. Rasmussen R, Claesson M, Stangerup S, et al. Fractionated stereotactic radiotherapy of vestibular schwannomas accelerates hearing loss. *Int J Radiat Oncol Biol Phys* 2012; 83(5):607–611.

47. Kapoor W, Batra S, Carson K, et al. Long-term outcomes of vestibular schwannomas treated with fractionated stereotactic radiotherapy: an institutional experience. *Int J Radiat Oncol Biol Phys* 2011; 81:647–653.

48. Plotkin SR, Merker VL, Halpin C, et al. Bevacizumab for progressive vestibular schwannoma in neurofibromatosis type 2: a retrospective review of 31 patients. *Otol Neurotol* 2012; 33(6):1046–1052.

49. Michel J, Fakhry N, Santini L, et al. Nasal and paranasal esthesioneuroblastomas: clinical outcomes. *Eur Ann Otorhinolaryngol Head Neck Dis* 2012; 129(5):238–243.

50. Ow TJ, Hanna EY, Roberts DB, et al. Optimization of long-term outcomes for patients with esthesioneuroblastoma. *Head Neck* 2014; 36(4):524–530.

51. Bradley PJ, Jones NS, Robertson I. Diagnosis and management of esthesioneuroblastoma. *Curr Opin Otolaryngol Head Neck Surg* 2003; 11:112–118.

52. Dias FL, Sa GM, Lima RA, et al. Patterns of failure and outcome in esthesioneuroblastoma. *Arch Otolaryngol Head Neck Surg* 2003; 129:1186–1192.

53. Gruber G, Laedrach K, Baumert B, et al. Esthesioneuroblastoma: irradiation alone and surgery alone are not enough. *Int J Radiat Oncol Biol Phys* 2002; 54:486–491.

54. Eich HT, Hero B, Staar S, et al. Multimodality therapy including radiotherapy and chemotherapy improves event-free survival in stage C esthesioneuroblastoma. *Strahlenther Onkol* 2003; 179:233–240.

55. Bak M, Wein RO. Esthesioneuroblastoma: a contemporary review of diagnosis and management. *Hematol Oncol Clin North Am* 2012; 26(6):1185–1207.

CHAPTER 11

Meningiomas

Rakesh Jalali, Patrick Y. Wen, and Takamitsu Fujimaki

Epidemiology

Meningiomas are the most common type of primary brain tumours in adults, accounting for 30% of the total (1, 2). The incidence of meningioma increases progressively with age. Meningiomas in children are rare, and usually associated with neurofibromatosis type 2 (NF2) or prior therapeutic radiation therapy (3, 4). Meningiomas are more common in women, with a female-to-male ratio of about 2:1 or 3:1 (3, 5). Spinal meningiomas, which account for 10% of all meningiomas, have an even higher female-to-male ratio of approximately 9:1. In contrast, the incidence in females is not significantly increased in atypical or anaplastic meningiomas, children, and radiation-induced meningiomas (4).

Pathological classification

The 2007 World Health Organization (WHO) classification of tumours of the central nervous system lists 15 subtypes of meningioma (Box 11.1) (6). Nine of them are purely benign (grade I) tumours, whereas atypical meningioma, clear cell meningioma, and chordoid meningioma are grade II, and papillary meningioma, anaplastic meningioma, and rhabdoid meningioma are grade III. Histologically, atypical meningiomas are defined as meningiomas with loss of architectural pattern, prominent nucleoli, nuclear pleomorphism, increased mitotic activity, necrosis, and hypercellularity. They may invade the brain or show malignant histology. These tumours have a more aggressive natural history than benign tumours. WHO grade III malignant meningiomas exhibit frank histological malignancy or 20 mitotic figures per 10 high-power fields. Brain invasion does not necessarily imply WHO grade III meningioma; in the absence of frank anaplasia (7), approximately 70–80% are WHO grade I, 5–35% are WHO grade II, and 1–3% are WHO grade III (8, 9). At the time of recurrence, most tumours retain the same histological pattern, but some exhibit a more advanced grade or a higher proliferative index (10).

Genetic factors

Approximately 50–75% of patients with NF2 have meningiomas, which are often multiple (11). NF2 is an autosomal dominant disorder caused by a mutation in the *NF2* gene on chromosome 22, a tumour suppressor gene which encodes a membrane cytoskeletal protein called merlin or schwannomin (12). Meningiomas may also occur in schwannomatosis, a condition characterized by multiple schwannomas and mutations in the *SMARCB1* tumour suppressor gene (13).

Hormonal factors

Because meningiomas are more common in women, especially during their reproductive years (14, 15), as well as the presence of progesterone and androgen receptors in two-thirds of patients (16, 17), there has been longstanding interest in the possible role of sex hormones in meningioma growth (18–20). Additionally, meningiomas may be more common among breast cancer patients (21). Epidemiological data (22, 23) and case reports (24) have suggested that exogenous oestrogens and progestins for hormone replacement therapy and contraceptive use may promote meningioma development or growth, but the associations are controversial (25, 26).

Risk factors

The most important risk factor for development of meningiomas is prior exposure to irradiation (26, 27). This may result from low doses used to treat tinea capitis (28), intermediate doses used for prophylactic irradiation to prevent central nervous system relapse in acute leukaemia, and high doses for treatment of central nervous system and head and neck tumours (29, 30). There are reports of increased incidence of meningiomas following childhood exposure to computed tomography (CT) scans (31), and dental X-rays (32), although the data is less conclusive. The latency of radiation-induced meningiomas ranges from 20 years or more. In general, radiation-induced meningiomas have greater atypia and are more likely to be multiple. There are also reports of an association between body mass index and meningiomas in women with an odds ratio of 1.4–2.1 (33). Associations with mobile phone use (26) and head injury (26, 34) have been reported but are not conclusive.

Clinical presentation

Increasingly, meningiomas are asymptomatic and discovered incidentally on a neuroimaging study or at autopsy. In one study, 0.9% of the population had an asymptomatic meningioma (35).

Symptoms caused by meningiomas are related to their location. Meningiomas can attach to the dura at any site in the nervous system. Most commonly they arise from cranial vault, and at sites of dural reflection such as the falx cerebri, tentorium cerebelli, and dura of the adjacent venous sinuses (36). Less commonly, they can occur along the optic nerve sheath, with ventricles or in the spine. The most common presenting symptom is a seizure, occurring in up to 40% of patients (37, 38). Seizures tend to be more common with convexity meningiomas (38) and tumours with peritumoural oedema. Other symptoms include headaches, focal deficits, and rarely, hydrocephalus caused by large posterior fossa tumours. Very

> **Box 11.1** The grading of meningiomas according to the 2007 WHO classification of tumours of the central nervous system
>
> **Grade I**
>
> Meningothelial
>
> Fibrous (fibroblastic)
>
> Transitional (mixed)
>
> Psammomatous
>
> Angiomatous
>
> Microcystic
>
> Secretory
>
> Lymphoplasmocyte-rich
>
> Metaplastic.
>
> **Grade II**
>
> Atypical
>
> Clear cell meningioma (intracranial)
>
> Chordoid.
>
> **Grade III**
>
> Papillary
>
> Anaplastic (malignant) meningioma
>
> Rhabdoid.
>
> Source data from Louis DN, Ohgaki H, Wiestler OD, Cavenee WK, Ellison DW, Figarella-Branger D, Perry A, Reifenberger G, Von Deimling A (Eds), *World Health Organization Classification of Tumours of the Central Nervous System*, Fourth Edition Revised, Copyright (2016), IARC Publications.

rarely, parasellar or subfrontal meningiomas may cause optic atrophy in one eye as a result of compression of the optic nerve and papilloedema in the other due to elevation of intracranial pressure, giving rise to the 'Foster–Kennedy syndrome' (39).

Treatment and management of meningioma patients

Medical management of meningioma patients

Patients who present with seizures should be treated with standard antiepileptic drugs (AEDs) such as levetiracetam, although other agents are also acceptable. For other types of brain tumours it is preferable to avoid AEDs that induce hepatic cytochrome P450 enzymes since this may interfere with the metabolism of chemotherapeutic agents used to treat the tumour. Given the lack of systemic agents for meningiomas, this concern is of less importance currently, although this may change in the future as new therapies are developed. Routine use of prophylactic AEDs for patients who have not experienced a seizure are not recommended (40). Atypical and malignant meningiomas may be associated with peritumoural oedema. In patients who are symptomatic, corticosteroids such as dexamethasone 2–4 mg twice daily may be used. In general, the lowest possible dose should be

used to avoid corticosteroid complications. Patients with meningiomas are at increased risk of thromboembolism, especially in the perioperative period, although this risk is diminishing with aggressive prophylaxis (41). In the immediate postoperative period when anticoagulation is contraindicated, inferior vena cava filters may be used. If there are no contraindications, anticoagulation, preferably with low-molecular-weight heparin is indicated.

Surgery

Surgery is the primary treatment for meningiomas in most instances. However, for surgical planning, an understanding of the growth pattern and biology of meningiomas is important.

Meningiomas arise from arachnoid cells and mostly become attached to the dura mater (Fig. 11.1a). They often invade into the overlying calvaria, and this sometimes results in thickening of the skull (6). Cranial nerves or important arteries may also become involved with the tumours, especially in cases of meningioma arising in the skull base. Adjacent to the dural attachment, thickening of the dura, or the 'dural tail sign', is often evident on gadolinium-enhanced magnetic resonance imaging (MRI) scans (Fig. 11.1b). Although tumour cells may not always invade into the whole dural tail or cause calvarial thickening, they do to some extent (42). As for the boundary between meningioma and the brain parenchyma, there is a clear surgical margin in most cases, and the pia mater remains intact. However in some meningiomas, especially WHO grade II or grade III meningiomas, the pia mater is destroyed and tumour cells invade into the brain parenchyma (Fig. 11.1d) (6).

In general, for WHO grade I meningiomas, total removal of the tumour together with the dural attachment and invasion to the bone can provide cure. However, when important arteries or cranial nerves are involved, it is not always easy to resect tumours without damaging these important structures. If the tumour has become attached to the superior sagittal sinus, the posterior two-thirds at least of which are not resectable, then total removal of the dural attachment is not possible. In these instances, partial removal may also be an option, since the growth of many meningiomas is relatively slow (43), and therefore any small residual tumour would not be a problem in many cases.

In the 1950s, Simpson proposed a classification system—the 'Simpson grading'—for the degree of resection (Box 11.2) (44). For example, in Simpson grade 1 resection, where the tumours were totally resected together with removal of the dural attachment and abnormal bone, recurrences were observed in 8.9% of patients. In contrast, for Simpson grade 3 resection, where tumours were removed totally without removal or coagulation of the dural attachment, recurrences were observed in 29.2% of patients. Since then, this grading system has been widely used.

In 2010, however, Sughrue et al. questioned the validity of this grading system, and demonstrated that there were no statistically significant differences in recurrence-free survival between Simpson grade 1, grade 2, grade 3, and grade 4 resections (45). They concluded that Simpson grade 1 or grade 2 resection provides no clear benefit (especially for skull base meningiomas). On the other hand, based on analysis of WHO grade I convexity meningiomas, Hasseleid et al. concluded that Simpson grade 1 resection is still a gold standard of care for convexity meningiomas with benign histology (46). The difference between the conclusions of these

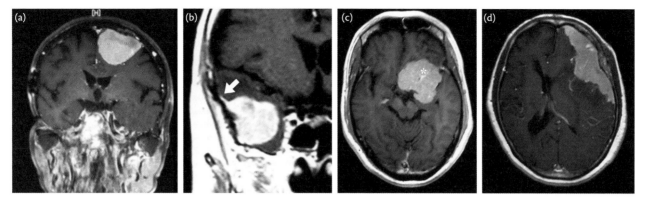

Fig. 11.1 Various types of meningiomas. T1-weighted gadolinium (Gd)-enhanced MRI scans. (a) A convexity meningioma. The tumour did not have attachment to the superior sagittal sinus nor the falx but attached to the dura of the convexity. (b) A convexity meningioma of the temporal area. The dural tail is evident (white arrow). (c) A giant skull base meningioma. The middle cerebral artery (*) was encased in the tumour. (d) An atypical meningioma. The boundary between the tumour and the cerebral cortex was obscure during surgery and the invasion was confirmed by histological examination. Postoperative irradiation was performed.

two articles might have been attributable to the difference between the patient populations studied. In an editorial for the *Journal of Neurosurgery*, Heros pointed out that there were several important differences between these two reports (47). One was that the series reported by Sughrue et al. contained more skull base meningiomas than is usual in the normal population: 50.6%, compared with 40% for the general population, according to the Brain Tumor Registry of Japan (Fig. 11.2) (2).

Meningiomas of the skull base are reported to grow at a slower rate than those in other locations (48). Therefore, radical resection might not be an important factor in any cohort that contains a higher proportion of skull base meningiomas, as was the case in Sughrue et al.'s series.

As for prediction of recurrence, histological examination of the tumour is also important. Several reports have indicated that measurement of proliferative activity by MIB-1 immunohistochemistry is useful for predicting the potential for recurrence of meningiomas (49, 50).

Generally, total removal with any dural or bony attachment should be attempted for meningiomas, but if the tumour is located in the skull base or involves important structures such as

arteries (Fig. 11.1c) or cranial nerves, then leaving a small amount of tumour is a treatment option (47).

Any remnant tumour should be observed closely, and reoperation or additional radiation treatment (described later) should be considered if re-growth occurs.

In recent years, with advances in interventional neuroradiology, preoperative embolization of tumour feeding arteries is sometimes performed. This reduces blood loss during surgery, shortens the operation time, and might lead to better surgical resection. However, the advantages of this procedure have not yet established, and further investigations are needed (51).

Radiotherapy for meningiomas

Radiotherapy was debated to have any role in meningiomas in the early part of this century as they were thought to be radioresistant. This was mainly due to theories presuming that radiation led to malignant degeneration of benign tumours or meningiomas can be even induced by radiation itself (previously described in the risk factors section) (52). The preconception that meningiomas are radioresistant tumours was proved to be wrong by large retrospective studies which showed a significant role of radiotherapy

---

Box 11.2 The Simpson grading system for removal of meningiomas

♦ Grade 1: macroscopically complete removal, with excision of dural attachment and of any abnormal bone. (Resection of the dural venous sinus.)

♦ Grade 2: macroscopically complete removal and, with coagulation of dural attachment.

♦ Grade 3: macroscopically complete removal, without resection or coagulation of dural attachment. (Without removal of invaded sinus or hyperostotic bone.)

♦ Grade 4: partial removal.

♦ Grade 5: simple decompression (with or without biopsy).

Source data from *J Neurol Neurosurg Psychiatry*, 20(1), Simpson D, The recurrence of intracranial meningiomas after surgical treatment, pp. 22–39, Copyright (1957), BMJ Publishing Group Ltd.

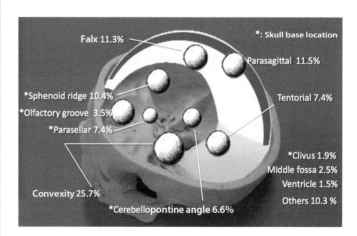

Fig. 11.2 Frequency of meningiomas of each localization according to the Brain Tumor Registry of Japan.

in local control and reducing recurrences in large meningiomas, either suboptimally excised or as the only treatment in inoperable tumours. Technological advancements in precise delivery of modern conformal radiotherapy like stereotactic radiotherapy and intensity-modulated radiotherapy (IMRT) aided in optimal dose delivery and reduction of normal tissue damage. Studies demonstrate higher local control rates and recurrence-free survival rates with conformal radiotherapy compared to conventional techniques used in the past.

The role of radiotherapy, indications, and guidelines for energy, dose, and fractionation of radiotherapy for meningioma are relatively lacking due to a lack of phase III randomized controlled trials. Available evidence for adjuvant or upfront radiotherapy for meningioma is based on large retrospective studies or non-randomized prospective studies showing excellent local control rates with stereotactic radiosurgery (SRS) and fractionated external beam radiotherapy (EBRT). Among various large studies, a review of nearly 50 studies involving more than 4500 patients by Mehta et al. showed merits and demerits of various forms of radiotherapy. SRS showed 5-year recurrence free survival of 75–100%, while fractionated radiotherapy showed 80–100% (53).

The natural history of benign meningiomas was described for 244 patients with benign meningiomas on serial surveillance MRI scans and at a follow-up of about 4 years, 74% showed growth on volumetric criteria (>8.2%) and 44% using linear criteria (2 mm), with 26.3% requiring treatment in this period (54).

Recurrence rates based on Simpson grading of excision of meningiomas (as described earlier in the surgery section) shows a certain number of patients experience recurrences after incomplete resection as well as grade 1 (theoretically complete) resection (44).

A retrospective study to identify clinical features associated with progression and death in atypical meningioma revealed that bone involvement is associated with increased tumour progression and decreased overall survival. Subtotal resection was associated with increased tumour progression while aggressive bone removal with wide-excision cranioplasty or adjuvant bone irradiation shows improvement in treatment outcome (55).

Indications for radiotherapy

1. Primary radiotherapy: medically inoperable or not amenable for surgical excision in symptomatic patients due to close proximity to critical structures.

2. Radiotherapy after subtotal excision for grade I tumours: subtotal excision alone may not be sufficient particularly at areas where re-excision will not be feasible due to close proximity to important structures, such as in a parasellar/skull base location, and will need postoperative radiotherapy to decrease the chance of recurrence.

3. Radiotherapy after subtotal resection for atypical and malignant lesions: recurrence rates of grade II and grade III are high. These tumours always need postoperative radiotherapy irrespective of location and size of the lesion.

4. Radiotherapy after gross total excision of grade II and grade III tumours: upfront radiotherapy may be withheld in grade II lesions which are totally excised, are amenable to close observation with contrast MRI scanning, and those which are amenable

for re-excision at recurrence. However, those situated at eloquent areas and grade III malignant lesions need postoperative radiotherapy after the first excision.

5. Radiotherapy at recurrence: radiotherapy alone or after excision of the recurrent lesion is effective for salvage of recurrent lesions.

Modalities of radiotherapy

Fractionated external beam radiotherapy

Compared to conventional radiotherapy and three-dimensional conformal radiotherapy, IMRT is useful in tumours close to critical areas, especially the skull base. IMRT provides better tumour coverage, better sparing of the normal structures, improves local control, and reduces toxicity. In the pre-IMRT era, patients were treated with fractionated stereotactic conformal radiotherapy (SCRT). Late toxicity rates after IMRT in literature are less than 5%. Improvements in outcome after IMRT are also related to advances in technology of treatment planning and delivery. IMRT delivered by segmental, dynamic, and arc-based IMRT and tomotherapy techniques seem to produce equivalent target coverage and avoidance of critical structures, although tomotherapy provides a marginally better coverage and normal tissue toxicity (56).

Radiosurgery (RS)

Radiosurgery (RS) is a preferred modality for recurrent, small, grade I lesions located in close proximity to critical structures or if the condition of the patient does not permit delivery of prolonged fractionated radiotherapy. Ideally in grade II or grade III lesions, RS is not practised as the target volume of RS will not encompass subclinical disease. However if the location of tumour is critical for re-excision and the residual disease is small, they can be considered for RS. RS can be delivered by LINAC, Gamma Knife®, or robotic radiosurgery system by CyberKnife®. A meningioma size of greater than 3.5 cm mean diameter, optic nerve/chiasm compression, or optic nerve sheath meningioma (ONSM) are cited as contraindications to single-fraction radiosurgery. For larger meningiomas, some groups have delivered RS for two to five fractions by CyberKnife® and reported good short-term progression-free survival (PFS) rates and low toxicity (57).

Proton therapy and heavy ions

Proton beam therapy is used as a boost treatment after EBRT with comparable results with photon therapy. One debatable advantage of proton therapy is the relatively low incidence of second malignancies due to reduced integral dose, although long-term follow-up results are not available. Carbon ion therapy has been used in the setting of re-irradiation. Early results of this were comparable to photon therapy (58).

Imaging for volume delineation and planning

Contrast-enhanced T1 MRI is the best imaging modality for all meningiomas and fat-suppressed sequences may be needed for a few skull base tumours. For bony structures, infiltration of cavernous sinus or other regions of the skull base, CT is better to demonstrate bone infiltration and osteolytic areas. Hence co-registration of CT/MRI may be helpful in many situations (59).

Positron emission tomography (PET) imaging, especially with amino-acid-PET or somatostatin-receptor-PET has been tested for volume delineation, mainly to distinguish tumour from inflammation and oedema. ^{11}C-methionine positron emission tomography (MET-PET) for gross tumour volume delineation in fractionated stereotactic radiotherapy of skull base meningiomas demonstrated that addition of MET-PET can lead to an increase, as well as a decrease in gross target volume (GTV). In addition, the inter-observer variability of target volume definition was reduced significantly when adding MET-PET to CT/MRI-based contouring.

^{68}Ga-DOTA-D Phe[1]-Tyr[3]-octreotide (DOTATOC)-PET has also been used in the treatment planning of meningiomas. In a study, ^{68}GaDOTATOC-PET/CT for radiation treatment planning provided additional information on tumour extension, median GTV was larger. Many more studies implementing ^{68}Ga-DOTATOC-PET/CT for volume delineation have shown adaptations even in the postoperative setting, or in regions of bony anatomy (60).

Modern imaging-based treatment planning such as CT/MRI-based target definition and appropriate immobilization has improved the results of modern conformal EBRT. Goldsmith and colleagues have shown that with MRI-based planning and appropriate immobilization the local control rate has improved from 77% to 98% (61).

Planning target volumes have varied from a 2–4 cm expansion around the GTV to about 5 mm in the modern SCRT techniques. Traditional definition of margins as defined by Milker-Zabel et al. was 1–2 mm against normal brain, 3 mm against osseous structures, and 5 mm along the dura (62). However, with lesser margins as in SCRT, marginal recurrences are unknown. The SCRT technique for skull base meningiomas demonstrated an impressive 5-year local control rate of 100% and actuarial survival rate of 91%. SCRT was well tolerated with minimal toxicity in terms of cranial neuropathy, pituitary dysfunction, and cognitive dysfunction was minimal (63).

A common feature with meningioma is its dural attachment with occasional invasion and also invasion of the overlying periosteum. The linear trailing enhancement noted adjacent to the meningioma is known as the 'dural tail', initially described by Borovich and Doron. Ahmadi et al. confirmed the enhancement histopathologically and identified two types: continuous and discontinuous. The continuous enhancements were found to contain only 'proliferation, inflammation and hypervascularity' of the arachnoid membrane but not invasion by the meningioma, while the discontinuous enhancements showed invasion by the dural tumour. Dural tail is only a radiological finding and the majority of the studies demonstrating efficacy of surgery alone have not excised the dural tail (64).

In the present context, identifying the tumour accurately is very critical in achieving maximum local control. Inclusion of the more suspicious, thick or nodular dural area adjoining the main meningeal tumour is vital.

Hyperostosis in the bone adjacent to a skull base meningioma is found to have tumour invasion and in order to achieve a complete resection, removal of the adjacent bone has been recommended by Pieper and colleagues. Simpson grade I resection needs removal of adjacent bone. If not removed during surgery, inclusion of the hyperostotic bone in the SRS or the EBRT volume has been shown to improve the local control, although in tumours located close to optic pathway or petrous ridge, this might increase the toxicity (65).

Perilesional oedema indicates a likelihood of brain invasion (for each centimetre of oedema, the probability of brain invasion increases by 20%) and has been shown to relate to tumour aggressiveness, correlating with a high meningioma MIB-1 index (66).

Results of fractionated external beam radiotherapy

Primary EBRT for optic nerve sheath meningioma

Optic nerve sheath meningiomas arising from the dura surrounding the optic nerve are ideal tumours for primary EBRT. Due to the relative rarity of these tumours, they were either observed or excised, both of which led to blindness in the affected eye. Optic nerve-sparing surgery can lead to damage to the blood vessels that surround the nerve in the sheath and eventually lead to blindness. Advances in neuroimaging have led to an increase in incidence of these tumours. Modern conformal radiotherapy has proved effective in preserving useful vision. ONSMs are presently managed on the basis of clinical and radiological findings.

Turbin et al. reported outcomes of 64 optic nerve sheath meningiomas (ONSM) patients with EBRT to a dose of 50–55 Gy and found that fractionated EBRT was better in vision preservation compared to surgery alone or observation. Available literature shows excellent efficacy of EBRT alone for ONSM with a local control of 98%, improved vision in 75%, and stable vision in an additional 21%. Only 4% of patients had visual deterioration either at recurrence or as a sequel to EBRT (67). The natural course of ONSM being gradual visual loss leading to blindness in the affected eye, an earlier treatment initiation is found to yield higher visual preservation rates, although this is debatable in patients with normal vision and incidentally detected tumours.

Primary EBRT for skull base meningioma

The proximity of these tumours to vital structures makes decision-making of treatment based on expertise of the treating clinician. With a growth rate of 1–3 mm per year, incidentally detected asymptomatic tumours, especially in elderly patients, just need observation alone by surveillance with contrast-enhanced MRI. Intervention is needed when tumour growth is documented or with clinical worsening. Fractionated stereotactic radiotherapy, IMRT, or image-guided radiotherapy techniques for these complex-shaped lesions in close vicinity to sensitive organs at risk by using multifield techniques or with intensity-modulated individual beams improves dose conformality and reduces dose to normal structures.

Nutting et al. demonstrated long-term efficacy of fractionated stereotactic radiotherapy in 222 patients with grade I meningioma, treated with doses of 50–55 Gy in 30–33 fractions. While the overall cohort had 5- and 10-year local control rates of 93% and 86% respectively, patients with cavernous sinus/parasellar region meningiomas had local control of 100%. Cranial nerve deficit occurred in 3.5% (68).

Postoperative external beam radiotherapy

Radical excision of meningiomas may not be feasible for many sites. Likelihood of progression after incomplete resection is shown to be nearly 35% at 5 years. Studies by Milker-Zabel and Henzel et al. have shown a 5-year PFS of about 95% after fractionated conformal radiotherapy in patients after subtotal resection (69, 70).

Results of radiosurgery

Studies involving radiosurgery either as sole treatment or after surgery to doses ranging from 10 to 14 Gy demonstrated 5-year recurrence-free survival of 75–100%. Various radiosurgery techniques are comparable with respect to clinical outcome and toxicity. The relationship between dose and volume on side effects after radiosurgery is well documented especially for cranial nerves and development of intracranial oedema. This forms the basis of limitation for radiosurgery for complex volumes adjacent to organs at risk and large size, while fractionated treatments are not associated with toxicity and dose, volume, or diameter of the tumour.

In patients with brainstem compression or in critical locations such as the foramen magnum, radiosurgery can be considered as a treatment alternative especially in older patients or patients with significant co-morbidities. Radiosurgery is recommended if the marginal doses are kept below 15 Gy (70).

Large data from the Pittsburgh group for radiosurgery for petroclival meningioma treated with the Gamma Knife® showed improvement in neurological status after radiosurgery with median dose to the tumour margin of 13 Gy. Overall 10-year PFS rate was 86% with radiation-related complications associated with convexity/falx tumours, not in the skull base region, and increasing tumour volume (71).

Toxicity after radiotherapy

Long-term toxicity is a concern for meningioma patients, as they usually have long life expectancies. Overall permanent toxicity rates of 0–18% and 2.5–23% have been reported with modern EBRT and radiosurgery techniques.

Toxicity after external beam radiotherapy

For EBRT, optic neuropathy and retinopathy are rare with doses of 54 and 45 Gy, respectively (<2 Gy per fraction) and rates of severe dry-eye syndrome, retinopathy, and optic neuropathy increase steeply after doses of 40, 50, and 60 Gy to related organs, respectively. Pituitary hormone insufficiency, seizures, hearing and other cranial nerve deficits, and necrosis are occasionally reported. Although an improvement of 38% in late effects after modern EBRT compared to traditional techniques has been shown by Al-Mefty et al. (10), grade III toxicity in terms of cranial neuropathy and deterioration of visual deficits has been shown to be about 1.7–2.2%. Soldà et al. showed that the rate of pituitary dysfunction and cognitive deficits after SCRT for skull base meningiomas is about 4% (72).

Toxicity after stereotactic radiosurgery

Cranial nerve deficits and vasogenic oedema are the most common side effects seen after SRS. The incidence of cranial deficits is about 8%, with the sensory nerves of the anterior visual pathway being most susceptible. Post-treatment vasogenic oedema was found to be most common in non-basal meningiomas particularly in parasagittal meningiomas, as they tend to have a large pial surface causing a larger part of the brain to be exposed. Basal meningiomas on the other hand are known to produce less oedema (73). Tumours more than 3 cm in size, doses greater than 15 Gy, and pretreatment oedema are all known to cause increased vasogenic oedema after SRS.

Recently, normal tissue tolerance and tolerance differences between select neural structures have been defined by various groups. For the optic pathway, the maximum dose in a single fraction should be below 10 Gy. Between 10 and 15 Gy, radiation-induced optic neuropathy was around 30% and approximately 80% with doses of 15 Gy or more, while doses of 12–16 Gy to only very small segments of the optic nerve were associated with acceptable toxicity (74).

Medical therapies for meningiomas

There is an important subgroup of patients with inoperable or high-grade tumours who develop recurrent disease following surgery and radiation therapy. The treatment options for these patients are currently inadequate and there is significant interest in finding more effective medical therapies for them (18, 75).

The evaluation of medical therapies has been complicated by the lack of data regarding the natural history of untreated meningiomas. Many chemotherapy studies report variable periods of disease stabilization, but it is difficult to know whether this represents an improvement since these tumours grow slowly and benign (WHO grade I) meningiomas especially may appear radiographically stable for prolonged periods (76, 77). Recently the Response Assessment in Neuro-Oncology (RANO) Working Group reviewed the historical benchmarks for medical therapy trials in surgery- and radiation-refractory meningioma and found a weighted 6-month progression-free survival (PFS6) of 29% for benign (WHO grade I) meningiomas, and 26% for atypical and malignant meningiomas (WHO grades II and III) (78).

Chemotherapy

Data from small clinical trials and case series suggest that most chemotherapeutic agents have minimal or no activity against meningiomas (3, 18, 19, 79–84). Most interest has focused on hydroxyurea, an oral ribonucleotide reductase inhibitor, which arrests meningioma cell growth in the S phase of the cell cycle and induces apoptosis (85). Although early reports suggested that hydroxyurea had activity in recurrent meningiomas (86), a large number of subsequent studies have failed to confirm these findings (87–93). Other agents that have been studied with negative results include chemotherapeutic regimens such as dacarbazine and Adriamycin®, or ifosfamide and mesna that have activity in other soft tissue tumours (37, 81, 94) as well as temozolomide (95), irinotecan (96), and alpha interferon (97, 98).

Hormonal therapy

Since oestrogen receptors are expressed in approximately 10% of meningiomas, while progesterone receptors and androgen receptors are present in approximately two-thirds of meningiomas (15, 18, 99–101), there has been extensive interest in hormonal therapy for meningiomas. However, studies of oestrogen (102, 103) and progesterone receptor inhibitors, including a large placebo-controlled phase II study of the antiprogesterone mifepristone failed to demonstrate any antitumour activity (104).

Somatostatin receptors, especially the sst2A subtype, are expressed in nearly 90% of meningiomas (105). In a pilot study of 16 patients with recurrent meningiomas treated with monthly injections of a sustained-release somatostatin analogue (Sandostatin LAR®), 31% experienced a response (106), suggesting that somatostatin analogues may have activity. However, a recently completed multicentre study of pasireotide (SOM230C), a somatostatin analogue with a wider somatostatin receptor spectrum (including subtypes 1, 2, 3, and 5) and higher affinity (particularly for subtypes 1, 3, and 5) than Sandostatin LAR® did not show any activity (107).

Targeted molecular agents

The importance of dysregulated cell signalling as a cause of neoplastic transformation is increasingly apparent. Emerging data have identified aberrant expression of critical signalling molecules in meningioma cells (84, 108), suggesting that drugs designed to target pathways involved in cell growth, proliferation, and angiogenesis may prove valuable in therapy. Unlike gliomas, where the blood–brain barrier limits the penetration of many therapeutic agents, the penetration of targeted agent in meningiomas is unlikely to be a major issue. However, in contrast to the extensive work on understanding the genetics of systemic cancers and gliomas, relatively little work has been conducted in understanding the growth factors and their receptors, and the signal transduction pathways that are critical to meningioma growth (80, 109–112).

Platelet-derived growth factor receptor

Meningiomas express both platelet-derived growth factor (PDGF)-AA and -BB and PDGF-beta receptors (113–116), raising the possibility of an autocrine signalling loop supporting meningioma cell growth and maintenance. Imatinib mesylate, an inhibitor of PDGFβ, was evaluated in a phase II study in 23 recurrent meningiomas by the North American Brain Tumor Consortium (NABTC). Although the treatment was generally well tolerated, the agent had minimal activity (117). More recently, imatinib has been combined with hydroxyurea and showed a PFS6 of 42.3% in grade II/III meningiomas, raising the possibility that this combination has some activity (118).

The epidermal growth factor receptor (EGFR) is also overexpressed in more than 60% of meningiomas (119–125). The NABTC conducted two small exploratory trials of the EGFR inhibitors erlotinib and gefitinib and found no objective responses. For grade I tumours, the PFS6 was 25%, while for grade II and III tumours, PFS6 was 29% (126).

Recently, evidence has emerged that the phosphatidylinositol-3-kinase/mammalian target of rapamycin (mTOR) pathway is activated in meningiomas and mTORC1 inhibitors such as temsirolimus have activities in orthotopic models (127). In addition to temsirolimus, a number of other mTOR inhibitors such as everolimus and sirolimus are clinically approved, and may have therapeutic potential in meningiomas.

Most promising are the results of recent deep sequencing studies of meningiomas which found *AKT1* E17K mutations in approximately 8%, and smoothened mutations (*SMO* W535L) in 5% of grade I meningiomas (128, 129). Since these are known oncogenic mutations for which there are available inhibitors, these findings have led to clinical trials of AKT and SMO inhibitors for meningiomas with these mutations.

Inhibition of angiogenesis

Meningiomas are highly vascular tumours. Vascular endothelial growth factor (VEGF) and VEGF receptors (VEGFRs) are expressed in meningiomas, and the level of expression increases with tumour grade (130–132). VEGF expression is increased two-fold in atypical meningiomas, and ten-fold in malignant meningiomas compared to benign meningiomas (130). VEGF also plays an important role in the formation of peritumoural oedema which adds to the morbidity of these tumours (131, 132). Inhibitors of VEGF and VEGFR have the potential not only to inhibit angiogenesis, but also to decrease peritumoural oedema.

Clinical trials of angiogenesis inhibitors for meningiomas are ongoing. A multicentre phase II study of sunitinib, a VEGFR/PDGFR inhibitor, was recently completed and appears to have activity with a PFS6 in grade II/III meningiomas of 42% (133). Phase II trials of vatalanib, another VEGFR/PDGFR inhibitor, and bevacizumab, a humanized monoclonal antibody, have completed accrual and results should become available in the near future. While these agents may have a modest effect on peritumoural oedema, and possibly tumour size, they are unlikely to represent a significant advance in therapy.

A recently identified potential biomarker for meningioma is TERT promoter mutation. The protein encoded by the *TERT* gene, telomerase reverse transcriptase, contributes essentially to the immortalization of cancer cells by extending their telomeres. Mutations in the promoter region at hotspots chromosome 5:1,295,228 (C228T) or chromosome 5:1,295,250 (C250T), result in new binding sites for members of the E-twenty-six (ETS) transcription factor family. Increased ETS-binding drives upregulation of *TERT* expression, and consecutively maintains telomere length of the proliferating cancer cells. Interestingly, increased *ETS-1* expression appears to be associated with aggressive course of meningioma. Median time to progression among mutant cases was 10.1 months compared with 179.0 months among wildtype cases. *TERT* promoter mutations are associated with higher meningioma grades and with early recurrence and may be a useful tool assisting in the grading of meningiomas (134).

Despite advances in surgery, radiation therapy, and radiosurgery, there is a small but important subset of patients with meningiomas who develop recurrent disease refractory to conventional therapies. Unfortunately, chemotherapies and hormonal therapies have so far shown minimal activity. Progress in identifying alternative forms of therapy for these patients with recurrent meningiomas has been limited by poor understanding of the molecular pathogenesis of meningiomas and the critical molecular changes driving tumour growth, and by the lack of meningioma cell lines and tumour models for preclinical studies. Nonetheless, progress in cancer genomics is providing molecular information about meningiomas at an increasing rate, helping to identify gene mutations such as in *AKT1* and *SMO* that may drive growth in a subset of tumours.

It is hoped that further advances in medical therapy based on understanding of the biology of this tumour will lead to more effective treatments for patients with meningiomas.

Conclusion

The gold standard for care for meningiomas is surgery, and radiation therapy and radiosurgery can be applied in some instances. The majority of meningiomas can be controlled by these modalities.

Acknowledgements

The authors thank Haruka Astumi (BS) and Wakae Fujimaki (MD, PhD) for their editorial assistance.

References

1. Central Brain Tumor Registry of the United States (CBTRUS). *CBTRUS Statistical Report (2010): Primary Brain and Central Nervous System Tumors Diagnosed in the United States in 2004-2006.* Hinsdale, IL: CBTRUS. http://www.cbtrus.org/2010-NPCR-SEER/CBTRUS-WEBREPORT-Final-3-2-10.pdf.

2. Japan, Committee of Brain Tumor Registry. Report of Brain Tumor Registry of Japan (1984–2000) 12th Ed. *Neurol Med Chir (Tokyo)* 2009; 49(Suppl):PS1–96.

3. Marosi C, Hassler M, Roessler K, et al. Meningioma. *Crit Rev Oncol Hematol* 2008; 67:153–171.

4. Banerjee J, Paakko E, Harila M, et al. Radiation-induced meningiomas: a shadow in the success story of childhood leukemia. *Neuro Oncol* 2009; 11:543–549.

5. Claus EB, Bondy ML, Schildkraut JM, et al. Epidemiology of intracranial meningioma. *Neurosurgery* 2005; 57:1088–1095.

6. Louis DN, Ohgaki H, Wiestler OD, et al. (eds) *WHO Classification of Tumours of the Central Nervous System.* Lyon: International Agency for Research on Cancer.

7. Maier H, Ofner D, Hittmair A, et al. Classic, atypical, and anaplastic meningioma: Three histopathological subtypes of clinical relevance. *J Neurosurg* 1992; 77:616–623.

8. Willis J, Smith C, Ironside JW, et al. The accuracy of meningioma grading: a 10-year retrospective audit. *Neuropathol Appl Neurobiol* 2005; 31:141–149.

9. Pearson BE, Markert JM, Fisher WS, et al. Hitting a moving target: evolution of a treatment paradigm for atypical meningiomas amid changing diagnostic criteria. *Neurosurg Focus* 2008; 24:E3.

10. Al-Mefty O, Kadri PA, Pravdenkova S, et al. Malignant progression in meningioma: documentation of a series and analysis of cytogenetic findings. *J Neurosurg* 2004; 101:210–218.

11. Goutagny S, Kalamarides M. Meningiomas and neurofibromatosis. *J Neurooncol* 2010; 99:341–347.

12. Rouleau GA, Merel P, Lutchman M, et al. Alteration in a new gene encoding a putative membrane-organizing protein causes neuro-fibromatosis type 2. *Nature* 1993; 363:515–521.

13. van den Munckhof P, Christiaans I, Kenter SB, et al. Germline SMARCB1 mutation predisposes to multiple meningiomas and schwannomas with preferential location of cranial meningiomas at the falxcerebri. *Neurogenetics* 2012; 13:1–7.

14. Klaeboe L, Lonn S, Scheie D, et al. Incidence of intracranial meningiomas in Denmark, Finland, Norway and Sweden, 1968–1997. *Int J Cancer* 2005; 117:996–1001.

15. Lamszus K. Meningioma pathology, genetics, and biology. *J Neuropathol Exp Neurol* 2004; 63:275–286.

16. Blankenstein MA, Verheijen FM, Jacobs JM, et al. Occurrence, regulation, and significance of progesterone receptors in human meningioma. *Steroids* 2000; 65:795–800.

17. Carroll RS, Zhang J, Dashner K, et al. Androgen receptor expression in meningiomas. *J Neurosurg* 1995; 82:453–460.

18. Norden AD, Wen PY. Chemotherapy and experimental medical therapies for meningiomas. In: Pamir N, Black P, Fahlbusch R (eds) *Meningiomas: A Comprehensive Text.* Philadelphia, PA: Elsevier, 2010; 667–679.

19. Dashti SR, Sauvageau E, Smith KA, et al. Nonsurgical treatment options in the management of intracranial meningiomas. *Front Biosci (Elite Ed)* 2009; 1:494–500.

20. Chargari C, Vedrine L, Bauduceau O, et al. Reapprasial of the role of endocrine therapy in meningioma management. *Endocr Relat Cancer* 2008; 15:931–941.

21. Schoenberg BS, Christine BW, Whisnant JP. Nervous system neoplasms and primary malignancies of other sites. The unique association between meningiomas and breast cancer. *Neurology* 1975; 25:705–712.

22. Blitshteyn S, Crook JE, Jaeckle KA. Is there an association between meningioma and hormone replacement therapy? *J Clin Oncol* 2008; 26:279–282.

23. Claus EB, Black PM, Bondy ML, et al. Exogenous hormone use and meningioma risk: what do we tell our patients? *Cancer* 2007; 110:471–476.

24. Gazzeri R, Galarza M, Gazzeri G. Growth of a meningioma in a transsexual patient after estrogen-progestin therapy. *N Engl J Med* 2007; 357:2411–2412.

25. Custer B, Longstreth WT, Jr, Phillips LE, et al. Hormonal exposures and the risk of intracranial meningioma in women: a population-based case-control study. *BMC Cancer* 2006; 6:152.

26. Wiemels J, Wrensch M, Claus EB. Epidemiology and etiology of meningioma. *J Neurooncol* 2010; 99:307–314.

27. Braganza MZ, Kitahara CM, Berrington de Gonzalez A, et al. Ionizing radiation and the risk of brain and central nervous system tumors: a systematic review. *Neuro Oncol* 2012; 14:1316–1324.

28. Ron E, Modan B, Boice JD, et al. Tumors of the brain and nervous system after radiotherapy in childhood. *N Engl J Med* 1988; 319:1033–1039.

29. Friedman DL, Whitton J, Leisenring W, et al. Subsequent neoplasms in 5-year survivors of childhood cancer: the Childhood Cancer Survivor Study. *J Natl Cancer Inst* 2010; 102:1083–1095.

30. Taylor AJ, Little MP, Winter DL, et al. Population-based risks of CNS tumors in survivors of childhood cancer: the British Childhood Cancer Survivor Study. *J Clin Oncol* 2010; 28:5287–5293.

31. Pearce MS, Salotti JA, Little MP, et al. Radiation exposure from CT scans in childhood and subsequent risk of leukaemia and brain tumors: a retrospective cohort study. *Lancet* 2012; 380:499–505.

32. Claus EB, Calvocoressi L, Bondy ML, et al. Dental x-rays and risk of meningioma. *Cancer* 2012; 118:4530–4537.

33. Jhawar BS, Fuchs CS, Colditz GA, et al. Sex steroid hormone exposures and risk for meningioma. *J Neurosurg* 2003; 99:848–853.

34. Preston-Martin S, Pogoda JM, Schlehofer B, et al. An international case-control study of adult glioma and meningioma: the role of head trauma. *Int J Epidemiol* 1998; 27:579–586.

35. Vernooij MW, Ikram MA, Tanghe HL, et al. Incidental findings on brain MRI in the general population. *N Engl J Med* 2007; 357:1821–1828.

36. Whittle I, Smith C, Navoo P, Collie D. Meningiomas. *Lancet* 2004; 363:1535–1543.

37. Chozick BS, Reinert SE, Greenblatt SH. Incidence of seizures after surgery for supratentorial meningiomas: a modern analysis. *J Neurosurg* 1996; 84:382–386.

38. Lieu AS, Howng SL. Intracranial meningiomas and epilepsy: incidence, prognosis and influencing factors. *Epilepsy Res* 2000; 38:45–52.

39. Kennedy F, Retrobulbar neuritis as an exact diagnostic sign of certain tumors and abscesses in the frontal lobe. *Am J Med Sci* 1991; 142:355–368.

40. Glantz MJ, Cole BF, Forsyth PA, et al. Practice parameter: anticonvulsant prophylaxis in patients with newly diagnosed brain tumors. Report of the Quality Standards Subcommittee of the American Academy of Neurology. *Neurology* 2000; 54:1886–1893.

41. Gerber DE, Segal JB, Salhotra A, et al. Venous thromboembolism occurs infrequently in meningioma patients receiving combined modality prophylaxis. *Cancer* 2007; 109:300–305.

42. Sotoudeh H. Yazdi HR, A review on dural tail sign. *World J Radiol* 2010; 2:188–192.

43. Nakaguchi H, Fujimaki T, Matsuno A, et al. Postoperative residual tumor growth of meningioma can be predicted by MIB-1 immunohistochemistry. *Cancer* 1999; 85:2249–2254.

44. Simpson D, The recurrence of intracranial meningiomas after surgical treatment. *J Neurol Neurosurg Psychiatry* 1957; 20:22–39.

45. Sughrue ME, Kane AJ, Shangari G, et al. The relevance of Simpson Grade I and II resection in modern neurosurgical treatment of World Health Organization Grade I meningiomas. *J Neurosurg* 2010; 113:1029–1035.

46. Hasseleid BF, Meling TR, Rønning P, et al. Surgery for convexity meningioma: Simpson Grade I resection as the goal. *J Neurosurg* 2012; 117:999–1006.

47. Heros RC. Editorial: Simpson grades. *J Neurosurg* 2012; 117:997–998.

48. Hashimoto N, Rabo CS, Okita Y, et al. Slower growth of skull base meningiomas compared with non-skull base meningiomas based on volumetric and biological studies. *J Neurosurg* 2012; 116:574–580.

49. Oya S, Kawai K, Nakatomi H, et al. Significance of Simpson grading system in modern meningioma surgery: integration of the grade with MIB-1 labeling index as a key to predict the recurrence of WHO Grade I meningiomas. *J Neurosurg* 2012; 117:121–128.

50. Ho DM, Hsu CY, Ting LT, Chiang H. Histopathology and MIB-1 labeling index predicted recurrence of meningiomas: a proposal of diagnostic criteria for patients with atypical meningioma. *Cancer* 2002; 94:1538–1547.

51. Singla A, Deshaies EM, Melnyk V, et al. Controversies in the role of preoperative embolization in meningioma management. *Neurosurg Focus* 2013; 35:E17.

52. Ron E, Modan B, Boice JD Jr, et al. Tumors of the brain and nervous system after radiotherapy in childhood. *N Engl J Med* 1988, 319:1033–1039.

53. Rogers L and Mehta M. Role of radiation therapy in treating intracranial Meningiomas. *Neurosurg Focus* 2007, 23:E4.

54. Oya S, Kim SH, Sade B, et al. The natural history of intracranial meningiomas. *J Neurosurg* 2011; 114:1250–1256.

55. Goyal L, Barnett G, et al. Local control and overall survival in atypical meningioma: a retrospective review. *Int J Radiat Oncol Biol Phys* 2000; 46:57–61.

56. Gupta T, Wadasadawala T, Master Z, et al. Encouraging early clinical outcomes with helical tomotherapy-based image-guided intensity-modulated radiation therapy for residual, recurrent, and/or progressive benign/low-grade intracranial tumors: a comprehensive evaluation. *Int J Radiat Oncol Phys Biol* 2012; 82:756–764.

57. Colombo F, Casentini L, Cavedon C, et al. Cyberknife radiosurgery for benign meningiomas: short-term results in 199 patients. *Neurosurgery* 2009; 64:A7–A13.

58. Weber DC, Lomax AJ, Rutz HP, et al. Swiss Proton Users Group. Spot-scanning proton radiation therapy for recurrent, residual or untreated intracranial meningiomas. *Radiother Oncol* 2004; 71:251–258.

59. Campbell BA, Jhamb A, Maguire JA, et al. Meningiomas in 2009: controversies and future challenges. *Am J Clin Oncol* 2009; 32:73–85.

60. Combs SE, Welzel T, Habermehl D, et al. Prospective evaluation of early treatment outcome in patients with meningiomas treated with particle therapy based on target volume definition with MRI and (68) GaDOTATOC-PET. *Acta Oncol* 2013; 52:514–520.

61. Goldsmith BJ, Larson DA. Conventional radiation therapy for skull base meningiomas. *Neurosurg Clin N Am* 2000; 11:605–615.

62. Milker-Zabel S, Zabel-du Bois A, Huber P, et al. Intensity-modulated radiotherapy for complex-shaped meningioma of the skull base: long-term experience of a single institution. *Int J Radiat Oncol Biol Phys* 2007; 68:858–863.

63. Jalali R, Loughrey C, Baumert B, et al. High precision focused irradiation in the form of fractionated stereotactic conformal radiotherapy (SCRT) for benign meningiomas predominantly in the skull base location. *Clin Oncol (R Coll Radiol)* 2002; 14:103–109.

64. Nägele T, Petersen D, Klose U, et al. The 'dural tail' adjacent to meningiomas studied by dynamic contrast-enhanced MRI: A comparison with histopathology. *Neuroradiology* 1994; 36:303–307.

65. Pieper DR, Al-Mefty O, Hanada Y, et al. Hyperostosis associated with meningioma of the cranial base: secondary changes or tumor invasion. *Neurosurgery* 1999; 44:742–747.

66. Mantle RE, Lach B, Delgado MR, et al. Predicting the probability of meningioma recurrence based on the quantity of peritumoral brain edema on computerized tomography scanning. *J Neurosurg* 1999; 91:375–383.

67. Bloch O, Sun M, Kaur S, et al. Fractionated radiotherapy for optic nerve sheath meningiomas. *J Clin Neurosci* 2012; 19:1210–1215.

68. Nutting C, Brada M, Brazil L, et al. Radiotherapy in the treatment of benign meningioma of the skull base. *J Neurosurg* 1999; 90:823–827.

69. Milker-Zabel S, Zabel A, Schultz-Ertner D, et al. Fractionated stereotactic radiotherapy in patients with benign or atypical intracranial meningiomas. *Int J Radiat Oncol Biol Phys* 2005; 61:809–816.

70. Henzel M, Gross MW, Hamm K, et al. Significant tumor volume reduction of meningiomas after stereotactic radiotherapy: results of prospective multicenter study. *Neurosurgery* 2006; 59:1188–1194.

71. Kondziolka D, Flickinger JC, Lunsford LD. Clinical research in stereotactic radiosurgery: lessons learned from over 10 000 cases. *Neurol Res* 2011; 33(8):792–802.

72. Soldà F, Wharram B, De Ieso PB, et al. Long-term efficacy of fractionated radiotherapy for benign meningiomas. *Radiother Oncol* 2013; 109:330–334.

73. Kondziolka D, Mathieu D, Lunsford LD, et al. Radiosurgery as definitive management of intracranial meningiomas. *Neurosurgery* 2008; 62:53–58.

74. Stafford S, Pollock B, Leavitt J, et al. A study on the radiation tolerance of the optic nerves and chiasm after stereotactic radiosurgery. *Int J Radiat Oncol Biol Phys* 2003; 55:1177–1181.

75. Wen PY, Quant E, Drappatz J, et al. Medical therapies for meningiomas. *J Neurooncol* 2010; 99:365–378.

76. Herscovici Z, Rappaport Z, Sulkes J, et al. Natural history of conservatively treated meningiomas. *Neurology* 2004; 63:1133–1134.

77. Zeidman LA, Ankenbrandt WJ, Paleologos N, et al. Analysis of growth rate in non-operated meningiomas. *Neurology* 2006; 66:A400.

78. Kaley T, Barani I, Chamberlain M, et al. Historical benchmarks for medical therapy trials in surgery- and radiation-refractory meningioma: a RANO review. *Neuro Oncol* 2014; 16(6):829–840.

79. Sioka C, Kyritsis AP. Chemotherapy, hormonal therapy, and immunotherapy for recurrent meningiomas. *J Neurooncol* 2009; 92:1–6.

80. McMullen KP, Stieber VW. Meningioma: current treatment options and future directions. *Curr Treat Options Oncol* 2004; 5:499–509.

81. Chamberlain MC, Blumenthal DT. Intracranial meningiomas: diagnosis and treatment. *Expert Rev Neurother* 2004; 4:641–648.

82. Chamberlain MC. Adjuvant combined modality therapy for malignant meningiomas. *J Neurosurg* 1996; 84:733–736.

83. Norden AD, Drappatz J, Wen PY. Advances in meningioma therapy. *Curr Neurol Neurosci Rep* 2009; 9:231–240.

84. Johnson MD, Sade B, Milano MT, et al. New prospects for management and treatment of inoperable and recurrent skull base meningiomas. *J Neurooncol* 2008; 86:109–122.

85. Schrell UM, Rittig MG, Anders M, et al. Hydroxyurea for treatment of unresectable and recurrent meningiomas. I. Inhibition of primary human meningioma cells in culture and in meningioma transplants by induction of the apoptotic pathway. *J Neurosurg* 1997; 86:845–852.

86. Schrell UM, Rittig MG, Anders M, et al. Hydroxyurea for treatment of unresectable and recurrent meningiomas. II. Decrease in the size of meningiomas in patients treated with hydroxyurea. *J Neurosurg* 1997; 86:840–844.

87. Mason WP, Gentili F, Macdonald DR, et al. Stabilization of disease progression by hydroxyurea in patients with recurrent or unresectable meningioma. *J Neurosurg* 2002; 97:341–346.

88. Newton HB, Scott SR, Volpi C. Hydroxyurea chemotherapy for meningiomas: enlarged cohort with extended follow-up. *Br J Neurosurg* 2004; 18:495–499.

89. Rosenthal MA, Ashley DL, Cher L. Treatment of high risk or recurrent meningiomas with hydroxyurea. *J Clin Neurosci* 2002; 9:156–158.

90. Loven D, Hardoff R, Sever ZB, et al. Non-resectable slow-growing meningiomas treated by hydroxyurea. *J Neurooncol* 2004; 67:221–226.

91. Cusimano MD. Hydroxyurea for treatment of meningioma. *J Neurosurg* 1998; 88:938–939.

92. Newton HB. Hydroxyurea chemotherapy in the treatment of meningiomas. *Neurosurg Focus* 2007; 23:E11.

93. Swinnen LJ, Rankin C, Rushing EJ, et al. Southwest Oncology Group S9811: a phase II study of hydroxyurea for unresectable meningioma. *J Clin Oncol* 2009; 27:15s.

94. Kyritsis AP. Chemotherapy for meningiomas. *J Neurooncol* 1996; 29:269–272.

95. Chamberlain MC, Tsao-Wei DD, Groshen S. Temozolomide for treatment-resistant recurrent meningioma. *Neurology* 2004; 62:1210–1212.

96. Chamberlain MC, Tsao-Wei DD, Groshen S. Salvage chemotherapy with CPT-11 for recurrent meningioma. *J Neurooncol* 2006; 78:271–276.

97. Kaba SE, DeMonte F, Bruner JM, et al. The treatment of recurrent unresectable and malignant meningiomas with interferon alpha-2B. *Neurosurgery* 1997; 40:271–275.

98. Chamberlain MC, Glantz MJ. Interferon-alpha for recurrent World Health Organization grade 1 intracranial meningiomas. *Cancer* 2008; 113:2146–2151.

99. Sanson M, Cornu P. Biology of meningiomas. *Acta Neurochir (Wien)* 2000; 142:493–505.

100. Hsu DW, Efird JT, Hedley-Whyte ET. Progesterone and estrogen receptors in meningiomas: prognostic considerations. *J Neurosurg* 1997; 86:113–120.

101. McCutcheon IE. The biology of meningiomas. *J Neurooncol* 1996; 29:207–216.

102. Goodwin JW, Crowley J, Eyre HJ, et al. A phase II evaluation of tamoxifen in unresectable or refractory meningiomas: a Southwest Oncology Group study. *J Neurooncol* 1993; 15:75–77.

103. Markwalder TM, Seiler RW, Zava DT. Antiestrogenic therapy of meningiomas – a pilot study. *Surg Neurol* 1985; 24:245–249.

104. Grunberg SM, Weiss MH, Russell CA, et al. Long-term administration of mifepristone (RU486): clinical tolerance during extended treatment of meningioma. *Cancer Invest* 2006; 24:727–733.

105. Arena S, Barbieri F, Thellung S, et al. Expression of somatostatin receptor mRNA in human meningiomas and their implication in in vitro antiproliferative activity. *J Neurooncol* 2004; 66:155–166.

106. Chamberlain MC, Glantz MJ, Fadul CE. Recurrent meningioma: salvage therapy with long-acting somatostatin analogue. *Neurology* 2007; 69:969–973.

107. Norden A, Hammond S, Drappatz J, et al. Phase II study of monthly pasireotide LAR (SOM230C) for recurrent or progressive meningioma. *Neuro-Oncology* 2015; 84(3):280–286.

108. Simon M, Bostrom JP, Hartmann C. Molecular genetics of meningiomas: from basic research to potential clinical applications. *Neurosurgery* 2007; 60:787–798.

109. Ragel B, Jensen RL. New approaches for the treatment of refractory meningiomas. *Cancer Control* 2003; 10:148–158.

110. Johnson M, Toms S. Mitogenic signal transduction pathways in meningiomas: novel targets for meningioma chemotherapy? *J Neuropathol Exp Neurol* 2005; 64:1029–1036.

111. Jagannathan J, Oskouian RJ, Yeoh HK, et al. Molecular biology of unreresectable meningiomas: implications for new treatments and review of the literature. *Skull Base* 2008; 18:173–187.

112. Riemenschneider MJ, Perry A, Reifenberger G. Histological classification and molecular genetics of meningiomas. *Lancet Neurol* 2006; 5:1045–1054.

113. Wang JL, Nister M, Hermansson M, et al. Expression of PDGF beta-receptors in human meningioma cells. *Int J Cancer* 1990; 46:772–778.

114. Yang SY, Xu GM. Expression of PDGF and its receptor as well as their relationship to proliferating activity and apoptosis of meningiomas in human meningiomas. *J Clin Neurosci* 2001; 8(Suppl 1):49–53.

115. Nagashima G, Asai J, Suzuki R, et al. Different distribution of c-myc and MIB-1 positive cells in malignant meningiomas with reference to TGFs, PDGF, and PgR expression. *Brain Tumor Pathol* 2001; 18:1–5.

116. Maxwell M, Galanopoulos T, Hedley-Whyte ET, et al. Human meningiomas co-express platelet-derived growth factor (PDGF) and PDGF-receptor genes and their protein products. *Int J Cancer* 1990; 46:16–21.

117. Wen PY, Yung WK, Lamborn KR, et al. Phase II study of imatinib mesylate for recurrent meningiomas (North American Brain Tumor Consortium study 01-08). *Neuro Oncol* 2009; 11:853–860.

118. Reardon DA, Desjardins A, Vredenburgh JJ, et al. Phase II study of Gleevec plus hydroxyurea in adults with progressive or recurrent low-grade glioma. *Cancer* 2012; 118:4759–4767.

119. Andersson U, Guo D, Malmer B, et al. Epidermal growth factor receptor family (EGFR, ErbB2-4) in gliomas and meningiomas. *Acta Neuropathol (Berl)* 2004; 108:135–142.

120. Weisman AS, Raguet SS, Kelly PA. Characterization of the epidermal growth factor receptor in human meningioma. *Cancer Res* 1987; 47:2172–2176.

121. Carroll RS, Black PM, Zhang J, et al. Expression and activation of epidermal growth factor receptors in meningiomas. *J Neurosurg* 1997; 87:315–323.

122. Jones NR, Rossi ML, Gregoriou M, et al. Epidermal growth factor receptor expression in 72 meningiomas. *Cancer* 1990; 66:152–155.

123. Johnson MD, Horiba M, Winnier AR, Arteaga CL. The epidermal growth factor receptor is associated with phospholipase C-gamma 1 in meningiomas. *Hum Pathol* 1994; 25:146–153.

124. Sanfilippo JS, Rao CV, Guarnaschelli JJ, et al. Detection of epidermal growth factor and transforming growth factor alpha protein in meningiomas and other tumors of the central nervous system in human beings. *Surg Gynecol Obstet* 1993; 177:488–496.

125. Linggood RM, Hsu DW, Efird JT, Pardo FS. TGF alpha expression in meningioma – tumor progression and therapeutic response. *J Neurooncol* 1995; 26:45–51.

126. Norden AD, Raizer JJ, Abrey LE, et al. Phase II trials of erlotinib or gefitinib in patients with recurrent meningioma. *J Neurooncol* 2010; 96:211–217.

127. Pachow D, Andrae N, Kliese N, et al. mTORC1 inhibitors suppress meningioma growth in mouse models. *Clin Cancer Res* 2013; 19:1180–1189.

128. Brastianos PK, Horowitz PM, Santagata S, et al. Genomic sequencing of meningiomas identifies oncogenic SMO and AKT1 mutations. *Nat Genet* 2013; 45:285–289.

129. Clark VE, Erson-Omay EZ, Serin A, et al. Genomic analysis of non-NF2 meningiomas reveals mutations in TRAF7, KLF4, AKT1, and SMO. *Science* 2013; 339:1077–1080.

130. Lamszus K, Lengler U, Schmidt NO, et al. Vascular endothelial growth factor, hepatocyte growth factor/scatter factor, basic fibroblast growth factor, and placenta growth factor in human meningiomas and their relation to angiogenesis and malignancy. *Neurosurgery* 2000; 46:938–947.

131. Provias J, Claffey K, delAguila L, et al. Meningiomas: role of vascular endothelial growth factor/vascular permeability factor in angiogenesis and peritumoral edema. *Neurosurgery* 1997; 40:1016–1026.

132. Goldman CK, Bharara S, Palmer CA, et al. Brain edema in meningiomas is associated with increased vascular endothelial growth factor expression. *Neurosurgery* 1997; 40:1269–1277.

133. Kaley T, Wen PY, Schiff D, et al. Phase II trial of sunitinib (SU011248) for recurrent meningioma. *Neuro-Oncology* 2010; 12(Suppl. 4):iv69–iv78.

134. Sahm F, Schrimpf D, Olar A, et al. TERT promoter mutations and risk of recurrence in meningioma. *J Natl Cancer Inst* 2015; 108(5):djv377.

CHAPTER 12

Other tumours of the meninges

M. Yashar S. Kalani, Sith Sathornsumetee,
and Charles Teo

Definition

Non-meningothelial tumours of the meninges constitute a rare but diverse group of pathologies (Box 12.1). This group consists of: (i) mesenchymal, non-meningothelial tumours including haemangiopericytomas, (ii) melanocytic lesions, and (iii) haemangioblastoma (1). The bulk of the literature on these tumours is limited to case reports or small series. As such, the discussion on the majority of this topic rests upon expert opinion and modification of treatment protocols for other diseases. Guidelines from the National Comprehensive Cancer Network (NCCN) and other professional organizations are not available.

Mesenchymal, non-meningothelial tumours

Mesenchymal, non-meningothelial tumours comprise benign and malignant tumours originating in the central nervous system (CNS) that histologically resemble extracranial tumours of soft tissue or bone. They range from benign tumours (World Health Organization (WHO) grade I) to malignant sarcomas (WHO grade IV) and can be classified according to their differentiated phenotypes. Haemangiopericytomas (WHO grade II and III) represent the most common mesenchymal, non-meningothelial tumours, which deserve discussion as a separate entity later in this chapter. In general, mesenchymal tumours can affect patients at any age without gender predilection. Rhabdomyosarcoma occurs primarily in children, whereas malignant fibrous histiocytoma and chondrosarcoma predominantly affect adults. No specific aetiology has been identified. However, cranial irradiation may serve as a risk factor for development of some mesenchymal tumours such as fibrosarcoma, chondrosarcoma, malignant fibrous histiocytoma, and osteosarcoma. Spontaneous regression of these tumours is rare.

Tumours of adipose tissue

Lipoma (8850/0)

Intracranial lipomas are quite rare and are mostly asymptomatic. They arise from the meninx primitiva and are located in the midline, involving the pericallosal structures in more than 50% of cases, the ambient and quadrigeminal cisterns in 25% of cases, the cerebellopontine angle in 10% of cases (Fig. 12.1), and the superior cerebellar, Sylvian and suprasellar cisterns (2–4). Spinal cord lipomas are less common, whereas intraventricular lipoma is rare (Fig. 12.2a). The incidence of lipomas has been postulated to be between 0.1% and 0.2% based on autopsy and radiological series (4).

More than half of the patients have other more serious brain malformations such as agenesis of the corpus callosum and they are rarely associated with congenital neurocutaneous disorders and vascular malformations including arteriovenous malformations and aneurysms (5). Occasionally, there is fibrous connection between soft or subcutaneous tissue and lipoma of central nervous system.

Other forms of lipomas include (i) *angiolipoma* (8861/0), a rare tumour commonly involving the spinal canal with mixed histology of adipose tissue and prominent vasculature underneath the tumour capsule; (ii) *hibernoma* (8880/0), an uncommon variant composed of brown fat; and (iii) *liposarcoma* (8850/3), an extremely rare but aggressive variant that may present with subdural haematoma or as a component in gliosarcoma.

Lipomas are generally asymptomatic with minimal mass effect on adjacent structures. Cases describing growth of lipomas in the setting of steroid use have been reported. Epidural lipomatosis is a non-neoplastic condition with diffuse hypertrophy of spinal epidural adipose tissue. It is frequently associated with chronic steroid administration, endocrinopathy with increased endogenous steroids, or prolonged use of protease inhibitors in AIDS patients (6, 7). The most common presentations of intracranial lipomas are seizures and headaches, although it is unclear if the seizures are caused by lipomas or the additional structural malformations present in the brains of these patients. Other presentations may be due to hydrocephalus (Fig. 12.2a, b), cranial nerve deficits, or crowding in the posterior fossa.

Although computed tomography (CT) may reveal calcifications present in some lipomas, magnetic resonance imaging (MRI) remains the gold-standard modality for diagnosis of these lesions. Lipomas have a high signal intensity on the T1-weighted sequences and intermediate to low signal intensity on T2-weighted sequences. Although the literature contains a small number of publications on the rare symptomatic lesion, the majority need no intervention.

Surgical resection may be associated with a high rate of morbidity for intracranial lipomas (8, 9). However, resection followed by radiation therapy may provide local control and clinical benefit for liposarcoma (10). Adjuvant chemotherapy may be considered but the efficacy has not been established. Surgical decompression may also be considered in patients with spinal cord lipoma, angiolipoma, or epidural lipomatosis, who present with myelopathy.

Surveillance should be performed with MRI annually for 1–2 years to confirm that the lesion does not exhibit growth or

Mesenchymal, non-meningothelial tumours

Solitary fibrous tumour/haemangiopericytoma

Grade 1 8815/0

Grade 2 8815/1

Grade 3 8815/3

Haemangioblastoma 9161/1

Haemangioma 9120/0

Epithelioid haemangioendothelioma 9133/3

Angiosarcoma 9120/3

Kaposi sarcoma 9140/3

Ewing sarcoma/PNET 9364/3

Lipoma 8850/0

Angiolipoma 8861/0

Hibernoma 8880/0

Liposarcoma 8850/3

Desmoid-type fibromatosis 8821/1

Myofibroblastoma 8825/0

Inflammatory myofibroblastic tumour 8825/1

Benign fibrous histiocytoma 8830/0

Fibrosarcoma 8810/3

Undifferentiated pleomorphic sarcoma/malignant fibrous histiocytoma 8802/3

Leiomyoma 8890/0

Leiomyosarcoma 8890/3

Rhabdomyoma 8900/0

Rhabdomyosarcoma 8900/3

Chondroma 9220/0

Chondrosarcoma 9220/3

Osteoma 9180/0

Osteosarcoma 9180/3

Osteochondroma 9210/0

Melanocytic tumours

Meningeal melanocytosis 8728/0

Meningeal melanocytoma 8728/1

Meningeal melanoma 8720/3

Meningeal melanomatosis 8728/3

Reproduced from Louis DN, Ohgaki H, Wiestler OD, Cavenee WK, Ellison DW, Figarella-Branger D, Perry A, Reifenberger G, Von Deimling A (Eds), *World Health Organization Classification of Tumours of the Central Nervous System*, Fourth Edition Revised, Copyright (2016), with permission from IARC Publications.

aggressive behaviour. In malignant tumours such as liposarcoma, MRI should be performed more frequently (i.e. every 3–6 months following definitive treatment). Symptomatic treatments such as antiepileptic drugs for seizures, vestibular suppressants and rehabilitation for vestibular symptoms, and cerebrospinal fluid (CSF) shunting for hydrocephalus should be provided for symptomatic patients.

Fibrous tumours

Solitary fibrous tumour (8815/0)

Solitary fibrous tumour (SFT) can arise from cranial or spinal meninges with potential to invade the skull base and CNS parenchyma. Extracranial SFT is usually classified in the same category with haemangiopericytoma. Historically, intracranial or intraspinal counterparts are described as separate entities. However, the 2016 WHO classification has defined SFT and haemangiopericytoma in the same diagnostic entity with grading according to the 2013 WHO classification of tumours of soft tissue and bone as grade I (8815/0), grade II (8815/1), and grade III (8815/3). Most SFTs in the CNS are benign with only 6% being malignant. Microscopically, SFT consists of spindle cells arranged in fascicles between bands of collagen with immunoreactivity against CD34, Bcl-2, ALDH1, and vimentin but not EMA or S-100 proteins (11). *NAB2–STAT6* gene fusion is consistently identified in meningeal SFT and haemangiopericytoma (12). This gene fusion resulted in strong nuclear expression of *STAT-6*. Therefore, STAT-6 immunohistochemistry is helpful to distinguish SFT from other histological mimics such as meningiomas (13). There is no gender predilection for SFT. The median age at diagnosis is 40–60 years old with less than 5% of cases under the age of 20. SFTs can arise from cranial and spinal meninges at various locations. The most common intracranial locations are tentorium cerebelli, frontal convexity, and cerebellopontine angle. Patients with intracranial SFTs presented with headache (50%) followed by gait disturbance (22%), weakness (19%), and visual defect (19%). CT often demonstrates hyperattenuated, solitary, and well-circumscribed lesions. Calcifications are uncommon. MRI reveals isointense or hypointense signals on both T1- and T2-weighted images with marked contrast enhancement (14). Restricted diffusion, an elevated peak of myoinositol, and increased perfusion are variable features on diffusion-weighted imaging, magnetic resonance spectroscopy, and perfusion MRI, respectively (15). Surgery is the mainstay treatment for SFT with gross total resection serving as a favourable prognostic factor (16, 17). Recurrence is more common in patients who had subtotal or partial resection. Radiation therapy may be considered for unresectable tumours but prospective studies with longer follow-up time are required to confirm the efficacy (18). Chemotherapy for SFT is discussed later in this chapter under 'Haemangiopericytoma, which has recently been designated as the same diagnosis.

Fibrosarcoma (8810/3)

Fibrosarcoma is a rare mesenchymal tumour composed of bundles of spindle cells arranged in a 'herringbone' pattern. It has high cellularity with increased mitotic activity and necrosis. Fibrosarcomas may present as discrete dural masses with frequent bone involvement or diffuse leptomeningeal disease. Fibrosarcoma may develop in the sellar region following radiation treatment for pituitary adenoma with the latency ranged from 5 to more than 10 years (19). Primary fibrosarcomas occur

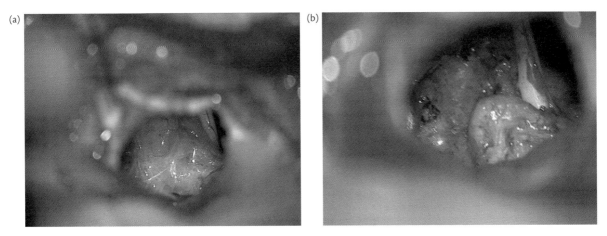

Fig. 12.1 (a) Intraoperative photograph showed a lipoma of the cerebellopontine angle. (b) Early stages of resection of the lipoma with preservation of the juxtaposed cranial nerve.

at any age with the most common ages between 30 and 50. Male to female ratio is roughly equal. Intracranial fibrosarcomas are generally aggressive tumours with the median survival of less than 1 year. Leptomeningeal seeding and systemic metastases are not uncommon. Symptoms and signs are dictated by size, location, and extent of the tumour. CT scans may demonstrate bone involvement. MRI typically shows a markedly enhancing lesion following contrast administration. There is no standard treatment for intracranial fibrosarcomas because of their rarity. Treatment should be individualized following multi-disciplinary discussion and may include surgical resection, chemotherapy and radiation therapy (20).

Undifferentiated pleomorphic sarcoma /malignant fibrous histiocytoma (8802/3)

Undifferentiated pleomorphic sarcoma /malignant fibrous histiocytoma involving the intracranial compartments is rare (Fig. 12.3). Given the rarity of these lesions it is difficult to comment on their epidemiology (21, 22). Tumours usually consist of atypical fibroblasts and histiocytes. The pathogenesis of these tumours is not well understood. These lesions may present with symptoms suggestive of mass effect and seizures. These lesions appear hyperintense on contrast-enhanced T1-weighted MRI sequence and may possess a 'dural tail' (23).

The mainstay of treatment for these tumours is aggressive microsurgical resection when possible. Given the rarity of these tumours, the role of chemoradiotherapy is not well defined. In aggressive/malignant variants, Camacho et al. recommend the use of a combination of carboplatin, 4'-epidoxorubicin and methotrexate combined with 60 Gy local adjuvant radiotherapy (24).

Myogenic tumours

Leiomyoma (8890/0) and leiomyosarcoma (8890/3)

Leiomyoma is a benign smooth muscle tumour composed of intersecting fascicles of spindle cells that lack mitotic activity, whereas leiomyosarcoma represents a malignant smooth muscle tumour. It displays immunoreactivity against smooth muscle actin and desmin. An angioleiomyoma variant has been reported. The most common location is cranial or spinal dura. However, the

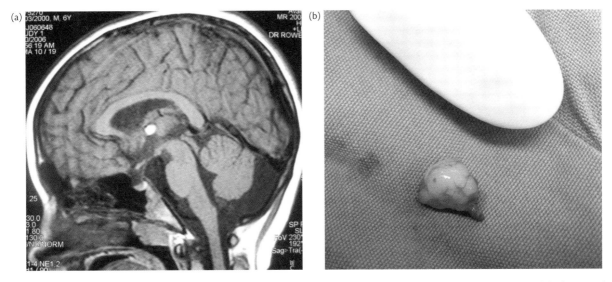

Fig. 12.2 (a) Mid-sagittal MRI demonstrated an intraventricular lipoma. This patient had mild ventriculomegaly and intermittent obstruction of the foramen of Monro. (b) Gross pathology of the tumour in (a) after en bloc resection.

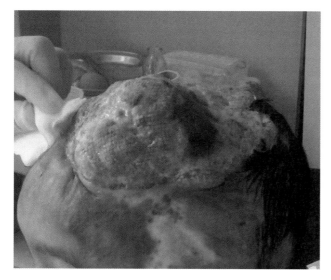

Fig. 12.3 Malignant fibrous histiocytoma showed extensive involvement of the calvarium and overlying scalp.

parasellar and pineal regions and parenchymal involvement have been described. Dural leiomyomas or leiomyosarcomas can be associated with Epstein–Barr virus infection in AIDS patients (25). Surgical resection is usually offered for patients with symptomatic tumours.

Rhabdomyoma (8900/0) and rhabdomyosarcoma (8900/3)

Rhabdomyoma is a tumour of well-differentiated striated muscle. It can originate from the trigeminal, facial, and vestibular cranial nerves (26–28). In addition, one case of meningeal rhabdomyomatosis has been reported (29). Although rhabdomyosarcomas represent the most common soft tissue paediatric sarcomas, they are exceedingly rare in the intracranial compartment (30). Reports of adult meningeal rhabdomyosarcomas are even rarer than those reported in children. Meningeal rhabdomyosarcomas must be distinguished from other pathologies including medullomyoblastoma, gliosarcoma, and germ cell tumours, all of which can exhibit skeletal muscle elements. Intracranial rhabdomyosarcoma may be associated with malformations of CNS.

The cell of origin of these tumours is postulated to be the pluripotent mesenchymal cells of the meninges. Although few cases have reported diffuse meningeal involvement, this pattern is associated with a worse prognosis (31, 32).

Presentation may be due to symptoms suggestive of raised intracranial pressure (Fig. 12.4a, b), cranial neuropathy, seizures, or headache. In contrast to other mesenchymal tumours, rhabdomyosarcomas are often infratentorial in location. Given the paucity of the literature on these lesions, it is difficult to quantify the contribution of each presentation.

The imaging workup for this tumour should be MRI of whole neuraxis. Positron emission tomography/CT may be considered to rule out an extracranial primary site. MRI usually demonstrates an enhancing mass on T1-weighted contrast sequences. Some centres utilize cerebrospinal fluid cytology to stage patients.

A review of 38 intracranial rhabdomyosarcomas reported a mean survival of 9.1 months (33). The majority of the reported cases have been managed with surgical resection (Fig. 12.4c, d) and adjuvant radiotherapy with a dose ranging from 2500 to 8200 cGy (34). The

utility of chemotherapy and the appropriate agent is a matter of debate and no guidelines have been reported on this topic. Recent case reports have demonstrated encouraging activity of concurrent temozolomide with radiotherapy and/or vincristine, actinomycin-D and cyclophosphamide (VAC), a standard chemotherapy regimen for systemic sarcoma (34).

Osteocartilaginous tumours

These are very rare tumours that mostly occur in and around the clivus and associated synchondroses. Conversely, osteomas and aneurysmal bone cysts, which are also included in this group, are much more common and are usually found in the calvarium and not the skull base. Osteocartilaginous tumours may derive from several origins including meningeal heterotopias, multipotent mesenchymal cells, mesenchymal differentiation of fibrous or fibrohistiocytic tumours, or teratoma.

Osteochondroma (9210/0)

The most common benign osteocartilaginous tumour is an osteochondroma of the long bones but these are rare in the craniofacial area. They are more commonly located in the mandibular condyle and coronoid process but have been documented in the skull base, foramen magnum, and frontotemporosphenoidal suture.

Imaging of benign bony tumours is best conducted with high-resolution CT scans. MRI is superior in ascertaining involvement of surrounding soft tissue structures. Benign bone tumours may be hot or cold on bone scans but malignant tumours are always hot. Presentation depends on their location and varies between being totally asymptomatic to cranial neuropathies and brainstem compression.

Treatment is directed by symptomatology. Incidental tumours may be left alone and followed with yearly clinic visits and MRI surveillance. Symptomatic tumours should be managed by consultation with specialized craniofacial and/or skull base teams to determine the best surgical or radiotherapeutic options. These slow-growing tumours are invariably cured with radical macroscopic resection.

Chondrosarcoma (9220/3)

Chondrosarcomas are rare tumours arising from the skull base, accounting for 6% of skull base and 0.1% of intracranial tumours (35). The most common locations for these tumours include the parasellar region (Fig. 12.5), cerebellopontine angle, and the convexity. These tumours commonly arise *de novo* but have been associated with Ollier's disease, Maffucci syndrome, Paget's disease, and osteochondroma. Chondrosarcomas have been described as conventional, mesenchymal, clear cell, and dedifferentiated subtypes, with the majority of intracranial tumours being conventional or mesenchymal.

The bones of the skull base develop via endochondral ossification and this mechanism of bony development has been linked to the pathogenesis of chondrosarcomas (36). Although poorly understood, several authors have postulated that chondrocytes within the rests of endochondral cartilage may serve as the cell of origin for these tumours while pluripotent mesenchymal cells of the skull base and mature fibroblasts have been cited as other sources (37–39).

Chondrosarcomas predominantly affect men during the second and third decades of life (40). These tumours commonly present with cranial neuropathies, symptoms suggestive of mass effect,

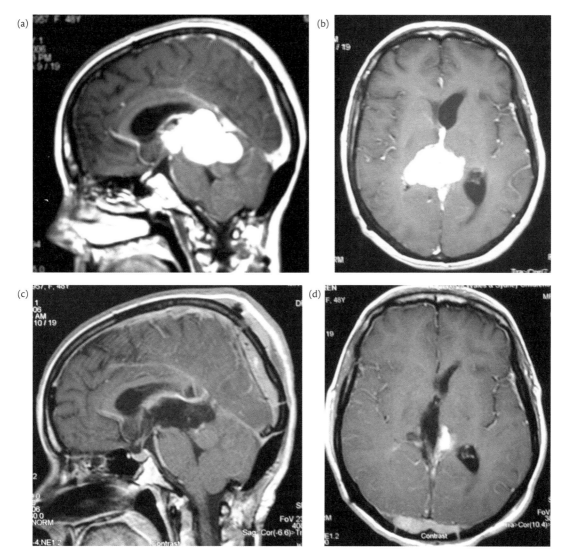

Fig. 12.4 (a, b) MRI findings of a third ventricular rhabdomyosarcoma in a 48-year-old woman who presented with reduced level of consciousness. The sagittal image showed extension into the posterior fossa and the axial image displayed the intimate involvement with the vein of Galen. (c, d) Brain MRI following a radical resection showed the residual tumour adherent to the vein of Galen.

or are incidentally identified. Despite an indolent course in most cases, rarely these tumours may exhibit rapid growth, causing morbidity, especially in the confines of the posterior fossa with its labyrinth of neurovascular structures.

Computed tomography frequently demonstrates a calcified mass; MRI demonstrates intermediate intensity on the T1-weighted sequences and heterogeneity on the T2-weighted sequences. These lesions enhance after the administration of contrast material.

Chondrosarcomas have been categorized based on degree of cellularity, nuclear atypia, and the amount of chondroid matrix into three grades. This grading system has clinical implications (41). The reported 5-year survival rates of chondrosarcomas are 90% for grade I, 81% for grade II, and 43% for grade III (42).

The mainstay of treatment for chondrosarcomas is aggressive microsurgical resection (40). With the improved visualization of the skull base with endoscopic, transnasal techniques, more radical and complete resections may be achieved with reduced morbidity (Fig. 12.6). Although the majority of the data on surgical management

of chondrosarcomas is represented as a pooled assessment, which sometimes includes chordomas, the prognosis of chondrosarcomas is much better than chordomas, and has been reported to be greater than 80% at 5 years (43).

Radiation as a stand-alone treatment for chondrosarcomas has been reported. Modalities include fractionated (photon) radiotherapy, proton beam therapy, and stereotactic radiosurgery. In the University of California at San Francisco (UCSF) experience, only 8% of patients received radiation as the sole modality (44). The 5-year rate of recurrence following treatment with radiation alone was 19%, which the authors noted was statistically lower than the recurrence rate of patients who received only surgical resection. This data is limited by its small sample size but suggests that in cases not amenable to aggressive surgical resection, biopsy followed by radiation therapy may be an acceptable alternative. In this UCSF series, grade I chondrosarcoma had a 15% chance of recurrence, and grades II and III demonstrated a recurrence rate of 16% and 33%, respectively (44). The range reported

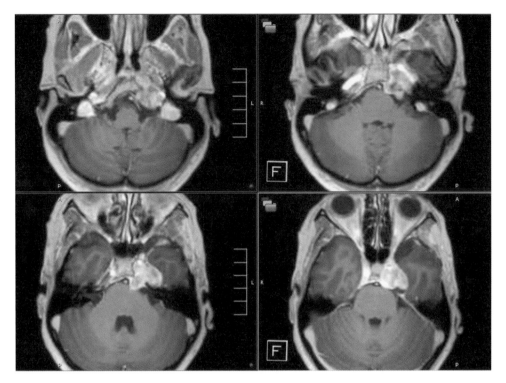

Fig. 12.5 Axial MRI demonstrated a left petrous apex, mildly enhancing, bony tumour in a 54-year-old woman who presented with cranial neuropathies. Pathology confirmed chondrosarcoma.

in the literature is 12–60% at a median follow-up of 1.9–30 years (40, 43).

Chemotherapy is not routinely administered for treatment of intracranial chondrosarcomas. However, several agents such as ifosfamide and doxorubicin have been used in selected cases owing to their activities in extracranial chondrosarcomas (45). In addition, targeted therapies directing at molecular abnormalities of chondrosarcomas may have a role in the future. Several deregulated signalling pathways such as PI3K, MEK-ERK, and integrins may represent promising therapeutic targets (46).

Osteosarcoma (9180/3)

Osteosarcoma arising from meninges is very rare. Occasionally it can present as a component of germ cell tumours or gliosarcoma.

Radiation-induced meningeal osteosarcomas have been reported (47, 48). The first-line treatment is surgical resection. Adjuvant radiotherapy and/or chemotherapy may be considered but with only limited evidence (49, 50).

Vascular tumours

Haemangioma (9120/0)

Most haemangiomas arise from bone. However, dural and CNS parenchymal origins have been rarely reported. Facial haemangioma may be associated with ipsilateral or contralateral leptomeningeal haemangioma. Histologically, haemangiomas can be classified into capillary or cavernous types. Intracranial capillary haemangioma can affect both sexes with the median ages of diagnosis of 4.8 and

(a)

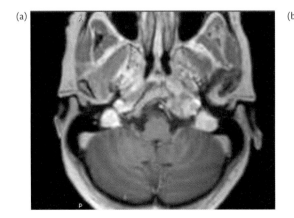

(b)

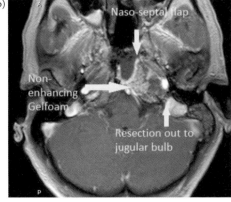

Fig. 12.6 (a) Pre- and (b) postoperative MRIs of chondrosarcoma showed a complete endoscopic endonasal resection of the tumour. The patient did extremely well without neurological deficits and resolution of preoperative cranial neuropathies.

22.5 years for men and women, respectively (51). The most common sites for capillary haemangiomas are extra-axial dura around major venous sinuses, whereas cavernous haemangiomas often involve dura of cavernous sinus, tentorium, and cerebellopontine angle (52). Intracranial dural haemangiomas are radiographically indistinguishable from meningiomas. Complete resection is the treatment of choice and is associated with favourable outcome.

Epithelioid haemangioendothelioma (9133/3)

Epithelioid haemangioendothelioma (EH) is a very rare vascular tumour of intermediate grade involving skull base, dura, and brain parenchyma. It affects infants to young adults and predominantly affects more males in childhood, whereas there is no gender predilection in adults (53). A study integrating genomic and cytogenetic evaluation of EH identified a characteristic gene fusion of WWTR1 (WW domain-containing transcription regulator 1) and CAMTA1 (calmodulin-binding transcription activator 1) derived from the t(1;3)(p36;q25) chromosomal translocation (54). This disease-defining gene fusion may serve as a new therapeutic target for EH. While EH has a low-to-intermediate proliferation index, it can exhibit aggressive clinical behaviour with local invasion in approximately one-third and distant metastases in 15% of cases. Gross total resection is recommended to prevent recurrence (55). Radiotherapy, chemotherapy, or both, may be offered in unresectable or partially removed tumours. Several chemotherapy regimens have been evaluated for extracranial EH. Antiangiogenic agents, particularly bevacizumab, have demonstrated promising efficacy in case series and a trial for EH and angiosarcoma (56).

Angiosarcoma (9120/3)

This malignant vascular tumour can arise primarily from brain parenchyma or meninges. Clinical course is usually rapid with progressive neurological symptoms. Brain MRI often demonstrates a well-demarcated tumour with avid enhancement following gadolinium administration. Complete resection is the primary treatment (57). Radiotherapy, chemotherapy, or both, may be considered as additional treatment in the adjuvant setting or salvage therapy for tumour recurrence. Some experts recommend temozolomide as the first-line agent because it crosses the blood–brain barrier and has activity against some sarcomas. Other agents include doxorubicin and paclitaxel but the activity in intracranial angiosarcoma has not been established. Antiangiogenic agents such as bevacizumab alone or in combination with radiotherapy or chemotherapy such as temozolomide have been used with some success in selected patients with intracranial angiosarcomas. In a recent open-label, multicentre, phase II study of 30 evaluable patients with metastatic or locally advanced, extracranial, angiosarcoma, or EH, bevacizumab was associated with 17% partial response, 50% stable disease, and a mean time to progression of 26 weeks (56). This promising activity warrants further investigation of bevacizumab and other antiangiogenic agents in intracranial angiosarcoma.

Kaposi sarcoma (9140/3)

Central nervous system involvement of Kaposi sarcoma is exceptionally rare. It can occur primarily in the brain or meninges or as a metastasis from extracranial sites in patients with AIDS. Kaposi sarcoma is invariably associated with human herpes virus type 8 (HHV8) infection. Subdural haematoma may be an initial presentation of dural Kaposi sarcoma (58). Antiretroviral treatment with or without chemotherapy may be considered.

Meningeal sarcomatosis

This is a very rare neoplastic condition with a predilection for the paediatric population (59). The gross appearance of the meninges is cloudy and thickened. Tumour cells may extend to the depths of sulci and nodular involvement of the subarachnoid space has been reported. Areas between the pia and arachnoid are filled with poorly differentiated spindle cells, suspended in a network of reticulin. Pathological re-evaluation with additional immunohistochemical stains of meningeal sarcomatosis demonstrated that most were in fact carcinoma, lymphoma, glioma, or primitive neuroectodermal tumours (PNETs).

Patients may present with symptoms suggestive of mass effect, seizures, cranial neuropathies, or other less specific symptoms (especially in children). The treatment paradigm for these tumours is not well established. Surgery may be attempted to relieve symptoms of mass effect. The role of adjuvant therapies including radiation and chemotherapy for this disease is evolving and made challenging due to the rarity of the tumour (60).

Ewing sarcoma/peripheral primitive neuroectodermal tumour (EWS-pPNET; 9364/3)

Ewing sarcoma/ peripheral primitive neuroectodermal tumour in the CNS is extremely rare and can occur as primary meningeal tumour or as local invasion from adjacent craniovertebral bony structures or soft tissues. It is most common during the second decade of life. Histologically, EWS/PNET displays small, round, undifferentiated cells with occasional Homer Wright rosettes and focal reactivity to neuronal markers such as synaptophysin or neuron-specific enolase. CD99 or Ewing sarcoma antigen is abundantly expressed on cell membranes, however, it is not specific. Therefore, the genetic test for characteristic translocations of chromosome 22 is recommended to confirm the diagnosis. The most common translocation is t(11;22)(q24;q12) resulting in fusion of the EWS gene on chromosome 22 and the FLI1 gene on chromosome 11 (61). A case of the rare translocation t(21;22)(q22;q12) has been reported (62). Treatment often includes surgical resection. Radiotherapy and/or chemotherapy may be considered as adjuvant or salvage treatments.

Haemangiopericytoma (8815)

Haemangiopericytoma or SFT (as discussed earlier in the chapter) is a rare tumour involving the meninges and arising from Zimmerman's pericytes, a modified smooth muscle cell (63). Historically, haemangiopericytoma was considered an aggressive subtype of meningioma (64). Haemangiopericytoma constitutes less than 1% of all intracranial tumours and approximately 2–4% of all meningeal tumours (65). These tumours are known for their aggressive growth (Fig. 12.7), high rate of local recurrence, and late distant metastases (66–68). SFT/haemangiopericytoma can be classified into grade I (8815/0), II (8815/1), and III (8815/3) according to the 2016 WHO classification. The WHO grade III SFT/haemangiopericytoma is associated with higher rates of recurrence than the grade II counterpart. However, overall survival may not be affected by tumour grade. The mean age of presentation ranges from 37 to 44 years (69–72). SFT/haemangiopericytoma affects men and women at similar rates with a slight male predominance in some series (73–75).

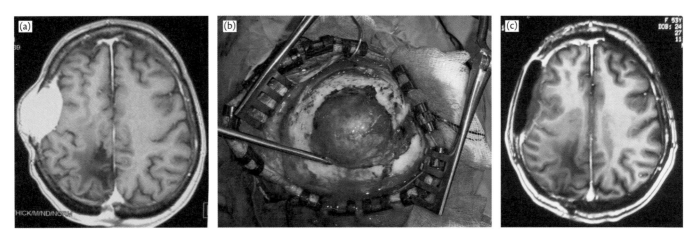

Fig. 12.7 (a) Axial contrast-enhanced T1-weighted MRI demonstrated the aggressive nature of a haemangiopericytoma that eroded through the dura and skull to involve the scalp. (b) Intraoperative photograph of the tumour in (a). (c) Postoperative MRI showed a complete resection of the tumour and involved dura, skull and sub-galeal soft tissue.

Symptoms and signs depend on the location of the tumour. The most common presentation in one of the largest series was headache (76). Other common causes of presentation include hydrocephalus, mass effect, seizures, nausea, and vomiting. Myelopathic symptoms can result from spinal disease due to metastases from primary intracranial tumour or rarely a primary spinal SFT/haemangiopericytoma that usually involves the cervical region (77). Acute neurological symptoms may arise from intratumoural haemorrhage.

SFT/haemangiopericytomas are multilobulated, heterogeneous extra-axial masses on both CT and MRI. They enhance avidly (Fig. 12.8) and heterogeneously following contrast administration

and may be associated with flow-related vascular malformations (78). Unlike meningiomas, hyperostosis and intratumoural calcification are usually not present (76). Angiography typically demonstrates dual blood supply from meningeal and cortical arteries with a corkscrew-like vascular pattern in the tumour. Preoperative embolization may reduce the risk of intraoperative bleeding and improve surgical outcome.

The mainstay of treatment for SFT/haemangiopericytoma is aggressive surgical resection (66, 73, 74). Profuse bleeding can occur during surgery. The UCSF group reviewed the literature on 563 patients with haemangiopericytoma. They determined an overall median survival of 13 years. The 1-, 5-, 10-, and 20-year survival rates were 95%, 82%, 60%, and 23%, respectively. Gross total resection alone resulted in a median survival of 13 years, whereas patients treated with subtotal resection alone had a median survival of 9.75 years (75). The addition of postoperative radiotherapy may increase disease-free and overall survival (79–85). An analysis of the Surveillance Epidemiology and End Results (SEER) database of 227 patients with CNS haemangiopericytoma demonstrated that the 5-year survival rate was 83% (81). Gross total resection in combination with adjuvant radiotherapy served as an independent favourable prognostic factor for overall survival in a multivariate analysis (81). In a review of the Queen's Square experience, the recurrence rates at 1, 5, and 15 years were 3.5%, 46%, and 92%, respectively. Stereotactic radiosurgery at the median marginal dose of 15 Gy after resection was associated with local control rate of 89% for grade II tumour and progression-free survival rates of 89%, 67%, and 0% at 1, 2, and 5 years, respectively, for grade III haemangiopericytoma (86). Single and repeated, Gamma Knife® or CyberKnife® radiosurgeries, exploited at higher marginal doses of 17 Gy or more, demonstrated improved local control rates of 95–100%, 71–85%, and 68–71% for 1, 2, and 5 years, respectively (87–89). Locoregional recurrence can occur at the primary site or as leptomeningeal seeding. Surgical resection is usually considered for recurrent local tumour, whereas stereotactic radiosurgery represents an important treatment option for small local recurrences (74). External beam radiotherapy, if not administered at the time of initial diagnosis, should be considered as a first-line salvage treatment (74). Distant metastases can develop in 20–25% of patients

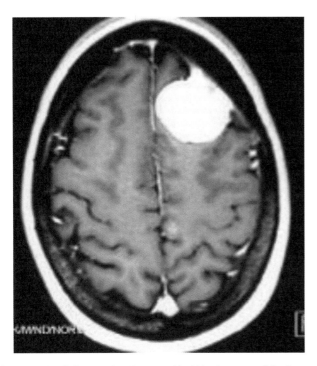

Fig. 12.8 MRI of a haemangiopericytoma with vivid enhancement following gadolinium administration.

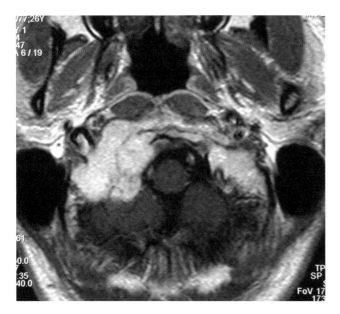

Fig. 12.9 Axial MRI showed bony metastases involving both occipital condyles approximately 4 years after resection of a tentorial haemangiopericytoma in a 26-year-old man.

and can occur many years following treatment of the primary site (Fig. 12.9) (66, 80). Unfortunately, the occurrences are not hampered by adjuvant radiotherapy. The most common sites of metastasis include bone, lung, liver, kidney, pancreas, and adrenals (65, 90). Multiple reports suggest that patients may continue to do well despite recurrence/metastasis and should be treated aggressively (74, 80).

Chemotherapy is not traditionally used for this tumour. Doxorubicin-containing regimens were administered in seven patients with recurrent haemangiopericytoma at the Mayo Clinic with only one partial response that lasted 8 months (91). Sequential chemotherapeutic regimens were studied in 15 patients with recurrent, radiation-refractory, haemangiopericytoma (92). The regimens were cyclophosphamide, doxorubicin, and vincristine (CAV) followed by alpha-interferon (IFNα) upon disease progression. Subsequent treatment with ifosfamide, carboplatin and etoposide (ICE) was applied when interferon failed to control tumour. Six patients had partial radiographic responses (two with CAV and four with IFNα) and fourteen patients had stable disease (nine with CAV and five with IFNα). The median survival was 14 months (92).

Haemangiopericytoma is a highly vascularized tumour with intense expression of VEGF and VEGFRs that may serve as therapeutic targets. A retrospective study of 14 patients with haemangiopericytoma or malignant solitary fibrous tumours from University of Texas MD Anderson Cancer Center demonstrated promising efficacy of bevacizumab (Avastin®), a humanized monoclonal antibody against VEGF, in combination with temozolomide, a DNA methylating agent (93). Temozolomide was orally administered at 150 mg/m^2 on days 1–8 and days 15–21 and bevacizumab was given intravenously at 5 mg/kg on day 8 and day 22 of a 28-day cycle. Using Choi's response criteria to evaluate tumour size and density by CT, partial responses were observed in 11 patients (79%) with a median time to response of 2.5 months. Two patients had stable disease and one patient developed progressive disease as

their best responses. With a median follow-up time of 34 months, the estimated progression-free survival was 9.7 months with a 6-month progression-free survival rate of 78.6%. Treatment was adequately tolerated with myelosuppression as the most frequent adverse event. A prospective trial of this regimen is ongoing.

Other cytotoxic chemotherapies and molecularly targeted agents have been used in selected cases. Trabectedin was reported to provide clinical benefit in a recurrent haemangiopericytoma patient who failed several prior therapies (94). Dasatinib (Sprycel®), an inhibitor of PDGFR, BCR/ABL, and SRC, showed disease control for over 2 years in a patient with recurrent heavily pretreated haemangiopericytoma with PDGFR overexpression (95). Sunitinib malate (Sutent®), a multitargeted kinase inhibitor against VEGFRs, PDGFRs, KIT, FMS-like tyrosine kinase (FLT-3), RET, and CSF-1 receptor, was associated with stable disease for more than 6–12 months in a few patients with metastatic haemangiopericytoma (96, 97).

Melanocytic lesions

Meningeal melanocytosis (8728/0)

The meningeal coverings can be affected by a range of melanocytic pathologies, including diffuse melanocytosis and melanomatosis, melanocytomas, and primary malignant melanomas (98). In diffuse melanocytosis, proliferating melanocytes involve the leptomeninges without frank invasion of the brain. Unequivocal invasion of brain parenchyma may indicate malignant transformation to melanomatosis. Diffuse meningeal melanomatosis is a very rare variant of primary malignant melanoma. This disease results from spread of malignant melanocytes into the Virchow–Robin spaces. This malignancy has been reported in both adults and children but appears to be more common in adults (98). A majority of meningeal melanocytosis cases are reported in children with neurocutaneous melanosis manifested as pigmented skin lesions and various CNS malformations such as Dandy–Walker malformation, lipoma, and syringomyelia.

The aetiology of diffuse melanocytosis is similar to that for primary malignant melanoma and is discussed below. Age of presentation is within the first two decades of life without gender and racial predilection. The most common sites of involvement include the cerebellum, pons, medulla and temporal lobes. The clinical presentation may be due to raised intracranial pressure, hydrocephalus caused by blockage of CSF absorption, or cranial neuropathies (99). Diffuse meningeal melanocytosis may clinically mimic other conditions including subacute meningitis, viral encephalitis, and idiopathic hypertrophic cranial pachymeningitis and may be identified during work-up for these pathologies (100, 101).

The clinical diagnosis of this pathology may be established by means of cytological examination of the CSF (100). MRI commonly reveals extensive leptomeningeal enhancement with focal or multifocal nodularity.

Optimal treatment for this rare tumour type is not established. Surgery for achieving the diagnosis and relieving mass effect may be attempted. Radiation and chemotherapy classically administered for melanoma have been used. Recently, temozolomide has been reported to provide clinical and radiographic improvement in a patient with meningeal melanocytosis (102). Prognosis for symptomatic patients is generally poor despite the lack of malignant histology.

Meningeal melanocytoma (8728/1)

Meningeal melanocytoma is a rare benign tumour of the lepto-meningeal melanocytes, cells that are derived from the neural crest. It accounts for 0.06–0.1% of brain tumours. Although these lesions can be found anywhere in the neuraxis, they have a pre-dilection for the foramen magnum, posterior fossa, and Meckel's cave (103). Spinal tumours often arise in the intradural extramedul-lary compartment of the cervical and thoracic spinal levels. Spinal intramedullary melanocytomas are very rare. The majority of cases of meningeal melanocytoma present in adults during the fourth or fifth decade, while paediatric presentation is exceedingly rare (104). Women are slightly more affected than men.

The clinical presentation is attributed to the location and size of the tumour. Patients may present with evidence of increased intracranial pressure, cranial nerve deficits, and rarely haemor-rhage (105, 106). Radiographically, melanocytomas present as well-defined, iso- to hyperdense, contrast-enhancing lesions on CT. The MRI signal abnormalities depend on the amount of melanin but most lesions are iso- to hyperintense on T1-weighted images and hypointense on T2-weighted images. These lesions are avidly contrast-enhancing on T1-weighted sequences.

Pathological evaluation reveals cells with fusiform, epithelial, polygonal, or spindle-like morphology with eosinophilic cyto-plasm. Grossly the lesions are well-circumscribed, darkly pig-mented masses.

The natural history of the majority of melanocytomas is benign. In rare cases, these tumours may transform into malignant mela-nomas (107). As such, the complete and aggressive microsurgical resection of these tumours should be the goal of treatment (108). In the setting of incomplete resection and without adjuvant radi-ation, these tumours have a 42% 5-year survival. In contrast, the 5-year survival rate for patients with incomplete resection but with adjuvant radiotherapy is 100% for cerebral melanocytoma and 59% for spinal meningeal melanocytoma (109, 110). Radiation doses of 45–55 Gy offered more local control than doses of less than 45 Gy (109). For spinal meningeal melanocytoma, a radiation dose of 50.4 Gy was associated with good local control and a low risk of radiation myelopathy (110). Despite complete resection, cases of tumour recurrence have been noted. This pattern of recurrence and the likelihood of malignant transformation have led some to recommend adjuvant radiation therapy for both completely and incompletely resected cases (111).

Malignant melanoma (8720/3)

Primary leptomeningeal melanoma is a rare disease, seen most commonly as a neurocutaneous syndrome in association with ocular melanosis in children (112, 113). In adults, these tumours are equally are but are not associated with neurocutaneous syn-dromes. Symptoms are generally non-specific and include cranial nerve deficits, seizures, hydrocephalus, or elevated intracranial pressure.

Pathologically these tumours present with cells infiltrating the subarachnoid space and occupying the Virchow–Robin spaces. As such, the diagnosis may be aided by CSF cytology. Radiographic evidence of tumour spread in the subarachnoid space may be noted on CT scan. Contrast administration will demonstrate enhance-ment of the meninges of the brainstem and the basilar cisterns. Rarely, and in advanced disease, the convexities may enhance. MRI

appearance of the tumour is variable and again dependent on the degree of melanin present.

Gross total resection when possible is associated with improved outcome. However, in many patients, the role of surgery is limited to achieving a diagnosis and relieving mass effect. Similar to melan-oma in other locations radiation is generally unsuccessful and the mainstay of treatment is palliative systemic therapy, although com-bination of whole-brain radiotherapy and systemic treatment may offer benefit in some cases (114). Systemic treatment options are similar to those for brain metastases from systemic malignant mel-anoma and are discussed in another chapter. In short, current treat-ment regimens may include: (i) immunotherapy with checkpoint inhibitors such as ipilimumab (anti-CTLA-4 antibody) and pem-brolizumab or nivolumab (anti-PD-1 antibodies) and interleukin-2 (IL-2); (ii) signal transduction inhibitors including BRAF inhibi-tors such as dabrafenib and vemurafenib, MEK inhibitors, and KIT inhibitors; and (iii) chemotherapy such as nitrosoureas, temozo-lomide, and intrathecal cytarabine for leptomeningeal melano-matosis (115). A recent report demonstrated that vemurafenib treatment was associated with improvement of symptoms, radio-graphic improvement, and CSF cytological remission in a patient with leptomeningeal melanomatosis (116).

Survival rates with this rare tumour are dismal with the majority of patients succumbing to the disease in 3–6 months. Rare surviv-als past 1 year have been reported but are the exception rather than the rule. However, the prognosis of patients with localized primary meningeal melanoma undergoing complete resection and without distant metastases is better than that of brain metastases from sys-temic malignant melanoma.

Haemangioblastoma (9161/1)

Meningeal haemangioblastoma is a rare tumour (117, 118). Leptomeningeal haemangioblastomatosis involving intracranial and spinal compartments is even rarer and more aggressive (119, 120). Haemangioblastomas can occur sporadically or in association with von Hippel–Lindau (VHL) disease, an autosomal dominant syndrome ascribed to mutations on chromosome 3 (121). VHL dis-ease and haemangioblastoma are discussed in Chapter 16. Briefly, haemangioblastomas are benign neoplasms and represent 1–2% of all primary central tumours (122). The presence of cerebellar hae-mangioblastoma is the most common initial manifestation, affect-ing 64% of patients with VHL and is the most important cause of mortality (123–125).

Meningeal haemangioblastoma can occur in supratentorial or, less commonly, infratentorial locations. Clinical manifestations of meningeal haemangioblastoma are similar to those of meningi-oma. The most common presenting symptoms of these tumours are symptoms suggestive of elevated intracranial pressure, headache, seizures, and cranial neuropathies. Given the rarity of these lesions, reliable epidemiological information is not available.

The imaging study of choice for the diagnosis of meningeal haemangioblastoma is gadolinium-enhanced MRI. Similar to haemangioblastomas in other locations, the tumour may appear isointense on T1-weighted images and demonstrate high signal on T2-weighted images. Contrast administration may result in focal enhancement although a mural nodule is usually not observed with meningeal haemangioblastoma. Meningeal haemangioblastomas may be highly vascular lesions with pathologically dilated vessels

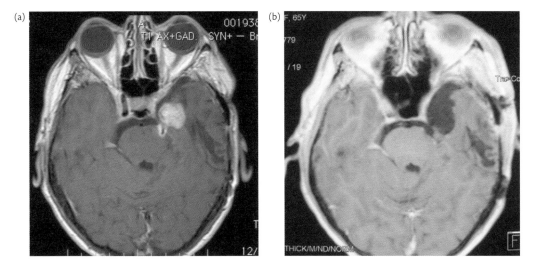

Fig. 12.10 (a, b) The preoperative MRI image showed a meningeal haemangioblastoma of the cavernous sinus. Although the postoperative image confirmed a complete resection, this patient suffered a recurrence 4 years later.

appearing hyperintense on flow-enhanced gadolinium studies (126). As such, angiography may be used to delineate the anatomy of the tumour as well as to selectively embolize the tumour prior to resection.

Haemangioblastomas, including the rare subset affecting the meninges, can be cured by surgical resection (Fig. 12.10) (127–131). Surgery can be combined with endovascular embolization to devascularize the tumour, aiding in its resection (132, 133). Other treatment modalities include radiation therapy and antiangiogenic agents, but these remain secondary modalities if surgery is not possible (134–137). Several antiangiogenic drugs, including IFNα2a; thalidomide; multitargeted angiogenic kinase inhibitors such as sunitinib, semaxanib, and pazopanib; and a monoclonal antibody against VEGF, bevacizumab, have demonstrated efficacy in single patients or case series with haemangioblastomas (138–146). These promising agents represent a reasonable option for surgically unresectable or refractory haemangioblastomas.

References

1. Louis DN, Ohgaki H, Wiestler OD, et al. The 2007 WHO classification of tumors of the central nervous system. *Acta Neuropathol* 2007; 114:97–109.

2. Jabot G, Stoquart-Elsankari S, Saliou G, et al. Intracranial lipomas: clinical appearances on neuroimaging and clinical significance. *J Neurol* 2009; 256:851–855.

3. Eghwrudjakpor PO, Kurisaka M, Fukuoka M, et al. Intracranial lipomas: current perspectives in their diagnosis and treatment. *Br J Neurosurg* 1992; 6:139–144.

4. Saatci I, Aslan C, Renda Y, Besim A. Parietal lipoma associated with cortical dysplasia and abnormal vasculature: case report and review of the literature. *AJNR Am J Neuroradiol* 2000; 21:1718–1721.

5. Canyigit M, Oguz KK. Epidermal nevus syndrome with internal carotid artery occlusion and intracranial and orbital lipomas. *AJNR Am J Neuroradiol* 2006; 27:1559–1561.

6. Al-Khawaja D, Seex K, Eslick GD. Spinal epidural lipomatosis--a brief review. *J Clin Neurosci* 2008; 15:1323–1326.

7. Vince GH, Brucker C, Langmann P, et al. Epidural spinal lipomatosis with acute onset of paraplegia in an HIV-positive patient treated with corticosteroids and protease inhibitor: case report. *Spine (Phila Pa 1976)* 2005; 30:E524–E527.

8. Gastaut H, Regis H, Gastaut JL, et al. Lipomas of the corpus callosum and epilepsy. *Neurology* 1980; 30:132–138.

9. Maiuri F, Cirillo S, Simonetti L, et al. Intracranial lipomas: diagnostic and therapeutic considerations. *J Neurosurg Sci* 1988; 32:161–167.

10. Mumert ML, Walsh MT, Jensen EM, et al. Pleomorphic liposarcoma originating from intracranial dura mater. *J Neurooncol* 2010; 97:149–153.

11. Bouvier C, Bertucci F, Métellus P, et al. ALDH1 is an immunohistochemical diagnostic marker for solitary fibrous tumors and hemangiopericytomas of the meninges emerging from gene profiling study. *Acta Neuropathol Commun* 2013; 1:10.

12. Schweizer L, Koelsche C, Sahm F, et al. Meningeal hemangiopericytoma and solitary fibrous tumors carry the NAB2-STAT6 fusion and can be diagnosed by nuclear expression of STAT6 protein. *Acta Neuropathol* 2013; 125:651–658.

13. Doyle LA, Vivero M, Fletcher CD, et al. Nuclear expression of STAT6 distinguishes solitary fibrous tumor from histologic mimics. *Mod Pathol* 2014; 27:390–395.

14. Wang XQ, Zhou Q, Li ST, et al. Solitary fibrous tumors of the central nervous system: clinical features and imaging findings in 22 patients. *J Comput Assist Tomogr* 2013; 37:658–665.

15. Clarençon F, Bonneville F, Rousseau A, et al. Intracranial solitary fibrous tumor: imaging findings. *Eur J Radiol* 2011; 80:387–394.

16. Bouvier C, Métellus P, de Paula AM, et al. Solitary fibrous tumors and hemangiopericytomas of the meninges: overlapping pathological features and common prognostic factors suggest the same spectrum of tumors. *Brain Pathol* 2012; 22:511–521.

17. Fargen KM, Opalach KJ, Wakefield D, et al. The central nervous system solitary fibrous tumor: a review of clinical, imaging and pathologic findings among all reported cases from 1996 to 2010. *Clin Neurol Neurosurg* 2011; 113:703–710.

18. Metellus P, Bouvier C, Guyotat J, et al. Solitary fibrous tumors of the central nervous system: clinicopathological and therapeutic considerations of 18 cases. *Neurosurgery* 2007; 60:715–722.

19. Berkmann S, Tolnay M, Hänggi D, et al. Sarcoma of the sella after radiotherapy for pituitary adenoma. *Acta Neurochir (Wien)* 2010; 152:1725–1735.

20. Chopra R, Bhardwaj M, Premsagar IC. Fibrosarcoma of the meninges. *Rare Tumors* 2010; 2:e3.

21. Berry AD 3rd, Reintjes SL, Kepes JJ. Intracranial malignant fibrous histiocytoma with abscess- like tumor necrosis. Case report. *J Neurosurg* 1988; 69:780–784.

22. Fujimura N, Sugita Y, Hirohata M, et al. Primary intracerebral malignant fibrous histiocytoma in a child. *Pediatr Neurosurg* 2002; 37:271–274.

23. Ozdemir M, Ozgural O, Bozkurt M, et al. Primary intracerebral malignant fibrous histiocytoma mimicking a meningioma. *Turk Neurosurg* 2012; 22:475–477.

24. Camacho FM, Moreno JC, Murga M, et al. Malignant fibrous histiocytoma of the scalp: multidisciplinary treatment. *J Eur Acad Dermatol Venereol* 1999; 13:175–182.

25. Bejjani GK, Stopak B, Schwartz A, et al. Primary dural leiomyosarcoma in a patient infected with human immunodeficiency virus: case report. *Neurosurgery* 1999; 44:199–202.

26. Zwick DL, Livingston K, Clapp L, et al. Intracranial trigeminal nerve rhabdomyoma/choristoma in a child: a case report and discussion of possible histogenesis. *Hum Pathol* 1989; 20:390–392.

27. Vandewalle G, Brucher JM, Michotte A. Intracranial facial nerve rhabdomyoma. Case report. *J Neurosurg* 1995; 83:919–922.

28. Harder A, Müller-Schulte E, Jeibmann A, et al. A 68-year old man with a cerebellopontine angle tumor. *Brain Pathol* 2013; 23:483–484.

29. Jarrell HR, Krous HF, Schochet SS Jr. Meningeal rhabdomyomatosis. *Arch Pathol Lab Med* 1981; 105:387.

30. Kobayashi S, Hirakawa E, Sasaki M, et al. Meningeal rhabdomyosarcoma. Report of a case with cytologic, immunohistologic and ultrastructural studies. *Acta Cytol* 1995; 39:428–434.

31. Korinthenberg R, Edel G, Palm D, et al. Primary rhabdomyosarcoma of the leptomeninx. Clinical, neuroradiological and pathological aspects. *Clin Neurol Neurosurg* 1984; 86:301–305.

32. Smith MT, Armbrustmacher VW, Violett TW. Diffuse meningeal rhabdomyosarcoma. *Cancer* 1981; 47:2081–2086.

33. Celli P, Cervoni L, Maraglino C. Primary rhabdomyosarcoma of the brain: observations on a case with clinical and radiological evidence of cure. *J Neurooncol* 1998; 36:259–267.

34. Palta M, Riedel RF, Vredenburgh JJ, et al. Primary meningeal rhabdomyosarcoma. *Sarcoma* 2011; 2011:312802.

35. Cianfriglia F, Pompili A, Occhipinti E. Intracranial malignant cartilaginous tumors. Report of two cases and review of literature. *Acta Neurochir (Wien)* 1978; 45:163–175.

36. Lau DP, Wharton SB, Antoun NM, et al. Chondrosarcoma of the petrous apex. Dilemmas in diagnosis and treatment. *J Laryngol Otol* 1997; 111:368–371.

37. Korten AG, ter Berg HJ, Spincemaille GH, et al. Intracranial chondrosarcoma: review of the literature and report of 15 cases. *J Neurol Neurosurg Psychiatry* 1998; 65:88–92.

38. Almefty K, Pravdenkova S, Colli BO, et al. Chordoma and chondrosarcoma: similar, but quite different, skull base tumors. *Cancer* 2007; 110:2457–2467.

39. Coltrera MD, Googe PB, Harris TJ, et al. Chondrosarcoma of the temporal bone. Diagnosis and treatment of 13 cases and review of the literature. *Cancer* 1986; 58:2689–2696.

40. Gay E, Sekhar LN, Rubinstein E, et al. Chordomas and chondrosarcomas of the cranial base: results and follow-up of 60 patients. *Neurosurgery* 1995; 36:887–896.

41. Neff B, Sataloff RT, Storey L, et al. Chondrosarcoma of the skull base. *Laryngoscope* 2002; 112:134–139.

42. Evans HL, Ayala AG, Romsdahl MM. Prognostic factors in chondrosarcoma of bone: a clinicopathologic analysis with emphasis on histologic grading. *Cancer* 1977; 40:818–831.

43. Bloch OG, Jian BJ, Yang I, et al. A systematic review of intracranial chondrosarcoma and survival. *J Clin Neurosci* 2009; 16:1547–1551.

44. Bloch OG, Jian BJ, Yang I, et al. Cranial chondrosarcoma and recurrence. *Skull Base* 2010; 20:149–156.

45. La Rocca RV, Morgan KW, Paris K, et al. Recurrent chondrosarcoma of the cranial base: a durable response to ifosfamide-doxorubicin chemotherapy. *J Neurooncol* 1999; 41:281–283.

46. Bloch O, Sughrue ME, Mills SA, et al. Signalling pathways in cranial chondrosarcoma: potential molecular targets for directed chemotherapy. *J Clin Neurosci* 2011; 18:881–885.

47. Ziewacz JE, Song JW, Blaivas M, et al. Radiation-induced meningeal osteosarcoma of tentorium cerebelli with intradural spinal metastases. *Surg Neurol Int* 2010; 1:14.

48. Utsuki S, Oka H, Sato K, et al. Radiation-induced osteosarcoma with a rhabdomyosarcoma component arising from the dura mater: a case report. *Clin Neuropathol* 2009; 28:96–100.

49. Setzer M, Lang J, Turowski B, et al. Primary meningeal osteosarcoma: case report and review of the literature. *Neurosurgery* 2002; 51:488–492.

50. Bar-Sela G, Tzuk-Shina T, Zaaroor M, et al. Primary osteogenic sarcoma arising from the dura mater: case report. *Am J Clin Oncol* 2001; 24:418–420.

51. Phi JH, Kim SK, Cho A, et al. Intracranial capillary hemangioma: extra-axial tumorous lesions closely mimicking meningioma. *J Neurooncol* 2012; 109:177–185.

52. Perry JR, Tucker WS, Chui M, et al. Dural cavernous hemangioma: an under-recognized lesion mimicking meningioma. *Can J Neurol Sci* 1993; 20:230–233.

53. Zheng J, Liu L, Wang J, et al. Primary intracranial epithelioid hemangioendothelioma: a low-proliferation tumor exhibiting clinically malignant behavior. *J Neurooncol* 2012; 110:119–127.

54. Tanas MR, Sboner A, Oliveira AM, et al. Identification of a disease-defining gene fusion in epithelioid hemangioendothelioma. *Sci Transl Med* 2011; 3:98ra82.

55. Parajón A, Vaquero J. Meningeal intracranial epithelioid hemangioendothelioma: case report and literature review. *J Neurooncol* 2008; 88:169–173.

56. Agulnik M, Yarber JL, Okuno SH, et al. An open-label, multicenter, phase II study of bevacizumab for the treatment of angiosarcoma and epithelioid hemangioendotheliomas. *Ann Oncol* 2013; 24:257–263.

57. Hackney JR, Palmer CA, Riley KO, et al. Primary central nervous system angiosarcoma: two case reports. *J Med Case Rep.* 2012; 6:251.

58. Ariza A, Kim JH. Kaposi's sarcoma of the dura mater. *Hum Pathol* 1988; 19:1461–1463.

59. Onofrio BM, Kernohan JW, Uihlein A. Primary meningeal sarcomatosis. A review of the literature and report of 12 cases. *Cancer* 1962; 15:1197–1208.

60. Cinalli G, Zerah M, Carteret M, et al. Subdural sarcoma associated with chronic subdural hematoma. Report of two cases and review of the literature. *J Neurosurg* 1997; 86:553–557.

61. Mazur MA, Gururangan S, Bridge JA, et al. Intracranial Ewing sarcoma. *Pediatr Blood Cancer* 2005; 45:850–856.

62. Antonelli M, Caltabiano R, Chiappetta C, et al. Primary peripheral PNET/Ewing's sarcoma arising in the meninges, confirmed by the presence of the rare translocation t(21; 22) (q22; q12). *Neuropathology* 2011; 31:549–555.

63. Stout AP, Murray MR. Hemangiopericytoma: a vascular tumor featuring Zimmermann's pericyte. *Ann Surg* 1942; 116:26–33.

64. Bailey P, Cushing H, Eisenhardt L. Angioblastic meningiomas. *Arch Pathol* 1928; 6:953–990.

65. Kumar N, Kumar R, Kapoor R, et al. Intracranial meningeal hemangiopericytoma: 10 years experience of a tertiary care Institute. *Acta Neurochir (Wien)* 2012; 154:1647–1651.

66. Mena H, Ribas JL, Pezeshkpour GH, et al. Hemangiopericytoma of the central nervous system: a review of 94 cases. *Hum Pathol* 1991; 22:84–91.

67. Goellner JR, Laws ER Jr, Soule EH, et al. Hemangiopericytoma of the meninges. Mayo Clinic experience. *Am J Clin Pathol* 1978; 70:375–380.

68. Guthrie BL, Ebersold MJ, Scheithauer BW, et al. Meningeal hemangiopericytoma: histopathological features, treatment, and long-term follow-up of 44 cases. *Neurosurgery* 1989; 25:514–522.

69. Jääskeläinen J, Servo A, Haltia M, et al. Intracranial hemangiopericytoma: radiology, surgery, radiotherapy, and outcome in 21 patients. *Surg Neurol* 1985; 23:227–236.

70. Pitkethly DT, Hardman JM, Kempe LG, et al. Angioblastic meningiomas; clinicopathologic study of 81 cases. *J Neurosurg* 1970; 32:539–544.

71. Kruse F Jr. Hemangiopericytoma of the meninges (angioblastic meningioma of Cushing and Eisenhardt). Clinico-pathologic aspects and follow-up studies in 8 cases. *Neurology* 1961; 11:771–777.

72. Osborne DR, Dubois P, Drayer B, et al. Primary intracranial meningeal and spinal hemangiopericytoma: radiologic manifestations. *AJNR Am J Neuroradiol* 1981; 2:69–74.

73. Rutkowski MJ, Jian BJ, Bloch O, et al. Intracranial hemangiopericytoma: clinical experience and treatment considerations in a modern series of 40 adult patients. *Cancer* 2012; 118:1628–1636.

74. Rutkowski MJ, Bloch O, Jian BJ, et al. Management of recurrent intracranial hemangiopericytoma. *J Clin Neurosci* 2011; 18:1500–1504.

75. Rutkowski MJ, Sughrue ME, Kane AJ, et al. Predictors of mortality following treatment of intracranial hemangiopericytoma. *J Neurosurg* 2010; 113:333–339.

76. Chiechi MV, Smirniotopoulos JG, Mena H. Intracranial hemangiopericytomas: MR and CT features. *AJNR Am J Neuroradiol* 1996; 17:1365–1371.

77. Liu HG, Yang AC, Chen N, et al. Hemangiopericytomas in the spine: clinical features, classification, treatment, and long-term follow-up in 26 patients. *Neurosurgery* 2013; 72:16–24.

78. Kalani MY, Martirosyan NL, Eschbacher JM, et al. Large hemangiopericytoma associated with arteriovenous malformations and dural arteriovenous fistulae. *World Neurosurg* 2011; 76:592.e7–e10.

79. Ghia AJ, Allen PK, Mahajan A, et al. Intracranial hemangiopericytoma and the role of radiation therapy: a population based analysis. *Neurosurgery* 2013; 72:203–209.

80. Schiariti M, Goetz P, El-Maghraby H, et al. Hemangiopericytoma: long-term outcome revisited. Clinical article *J Neurosurg* 2011; 114:747–755.

81. Sonabend AM, Zacharia BE, Goldstein H, et al. The role for adjuvant radiotherapy in the treatment of hemangiopericytoma: a Surveillance, Epidemiology, and End Results analysis. *J Neurosurg* 2014; 120:300–308.

82. Staples JJ, Robinson RA, Wen BC, et al. Hemangiopericytoma--the role of radiotherapy. *Int J Radiat Oncol Biol Phys* 1990; 19:445–451.

83. Jha N, McNeese M, Barkley HT Jr, et al. Does radiotherapy have a role in hemangiopericytoma management? Report of 14 new cases and a review of the literature. *Int J Radiat Oncol Biol Phys* 1987; 13:1399–1402.

84. Bastin KT, Mehta MP. Meningeal hemangiopericytoma: defining the role for radiation therapy. *J Neurooncol* 1992; 14:277–287.

85. Borg MF, Benjamin CS. A 20-year review of haemangiopericytoma in Auckland, New Zealand. *Clin Oncol (R Coll Radiol)* 1994; 6:371–376.

86. Kano H, Niranjan A, Kondziolka D, et al. Adjuvant stereotactic radiosurgery after resection of intracranial hemangiopericytomas. *Int J Radiat Oncol Biol Phys* 2008; 72:1333–1339.

87. Kim JW, Kim DG, Chung HT, et al. Gamma Knife stereotactic radiosurgery for intracranial hemangiopericytomas *J Neurooncol* 2010; 99:115–122.

88. Olson C, Yen CP, Schlesinger D, et al. Radiosurgery for intracranial hemangiopericytomas: outcomes after initial and repeat Gamma Knife surgery. *J Neurosurg* 2010; 112:133–139.

89. Veeravagu A, Jiang B, Patil CG, et al. CyberKnife stereotactic radiosurgery for recurrent, metastatic, and residual hemangiopericytomas *J Hematol Oncol* 2011; 4:26.

90. Pitkethly DT, Hardman JM, Kempe LG, et al. Angioblastic meningiomas; clinicopathologic study of 81 cases. *J Neurosurg* 1970; 32:539–544.

91. Galanis E, Buckner JC, Scheithauer BW, et al. Management of recurrent meningeal hemangiopericytoma. *Cancer* 1998; 82:1915–1920.

92. Chamberlain MC, Glantz MJ. Sequential salvage chemotherapy for recurrent intracranial hemangiopericytoma. *Neurosurgery* 2008; 63:720–726.

93. Park MS, Patel SR, Ludwig JA, et al. Activity of temozolomide and bevacizumab in the treatment of locally advanced, recurrent, and metastatic hemangiopericytoma and malignant solitary fibrous tumor. *Cancer* 2011; 117(21):4939–4947.

94. Martinez-Trufero J, Alfaro J, Felipo F, et al. Response to trabectedin treatment in a highly pretreated patient with an advanced meningeal hemangiopericytoma. *Anticancer Drugs* 2010; 21:795–798.

95. Peters KB, McLendon R, Morse MA, et al. Treatment of recurrent intracranial hemangiopericytoma with SRC-related tyrosine kinase targeted therapy: a case report. *Case Rep Oncol* 2010; 3:93–97.

96. Delgado M, Pérez-Ruiz E, Alcalde J, et al. Anti-angiogenic treatment (sunitinib) for disseminated malignant haemangiopericytoma: a case study and review of the literature. *Case Rep Oncol* 2011; 4:55–59.

97. Domont J, Massard C, Lassau N, et al. Hemangiopericytoma and antiangiogenic therapy: clinical benefit of antiangiogenic therapy (sorafenib and sunitinib) in relapsed malignant hemangiopericytoma/solitary fibrous tumor. *Invest New Drugs* 2010; 28:199–202.

98. Liubinas SV, Maartens N, Drummond KJ. Primary melanocytic neoplasms of the central nervous system. *J Clin Neurosci* 2010; 17:1227–1232.

99. Pirini MG, Mascalchi M, Salvi F, et al. Primary diffuse meningeal melanomatosis: radiologic-pathologic correlation *AJNR Am J Neuroradiol* 2003; 24:115–118.

100. Nicolaides P, Newton RW, Kelsey A. Primary malignant melanoma of meninges: atypical presentation of subacute meningitis. *Pediatr Neurol* 1995; 12:172–174.

101. Grant DN. Primary meningeal melanomatosis: limitations of current diagnostic techniques. *J Neurol Neurosurg Psychiatry* 1983; 46:874–875.

102. Miró J, Velasco R, Majós C, et al. Meningeal melanocytosis: a possibly useful treatment for a rare primary brain neoplasm. *J Neurol* 2011; 258:1169–1171.

103. Czarnecki EJ, Silbergleit R, Gutierrez JA. MR of spinal meningeal melanocytoma. *AJNR Am J Neuroradiol* 1997; 18:180–182.

104. Xie ZY, Hsieh KL, Tsang YM, et al. Primary leptomeningeal melanoma. *J Clin Neurosci* 2014; 21(6):1051–1052.

105. Shinoda K, Hayasaka S, Nagaki Y, et al. Melanocytoma of the left optic nerve head and right retrobulbar optic neuropathy compressed by a tuberculum sellae meningioma. *Ophthalmologica* 2000; 214:161–163.

106. Hino K, Nagane M, Fujioka Y, et al. Meningeal melanocytoma associated with ipsilateral nevus of Ota presenting as intracerebral hemorrhage: case report. *Neurosurgery* 2005; 56:E1376.

107. Wang F, Qiao G, Lou X, et al. Malignant transformation of intracranial meningeal melanocytoma. Case report and review of the literature. *Neuropathology*. 2011; 31:414–420.

108. O'Brien DF, Crooks D, Mallucci C, et al. Meningeal melanocytoma. *Childs Nerv Syst* 2006; 22(6):556–561.

109. Rades D, Schild SE, Tatagiba M, et al. Therapy of meningeal melanocytomas. *Cancer* 2004; 100:2442–2447.

110. Rades D, Schild SE. Dose-response relationship for fractionated irradiation in the treatment of spinal meningeal melanocytomas: a review of the literature. *J Neurooncol* 2006; 77:311–314.

111. Lin B, Yang H, Qu L, et al. Primary meningeal melanocytoma of the anterior cranial fossa: a case report and review of the literature. *World J Surg Oncol* 2012; 10:135.

112. Allcutt D, Michowiz S, Weitzman S, et al. Primary leptomeningeal melanoma: an unusually aggressive tumor in childhood *Neurosurgery* 1993; 32:721–729.

113. Nicolaides P, Newton RW, Kelsey A. Primary malignant melanoma of meninges: atypical presentation of subacute meningitis. *Pediatr Neurol* 1995; 12:172–174.

114. Bot I, Blank CU, Brandsma D. Clinical and radiological response of leptomeningeal melanoma after whole brain radiotherapy and ipilimumab. *J Neurol* 2012; 259:1976–1978.

115. Fonkem E, Uhlmann EJ, Floyd SR, et al. Melanoma brain metastasis: overview of current management and emerging targeted therapies. *Expert Rev Neurother* 2012; 12:1207–1215.

116. Schäfer N, Scheffler B, Stuplich M, et al. Vemurafenib for leptomeningeal melanomatosis. *J Clin Oncol* 2013; 31:e173–e174.

117. Tsugu H, Fukushima T, Ikeda K, et al. Hemangioblastoma mimicking tentorial meningioma: preoperative embolization of the meningeal

arterial blood supply--case report. *Neurol Med Chir (Tokyo)* 1999; 39:45–48.

118. Takeuchi H, Hashimoto N, Kitai R, et al. A report of supratentorial leptomeningeal hemangioblastoma and a literature review. *Neuropathology* 2008; 28:98–102.

119. Zhang Q, Ma L, Li WY, et al. Von Hippel-Lindau disease manifesting disseminated leptomeningeal hemangioblastomatosis: surgery or medication? *Acta Neurochir (Wien)* 2011; 153:48–52.

120. Courcoutsakis NA, Prassopoulos PK, Patronas NJ. Aggressive leptomeningeal hemangioblastomatosis of the central nervous system in a patient with von Hippel-Lindau disease. *AJNR Am J Neuroradiol* 2009; 30:758–760.

121. Butman JA, Linehan WM, Lonser RR. Neurologic manifestations of von Hippel-Lindau disease. *JAMA* 2008; 300:1334–1342.

122. Couch V, Lindor NM, Karnes PS, et al. von Hippel-Lindau disease. *Mayo Clin Proc* 2000; 75:265–272.

123. Conway JE, Chou D, Clatterbuck RE, et al. Hemangioblastomas of the central nervous system in von Hippel-Lindau syndrome and sporadic disease. *Neurosurgery* 2001; 48:55–62.

124. Neumann HP, Eggert HR, Weigel K, et al. Hemangioblastomas of the central nervous system. A 10-year study with special reference to von Hippel-Lindau syndrome. *J Neurosurg* 1989; 70:24–30.

125. Constans JP, Meder F, Maiuri F, et al. Posterior fossa hemangioblastomas. *Surg Neurol* 1986; 25:269–275.

126. Ho VB, Smirniotopoulos JG, Murphy FM, et al. Radiologic-pathologic correlation: hemangioblastoma. *AJNR Am J Neuroradiol* 1992; 13:1343–1352.

127. Yasargil MG, Antic J, Laciga R, et al. The microsurgical removal of intramedullary spinal hemangioblastomas. Report of twelve cases and a review of the literature. *Surg Neurol* 1976; 3:141–148.

128. Murota T, Symon L. Surgical management of hemangioblastoma of the spinal cord: a report of 18 cases. *Neurosurgery* 1989; 25:699–707.

129. Brotchi J, Fischer G. Haemangioblastoma. In: Fischer G, Brotchi J (eds) *Intramedullary Spinal Cord Tumors*. Stuttgart: Thieme Medical Publishers; 1996:72–77.

130. Roonprapunt C, Silvera VM, Setton A, et al. Surgical management of isolated hemangioblastomas of the spinal cord. *Neurosurgery* 2001; 49:321–327.

131. Constans JP, Meder F, Maiuri F, et al. Posterior fossa hemangioblastomas. *Surg Neurol* 1986; 25:269–275.

132. Eskridge JM, McAuliffe W, Harris B, et al. Preoperative endovascular embolization of craniospinal hemangioblastomas. *AJNR Am J Neuroradiol* 1996; 17:525–531.

133. Takeuchi S, Tanaka R, Fujii Y, et al. Surgical treatment of hemangioblastomas with presurgical endovascular embolization. *Neurol Med Chir (Tokyo)* 2001; 41:246–251.

134. Chang SD, Meisel JA, Hancock SL, et al. Treatment of hemangioblastomas in von Hippel-Lindau disease with linear accelerator-based radiosurgery. *Neurosurgery* 1998; 43:28–34.

135. Patrice SJ, Sneed PK, Flickinger JC, et al. Radiosurgery for hemangioblastoma: results of a multiinstitutional experience. *Int J Radiat Oncol Biol Phys* 1996; 35:493–499.

136. Pan L, Wang EM, Wang BJ, et al. Gamma knife radiosurgery for hemangioblastomas. *Stereotact Funct Neurosurg* 1998; 70(Suppl 1):179–186.

137. Niemela M, Lim YJ, Soderman M, et al. Gamma knife radiosurgery in 11 hemangioblastomas. *J Neurosurg* 1996; 85:591–596.

138. Capitanio JF, Mazza E, Motta M, et al. Mechanisms, indications and results of salvage systemic therapy for sporadic and von Hippel-Lindau related hemangioblastomas of the central nervous system. *Crit Rev Oncol Hematol* 2013; 86:69–84.

139. Madhusudan S, Deplanque G, Braybrooke JP, et al. Antiangiogenic therapy for von Hippel-Lindau disease. *JAMA* 2004; 291:943–944.

140. Niemelä M, Mäenpää H, Salven P, et al. Interferon alpha-2a therapy in 18 hemangioblastomas. *Clin Cancer Res* 2001; 7:510–516.

141. Piribauer M, Czech T, Dieckmann K, et al. Stabilization of a progressive hemangioblastoma under treatment with thalidomide. *J Neurooncol* 2004; 66:295–299.

142. Schuch G, de Wit M, Höltje J, et al. Case 2. Hemangioblastomas: diagnosis of von Hippel-Lindau disease and antiangiogenic treatment with SU5416. *J Clin Oncol* 2005; 23:3624–3626.

143. Reyes-Botero G, Gállego Pérez-Larraya J, Sanson M. Sporadic CNS hemangioblastomatosis, response to sunitinib and secondary polycythemia. *J Neurooncol* 2012; 107:439–440.

144. Kim BY, Jonasch E, McCutcheon IE. Pazopanib therapy for cerebellar hemangioblastomas in von Hippel-Lindau disease: case report. *Target Oncol* 2012; 7:145–149.

145. Riklin C, Seystahl K, Hofer S, et al. Antiangiogenic treatment for multiple CNS hemangioblastomas. *Onkologie* 2012; 35:443–445.

146. Seystahl K, Weller M, Bozinov O, et al. Neuropathological characteristics of progression after prolonged response to bevacizumab in multifocal hemangioblastoma. *Oncol Res Treat* 2014; 37:209–212.

CHAPTER 13

Tumours of the haematopoietic system

Tracy T. Batchelor, Oussama Abla, Zhong-ping Chen, Dennis C. Shrieve, and Samar Issa

Primary central nervous system lymphoma

Definition

Primary central nervous system lymphoma (PCNSL) is an extranodal non-Hodgkin's lymphoma (NHL) confined to the brain, leptomeninges, eyes, and/or spinal cord (1). The prognosis of PCNSL is inferior to that of other NHL subtypes including other organ-specific subtypes of extranodal NHL. The 5- and 10-year survival proportions for PCNSL are 29.3% and 21.6%, respectively (2). The diagnosis and management of PCNSL differs from that of other primary brain cancers and NHL in other parts of the body.

Epidemiology

Primary CNS lymphoma is a rare brain tumour and subtype of NHL. An estimated 1425 cases of PCNSL were diagnosed each year in the United States from 2007 to 2011 and the number of cases is expected to increase further with the ageing of the US population (2). The median age at diagnosis is 65 and PCNSL is slightly more common among males. PCNSL accounted for approximately 2.1% of total and 6.2% of malignant primary CNS tumours diagnosed each year in the United States between 2007 and 2011. Between 1970 and 2000, the incidence of PCNSL increased, largely due to the human immunodeficiency virus (HIV) pandemic. Since 2000, there has been a further increase in the incidence of PCNSL, especially in the elderly.

Aetiology

Acquired or congenital immunodeficiency is the major risk factor for the development of PCNSL. Infection with HIV increases the risk of PCNSL by 3600-fold, and this is thought to have accounted for the increased incidence from 1970 to 2000. However, the incidence of PCNSL has decreased in the era of highly active antiretroviral therapy (HAART) (3). Central nervous system post-transplant lymphoproliferative disorder is the second most common malignancy to be diagnosed in organ transplant recipients after skin cancer (4). The time of appearance of PCNSL following transplantation ranges from 3 weeks to 21 years, with a mean time of 33 months. Almost half of cases of PCNSL occur within 1 year of transplant. Patients with congenital immunodeficiencies have a 4% risk of developing PCNSL. Immunosuppressive conditions such as

systemic lupus erythematosus, vasculitis, and idiopathic thrombocytopenic purpura also increase the risk of PCNSL. Second malignancies are not uncommon in patients with PCNSL. In a study of 129 PCNSL patients with a median follow-up of 44.8 months, 30 second malignancies were identified in 28 patients for a second malignancy proportion of 22.2%. Twenty (15.5%) were prior or synchronous malignancies and 10 (7.7%) were subsequent malignancies. The most common second malignancies were skin, prostate, and gastrointestinal cancers (5).

Pathogenesis

Approximately 90% of PCNSL cases are diffuse large B-cell lymphomas (DLBCL), with the remainder consisting of T-cell lymphomas, poorly characterized low-grade lymphomas, or Burkitt's lymphomas (6). Histologically, primary CNS DLBCL is composed of centroblasts or immunoblasts typically clustered in the perivascular space, with reactive small lymphocytes, macrophages and activated microglial cells intermixed with the tumour cells. Most tumours express pan-B-cell markers including CD19, CD20, CD22, and CD79a. The molecular mechanisms underlying transformation and localization to the CNS are poorly understood (7). Limitations in molecular studies of PCNSL include the rarity of the disease and the limited availability of tissue since the diagnosis is most often made with stereotactic needle biopsy. Like systemic DLBCL, PCNSL harbours chromosomal translocations of the *BCL6* gene, deletions in 6q, and aberrant somatic hypermutation in proto-oncogenes including *MYC* and *PAX5*. Inactivation of *CDKN2A* is also commonly observed in both entities. Similar to DLBCL, PCNSL can be classified into three molecular subclasses by gene expression profiling: type 3 large B-cell lymphoma, germinal centre B-cell (GCB) lymphoma, and post-germinal centre activated B-cell lymphoma (ABC). In DLBCL cases, the ABC gene expression profile is associated with an inferior prognosis versus the GCB profile. The ABC subclass accounted for greater than 95% of primary CNS DLBCL cases in one series (8). This higher prevalence of the ABC gene expression profile subtype in PCNSL is likely to account for the relatively inferior prognosis of this lymphoma versus systemic DLBCL. Moreover, there are other molecular features that distinguish primary CNS DLBCL from systemic DLBCL. Gene expression profiles demonstrate that PCNSL is characterized by differential expression of genes related to adhesion and extracellular matrix pathways, including *MUM1, CXCL13*, and *CHI3L1*. The ongoing somatic hypermutation with biased use of V_H gene segments that has been observed in PCNSL is suggestive of an antigen-dependent proliferation. These observations are consistent with the hypothesis that PCNSL arises following antigen-dependent activation of circulating B cells, which subsequently localize to the CNS by expression of various adhesion and extracellular-matrix related genes. However, further molecular studies to investigate the transforming events and the subsequent events responsible for CNS tropism in PCNSL are needed. Genomic analysis of 19 tumour specimens obtained from 19 immunocompetent PCNSL patients demonstrated a high prevalence of *MYD88* mutations and other genetic alterations consistent with activation of the B-cell receptor (BCR), toll-like receptor (TLR), and nuclear factor-kappa beta (NF-κB) pathways in greater than 90% of cases. These observations provide insight into potential therapeutic targets for future clinical trials in PCNSL (7, 9).

Clinical presentation

The presenting symptoms and signs of PCNSL are variable. In 248 immunocompetent patients with this tumour, 43% had neuropsychiatric signs, 33% had symptoms of increased intracranial pressure, 14% had seizures, and 4% had ocular symptoms (10). Seizures are less common than with other types of brain tumours probably because PCNSL involves predominantly subcortical white matter rather than epileptogenic grey matter. Unlike patients with systemic NHL, PCNSL patients rarely manifest B symptoms such as weight loss, fevers, or night sweats.

The International PCNSL Collaborative Group (IPCG) has developed guidelines to determine extent of disease (11). A gadolinium-enhanced brain magnetic resonance imaging (MRI) scan is the most sensitive radiographic study for the detection of PCNSL. Most PCNSL patients present with a single brain mass. The diagnosis of PCNSL is typically made by stereotactic brain biopsy. Occasionally, if a brain biopsy cannot be performed the diagnosis can be made by cerebrospinal fluid (CSF) analysis, or by analysis of vitreous fluid aspirate in patients with ocular involvement. However, given the possible delay in diagnosis and treatment with the latter two methods, prompt stereotactic biopsy is advised in almost all cases that are surgically accessible. Concurrent leptomeningeal and ocular involvement occurs in approximately 15–20% and 5–25% of PCNSL patients, respectively. While leptomeningeal dissemination of PCNSL does not appear to negatively impact prognosis, ocular involvement was associated with an inferior progression-free (PFS) and overall survival (OS) in one prospective study (12). Presenting symptoms of ocular involvement include eye pain, blurred vision, and floaters (13). A thorough diagnostic evaluation is needed to establish the extent of the lymphoma and to confirm localization to the CNS. Physical examination should consist of lymph node examination, a testicular examination in men, and a comprehensive neurological examination. A lumbar puncture should be performed if not contraindicated, and CSF should be assessed by flow cytometry, cytology, and immunoglobulin heavy-chain gene rearrangement. Because extra-neural disease must be excluded to establish a diagnosis of *primary* CNS lymphoma, computerized tomography/positron emission tomography (CT/PET) scans of the chest, abdomen, and pelvis, and a bone marrow aspirate and biopsy are advised to exclude occult systemic disease. Involvement of the optic nerve, retina, or vitreous humour should be excluded with a comprehensive eye evaluation by an ophthalmologist that includes a slit-lamp examination. Blood tests should include a complete blood count, a basic metabolic panel, serum lactate dehydrogenase, and HIV serology (11).

Two prognostic scoring systems have been developed specifically for PCNSL (14, 15). In a retrospective review of 105 PCNSL patients, the International Extranodal Lymphoma Study Group (IELSG) identified age over 60 years, Eastern Cooperative Oncology Group (ECOG) performance status greater than 1, elevated serum lactate dehydrogenase level, elevated CSF protein concentration, and involvement of deep regions of the brain as independent predictors of poor prognosis. In patients with 0–1 factors (low risk), 2–3 factors (intermediate risk), and 4–5 factors (high risk) the 2-year survival proportions were 80%, 48%, and 15%, respectively. In another prognostic model, PCNSL patients were divided into three groups based on age and performance status: (i) less than 50 years old; (ii) 50 years old or older with a Karnofsky performance score (KPS) of 70 or higher; (iii) 50 years old or older with a KPS less than 70. Based on these three divisions significant differences in overall and failure-free survival were observed. There is no formal staging system that correlates with prognosis or response to treatment in PCNSL. However, as PCNSL is a multicompartmental disease potentially involving the brain, spinal cord, eye, and CSF, the IPCG recommends an extent of disease evaluation, as noted above, that will enable clinicians to follow the response to therapy (11).

Imaging

Contrast-enhanced brain MRI is the imaging modality of choice in evaluating a patient with a suspected diagnosis of PCNSL. If MRI is not possible or is contraindicated, a contrast-enhanced brain CT scan is advised. The mass is typically isointense to hyperintense on T2-weighted MRI sequences and homogeneously enhancing on post-contrast images (Fig. 13.1).

Since PCNSL is characterized by a high nuclear:cytoplasmic ratio and high cell density, there may be regions of restricted diffusion observed on diffusion-weighted MRI sequences and apparent diffusion coefficient imaging may be useful as a biomarker of response to chemotherapy (16).

In immunocompetent PCNSL patients, lesions are solitary in 65% of cases and are located in a cerebral hemisphere (38%), thalamus/basal ganglia (16%), corpus callosum (14%), periventricular region (12%), or cerebellum (9%) (17). Isolated spinal cord involvement is rare and observed in less than 1% of cases so spinal imaging is only necessary if warranted based on clinical suspicion or to screen for leptomeningeal involvement if lumbar puncture cannot be performed.

Treatment: adults

Treatment for newly diagnosed PCNSL consists of a remission-induction (induction) phase and a remission-consolidation (consolidation) phase. Typically, induction consists of chemotherapy with the objective of achieving a complete response/remission. Once this response/remission is achieved a different chemotherapy regimen or whole-brain radiation therapy (WBRT) is administered to 'consolidate' the response/remission. Defining response to treatment in PCNSL requires assessment of all documented sites (brain, CSF, eye) of involvement on the baseline assessment. The IPCG has

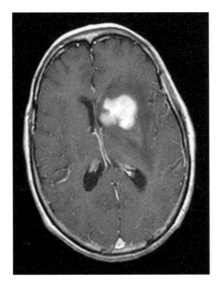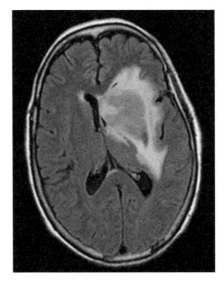

Fig. 13.1 Magnetic resonance images from a patient with PCNSL. A T1-weighted, axial, post-contrast, scan (left) demonstrates intense, homogenous enhancement of the tumour in the region of the left caudate nucleus. An axial T2/FLAIR scan at the same anatomical level (right) demonstrates hyperintense signal surrounding the tumour, reflecting vasogenic cerebral oedema.

Images courtesy of Priscilla K. Brastianos, M.D.

established response criteria that have been adopted into most prospective clinical trials of PCNSL (Table 13.1) (11).

Surgery

Surgical resection is not part of the standard treatment approach for PCNSL given the multifocal nature of this tumour (18). Although in one report a possible benefit of gross total resection in PCNSL patients was suggested, this was a retrospective, subset analysis likely confounded by selection bias (19). Other reports demonstrate no clear benefit. Median survival following surgery alone is 1–4 months (20). The role of neurosurgery in PCNSL is to establish a diagnosis via stereotactic biopsy.

Corticosteroids

Corticosteroids decrease tumour-associated oedema and may result in partial radiographic regression of PCNSL. However, after

an initial response to corticosteroids, almost all patients quickly relapse. Corticosteroids should be avoided if possible prior to a stereotactic brain biopsy, given the risk of disrupting cellular morphology, resulting in a non-diagnostic pathological specimen. Nevertheless, initial radiographic response to corticosteroids in newly diagnosed PCNSL patients is a favourable prognostic marker with survival of 117 months in responders versus 5.5 months in non-responders in one study (21).

Radiation

Historically, PCNSL was treated only with WBRT at doses ranging from 36 to 45 Gy, which resulted in a high proportion of radiographic responses but also early relapse. In a multicentre, phase II trial, 41 patients were treated with WBRT to 40 Gy plus a 20 Gy tumour boost and achieved a median OS of 12 months (22). Given the lack of durable responses to radiation and the risk of

Table 13.1 International PCNSL Collaborative Group consensus guidelines for the assessment of response in PCNSL

Response	Brain imaging	Steroid dose	Ophthalmologic examination	CSF cytology
Complete response	No contrast enhancing disease	None	Normal	Negative
Unconfirmed complete response	No contrast enhancing disease	Any	Normal	Negative
	Minimal enhancing disease	Any	Minor RPE abnormality	Negative
Partial response	50% decrease in enhancement	NA	Normal or minor RPE abnormality	Negative
	No contrast enhancing disease	NA	Decrease in vitreous cells or retinal infiltrate	Persistent or suspicious
Progressive disease	25% increase in enhancing disease	NA	Recurrent or new disease	Recurrent or positive
	Any new site of disease			
Stable disease	All scenarios not covered by responses above			

CSF, cerebrospinal fluid; RPE, retinal pigment epithelium; NA, not applicable.

Reproduced from *J Clin Oncol*, 23(22), Abrey LE, Batchelor TT, Ferreri AJ, Gospodarowicz M, Pulczynski EJ, Zucca E, et al., Report of an international workshop to standardize baseline evaluation and response criteria for primary CNS lymphoma, pp. 5034–5043, Copyright (2005), with permission from American Society of Clinical Oncology.

neurotoxicity associated with this modality of therapy, WBRT alone is no longer a recommended treatment for patients with newly diagnosed PCNSL. Moreover, as PCNSL is an infiltrative, multifocal disease, focal radiation or radiosurgery is not typically advised.

Chemoradiation

Prior to the establishment of methotrexate as the foundation of chemotherapy for PCNSL, regimens that were standardized in other forms of NHL were utilized. A randomized trial of WBRT versus WBRT plus cyclophosphamide, doxorubicin, vincristine, and prednisone (CHOP) was terminated early due to poor accrual although results suggested that WBRT and CHOP was not superior to WBRT alone (23). Given that the agents in the CHOP regimen poorly penetrate the blood–brain barrier, this was not a surprising result and this treatment regimen was abandoned for patients with CNS lymphoma.

Combined modality therapy for PCNSL consists of WBRT and chemotherapy. The most effective chemotherapeutic for PCNSL at this time is intravenous, high-dose methotrexate (HD-MTX) at variable doses ($1–8$ g/m^2), typically utilized in combination with other chemotherapeutic agents or WBRT, or both. However, there is no consensus on the optimal dose of HD-MTX or on the role of WBRT in combination with methotrexate in the management of PCNSL. A number of randomized trials have been developed to address these issues. Doses of methotrexate greater or equal to 3 g/m^2 result in therapeutic concentrations in the brain parenchyma and CSF, and when combined with WBRT lead to more durable treatment responses (24–26). In a phase II trial, 79 PCNSL patients were randomized to receive induction therapy with either (i) HD-MTX (3.5 g/m^2, day 1) versus (ii) HD-MTX (3.5 g/m^2, day 1) + cytarabine (2 g/m^2 twice daily, days 2–3). Each chemotherapy cycle was 21 days. All patients underwent consolidative WBRT after induction chemotherapy. The HD-MTX + cytarabine arm had a higher proportion of complete radiographic responses (46% versus 18%) and a superior 3-year OS (27). However, it is now recognized that there is a high incidence of neurotoxicity with combined modality treatment that includes WBRT, especially in elderly patients (28). Moreover, higher doses of consolidative WBRT, which are associated with higher risk of neurotoxicity, do not improve outcome. In a non-randomized study of 33 PCNSL patients in complete radiographic response after methotrexate-based chemotherapy, WBRT doses greater than 40 Gy were not associated with improved disease control but were associated with cognitive impairment (29). These observations have prompted studies utilizing *lower doses* of consolidative WBRT. In a multicentre, phase II study, no significant neurocognitive decline was observed after consolidative reduced-dose WBRT (23.4 Gy) and cytarabine in patients who had achieved a complete response to induction chemotherapy including HD-MTX (30). However, further study and longer neuropsychological follow-up of these patients is necessary to definitively assess the safety of this regimen as numerous studies have demonstrated the delayed neurotoxic effects of WBRT in the PCNSL population and the reduced risk of neurotoxicity in regimens consisting of chemotherapy alone (31, 32).

Chemotherapy

Given the risk of treatment-related neurotoxicity in regimens that include WBRT, many experts advise deferral of WBRT and the application of chemotherapy induction and consolidative approaches for newly diagnosed PCNSL patients. These approaches are based on a foundation of HD-MTX. Variable doses and schedules of HD-MTX have been utilized in these approaches, but in general, doses greater than or equal to 3 g/m^2 delivered as an initial bolus followed by an infusion over 3 hours, administered every 10–21 days is recommended for optimal outcomes and adequate CSF concentrations (25). Multiple, phase II studies have demonstrated the safety, efficacy, and relatively preserved cognition of HD-MTX-based chemotherapy regimens (33, 34). Moreover, longer duration of induction chemotherapy with HD-MTX (greater than six cycles) results in higher complete response proportions (30, 33).

In a multicentre study of 25 patients treated with intravenous methotrexate (8 g/m^2) monotherapy, 52% of patients achieved a complete response (CR), the median PFS was 12.8 months, the median OS was 55.4 months, and median disease-specific survival had not been reached at 72.3 months (35). In this study, 5 of the 25 patients treated with methotrexate alone achieved a CR and have not relapsed after a median follow-up of 6.8 years.

While methotrexate monotherapy may be effective for a small subset of patients, patients will generally require combination chemotherapy to achieve a durable response. In patients over 60 years of age, a regimen consisting of methotrexate, CCNU, procarbazine, methylprednisolone, intrathecal methotrexate, and intrathecal Ara-C was associated with a median OS of 14.3 months and a decreased risk of neurotoxicity relative to historical controls (36). Another regimen including methotrexate, Ara-C, vincristine, ifosfamide, cyclophosphamide, and intrathecal methotrexate/Ara-C/prednisolone was associated with a 71% overall response rate and a median OS of 50 months. Despite these promising results, however, 6 patients died from treatment-related complications and 12 patients had Ommaya reservoir infections (37). The combination of methotrexate, temozolomide, and rituximab (MTR) induction followed by consolidation with etoposide and cytarabine has been utilized successfully in the multicentre setting as induction therapy in PCNSL (34). Each agent in the MTR regimen has been studied as monotherapy in PCNSL patients with activity of each agent demonstrated (33, 38, 39). In this study, 66% of patients treated with MTR induction achieved a complete radiographic response and the median PFS was 2.4 years. However, these preliminary results from non-randomized, uncontrolled studies must be confirmed in prospective, randomized clinical trials.

The IELSG conducted a follow-up, randomized, phase II trial in newly diagnosed PCNSL patients utilizing the MTX + cytarabine combination from the IELSG20 study as a control arm. In this study, IELSG32, three different induction chemotherapy regimens were compared: arm A, MTX + cytarabine; arm B, MTX + cytarabine + rituximab; arm C, MTX + cytarabine + rituximab + thiotepa (MATRix). In this study the combination of the four drugs (arm C, MATRix) was superior to the other arms in terms of complete response and overall response proportions (40). There are other induction chemotherapy regimens currently under study in randomized, multicentre trials including the methotrexate, temozolomide, rituximab (MTR) regimen (34); the rituximab, procarbazine, methotrexate, vincristine (R-MPV) regimen (30); and the rituximab, methotrexate, teniposide, BCNU, prednisolone (R-MBVP) regimen (41). In addition to different chemotherapeutic agents these different induction regimens also include different doses and schedules of methotrexate. As there have been no head-to-head comparisons of these induction chemotherapy regimens in

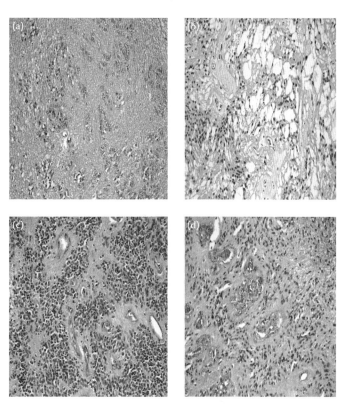

Fig. 5.1 Histology of ependymoma. (a) Ependymoma (WHO grade II). (b) Anaplastic ependymoma (WHO grade III). (c) Subependymoma (WHO grade I). (d) Myxopapillary ependymoma (WHO grade I).

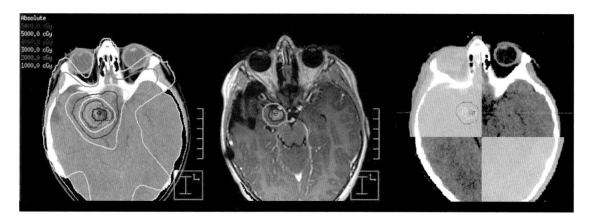

Fig. 8.3 Radiation plan for a 12-year-old boy with recurrent ganglioglioma, prescription dose was 5400 cGy in 30 fractions (left panel). Fusion of the diagnostic MRI (middle panel) allows the delineation of the gross tumour volume (GTV, blue line) and planning target volume (PTV, green line) that incorporates a safety margin for tumour infiltration and daily setup variation. CT acquisition on the linear accelerator (right panel) allows co-registration and comparison of the 'CT of the day' (light grey checker) with the planning CT (dark grey checker) to detect and correct positioning variation with millimetre accuracy.

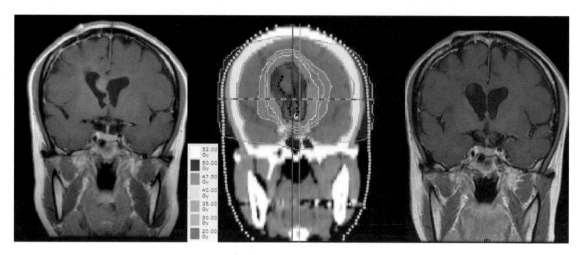

Fig. 8.5 Pre-radiation coronal T1-enhanced MRI of a 38-year-old woman with recurrent central neurocytoma (left panel) treated with image-guided conformal radiotherapy (middle panel) and with a near total radiographic response to treatment and subsequently stable disease 5 years post radiation (right panel).

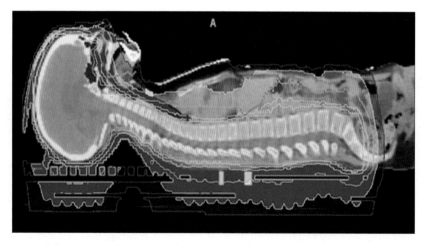

Fig. 9.4 Tomotherapy plan for craniospinal radiotherapy.

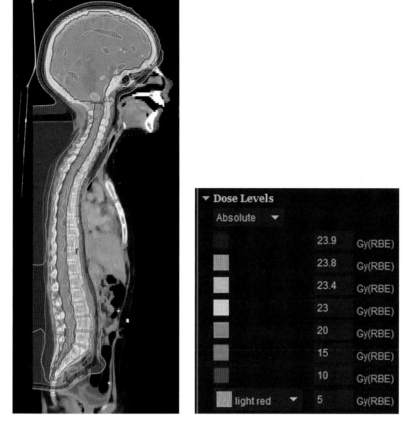

▼ **Dose Levels**		
Absolute ▼		
	23.9	Gy(RBE)
	23.8	Gy(RBE)
	23.4	Gy(RBE)
	23	Gy(RBE)
	20	Gy(RBE)
	15	Gy(RBE)
	10	Gy(RBE)
light red ▼	5	Gy(RBE)

Fig. 9.5 Pencil beam scanning dose distribution for craniospinal irradiation in a child with medulloblastoma.

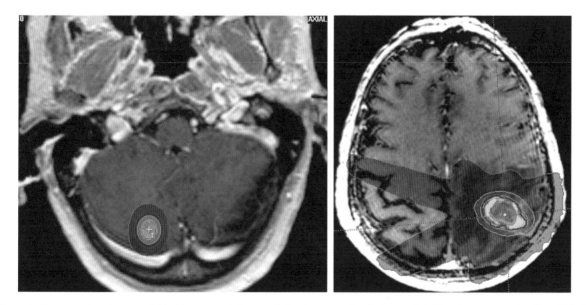

Fig. 19.1 Example of stereotactic radiosurgery (left) with an arc technique applied, and stereotactic radiotherapy (right) for a larger metastasis with multiple fixed convergent beams. Light blue colour: high-dose area, purple colour: low-dose area.

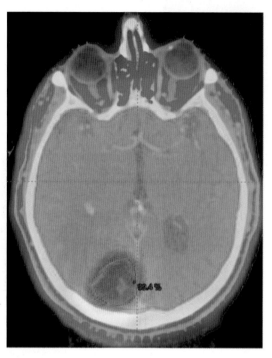

Fig. 19.2 Example of simultaneous integrated boost technique with whole-brain radiotherapy (WBRT). Green colour: dose for WBRT, red colour: a higher dose delivered at the same time as WBRT during the same daily radiotherapy session, for example, a total dose of 30 Gy for the whole brain and 60 Gy to the metastases.

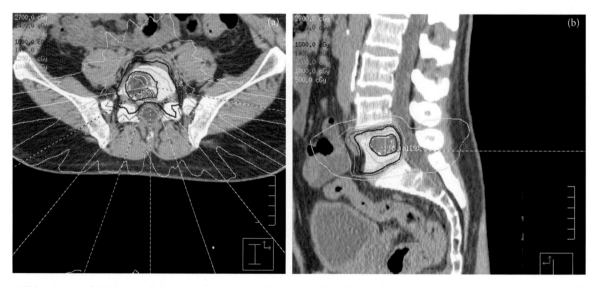

Fig. 20.2 Axial (a) and sagittal (b) MRI views of a L5 metastasis from renal cell carcinoma. The SBRT treatment plan is included. Note the rapid dose fall-off from the 24 Gy isodose line (red) to the 10 Gy isodose line (light blue) at the anterior edge of the spinal canal.

randomized trials for newly diagnosed PCNSL, there is no compelling rationale at this time to select one over the other. Future randomized trials will likely test these different induction regimens against one another to identify the optimal chemotherapy combination to use in patients with newly diagnosed PCNSL.

Rituximab, a chimeric monoclonal antibody targeting the CD20 antigen on B lymphocytes, improves response rate and prolongs event-free survival and OS in systemic DLBCL. It is being incorporated in combination induction chemotherapy regimens for PCNSL. When rituximab is administered intravenously at doses of 375–800 mg/m^2, CSF levels from 0.1% to 4.4% of serum levels are achieved. Despite limited CSF penetration, radiographic responses have been observed in relapsed PCNSL patients treated with rituximab monotherapy and this antibody has been incorporated into contemporary regimens for PCNSL (42). Moreover, in historical comparisons the complete radiographic response rates are higher with induction regimens that include rituximab versus those in which there is no rituximab (43).

The optimal consolidative therapy for PCNSL has not been identified. Options include WBRT, chemotherapy, or high-dose-chemotherapy followed by autologous stem cell transplantation (HDT/ASCT). Given the risk of clinical neurotoxicity, several trials have assessed whether WBRT can be *eliminated* from the management of PCNSL. In a multicentre, phase III trial, patients were randomized to receive HD-MTX-based chemotherapy with or without consolidative WBRT (44, 45). Five hundred and fifty-one patients were enrolled of whom 318 were treated per protocol. Intent-to-treat analysis revealed that patients treated in the combined modality arm (chemotherapy + WBRT) achieved use improved PFS but no improvement was observed in OS, demonstrating that the elimination of WBRT from the treatment regimen did not compromise OS. There are also efforts to reduce the dose of consolidative WBRT in an effort to mitigate the risk of neurotoxicity as noted above (30). Employing chemotherapy alone in the consolidation phase of therapy is also being studied. In a cooperative group, multicentre, phase II study, 44 PCNSL patients were treated with induction chemotherapy consisting of HD-MTX at 8 g/m^2 (day 1), rituximab at 375 mg/m^2 (day 3), and temozolomide at 150 mg/m^2 (days 7–11) (34). This induction chemotherapy was followed by consolidative chemotherapy consisting of intravenous etoposide 5 mg/kg as a continuous infusion over 96 hours and cytarabine at 2 g/m^2 every 12 hours for eight doses. Sixty-six per cent of these patients achieved CR to induction chemotherapy, median PFS of the entire group was 2.4 years, and median OS was not observed at the time of publication. These results are comparable to regimens that *include* consolidative WBRT. It is noteworthy that in this study PFS was significantly shorter in PCNSL patients in whom chemotherapy was delayed for more than 1 month after diagnosis compared to those patients who promptly initiated chemotherapy (3-year PFS of 20% versus 59%, respectively). This observation highlights the importance of early diagnosis and prompt initiation of chemotherapy in PCNSL patients. Given the success of high-dose chemotherapy HDT/ASCT in relapsed or refractory systemic NHL and PCNSL there is also interest in this approach as consolidative therapy for newly diagnosed PCNSL (46). Conditioning regimens including thiotepa have demonstrated the most encouraging results. In a multicentre, phase II study, 79 patients were treated with induction HD-MTX, cytarabine, rituximab, and thiotepa, followed by carmustine and thiotepa conditioning prior to ASCT. The overall response rate was 91%, 2-year OS was 87%, and treatment-related deaths occurred in less than 10% of enrolled patients. The toxicities, mostly cytopenias, were manageable. There are four ongoing, multicentre, randomized trials comparing the efficacy of consolidative HDT/ASCT versus chemotherapy or WBRT for newly diagnosed PCNSL (Table 13.2).

Intrathecal chemotherapy

Several first-generation chemotherapy regimens for PCNSL included intrathecal chemotherapy. However, a number of non-randomized studies that included intrathecal chemotherapy did not improve outcomes in PCNSL relative to regimens that did not include intrathecal injections of chemotherapy (47, 48). Moreover, the ability to consistently achieve micromolar concentrations of MTX in the CSF at least at doses of 8 g/m^2 has led to the elimination of intrathecal chemotherapy from most of the induction chemotherapy regimens currently in use. However, the question regarding the role of intrathecal chemotherapy in the management of PCNSL should ultimately be addressed in a randomized trial.

Treatment in the elderly

Elderly patients account for more than half of all the subjects diagnosed with PCNSL (2). The risk of neurotoxicity is highest in this population, and in general, chemotherapy alone is the preferred option for this subgroup. The majority of PCNSL patients over 60 years of age develop clinical neurotoxicity after treatment with a WBRT-containing regimen and some of these patients die of treatment-related complications, rather than recurrent disease (49). Several studies have indicated that HD-MTX at doses of 3.5–8 g/m^2 is generally well tolerated in elderly patients with manageable grade 3 or 4 renal and haematological toxicity (50, 51). A meta-analysis of 783 PCNSL patients over 60 years of age demonstrated that regimens including HD-MTX are associated with improved survival. While WBRT alone was also associated with improved survival it was also associated with an increased risk of neurological side effects (odds ratio, 5.23) (52). In a multicentre, randomized, phase II trial of chemotherapy alone in elderly patients with PCNSL, 98 patients were randomized to receive three 28-day cycles of either MPV-A (methotrexate 3.5 g/m^2, days 1,15; procarbazine 100 mg/m^2, days 1–7; vincristine 1.4 mg/m^2, days 1 and 15) or MT (methotrexate 3.5 g/m^2, days 1 and 15; temozolomide 100–150 mg/m^2, days 1–5, 15–19) with one additional cycle of cytarabine (3 g/m^2/day for 2 consecutive days) in the MPV arm only. While trends favoured the MPV-A regimen over the simpler, less toxic MT regimen with respect to CR rate, PFS and OS, none of these differences reached statistical difference (53). Subsequent studies suggest that the addition of rituximab to both MPV and MT could increase the radiographic response rate. Other non-randomized studies have demonstrated the feasibility of HD-MTX (8 g/m^2) and multi-agent, immunochemotherapy consisting of rituximab, methotrexate, procarbazine, and lomustine for elderly patients with newly diagnosed PCNSL (51, 54, 55). There is no standard of care established for elderly patients (>60 years of age) with newly diagnosed PCNSL but deferral of WBRT and utilization of chemotherapeutic approaches is the primary approach recommended by most experts.

Refractory and relapsed lymphoma

Despite aggressive first-line treatment, the majority of patients with PCNSL will progress or relapse and require salvage therapy.

Table 13.2 Randomized trials in primary central nervous system lymphoma

Induction	Consolidation
Completed trials	
Medical Research Council Phase II, *n* = 53 (stopped early) (MUST INCLUDE RITUXIMAB) *CHOP versus WBRT followed by CHOP* (23)	**G-PCNSL-SG-1 – NCT00153530** Phase III, *n* = 551, age ≥ 18 years *Arm 1: methotrexate ± ifosfamide => WBRT* *Arm 2: methotrexate ± ifosfamide* (44)
IELSG 20—NCT00210314 Phase II; *n* = 79, ages 18–75 years *Induction arm 1: methotrexate + cytarabine => WBRT* *Induction arm 2: methotrexate => WBRT* (27)	
ANOCEF-GOELAMS—NCT00503594 Phase 2, *n* = 95, age ≥ 60 years *Arm 1: methotrexate, procarbazine, vincristine, cytarabine* *Arm 2: methotrexate, temozolomide* (53)	
IESLG 32—NCT01011920 Phase 2, *n* = 227, ages 18–70 years *Induction arm 1: methotrexate, cytarabine* *Induction arm 2: methotrexate, cytarabine, rituximab* *Induction arm 3: methotrexate, cytarabine, rituximab, thiotepa* (40)	
Ongoing trials	
ALLG/HOVON—EudraCT 2009-014722-42 Phase 3, *n* = 200, ages 18–70 years rituximab, methotrexate, BCNU, teniposide, prednisone *Arm 1: rituximab, methotrexate, BCNU, teniposide, prednisone => cytarabine, WBRT* *Arm 2: methotrexate, BCNU, teniposide, prednisone => cytarabine, WBRT*	**IESLG 32—NCT01011920** Phase 2, n = 104, ages 18–70 years *Consolidation arm 1: WBRT* *Consolidation arm 1: HDT/ASCT*
	ANOCEF-GOELAMS—NCT00863460 Phase 2, *n* = 100, ages 18–60 years R-MBVP => *Consolidation arm 1: HDT/ASCT* *Consolidation arm 2: WBRT*
	RTOG 1114—NCT01399372 Phase 2, *n* = 84, age ≥18 years Methotrexate, procarbazine, vincristine, rituximab => *Consolidation arm 1: WBRT (lower dose) => cytarabine* *Consolidation arm 2: cytarabine*
	Alliance 51101—NCT01511562 Phase 2, *n* = 110, ages 18–75 years Methotrexate, temozolomide, rituximab, cytarabine => *Consolidation arm 1: HDT/ASCT* *Consolidation arm 2: etoposide, cytarabine*
	MATRix/IELSG43 Phase 2, *n* = 220, ages 18–70 years Methotrexate, cytarabine, thiotepa, rituximab (MATRix) => *Consolidation arm 1: HDT/ASCT* *Consolidation arm 2: dexamethasone, ifosfamide, VP-16, carboplatin (DEViC)*

ALLG: Australasian Leukaemia and Lymphoma Group; ANOCEF, Association des Neuro-Oncologue d'Expression Française; GOELAMS, Groupe Ouest Est d'Etude des Leucémies et Autres Maladies du Sang; G-PCNSL-SG, German Primary CNS Lymphoma Study Group; HDT/ASCT, high-dose chemotherapy and autologous stem cell transplantation; HOVON, Stichting Hemato-Oncologie voor Volwassenen Nederland (Dutch-Belgian Cooperative Trial Group for Hematology Oncology); IELSG, International Extranodal Lymphoma Study Group; NCT, national clinical trial; RTOG, Radiation Therapy Oncology Group; WBRT, whole brain radiation therapy.

Optimal management of relapsed or refractory PCNSL has yet to be determined and has only been studied in relatively small studies using heterogeneous therapies. Despite high initial response rates with HD-MTX-based induction therapy, most patients with PCNSL relapse. Moreover, there is a subset of patients who have HD-MTX-refractory disease. In general, prognosis for patients with relapsed or progressive PCNSL is poor with a median survival of approximately 4.5 months (56). In a study of 256 PCNSL patients with relapsed or refractory disease after initial therapy, relapse was asymptomatic in 25% of patients and was identified on serial surveillance imaging. This highlights the importance of surveillance imaging as recommended by the IPCG. Survival was worse in those patients who had refractory PCNSL or who relapsed within 1 year versus those who relapsed after 1 year (57). Although relapses in PCNSL are predominantly within the CNS, relapses in extraneural organs are reported in up to 17% of patients (58). Late relapses also appear to occur more commonly in primary CNS DLBCL versus systemic DLBCL. In one long-term follow-up study, 26% of all relapses were after 5 years and 1.7% were after 10 years (58). Re-challenge with HD-MTX can be effective in patients who had previously responded to this agent. In a multicentre, retrospective study of 22 relapsed PCNSL patients with a history of prior response to HD-MTX, 91% had a radiographic response to the first salvage treatment with HD-MTX, and 100% to a second salvage. The median OS from the first salvage was 61.9 months (59). In patients who have not previously been treated with HDT/ASCT this is also an option at the time of relapse. In a phase II trial of 43 patients with relapsed or refractory PCNSL, salvage therapy with high-dose cytarabine and etoposide was followed by HDT/ASCT with a conditioning regimen consisting of thiotepa, busulfan, and cyclophosphamide. Twenty-seven patients ultimately proceeded to transplantation. Twenty-six of 27 patients had a CR and the median PFS and OS in this group were 41.1 and 58.6 months, respectively (60). It is also noteworthy that in a small series of patients with relapsed PCNSL after initial HDT/ASCT a second autotransplantation was successful as salvage treatment (61). WBRT in patients who have not received radiation as a part of their initial treatment is an effective option in the relapsed PCNSL setting, although the risk of neurotoxicity remains high (62, 63). Many clinicians reserve WBRT for those patients with chemotherapy-refractory disease or at the time of relapse. In a series of 27 relapsed or refractory PCNSL patients treated with WBRT (median dose 36 Gy), 74% achieved an overall radiographic response and the median OS was 10.6 months. Delayed neurotoxicity rates of 15% were noted at doses greater than 36 Gy even in this setting of short survival. Novel therapeutic agents currently under study for primary CNS DLBCL include ibrutinib, lenalidomide, pomalidomide, buparlisib, pemetrexed, everolimus, pemetrexed, and bendamustine (7). In light of the fact that more than 90% of primary CNS DLBCL cases are of the poor prognosis ABC subtype and the importance of BCR signalling in these tumours, a treatment regimen designed to target BCR signal transduction using the Bruton's tyrosine kinase (BTK) inhibitor, ibrutinib is noteworthy. In six patients treated with temozolomide, etoposide, doxil, dexamethasone, ibrutinib, and rituximab (TEDDI-R), it was observed that all patients had tumour regression with three achieving CR and one achieving PR (64). Lenalidomide, an oral, immunomodulatory agent has antiproliferative properties and is the subject of several ongoing, prospective clinical trials in relapsed and refractory PCNSL. In one report of six patients with relapsed PCNSL, two patients (33%) achieved a CR including duration of 24+ months in one subject (65). In a phase I study of dose-escalating lenalidomide, nine patients with relapsed or refractory CNS lymphoma (seven PCNSL, two secondary central nervous system lymphomas (SCNSL)) were treated and eight out of eight evaluable subjects achieved objective responses (four CR, four PR) after 1 month of lenalidomide monotherapy. In a separate cohort of ten patients from the same study with relapsed or refractory CNS lymphoma (eight PCNSL, two SCNSL), lenalidomide (5–10 mg) was administered as maintenance therapy after first-line salvage treatment and five patients maintained durable responses for 2 or more years suggesting that this agent should be further investigated as a potential maintenance or consolidative therapy (66). Clinical trials of lenalidomide plus rituximab for relapsed or refractory PCNSL are ongoing.

Neurotoxicity

The most frequent complication in long-term PCNSL survivors is delayed neurotoxicity. Although this risk is high, the exact incidence of delayed neurotoxicity is unclear, as most studies have not systematically assessed neurocognitive function with serial neuropsychological testing. The elderly are at highest risk for this complication, with the majority of patients aged over 60 developing clinical neurotoxicity following combined modality therapy. Treatment with WBRT has been identified as the major risk factor for the development of late neurotoxicity. Common symptoms and signs include deficits in attention, memory, executive function, gait ataxia, and incontinence. These deficits have a detrimental impact on quality of life. Radiographic findings include periventricular white matter changes, ventricular enlargement, and cortical atrophy. Pathological studies reveal demyelination, hippocampal neuronal loss, and large-vessel atherosclerosis (67). Although the pathophysiology is unclear and likely multifactorial, damage to neural progenitor cells has been implicated as playing an important role in radiation-related neurotoxicity (68). Currently, there are no treatments to reverse these delayed neurotoxic effects. Neuropsychological function was maintained in one long-term follow-up study of PCNSL patients treated with chemotherapy alone. It is critical that serial neuropsychological and quality-of-life assessments be incorporated into clinical trials of patients with PCNSL, as cognitive outcome is a critical endpoint. The IPCG has developed an instrument for this purpose, which is composed of quality-of-life questionnaires and standardized neuropsychological tests that include assessment of executive function, attention, memory, and psychomotor speed (28).

Monitoring and follow-up

As treatment improves for PCNSL more patients are living longer, emphasizing the need to optimize neurocognitive function and quality of life. The IPCG recommends a schedule of follow-up neuroimaging studies and cognitive assessments in PCNSL survivors (11).

PCNSL in children

Primary CNS lymphoma is rare in childhood, accounting for approximately 1% of all PCNSL cases diagnosed from 1973 to 1998 in the United States (69). Fewer than 100 cases have been reported with the largest series consisting of 29 cases. Although most reported cases were in immunocompetent hosts, both acquired and congenital immunodeficiency increase the risk of PCNSL in the paediatric population. As with PCNSL in adults, the majority of cases consist of the diffuse large B-cell type. In the largest series reported the median age at diagnosis was 14 years. Although paediatric PCNSL may have a better prognosis and treatment outcome compared to the adult population the small number of cases and the lack of any prospective clinical trials make such a conclusion speculative (69).

As with adults, it is very unlikely that resection confers any benefit to children with PCNSL given the multifocal nature of the disease. In an older series of paediatric PCNSL patients treated with WBRT alone or in combination with chemotherapy, the median OS was 17 months. Subsequent series of children with PCNSL treated with methotrexate and/or cytarabine containing chemotherapy regimens suggests better outcomes with event-free survival of 70% in one series. In the largest series of 29 children with PCNSL the treatment regimens were heterogeneous although 20/29 were initially treated with chemotherapy approaches and 15/29 subjects received high-dose methotrexate and cytarabine as a component of their induction chemotherapy. The 3-year OS for the entire group was 80% with 10/29 patients experiencing relapse. Five of the six patients who relapsed after chemotherapy alone were successfully salvaged. Four patients treated with HDT/ASCT at the time of relapse achieved CR and none had relapsed at the time of the report. Unfortunately, long-term follow-up was available for only seven patients in this study with three out of seven manifesting learning disabilities. Given the potential for long-term survival and the well-characterized risks of neurotoxicity with WBRT in children the authors of this report suggest the use of methotrexate-based chemotherapy approaches without WBRT as initial therapy (69).

Other types of PCNSL

Primary vitreoretinal lymphoma

Primary vitreoretinal lymphoma (PVRL), also referred to as primary intraocular lymphoma, is a rare form of DLBCL usually presenting as a posterior uveitis and with a unique tropism for the retina (70). As noted previously, 5–25% of patients with PCNSL will have concurrent ocular involvement and such patients have an inferior prognosis. PVRL is less common than concurrent brain and ocular lymphoma with an estimated 380 cases diagnosed each year in the United States. It is estimated that 65–95% of patients with PVRL will subsequently develop CNS lymphoma, which may account for the relatively poor prognosis of PVRL. Delay in diagnosis is common as patients most commonly present with non-specific ocular symptoms such as blurred vision, decreased visual acuity, and floaters. The most common findings are vitreous cell infiltration (lymphomatous and inflammatory cells) and subretinal tumour infiltration as noted on dilated funduscopy, fluorescent angiography, and optical coherent tomography. The gold standard for PVRL diagnosis is the identification of PVRL cells in the eye achieved by aqueous aspiration, vitrectomy, retinal or chorioretinal biopsy, and, rarely, enucleation. Cytology and histopathology are required for pathological diagnosis. Optimal treatment for PVRL is not defined and consists of local (intravitreal therapy, radiation) or systemic (intravenous chemotherapy) approaches. Micromolar (i.e. cytotoxic) doses of methotrexate can be achieved in the aqueous and vitreous humour with a dose of 8 g/m^2 (71). In a retrospective study of 83 immunocompetent patients with PVRL with a

median age of 65 years, the median time to diagnosis was 6 months (72). Diagnosis was achieved by vitrectomy in 74/83 patients and 55 of the cases were large B-cell. Nine of 60 (15%) patients had concurrent CSF involvement by lymphoma. Treatment consisted of local therapy (intravitreal methotrexate, ocular radiation) in 23 patients and extensive therapy (systemic chemotherapy, WBRT) in 53 patients. Forty-seven patients relapsed in the brain (47%), eyes (30%), brain and eyes (15%), and systemically (8%) at a median time of 19 months. Local therapy did not increase the risk of brain-specific or overall relapse. The median PFS and OS were 29.6 months and 58 months, respectively and were unaffected by treatment type. Ocular complications, including decreased visual acuity and cataracts, occurred in 32% and 36% of patients receiving local radiation or intravitreal chemotherapy, respectively. Based on observations from this, albeit retrospective, study there is no compelling evidence to recommend local versus systemic therapy for PVRL. It is not clear whether systemic chemotherapy might reduce the risk of subsequent CNS involvement (70, 72).

Primary leptomeningeal lymphoma

Primary leptomeningeal lymphoma (PLL) is defined as lymphoma confined to the leptomeninges (CSF) without involvement of brain, spinal cord, eye, or other extraneural organs (73). PLL is rare, accounting for approximately 7% of all PCNSL cases with only case reports or small case series reported. The IPCG summarized the largest, retrospective series of PLL consisting of 48 cases from 12 centres from 1981 to 2011 (73). In this series the median age at diagnosis was 51. Most cases consisted of DLBCL although 9/48 (19%) were primary leptomeningeal T-cell lymphomas. Consistent with other forms of leptomeningeal cancer, most (68%) patients presented with multifocal neurological symptoms and signs including cranial neuropathies, weakness, bowel or bladder dysfunction, or pain. Brain or spine imaging was abnormal in 81%, most commonly leptomeningeal enhancement in the brain and spinal cord. Diagnosis was established by CSF cytology in 67% of patients although meningeal biopsy was required to make the diagnosis in 33% of patients. In the patients with diagnostic CSF, a median of three lumbar punctures was required to make the diagnosis. Treatment in this retrospective series was variable including systemic chemotherapy and intrathecal chemotherapy and radiation. However, most patients (68%) received intravenous methotrexate as part of their treatment. Most patients achieved either complete or partial responses based on imaging and CSF analysis. The median time to progression was 8 months and the median OS was 24 months. Eleven patients were alive at a median of 50 months of follow-up and were potentially cured with treatment. Given the retrospective nature of this study, firm conclusions regarding the optimal therapeutic approach to PLL are not possible (73, 74).

Primary intramedullary spinal cord lymphoma

Primary intramedullary spinal cord lymphoma (PISCL) is another rare variant of PCNSL with the published experience consisting of case reports and one case series (75). The case series consisted of 14 patients with PISCL from a single institution. The median age at diagnosis in this case series was 62.5 years. Most patients were presumed to have demyelinating disease at presentation and delay in diagnosis was common with a median time to PISCL diagnosis of 8 months. Patients presented with multifocal symptoms and signs and MRI demonstrated multifocal intramedullary spinal cord enhancement with 8/14 demonstrating radiographic involvement of the conus medullaris, cauda equina or both. Concurrent brain involvement occurred in 9/14 patients. Diagnosis was made by biopsy (ten patients), CSF analysis (one), or at autopsy (one). Methotrexate was the most commonly utilized initial treatment approach (9/12). However, relapses occurred in most patients, 50% of patients were wheelchair-dependent by 10 months and the 2-year survival was only 36% (75).

Intravascular large B-cell lymphoma of the central nervous system

Intravascular large B-cell lymphoma (IVLBCL) is a rare form of lymphoma, mainly encountered in elderly patients (76). Pleomorphic large lymphoid cells are confined within small arteries, veins, and capillaries. The CNS and skin are the most frequently involved organs and isolated CNS cases have been reported. Clinical manifestations are variable although fever, rash, and encephalopathy are common. Cerebral ischaemic lesions occur in approximately 50% of IVLBCL cases and may be the initial neurological presentation of IVLBCL. The lack of underlying vascular risk factors may be suggestive of this diagnosis in a patient presenting with multiple cerebral infarcts. Diagnosis of IVLBCL is difficult due to the non-specific systemic and neurological manifestations of the disease. In one report, approximately half of the IVLBCL diagnoses were made on postmortem analysis. Brain biopsy is necessary to make the diagnosis of CNS-IVLBCL. Outcomes are generally poor with greater than 80% mortality in one report, possibly due to delayed diagnosis and treatment. However, early diagnosis and treatment might be effective in some patients. Regimens that include high-dose methotrexate and rituximab have been successful in the management of some patients with isolated CNS-IVLBCL. Combinations of high-dose methotrexate-based and anthracycline-based regimens (e.g. R-CHOP) are necessary for patients with systemic and CNS involvement (77).

Lymphomatoid granulomatosis of the central nervous system

Lymphomatoid granulomatosis (LYG) is a rare angiocentric and angiodestructive B-cell proliferative process often associated with a reactive T-cell infiltration (78). Underlying immunodeficiencies are common in LYG and patients with systemic LYG are Epstein–Barr virus positive (EBV+). LYG typically involves the lungs but may also occur in extra-pulmonary sites including the CNS. A grading system from I to III has been proposed to classify LYG based on the presence of atypical lymphocytes, EBV+ B cells, and necrosis (79). Grade III LYG is considered a monoclonal, malignant lymphoma. Concurrent systemic and CNS-LYG occurs in 22.5–52% of cases. Isolated CNS involvement has been reported in approximately 20 cases in the literature. In a summary of these published cases, the mean age at diagnosis was 45 years and CNS-LYG was more common in males. Radiographic features include discrete, ring-enhancing brain parenchymal masses or diffuse, infiltrative lesions. A multifocal, punctate, and linear enhancing radiographic pattern is most common. Due to the non-specific radiographic features, biopsy or resection is required for a specific histopathological diagnosis. Treatment of systemic LYG involves steroids, interferon, cyclosprine A, rituximab, chemotherapy, or HDT/ASCT. Treatment of CNS-LYG has mainly consisted of steroids, radiation, and chemotherapy. In the subgroup of CNS-LYG patients with discrete brain masses resection is anecdotally associated with improved survival. Although also anecdotal, it is possible that less aggressive therapy is necessary for grade I CNS-LYG while chemotherapy alone or in combination with radiation is required for grade II or grade III CNS-LYG. Prognosis is variable but CNS involvement is considered a poor prognostic marker. However, aggressive treatment may lead to long-term survival in some cases of CNS-LYG.

PCNSL in the immunocompromised host: acquired immunodeficiency syndrome

The incidence of AIDS-related PCNSL has significantly decreased in the era of HAART. Studies have shown a survival benefit in patients with AIDS-related PCNSL who receive HAART compared to WBRT alone, and there have been case reports of radiographic regression of PCNSL following HAART alone. An increase in the CD4+ count to above 50 cells/μL, and a decrease in HIV viral load are associated with improved survival. Standard treatment in this setting is currently HAART with WBRT. However, the neurotoxicity associated with WBRT has generated interest in studies of high-dose methotrexate alone, which have yielded promising results (80).

PCNSL in the immunocompromised host: primary CNS post-transplant lymphoproliferative disease

Primary CNS post-transplant lymphoproliferative disease (PCNSPTLD) occurs in the setting of solid organ transplantation, is typically diagnosed years after transplant in the setting of immunosuppressive therapy, and is associated with a high frequency (>90%) of EBV+ (4). The largest series of PCNSPTLD included 84 cases of solid organ transplant recipients (79% kidney) (81). The median time to diagnosis of PCNSPTLD was 54 months but 25/84 of cases presented more than 10 years after solid organ transplantation. The pathological diagnosis was monomorphic histology (83%) and 93% of tumour specimens were EBV+. In this series, CSF involvement was diagnosed in 10% of subjects while ocular involvement was not noted in any subject. Initial treatment consisted of reduction of immunosuppression in 93% of subjects. Additional treatment consisted of high-dose methotrexate (48%), high-dose cytarabine (33%), WBRT (24%), and/or rituximab (44%). Sixty per cent of patients responded to first-line treatments as outlined above although treatment-related mortality was 13%. The 3-year PFS and OS rates were 32% and 43%, respectively. Lack of response to first-line therapy was a poor prognostic sign.

Primary T-cell central nervous system lymphoma

Primary CNS T-cell lymphoma (TPCNSL) is a rare subtype of PCNSL with an estimated incidence of less than 4% of PCNSL cases in Western countries but up to 8% of PCNSL cases in Japan. There are fewer than 100 cases reported in the literature. Most are classified as peripheral T-cell lymphomas (PTCLs), not otherwise specified. The largest series of TPCNSL contained 45 cases collected over 23 years from different medical centres from around the world (82). Based on the long time interval for case ascertainment, the variable treatments and multiple different sites definitive comparison to primary CNS DLBCL is not possible. However, it can be stated that the clinical features of these 45 TPCNSL cases were generally similar to those reported in patients with primary CNS DLBCL. The median age at diagnosis was 59.5, there was a male preponderance, 19% had positive CSF cytology, 4% had ocular involvement, and 29% had multiple brain lesions. Treatment was heterogeneous. Twenty-four out of 45 patients received chemotherapy followed by irradiation, 7/45 received chemotherapy alone, 2/45 received intra-arterial chemotherapy, and 11/45 received irradiation alone. Methotrexate was the most commonly used chemotherapeutic agent (29/45). Performance status at diagnosis and use of methotrexate were associated with disease-specific survival in a multivariate model. The median PFS and OS durations in this case series were 22 months and 25 months, respectively (82).

Primary central nervous system anaplastic large T-cell lymphoma

Primary CNS anaplastic large T-cell lymphoma (ALCL) is a rare entity with approximately 25 cases reported in the literature (83). In the cases reported with ALK status, 13 patients were ALK-positive and 10 patients were ALK-negative. Leptomeningeal involvement is not uncommon in primary CNS-ALCL, occurring in 10/24 reported cases. Clinical symptoms and signs are often related to leptomeningeal or dural involvement. ALK-positive patients are younger and may have a more favourable prognosis. Leptomeningeal involvement does not appear to confer an inferior prognosis although the number of reported cases is too small to draw firm conclusions.

Primary central nervous system natural killer/T-cell lymphoma

Natural killer/T-cell lymphomas (NK/TCLs) are a rare group of NHLs arising from post-thymic T cells. These lymphomas are more common in Asian and South American populations (84). Systemic NK/TCL rarely disseminates to the nervous system. Extranodal, primary CNS-NK/TCL of the nasal type is a rare entity with fewer than ten cases reported in the literature (85). Only one female case has been reported. Five of the six reported primary CNS-NK/TCL cases involved brain parenchyma while one was confined to the leptomeninges. Five of the six cases were positive for EBV suggesting a pathogenic role for this infectious agent in primary CNS-NK/TCL. All cases experienced a rapidly progressive course and poor outcome with survival ranging from 1–18 months. Radiation and multiagent chemotherapy have been utilized but no standard of care exists for this very rare malignancy.

Low-grade primary central nervous system lymphoma

Low-grade primary CNS lymphomas of the brain parenchyma are extremely rare. The largest series consisted of 40 subjects collected from 18 centres in 5 countries (86). These 40 tumours consisted mainly of non-classifiable small cell lymphomas although there were 11 cases of lymphoplasmacytic lymphoma and 1 case of follicular lymphoma. The median age at diagnosis was 60. Treatment was variable with chemoradiation in 15 patients, irradiation alone

in 12 patients, chemotherapy alone in 10 patients, tumour resection alone in 2 patients, and no treatment in 1 patient. The median PFS, disease-free survival, and OS durations were 61.5 months, 130 months, and 79 months, respectively. Older age was the only variable that was associated with inferior PFS and OS in multivariate analysis.

Mucosa-associated lymphoid tissue lymphoma of the dura

Mucosa-associated lymphoid tissue (MALT) lymphomas are a subtype of marginal zone lymphoma and may arise in multiple organs. The pathogenesis of these lymphoid tumours is related to chronic infection and autoimmune disease. MALT lymphoma of the dura is a rare lymphoid tumour with approximately 100 cases reported in the literature. In a review of 91 patients with MALT lymphoma of the dura, the median age at diagnosis was 52 and female gender predominated (79%) (87). Symptoms and signs are often subtle and slowly progressive. Most patients present with headaches (43%) or seizures (38%) and single intracranial dural lesions are more common (84%). Radiographic features are similar to meningiomas including extra-axial location and contrast enhancement. However, restricted diffusion may be present and while typical for lymphoma would be unusual for meningioma. Transient radiographic response to corticosteroids is also suggestive of lymphoma rather than meningioma (88). In the series of 91 patients with MALT lymphomas of the dura, treatment consisted of either surgery, radiation, chemotherapy, or combinations of these modalities. Outcomes were uniformly good irrespective of treatment modality or unifocality versus multifocality with 94% of patients alive at the time of the report.

Central nervous system Hodgkin's lymphoma

Hodgkin's lymphoma (HL) rarely involves the CNS with an incidence of 0.02–0.5% reported (89). The largest case series reported consists of 16 cases of CNS-HL collected from 13 centres in 6 countries (90). In this series, eight patients presented with CNS-HL at the time of initial HL diagnosis, two of whom had isolated CNS-HL, and eight patients presented with CNS-HL at the time of HL relapse. In the eight patients who presented at the time of disease relapse the median time to diagnosis of CNS-HL was 11.7 months (range 6.9–189 months) and five of the eight had isolated CNS disease. The median age at diagnosis of CNS-HL was 45 years. Presenting neurological symptoms were variable including headaches, seizures, encephalopathy, motor, and sensory symptoms. Ten of the 16 cases presented with brain parenchymal disease, 5 presented with isolated leptomeningeal or dural disease, and 1 presented with brain and leptomeningeal disease. Fifteen patients had histological confirmation of CNS-HL by biopsy, resection, or autopsy and 1 patient had diagnosis of CNS-HL by CSF. All 16 cases had classical HL according to WHO criteria including 7 with classical HL, NOS; 7 with nodular sclerosis; and 2 with mixed cellularity. Nine patients underwent lumbar puncture for CSF analysis with two of these nine demonstrating 'atypical cells' in the CSF. Treatment was variable and included surgery or radiation alone, chemotherapy and radiation, or chemotherapy alone. The median OS for these 16 CNS-HL patients was 60.9 months from the first diagnosis of HL and 43.8 months from the diagnosis of CNS-HL.

Long-term survival was observed in patients who achieved a complete response to treatment.

PCNSL management guidelines

The National Comprehensive Cancer Network (NCCN) and the European Association of Neuro-Oncology (EANO) have published management/treatment guidelines for PCNSL although there is only limited data available from randomized clinical trials (91, 92). The IPCG has established consensus-based response criteria and a neurocognitive battery for incorporation into clinical trials (11, 28). The IPCG criteria may also be useful for the assessment of patient outcomes in clinical practice.

Post-treatment surveillance

As treatment improves for PCNSL, more patients are living longer, emphasizing the need to optimize neurocognitive function and quality of life. The IPCG recommends a schedule of follow-up neuroimaging studies and cognitive assessment in PCNSL survivors (11).

Current research topics

Preclinical research studies include efforts to elucidate the underlying genetic drivers of primary CNS DLBCL utilizing whole-exome or whole-genome sequencing. As noted previously, preliminary studies have identified mutations and activation of signal transduction pathways, which appear to be unique to primary CNS DLBCL versus other types of nodal and extranodal DLBCL. Identification of predictive imaging markers is also of interest in order to identify PCNSL patients most likely to benefit from chemotherapy. Medical therapies focused on targeting the relevant pathways of the ABC subtype of DLBCL are also under development. Finally, despite the rarity of PCNSL there are an increasing number of randomized trials (see Table 13.2) either completed or under development that will provide future guidance in the management of this lymphoma subtype.

Histiocytic tumours of the central nervous system

Definition

Histiocytoses are a diverse group of proliferative disorders involving dendritic cells and macrophages. They represent a spectrum of diseases ranging from a reactive inflammatory accumulation of cells, pathological immune activation, or neoplastic clonal proliferation (93). The most common types of histiocytoses are Langerhans cell histiocytosis (LCH), haemophagocytic lymphohistiocytosis (HLH), and the non-LCH disorders.

The WHO classification of histiocytic tumours include LCH and non-LCH disorders such as Erdheim–Chester disease (ECD), Rosai–Dorfman disease (RDD), juvenile xanthogranuloma (JXG), and histiocytic sarcoma (HS). This section will focus on the CNS presentations of these histiocytic neoplasms.

Langerhans cell histiocytosis

Langerhans cell histiocytosis is a dendritic cell (DC) neoplasm defined by the presence in the lesion of pathological Langerhans cells (LCH cells) that are positive for CD1a, CD207 (langerin), and S100. Although LCH was once considered a disorder of immune regulation, the identification of activating mutations in the proto-oncogene *BRAF* V600E in 50–60% of cases, and MEK and ERK phosphorylation in 100% of examined cases, has changed the definition of LCH to a dendritic cell neoplasm with a strong inflammatory component (94).

Clinically, LCH has a diverse clinical behaviour ranging from benign single system disease (SS) that can regress spontaneously to multisystem (MS) disease that can be life-threatening or a chronically reactivating form of disease that has the potential to result in significant permanent sequelae such as diabetes insipidus (DI), growth retardation, bone pain, hearing loss, sclerosing cholangitis, and CNS neurodegenerative disease (CNS-ND) (95). LCH can occur at any age but is more common in children, of whom two-thirds have SS-LCH predominantly in bone followed by skin. In adults, the mean age at diagnosis is 35 years with 10% being older than 55 years. Most adults with LCH have MS-LCH with skin and lung involvement in 51% and 62%, respectively (96). MS-LCH, involving two or more systems, can be associated with a poor survival when there is risk of organ involvement (RO$^+$) such as liver, spleen, or bone marrow. Patients with MS-LCH who are RO$^-$ have better survival and are usually treated with systemic chemotherapy (vinblastine/prednisone) in an attempt to reduce reactivations and prevent permanent sequelae (95). The Histiocyte Society LCH-III trial demonstrated that prolongation of induction therapy to 12 weeks in patients who did not achieve a complete response by week 6, and an early switch to salvage therapy for those with progressive disease on week 6, appeared to significantly decrease mortality in MS-LCH patients (97). Central nervous system disease in LCH can manifest either as DI, CNS-ND, or as parenchymal CNS mass lesions. DI is the most common neuroendocrine manifestation of LCH with an incidence of 8–12% (97). The differential diagnosis in children with isolated DI and pituitary stalk thickening includes LCH, germinoma, or lymphoma. Craniofacial bone lesions, particularly in the ear, eye, and oral region, have been found to be associated with a three-fold greater risk for DI independent of the extent of disease, and therefore these lesions are termed CNS-risk lesions (98). Patients with LCH and coexisting DI carry a higher risk of anterior pituitary dysfunction and CNS-ND (99). Development of DI during or after treatment of another site is considered reactivation and can be treated with LCH-directed therapy for an additional year with single-agent cytarabine (100) or with cytarabine/vincristine/prednisone therapy (101). In adults with isolated DI, the differential diagnosis may also include Erdheim–Chester disease (ECD). In the absence of other sites of disease in a patient in whom a pituitary biopsy is not possible, checking for *BRAF* V600E in peripheral blood or CSF may support the diagnosis and identify a potential for targeted therapy (100). Clofarabine is also a reasonable alternative therapy for both LCH and ECD in adults with isolated pituitary lesions (102).

The second most common CNS finding in LCH is CNS-ND, which is a devastating and irreversible complication that may occur even 10 years after resolution of LCH lesions. It is characterized by a cerebellar syndrome or learning difficulties, with bilateral symmetric lesions in the dentate nucleus of the cerebellum or basal ganglia on neuroimaging (103). Patients may develop clinical symptoms of dysarthria, ataxia, dysmetria, and behavioural changes. The diagnostic radiological findings may precede clinical symptoms by several years (104), and it is unknown when is the best time to treat these patients. Patients with CNS-risk lesions and with radiographic CNS-ND should be routinely monitored with regular neurological examinations and the Ataxia Rating Scale to document early changes in tremor, speech, visual abilities, and motor function (100). A score increase of 5 points indicates clinical deterioration, which together with progressive changes on MRI, should merit starting empirical systemic therapy. Similarly, annual brain MRI should be performed on patients with DI to screen for the development of CNS-ND. Early treatment in patients with worsening symptoms is essential. Intravenous gamma-globulin and retinoic acid have been reported to stabilize progression of CNS-ND (105, 106). In one series, vincristine/cytarabine was associated with improvement in clinical symptoms and MRI findings in six out of eight patients (107). Some patients fail to respond to these therapies and have a gradual decline in neurological function over the course of years. More recently, an anecdotal response to vemurafenib (*BRAF* V600E inhibitor) has been reported in a 3-year-old boy with progressive CNS-ND LCH (108). Phase I/II trials are ongoing in paediatric patients of the BRAF inhibitor, dabrafenib (NCT01677741).

Parenchymal mass lesions of the brain secondary to LCH may respond to vinblastine/prednisone, cladribine, cytarabine, or clofarabine (102, 107, 109, 110). Although there is no supportive evidence from a randomized trial, cytarabine has been effective in a majority of patients and has shown possible benefit against CNS-ND LCH (107). Vinblastine/prednisone is an alternative frontline treatment of pituitary/hypothalamic lesions based on established protocols for multisystem LCH (97).

Erdheim–Chester disease

Erdheim–Chester disease, a rare non-LCH disorder, appears to be morphologically and immunohistochemically a member of the JXG family that involves the long bones in a bilateral fashion. ECD can be distinguished from LCH by the characteristic XG immunostaining, which is factor XIIIa+/CD68+/CD163+/fascin+ and S100−/CD1a−/Langerin−/Birbeck granules (111, 112). ECD occurs predominantly in adults between the ages of 40 and 70 years (mean age 55 years), and is more frequently diagnosed in males (113). Paediatric cases of ECD have rarely been described (114).

The aetiology of ECD has been a matter of debate, as it has been considered either an inflammatory disorder or a clonal neoplastic disease. The recent discovery of *BRAF* V600E mutations and MAP kinase pathway mutations in ECD cases, as well as the high frequency of association between LCH and ECD, may re-define ECD as an inflammatory myeloid neoplasia (115, 116).

The diagnosis of ECD is based on histopathological findings in the appropriate clinical and radiological context. The radiographic finding of bilateral and symmetric diaphyseal and metaphyseal osteosclerosis in the legs is present in almost all patients. ECD is a true multisystemic disease, as almost all organs can be involved. Patients may present with skeletal involvement with bone pain, DI, exophthalmos, xanthelasma, interstitial lung disease, bilateral adrenal enlargement, retroperitoneal fibrosis with perirenal and/or ureteral obstruction, renal impairment, testis infiltration, and involvement of the cardiovascular system (113). CNS involvement occurs in 40% of ECD patients. Cerebellar and pyramidal syndromes are the most frequent neurological complications, but seizures, headaches, neuropsychiatric signs or cognitive impairment, sensory disturbances, cranial nerve paralysis, and asymptomatic

lesions can also occur. Neurological involvement leads to severe functional disability in almost all patients. CNS involvement is a major prognostic factor in ECD, as studies have identified this factor as an independent predictor of death. The most devastating neurological complication of ECD is neurodegenerative involvement of the cerebellum, which is present in 17% of patients and is extremely difficult to treat (113).

There is no standard therapy for patients with ECD and response to treatment is variable. The prognosis of ECD is guarded with more than half of patients dying of their disease within 3 years from diagnosis. Interferon alpha (IFNα) appears to be the best choice for the initial treatment of ECD. Rapid and persistent regression of retro-orbital infiltration and a progressive improvement of bone lesions, pain, and DI have been reported in three ECD patients given IFNα (117). However, in eight patients with ECD treated with low-dose IFNα (3 MU × 3/week), the efficacy differed between the sites involved (118). In some cases, the symptoms failed to respond to such low doses of IFNα, particularly in patients with severe multisystemic forms of ECD (CNS and cardiovascular involvement) (119). Therefore, higher doses of IFNα (9 MU × 3/week) are recommended since they might be more effective against meningeal infiltrations, sub- and retrosellar masses, and pericardial and pseudo-atrial infiltrations (113). However, IFNα is not effective against neurodegenerative ECD. Survival analysis of 53 ECD patients showed that treatment with IFNα and/or pegylated IFNα was a major independent predictor of survival (119). Therefore, it is generally recommended to start treatment with pegylated forms of IFNα since they are better tolerated than IFNα in the long term.

In a pilot study of vemurafenib (*BRAF* V600E inhibitor) for three patients with multisystemic and refractory ECD who carried the *BRAF* V600E mutation, two of whom also had skin or lymph node LCH, vemurafenib led to rapid, substantial clinical and biological improvement of all three patients (120). Subsequently, five other patients were treated with vemurafenib and the drug was associated with long-term efficacy. One patient developed squamous cell carcinoma after 6 months of treatment, but no major adverse effects were reported in the others (121). Long-term remissions have also been anecdotally reported in ECD patients treated with cladribine, anakinra, or imatinib mesylate, although mixed responses have also been observed (122–124). Radiotherapy to ECD lesions has been reported but mainly as short-term palliation, with disease progression occurring within months. Surgical debulking is limited in ECD to severe orbital lesions or resectable intracranial lesions (113).

The prognosis of ECD is poor, with 43% of patients alive after an average follow-up of 32 months. Recent reports describing survival of ECD patients treated with interferon therapy describe a 5-year OS of 68% (113). The promising results obtained with vemurafenib in ECD patients will likely lead to better long-term outcomes in the future, however, larger studies are urgently needed.

Rosai–Dorfman disease

Rosai–Dorfman disease, or sinus histiocytosis with massive lymphadenopathy, is another rare non-LCH disorder characterized by a benign proliferation of S100-positive histiocytes within the sinus of the lymph nodes and the lymphatic vessels of internal organs. Initially described by Rosai and Dorfman in 1969, RDD is defined as a non-neoplastic, polyclonal, and self-limited disease. RDD cells are CD14+, HLA-DR+, CD68+, CD163+, S100+, and fascin+ macrophages, and they are typically negative for CD1a and langerin (125).

RDD is most frequently seen in children and young adults, but can occur at any age. Patients presenting with isolated intracranial disease tend to be older. The disease is more common in males and in individuals of African descent (126). The aetiology of RDD remains unknown, and no *BRAF* V600E mutations have been identified (127). However, RDD has been reported following bone marrow transplant for precursor-B acute lymphoblastic leukaemia, concurrently with HL and NHL or with other histiocytic disorders such as LCH and HS. RDD has also been associated with autoimmune diseases such as autoimmune lymphoproliferative syndrome, autoimmune haemolytic anaemia, systemic lupus erythematous, and juvenile idiopathic arthritis (93).

The most common presentation of RDD is bilateral, painless, massive cervical lymphadenopathy associated with fever, night sweats, fatigue, and weight loss. Mediastinal, inguinal, and retroperitoneal lymph nodes may also be involved. Extranodal involvement by RDD has been documented in 43% of cases with the most frequent sites being skin, soft tissue, upper respiratory tract, multifocal bone, eye, and retro-orbital tissue (126). Other reported sites include the urogenital tract, breast, gastrointestinal tract, liver, pancreas, and lungs. Head and neck involvement has been reported in 22% of cases, most commonly the nasal cavity followed by the parotid gland. The CNS, mainly the meninges, is involved in less than 5% of cases and this usually occurs without extracranial lymphadenopathy. Most intracranial lesions are attached to the dura with only a few extending into the parenchyma. CNS disease can present clinically and radiologically like meningioma, but the presence of emperipolesis in the CSF is usually diagnostic of CNS RDD (93, 126).

In a review of 111 RDD cases with involvement of the CNS, 15% of patients showed relapses or had died, but only 19 of them had been followed for more than 3 years (128). Subsequent cases have been published mainly describing stable results after surgery, sometimes combined with corticosteroids or azathioprine (129). Partial resection followed by adjuvant chemotherapy has been recommended, especially for difficult sites (129). However, progression to blindness and deafness has been reported (130), as well as mixed responses with an enlargement of the intracranial lesion, but resolution of extracranial manifestations, following treatment with steroids (131). In a retrospective study of 13 patients, 6 patients with involvement of the CNS, Zhu et al. observed stable conditions in only half of their cases (132). The treatment of CNS RDD is not well established, but surgical resection seems to be the most effective strategy. Treatment of relapsed or refractory RDD cases with cladribine (133) or clofarabine (102), both of which can penetrate the blood–brain barrier, is promising. Long-term remissions of intracranial RDD have also been reported after post-surgical maintenance with CHOP-like regimens (134). Further, the efficacy of the anti-CD20 monoclonal antibody, rituximab, has been anecdotally described in refractory cases (135). Lastly, one report described a patient with systemic RDD who demonstrated a rapid and complete response to the tyrosine kinase inhibitor imatinib mesylate. The patients' histiocytes were positive for the imatinib target proteins 'platelet-derived growth factor-receptor β (PDGFRB)' and 'KIT'. The disease completely responded to treatment with 400–600 mg daily of imatinib for more than 7 months (136).

Juvenile xanthogranuloma

Juvenile xanthogranuloma, the most common form of non-LCH disorders, is a benign proliferative disorder that usually resolves spontaneously. It affects the skin in 80% of cases and occurs predominantly in early childhood, although adults may also be affected. JXG has been associated with neurofibromatosis type 1 (NF1) and juvenile myelomonocytic leukaemia (JMML). In these patients, the JXG usually precedes or occurs concurrently with JMML. Children with JXG and NF1 have a 20–32-fold increased risk of JMML than patients with NF1 alone. JXG diagnosis is confirmed by biopsy to rule out LCH or other benign histiocytoses. Typical histopathological features of JXG are giant cells with a ring of nuclei (Touton giant cells), which are also characteristic of ECD. Immunohistochemistry is classically positive for factor XIIIa, fascin, CD14, CD68, and CD163 and negative for Langerin, CD1a, and the S100 protein (114).

The pathogenesis of JXG is unknown, but recent whole-exome sequencing studies suggest a role of pathological ERK activation. One study identified 17 somatic mutations by whole-exome sequencing in four JXG lesions, and although no *BRAF* V600E mutations were identified in these lesions, a *PI3KCD* mutation was identified in one patient and a germline *NF1* mutation was found in another one with NF1 and JXG (127).

Systemic JXG is rare (4–10%) and has been reported in the soft tissues, orbits, CNS, heart, lungs, bone, and bone marrow (137). Isolated intracranial JXG is rare, and most patients have multiple intracranial or spinal cord lesions or leptomeningeal involvement. The disease may cause significant neurological problems such as seizures, DI, blindness, and subdural effusions (138). Further, fatalities due to CNS JXG and malignant transformation to a clonal histiocytic neoplasm have been reported (139).

The standard treatment for solitary and symptomatic CNS JXG is surgical resection, provided that surgery is feasible. Patients with unresectable or multifocal cranial JXG have been successfully treated with cladribine (140), clofarabine (102), and vinblastine (141). A review suggested that symptomatic cases of multisystem JXG, including CNS disease, can successfully be treated with LCH-based regimens that include corticosteroids and vinca alkaloids (142). Cranial radiation therapy can be considered for unresectable and refractory CNS disease; however, due to its severe side effects in young children, it is preferable to reserve this option as the last therapeutic attempt.

Histiocytic sarcoma

Histiocytic sarcoma is a very rare non-Langerhans cell histiocytic neoplasm that arises from antigen-processing phagocytes (or mature histiocytes). The aetiology of HS remains unknown, but some cases have been diagnosed in patients with mediastinal germ cell tumours, follicular lymphoma, myelodysplastic syndrome, and acute lymphoblastic leukaemia (143). More recent Sanger sequencing data showed a high rate of *BRAF* V600E mutations (62.5%, five of eight) in histiocytic sarcoma cases (144), which suggests a central role of the BRAF pathway in the pathogenesis or malignant transformation of histiocytic and dendritic cell neoplasms. HS has been reported in all age groups but is more commonly observed in adults, with a median age of 46–55 years, and predominantly in males. Clinically, HS presents with single or multifocal extranodal tumours, most commonly in the bowels, skin, or soft tissue. Diffuse lymphadenopathy, fever, weight loss, small bowel obstruction, and bone marrow involvement with cytopenias have been reported (143). Rarely, HS can involve any site within the CNS, including the brain parenchyma, spinal cord, and meninges. Patients can present with headaches or neurological deficits, which can sometimes be misdiagnosed as demyelinating disease (145). Excisional biopsy usually shows large cells with abundant eosinophilic cytoplasm, ovoid nuclei, and one or more nucleoli. Immunohistochemistry is positive for histiocytic markers like CD163, CD68, CD45, and lysozyme. CD1a staining is classically negative which differentiates HS from LCH. S100 can be weakly positive while Ki67 is variable (143).

Treatment strategies for HS include surgical resection, steroids, chemotherapy, and radiotherapy. Most CNS HS tumours are unresectable due to their location and number. Total excision, if possible, should always be considered as it may provide a better prognosis with survival up to 1 year after complete resection (146). Steroids may relieve the symptoms temporarily by their antioedematous and oncolytic effects, but should be avoided before a biopsy as they may interfere with an accurate pathological diagnosis (145). Chemotherapy for HS has historically been unsuccessful (147). High doses of MTX and Ara-C were found to be ineffective in one case report of a CNS HS (145). However, long-term remissions with thalidomide (148, 149), alemtuzumab (150), or the MAID (mesna, doxorubicin, ifosfamide, and dacarbazine) regimen (151) have been reported in systemic HS. Some investigators recommend consolidation with haematopoietic stem cell transplant (152), although it remains controversial whether this prolongs survival. Dramatic response to vemurafenib has been reported in a *BRAF* V600E-mutated primary CNS HS (153). Whole-brain radiotherapy in CNS HS may improve the response to chemotherapy and may decrease local recurrence rates, but it is not curative and the rate of neurotoxicity is high (143, 145). Regardless of the treatment, the prognosis of HS is very poor and most patients die within months from the diagnosis. Patients with localized disease have a better prognosis than those with intracranial or metastatic disease. Due to the rarity of this disease in adults and children, the optimal treatment approach has yet to be determined. In the meantime, patients should be referred for clinical trials or treated at tertiary care centres with experience in histiocytic sarcomas.

The Histiocyte Society has recently opened an international registry for the rare histiocytic disorders (IRHDR) to better understand the natural history, clinicopathological features, and the most effective therapeutic strategies for all of the non-LCH disorders, including histiocytic sarcomas and other malignant histiocytoses.

References

1. Batchelor TT, DeAngelis LM (eds). *Lymphoma and Leukemia of the Nervous System* (2nd edn). New York: Springer; 2013.

2. Ostrom QT, Gittleman H, Liao P, et al. CBTRUS statistical report: primary brain and central nervous system tumors diagnosed in the United States in 2007-2011. *Neuro Oncol* 2014; 16 Suppl 4:iv1–63.

3. Matinella A, Lanzafame M, Bonometti MA, et al. Neurological complications of HIV infection in pre-HAART and HAART era: a retrospective study. *J Neurol* 2015; 262(5):1317–1327.

4. Cavaliere R, Petroni G, Lopes MB, et al. Primary central nervous system post-transplantation lymphoproliferative disorder: an International Primary Central Nervous System Lymphoma Collaborative Group Report. *Cancer* 2010; 116(4):863–870.

5. Wang J, Pulido JS, O'Neill BP, et al. Second malignancies in patients with primary central nervous system lymphoma. *Neuro Oncol* 2015; 17(1):129–135.

6. Swerdlow SH, Campo E, Harris NL, et al. (eds) *WHO Classification of Tumours of Haematopoietic and Lymphoid Tissues*. Lyon: International Agency for Research on Cancer, 2008.

7. Ponzoni M, Issa S, Batchelor TT, et al. Beyond high-dose methotrexate and brain radiotherapy: novel targets and agents for primary CNS lymphoma. *Ann Oncol* 2014; 25(2):316–322.

8. Camilleri-Broet S, Criniere E, Broet P, et al. A uniform activated B-cell-like immunophenotype might explain the poor prognosis of primary central nervous system lymphomas: analysis of 83 cases. *Blood* 2006; 107(1):190–196.

9. Braggio E, Van Wier S, Ojha J, et al. Genome-wide analysis uncovers novel recurrent alterations in primary central nervous system lymphomas. *Clin Cancer Res* 2015; 21(17):3986–3994.

10. Bataille B, Delwail V, Menet E, et al. Primary intracerebral malignant lymphoma: report of 248 cases. *J Neurosurg* 2000; 92(2):261–266.

11. Abrey LE, Batchelor TT, Ferreri AJ, et al. Report of an international workshop to standardize baseline evaluation and response criteria for primary CNS lymphoma. *J Clin Oncol* 2005; 23(22):5034–5043.

12. Kreher S, Strehlow F, Martus P, et al. Prognostic impact of intraocular involvement in primary CNS lymphoma: experience from the G-PCNSL-SG1 trial. *Ann Hematol* 2015; 94(3):409–414.

13. Grimm SA, Pulido JS, Jahnke K, et al. Primary intraocular lymphoma: an International Primary Central Nervous System Lymphoma Collaborative Group Report. *Ann Oncol* 2007; 18(11):1851–1855.

14. Abrey LE, Ben-Porat L, Panageas KS, et al. Primary central nervous system lymphoma: the Memorial Sloan-Kettering Cancer Center prognostic model. *J Clin Oncol* 2006; 24(36):5711–5715.

15. Ferreri AJ, Blay JY, Reni M, et al. Prognostic scoring system for primary CNS lymphomas: the International Extranodal Lymphoma Study Group experience. *J Clin Oncol* 2003; 21(2):266–272.

16. Barajas RF, Jr, Rubenstein JL, Chang JS, et al. Diffusion-weighted MR imaging derived apparent diffusion coefficient is predictive of clinical outcome in primary central nervous system lymphoma. *AJNR Am J Neuroradiol* 2010; 31(1):60–66.

17. Kuker W, Nagele T, Korfel A, et al. Primary central nervous system lymphomas (PCNSL): MRI features at presentation in 100 patients. *J Neurooncol* 2005; 72(2):169–177.

18. Bellinzona M, Roser F, Ostertag H, et al. Surgical removal of primary central nervous system lymphomas (PCNSL) presenting as space occupying lesions: a series of 33 cases. *Eur J Surg Oncol* 2005; 31(1):100–105.

19. Weller M, Martus P, Roth P, et al. Surgery for primary CNS lymphoma? Challenging a paradigm. *Neuro Oncol* 2012; 14(12):1481–1484.

20. Batchelor T, Loeffler JS. Primary CNS lymphoma. *J Clin Oncol* 2006; 24(8):1281–1288.

21. Mathew BS, Carson KA, Grossman SA. Initial response to glucocorticoids. *Cancer* 2006; 106(2):383–387.

22. Nelson DF, Martz KL, Bonner H, et al. Non-Hodgkin's lymphoma of the brain: can high dose, large volume radiation therapy improve survival? Report on a prospective trial by the Radiation Therapy Oncology Group (RTOG): RTOG 8315. *Int J Radiat Oncol Biol Phys* 1992; 23(1):9–17.

23. Mead GM, Bleehen NM, Gregor A, et al. A medical research council randomized trial in patients with primary cerebral non-Hodgkin lymphoma: cerebral radiotherapy with and without cyclophosphamide, doxorubicin, vincristine, and prednisone chemotherapy. *Cancer* 2000; 89(6):1359–1370.

24. DeAngelis LM, Seiferheld W, Schold SC, et al. Combination chemotherapy and radiotherapy for primary central nervous system lymphoma: Radiation Therapy Oncology Group Study 93–10. *J Clin Oncol* 2002; 20(24):4643–4648.

25. Ferreri AJ, Guerra E, Regazzi M, et al. Area under the curve of methotrexate and creatinine clearance are outcome-determining factors in primary CNS lymphomas. *Br J Cancer* 2004; 90(2):353–358.

26. Glantz MJ, Cole BF, Recht L, et al. High-dose intravenous methotrexate for patients with nonleukemic leptomeningeal cancer: is intrathecal chemotherapy necessary? *J Clin Oncol* 1998; 16(4):1561–1567.

27. Ferreri AJ, Reni M, Foppoli M, et al. High-dose cytarabine plus high-dose methotrexate versus high-dose methotrexate alone in patients with primary CNS lymphoma: a randomised phase 2 trial. *Lancet* 2009; 374(9700):1512–1520.

28. Correa DD, Maron L, Harder H, et al. Cognitive functions in primary central nervous system lymphoma: literature review and assessment guidelines. *Ann Oncol* 2007; 18(7):1145–1151.

29. Ferreri AJ, Verona C, Politi LS, et al. Consolidation radiotherapy in primary central nervous system lymphomas: impact on outcome of different fields and doses in patients in complete remission after upfront chemotherapy. *Int J Radiat Oncol Biol Phys* 2011; 80(1):169–175.

30. Morris PG, Correa DD, Yahalom J, et al. Rituximab, methotrexate, procarbazine, and vincristine followed by consolidation reduced-dose whole-brain radiotherapy and cytarabine in newly diagnosed primary CNS lymphoma: final results and long-term outcome. *J Clin Oncol* 2013; 31(31):3971–3979.

31. Doolittle ND, Korfel A, Lubow MA, et al. Long-term cognitive function, neuroimaging, and quality of life in primary CNS lymphoma. *Neurology* 2013; 81(1):84–92.

32. Juergens A, Pels H, Rogowski S, et al. Long-term survival with favorable cognitive outcome after chemotherapy in primary central nervous system lymphoma. *Ann Neurol* 2010; 67(2):182–189.

33. Batchelor T, Carson K, O'Neill A, et al. Treatment of primary CNS lymphoma with methotrexate and deferred radiotherapy: a report of NABTT 96-07. *J Clin Oncol* 2003; 21(6):1044–1049.

34. Rubenstein JL, Hsi ED, Johnson JL, et al. Intensive chemotherapy and immunotherapy in patients with newly diagnosed primary CNS lymphoma: CALGB 50202 (Alliance 50202). *J Clin Oncol* 2013; 31(25):3061–3068.

35. Gerstner ER, Carson KA, Grossman SA, et al. Long-term outcome in PCNSL patients treated with high-dose methotrexate and deferred radiation. *Neurology* 2008; 70(5):401–402.

36. Hoang-Xuan K, Taillandier L, Chinot O, et al. Chemotherapy alone as initial treatment for primary CNS lymphoma in patients older than 60 years: a multicenter phase II study (26952) of the European Organization for Research and Treatment of Cancer Brain Tumor Group. *J Clin Oncol* 2003; 21(14):2726–2731.

37. Pels H, Schmidt-Wolf IG, Glasmacher A, et al. Primary central nervous system lymphoma: results of a pilot and phase II study of systemic and intraventricular chemotherapy with deferred radiotherapy. *J Clin Oncol* 2003; 21(24):4489–4495.

38. Reni M, Mason W, Zaja F, et al. Salvage chemotherapy with temozolomide in primary CNS lymphomas: preliminary results of a phase II trial. *Eur J Cancer* 2004; 40(11):1682–1688.

39. Batchelor TT, Grossman SA, Mikkelsen T, et al. Rituximab monotherapy for patients with recurrent primary CNS lymphoma. *Neurology* 2011; 76(10):929–930.

40. Ferreri AJ, Cwynarski K, Pulczynski E, et al. Addition of thiotepa and rituximab to antimetabolites significantly improves outcome in primary CNS lymphoma: first randomization of the IELSG32 trial. *Hematol Oncol* 2015; 33:103 (Abstr 9).

41. Poortmans PM, Kluin-Nelemans HC, Haaxma-Reiche H, et al. High-dose methotrexate-based chemotherapy followed by consolidating radiotherapy in non-AIDS-related primary central nervous system lymphoma: European Organization for Research and Treatment of Cancer Lymphoma Group Phase II Trial 20962. *J Clin Oncol* 2003; 21(24):4483–4488.

42. Rubenstein JL, Combs D, Rosenberg J, et al. Rituximab therapy for CNS lymphomas: targeting the leptomeningeal compartment. *Blood* 2003; 101(2):466–468.

43. Holdhoff M, Ambady P, Abdelaziz A, et al. High-dose methotrexate with or without rituximab in newly diagnosed primary CNS lymphoma. *Neurology* 2014; 83(3):235–239.

44. Thiel E, Korfel A, Martus P, et al. High-dose methotrexate with or without whole brain radiotherapy for primary CNS lymphoma (G-PCNSL-SG-1): a phase 3, randomised, non-inferiority trial. *Lancet Oncol* 2010; 11(11):1036–1047.

45. Korfel A, Thiel E, Martus P, et al. Randomized phase III study of whole-brain radiotherapy for primary CNS lymphoma. *Neurology* 2015; 84(12):1242–1248.

46. Illerhaus G, Fritsch K, Egerer G, et al. Sequential high dose immuno-chemotherapy followed by autologous peripheral blood stem cell transplantation for patients with untreated primary central nervous system lymphoma—a multicentre study by the Collaborative PCNSL Study Group Freiburg. *Blood* 2012, 120: abst 302.

47. Khan RB, Shi W, Thaler HT, et al. Is intrathecal methotrexate necessary in the treatment of primary CNS lymphoma? *J Neurooncol* 2002; 58(2):175–178.

48. Sierra Del Rio M, Ricard D, Houillier C, et al. Prophylactic intrathecal chemotherapy in primary CNS lymphoma. *J Neurooncol* 2012; 106(1):143–146.

49. Nayak L, Batchelor TT. Recent advances in treatment of primary central nervous system lymphoma. *Curr Treat Options Oncol* 2013; 14(4):539–552.

50. Jahnke K, Korfel A, Martus P, et al. High-dose methotrexate toxicity in elderly patients with primary central nervous system lymphoma. *Ann Oncol* 2005; 16(3):445–449.

51. Zhu JJ, Gerstner ER, Engler DA, et al. High-dose methotrexate for elderly patients with primary CNS lymphoma. *Neuro Oncol* 2009; 11(2):211–215.

52. Kasenda B, Ferreri AJ, Marturano E, et al. First-line treatment and outcome of elderly patients with primary central nervous system lymphoma (PCNSL)-a systematic review and individual patient data meta-analysis. *Ann Oncol* 2015; 26(7):1305–1313.

53. Omuro A, Chinot O, Taillandier L, et al. Multicenter randomized phase II trial of methotrexate (MTX) and temozolomide (TMZ) versus MTX, procarbazine, vincristine, and cytarabine for primary CNS lymphoma (PCNSL) in the elderly: An Anocef and Goelams Intergroup study. *J Clin Oncol* 2013; 31(Suppl): abstr 2032.

54. Kasenda B, Fritsch K, Schorb E, et al. Rituximab, methotrexate, procarbazine and lomustine for elderly primary CNS lymphoma patients—the PRIMAIN study by the German Cooperative PCNSL Group. *Hematol Oncol* 2015; 33:173 (Abstr 134).

55. Fritsch K, Kasenda B, Hader C, et al. Immunochemotherapy with rituximab, methotrexate, procarbazine, and lomustine for primary CNS lymphoma (PCNSL) in the elderly. *Ann Oncol* 2011; 22(9):2080–2085.

56. Jahnke K, Thiel E, Martus P, et al. Relapse of primary central nervous system lymphoma: clinical features, outcome and prognostic factors. *J Neurooncol* 2006; 80(2):159–165.

57. Langner-Lemercier S, Houillier C, Soussain C, et al. Management of outcome of primary CNS lymphoma at first relapse/progression: analysis of 256 patients from the French LOC Network. *Hematol Oncol* 2015; 33:173–174 (Abstr 135).

58. Wang N, Gill C, Betensky RA, et al. Relapse patterns in primary CNS diffuse large B-cell lymphoma. *Neurology* 2015; 84(14S):P3.1437.

59. Plotkin SR, Betensky RA, Hochberg FH, et al. Treatment of relapsed central nervous system lymphoma with high-dose methotrexate. *Clin Cancer Res* 2004; 10(17):5643–5646.

60. Soussain C, Hoang-Xuan K, Taillandier L, et al. Intensive chemotherapy followed by hematopoietic stem-cell rescue for refractory and recurrent primary CNS and intraocular lymphoma: Societe Francaise de Greffe de Moelle Osseuse-Therapie Cellulaire. *J Clin Oncol* 2008; 26(15):2512–2518.

61. Kasenda B, Schorb E, Fritsch K, et al. Primary CNS lymphoma—radiation-free salvage therapy by second autologous stem cell transplantation. *Biol Blood Marrow Transplant* 2011; 17(2):281–283.

62. Nguyen PL, Chakravarti A, Finkelstein DM, et al. Results of whole-brain radiation as salvage of methotrexate failure for immunocompetent patients with primary CNS lymphoma. *J Clin Oncol* 2005; 23(7):1507–1513.

63. Hottinger AF, DeAngelis LM, Yahalom J, et al. Salvage whole brain radiotherapy for recurrent or refractory primary CNS lymphoma. *Neurology* 2007; 69(11):1178–1182.

64. Dunleavey K, Lai C, Roschewski, et al. Phase I/II study of TEDDI-R with Ibrutinib in untreated and relapsed/refractory primary CNS lymphoma. *Hematol Oncol* 2015; 33:174–175 (Abstr 136).

65. Houillier C, Choquet S, Touitou V, et al. Lenalidomide monotherapy as salvage treatment for recurrent primary CNS lymphoma. *Neurology* 2015; 84(3):325–326.

66. Rubenstein JL, Formaker P, Wang X, et al. Lenalidomide is highly active in recurrent CNS lymphomas: phase I investigation of lenalidomide plus rituximab and outcomes of lenalidomide as maintenance monotherapy. *Hematol Oncol* 2015; 33:175 (Abstr 137).

67. Lai R, Abrey LE, Rosenblum MK, et al. Treatment-induced leukoencephalopathy in primary CNS lymphoma: a clinical and autopsy study. *Neurology* 2004; 62(3):451–456.

68. Monje ML, Vogel H, Masek M, et al. Impaired human hippocampal neurogenesis after treatment for central nervous system malignancies. *Ann Neurol* 2007; 62(5):515–520.

69. Abla O, Weitzman S, Blay JY, et al. Primary CNS lymphoma in children and adolescents: a descriptive analysis from the International Primary CNS Lymphoma Collaborative Group (IPCG). *Clin Cancer Res* 2011; 17(2):346–352.

70. Chan CC, Rubenstein JL, Coupland SE, et al. Primary vitreoretinal lymphoma: a report from an International Primary Central Nervous System Lymphoma Collaborative Group symposium. *Oncologist* 2011; 16(11):1589–1599.

71. Batchelor TT, Kolak G, Ciordia R, et al. High-dose methotrexate for intraocular lymphoma. *Clin Cancer Res* 2003; 9(2):711–715.

72. Grimm SA, McCannel CA, Omuro AM, et al. Primary CNS lymphoma with intraocular involvement: International PCNSL Collaborative Group Report. *Neurology* 2008; 71(17):1355–1360.

73. Taylor JW, Flanagan EP, O'Neill BP, et al. Primary leptomeningeal lymphoma: International Primary CNS Lymphoma Collaborative Group report. *Neurology* 2013; 81(19):1690–1696.

74. Lachance DH, O'Neill BP, Macdonald DR, et al. Primary leptomeningeal lymphoma: report of 9 cases, diagnosis with immunocytochemical analysis, and review of the literature. *Neurology* 1991; 41(1):95–100.

75. Flanagan EP, O'Neill BP, Porter AB, et al. Primary intramedullary spinal cord lymphoma. *Neurology* 2011; 77(8):784–791.

76. Cruto C, Taipa R, Monteiro C, et al. Multiple cerebral infarcts and intravascular central nervous system lymphoma: a rare but potentially treatable association. *J Neurol Sci* 2013; 325(1–2):183–185.

77. Kebir S, Kuchelmeister K, Niehusmann P, et al. Intravascular CNS lymphoma: Successful therapy using high-dose methotrexate-based polychemotherapy. *Exp Hematol Oncol* 2012; 1(1):37.

78. Gonzalez-Darder JM, Vera-Roman JM, Pesudo-Martinez JV, et al. Tumoral presentation of primary central nervous system

lymphomatoid granulomatosis. *Acta Neurochir (Wien)* 2011; 153(10):1963–1970.

79. Lucantoni C, De Bonis P, Doglietto F, et al. Primary cerebral lymphomatoid granulomatosis: report of four cases and literature review. *J Neurooncol* 2009; 94(2):235–242.

80. Gonzalez-Aguilar A, Soto-Hernandez JL. The management of primary central nervous system lymphoma related to AIDS in the HAART era. *Curr Opin Oncol* 2011; 23(6):648–653.

81. Evens AM, Choquet S, Kroll-Desrosiers AR, et al. Primary CNS posttransplant lymphoproliferative disease (PTLD): an international report of 84 cases in the modern era. *Am J Transplant* 2013; 13(6):1512–1522.

82. Shenkier TN, Blay JY, O'Neill BP, et al. Primary CNS lymphoma of T-cell origin: a descriptive analysis from the international primary CNS lymphoma collaborative group. *J Clin Oncol* 2005; 23(10):2233–2239.

83. Menon MP, Nicolae A, Meeker H, et al. Primary CNS T-cell lymphomas: a clinical, morphologic, immunophenotypic, and molecular analysis. *Am J Surg Pathol* 2015; 39(12):1719–1729.

84. Liao B, Kamiya-Matsuoka C, Gong Y, et al. Primary natural killer/T-cell lymphoma presenting as leptomeningeal disease. *J Neurol Sci* 2014; 343(1–2):46–50.

85. Prajapati HJ, Vincentelli C, Hwang SN, et al. Primary CNS natural killer/T-cell lymphoma of the nasal type presenting in a woman: case report and review of the literature. *J Clin Oncol* 2014; 32(8):e26–e29.

86. Jahnke K, Korfel A, O'Neill BP, et al. International study on low-grade primary central nervous system lymphoma. *Ann Neurol* 2006; 59(5):755–762.

87. Beltran BE, Kuritzky B, Quinones P, et al. Extranodal marginal zone lymphoma of the cranial dura mater: report of three cases and systematic review of the literature. *Leuk Lymphoma* 2013; 54(10):2306–2309.

88. Sebastian C, Vela AC, Figueroa R, et al. Primary intracranial mucosa-associated lymphoid tissue lymphoma. A report of two cases and literature review. *Neuroradiol J* 2014; 27(4):425–430.

89. Kresak JL, Nguyen J, Wong K, et al. Primary Hodgkin lymphoma of the central nervous system: two case reports and review of the literature. *Neuropathology* 2013; 33(6):658–662.

90. Gerstner ER, Abrey LE, Schiff D, et al. CNS Hodgkin lymphoma. *Blood* 2008; 112(5):1658–1661.

91. NCCN Clinical Practice Guidelines in Oncology (NCCN Guidelines®). *National Comprehensive Cancer Network. Central Nervous System Cancers.* Version 1.2015. 2015. http://www.nccn.org/professionals/physician_gls/f_guidelines.asp#cns.

92. Hoang-Xuan K, Bessell E, Bromberg J, et al. Diagnosis and treatment of primary CNS lymphoma in immunocompetent patients: guidelines from the European Association for Neuro-Oncology. *Lancet Oncol* 2015; 16(7):e322–e332.

93. Vaiselbuh SR, Bryceson YT, Allen CE, et al. Updates on histiocytic disorders. *Pediatr Blood Cancer* 2014; 61(7):1329–1335.

94. Berres ML, Lim KP, Peters T, et al. BRAF-V600E expression in precursor versus differentiated dendritic cells defines clinically distinct LCH risk groups. *J Exp Med* 2015; 212(2):281.

95. Abla O, Egeler RM, Weitzman S. Langerhans cell histiocytosis: current concepts and treatments. *Cancer Treat Rev* 2010; 36(4):354–359.

96. Arico M, Girschikofsky M, Genereau T, et al. Langerhans cell histiocytosis in adults. Report from the International Registry of the Histiocyte Society. *Eur J Cancer* 2003; 39(16):2341–2348.

97. Gadner H, Minkov M, Grois N, et al. Therapy prolongation improves outcome in multisystem Langerhans cell histiocytosis. *Blood* 2013; 121(25):5006–5014.

98. Grois N, Potschger U, Prosch H, et al. Risk factors for diabetes insipidus in Langerhans cell histiocytosis. *Pediatr Blood Cancer* 2006; 46(2):228–233.

99. Donadieu J, Rolon MA, Thomas C, et al. Endocrine involvement in pediatric-onset Langerhans' cell histiocytosis: a population-based study. *J Pediatr* 2004; 144(3):344–350.

100. Allen CE, Ladisch S, McClain KL. How I treat Langerhans cell histiocytosis. *Blood* 2015; 126(1):26–35.

101. Egeler RM, de Kraker J, Voute PA. Cytosine-arabinoside, vincristine, and prednisolone in the treatment of children with disseminated Langerhans cell histiocytosis with organ dysfunction: experience at a single institution. *Med Pediatr Oncol* 1993; 21(4):265–270.

102. Simko SJ, Tran HD, Jones J, et al. Clofarabine salvage therapy in refractory multifocal histiocytic disorders, including Langerhans cell histiocytosis, juvenile xanthogranuloma and Rosai-Dorfman disease. *Pediatr Blood Cancer* 2014; 61(3):479–487.

103. Barthez MA, Araujo E, Donadieu J. Langerhans cell histiocytosis and the central nervous system in childhood: evolution and prognostic factors. Results of a collaborative study. *J Child Neurol* 2000; 15(3):150–156.

104. Grois N, Prayer D, Prosch H, et al. Course and clinical impact of magnetic resonance imaging findings in diabetes insipidus associated with Langerhans cell histiocytosis. *Pediatr Blood Cancer* 2004; 43(1):59–65.

105. Idbaih A, Donadieu J, Barthez MA, et al. Retinoic acid therapy in 'degenerative-like' neuro-Langerhans cell histiocytosis: a prospective pilot study. *Pediatr Blood Cancer* 2004; 43(1):55–58.

106. Imashuku S. High dose immunoglobulin (IVIG) may reduce the incidence of Langerhans cell histiocytosis (LCH)-associated central nervous system involvement. *CNS Neurol Disord Drug Targets* 2009; 8(5):380–386.

107. Allen CE, Flores R, Rauch R, et al. Neurodegenerative central nervous system Langerhans cell histiocytosis and coincident hydrocephalus treated with vincristine/cytosine arabinoside. *Pediatr Blood Cancer* 2010; 54(3):416–423.

108. Donadieu J, Armari-Alla C, Templier I, et al. First use of vemurafenib in children LCH with neurodegenerative LCH. In: *30th Annual Histiocyte Society Meeting, Toronto, Canada;* October 28–30 2014; 35 (Abstr 3).

109. Dhall G, Finlay JL, Dunkel IJ, et al. Analysis of outcome for patients with mass lesions of the central nervous system due to Langerhans cell histiocytosis treated with 2-chlorodeoxyadenosine. *Pediatr Blood Cancer* 2008; 50(1):72–79.

110. Ng Wing Tin S, Martin-Duverneuil N, Idbaih A, et al. Efficacy of vinblastine in central nervous system Langerhans cell histiocytosis: a nationwide retrospective study. *Orphanet J Rare Dis* 2011; 6:83.

111. Chester W. Über Lipoidgranulomatose. *Virchows Arch Pathol Anat* 1930; 279(2):561–602.

112. Veyssier-Belot C, Cacoub P, Caparros-Lefebvre D, et al. Erdheim-Chester disease. Clinical and radiologic characteristics of 59 cases. *Medicine (Baltimore)* 1996; 75(3):157–169.

113. Diamond EL, Dagna L, Hyman DM, et al. Consensus guidelines for the diagnosis and clinical management of Erdheim-Chester disease. *Blood* 2014; 124(4):483–492.

114. Weitzman S, Jaffe R. Uncommon histiocytic disorders: the non-Langerhans cell histiocytoses. *Pediatr Blood Cancer* 2005; 45(3):256–264.

115. Emile JF, Diamond EL, Helias-Rodzewicz Z, et al. Recurrent RAS and PIK3CA mutations in Erdheim-Chester disease. *Blood* 2014; 124(19):3016–3019.

116. Hervier B, Haroche J, Arnaud L, et al. Association of both Langerhans cell histiocytosis and Erdheim-Chester disease linked to the BRAFV600E mutation. *Blood* 2014; 124(7):1119–1126.

117. Braiteh F, Boxrud C, Esmaeli B, et al. Successful treatment of Erdheim-Chester disease, a non-Langerhans-cell histiocytosis, with interferon-alpha. *Blood* 2005; 106(9):2992–2994.

118. Haroche J, Amoura Z, Trad SG, et al. Variability in the efficacy of interferon-alpha in Erdheim-Chester disease by patient and site of involvement: results in eight patients. *Arthritis Rheum* 2006; 54(10):3330–3336.

119. Arnaud L, Hervier B, Neel A, et al. CNS involvement and treatment with interferon-alpha are independent prognostic factors in

Erdheim-Chester disease: a multicenter survival analysis of 53 patients. *Blood* 2011; 117(10):2778–2782.

120. Haroche J, Cohen-Aubart F, Emile JF, et al. Dramatic efficacy of vemurafenib in both multisystemic and refractory Erdheim-Chester disease and Langerhans cell histiocytosis harboring the BRAF V600E mutation. *Blood* 2013; 121(9):1495–1500.

121. Haroche J, Cohen-Aubart F, Emile JF, et al. Reproducible and sustained efficacy of targeted therapy with vemurafenib in patients with BRAF(V600E)-mutated Erdheim-Chester disease. *J Clin Oncol* 2015; 33(5):411–418.

122. Courcoul A, Vignot E, Chapurlat R. Successful treatment of Erdheim-Chester disease by interleukin-1 receptor antagonist protein. *Joint Bone Spine* 2014; 81(2):175–177.

123. Janku F, Amin HM, Yang D, et al. Response of histiocytoses to imatinib mesylate: fire to ashes. *J Clin Oncol* 2010; 28(31):e633–e636.

124. Myra C, Sloper L, Tighe PJ, et al. Treatment of Erdheim-Chester disease with cladribine: a rational approach. *Br J Ophthalmol* 2004; 88(6):844–847.

125. Rosai J, Dorfman RF. Sinus histiocytosis with massive lymphadenopathy. A newly recognized benign clinicopathological entity. *Arch Pathol* 1969; 87(1):63–70.

126. Foucar E, Rosai J, Dorfman R. Sinus histiocytosis with massive lymphadenopathy (Rosai-Dorfman disease): review of the entity. *Semin Diagn Pathol* 1990; 7(1):19–73.

127. Chakraborty R, Hampton OA, Shen X, et al. Mutually exclusive recurrent somatic mutations in MAP2K1 and BRAF support a central role for ERK activation in LCH pathogenesis. *Blood* 2014; 124(19):3007–3015.

128. Adeleye AO, Amir G, Fraifeld S, et al. Diagnosis and management of Rosai-Dorfman disease involving the central nervous system. *Neurol Res* 2010; 32(6):572–578.

129. Le Guenno G, Galicier L, Uro-Coste E, et al. Successful treatment with azathioprine of relapsing Rosai-Dorfman disease of the central nervous system. *J Neurosurg* 2012; 117(3):486–489.

130. Nalini A, Jitender S, Anantaram G, et al. Rosai Dorfman disease: case with extensive dural involvement and cerebrospinal fluid pleocytosis. *J Neurol Sci* 2012; 314(1–2):152–154.

131. Walker RN, Nickles TP, Lountzis NI, et al. Rosai-Dorfman disease with massive intracranial involvement: asymmetric response to conservative therapy. *J Neuroimaging* 2011; 21(2):194–196.

132. Zhu F, Zhang JT, Xing XW, et al. Rosai-Dorfman disease: a retrospective analysis of 13 cases. *Am J Med Sci* 2013; 345(3):200–210.

133. Konca C, Ozkurt ZN, Deger M, et al. Extranodal multifocal Rosai-Dorfman disease: response to 2-chlorodeoxyadenosine treatment. *Int J Hematol* 2009; 89(1):58–62.

134. Rivera D, Perez-Castillo M, Fernandez B, et al. Long-term follow-up in two cases of intracranial Rosai-Dorfman Disease complicated by incomplete resection and recurrence. *Surg Neurol Int* 2014; 5:30.

135. Petschner F, Walker UA, Schmitt-Graff A, et al. 'Catastrophic systemic lupus erythematosus' with Rosai-Dorfman sinus histiocytosis. Successful treatment with anti-CD20/rutuximab. *Dtsch Med Wochenschr* 2001; 126(37):998–1001.

136. Utikal J, Ugurel S, Kurzen H, et al. Imatinib as a treatment option for systemic non-Langerhans cell histiocytoses. *Arch Dermatol* 2007; 143(6):736–740.

137. Dehner LP. Juvenile xanthogranulomas in the first two decades of life: a clinicopathologic study of 174 cases with cutaneous and extracutaneous manifestations. *Am J Surg Pathol* 2003; 27(5):579–593.

138. Freyer DR, Kennedy R, Bostrom BC, et al. Juvenile xanthogranuloma: forms of systemic disease and their clinical implications. *J Pediatr* 1996; 129(2):227–237.

139. Orsey A, Paessler M, Lange BJ, et al. Central nervous system juvenile xanthogranuloma with malignant transformation. *Pediatr Blood Cancer* 2008; 50(4):927–930.

140. Rajendra B, Duncan A, Parslew R, et al. Successful treatment of central nervous system juvenile xanthogranulomatosis with cladribine. *Pediatr Blood Cancer* 2009; 52(3):413–415.

141. Auvin S, Cuvellier JC, Vinchon M, et al. Subdural effusion in a CNS involvement of systemic juvenile xanthogranuloma: a case report treated with vinblastin. *Brain Dev* 2008; 30(2):164–168.

142. Stover DG, Alapati S, Regueira O, et al. Treatment of juvenile xanthogranuloma. *Pediatr Blood Cancer* 2008; 51(1):130–133.

143. Dalia S, Shao H, Sagatys E, et al. Dendritic cell and histiocytic neoplasms: biology, diagnosis, and treatment. *Cancer Control* 2014; 21(4):290–300.

144. Go H, Jeon YK, Huh J, et al. Frequent detection of BRAF(V600E) mutations in histiocytic and dendritic cell neoplasms. *Histopathology* 2014; 65(2):261–272.

145. So H, Kim SA, Yoon DH, et al. Primary histiocytic sarcoma of the central nervous system. *Cancer Res Treat* 2015; 47(2):322–328.

146. Bell SL, Hanzely Z, Alakandy LM, et al. Primary meningeal histiocytic sarcoma: a report of two unusual cases. *Neuropathol Appl Neurobiol* 2012; 38(1):111–114.

147. Feldman AL, Arber DA, Pittaluga S, et al. Clonally related follicular lymphomas and histiocytic/dendritic cell sarcomas: evidence for transdifferentiation of the follicular lymphoma clone. *Blood* 2008; 111(12):5433–5439.

148. Abidi MH, Tove I, Ibrahim RB, et al. Thalidomide for the treatment of histiocytic sarcoma after hematopoietic stem cell transplant. *Am J Hematol* 2007; 82(10):932–933.

149. Bailey KM, Castle VP, Hummel JM, et al. Thalidomide therapy for aggressive histiocytic lesions in the pediatric population. *J Pediatr Hematol Oncol* 2012; 34(6):480–483.

150. Shukla N, Kobos R, Renaud T, et al. Successful treatment of refractory metastatic histiocytic sarcoma with alemtuzumab. *Cancer* 2012; 118(15):3719–3724.

151. Uchida K, Kobayashi S, Inukai T, et al. Langerhans cell sarcoma emanating from the upper arm skin: successful treatment by MAID regimen. *J Orthop Sci* 2008; 13(1):89–93.

152. Mainardi C, D'Amore ES, Pillon M, et al. A case of resistant pediatric histiocytic sarcoma successfully treated with chemo-radiotherapy and autologous peripheral blood stem cell transplant. *Leuk Lymphoma* 2011; 52(7):1367–1371.

153. Idbaih A, Mokhtari K, Emile JF, et al. Dramatic response of a BRAF V600E-mutated primary CNS histiocytic sarcoma to vemurafenib. *Neurology* 2014; 83(16):1478–1480.

CHAPTER 14

Germ cell tumours

Claire Alapetite, Takaaki Yanagisawa, and Ryo Nishikawa

Definition (histology)

Histological classification of intracranial germ cell tumours (iGCTs) consists of germinoma, mature and immature teratoma, teratoma with malignant transformation, yolk sac tumour, embryonal carcinoma, choriocarcinoma (1), and mixed tumours of these components. A clinically practical classification into two subgroups, that is, germinoma and non-germinomatous GCTs (NGGCTs), is widely accepted. However, there are controversies: for example, immature teratoma and choriocarcinoma are both included in the NGGCT category, but the strength of treatment for those tumours should be different (2). There used to be another classification: secreting GCTs and non-secreting GCTs. However, not only germinomas but also most teratomas and some of the embryonal carcinomas would be categorized as non-secreting, which would not be reasonable from the therapeutic view. A Japanese group proposes a three-group classification based on prognosis: the good prognosis group consists of germinoma and mature teratoma; the intermediate prognosis group consists of immature teratoma, teratoma with malignant transformation, and mixed tumours of mainly germinoma and/or teratomatous components; and the poor prognosis group consists of choriocarcinoma, yolk sac tumour, embryonal carcinoma, and mixed tumours of mainly those malignant components (2).

Epidemiology

Geographic incidence has been considered to vary substantially. In far-east Asia, iGCT accounted for 2–3% of primary brain tumours—2.3% in Japan (3) and 1.8% in Korea (4)—while in the United States, iGCT accounts for 0.4% of primary brain tumours (5). A population-based study in a district of Japan reported the age-adjusted annual incidence of iGCTs as 0.62 per 100,000 (male (M) = 0.93, female (F) = 0.09) (6), while an age-adjusted incidence of 0.10 per 100,000 person-years (M = 0.14, F = 0.06) has been reported in the United States (5). However, the age-adjusted annual incidence of iGCT calculated from the Japan Cancer Surveillance Research Group in 14 population-based registries in Japan recently showed the annual incidence of 0.096 per 100,000 (M = 0.143, F = 0.046) (7). This group also reported the incidence of iGCTs in a district of Japan decreased over time, especially in males (8). Male dominance in pineal GCTs and histological distribution (about 40% are germinoma) are similar in the United States and Japan (7).

Molecular pathogenesis

The genetics of GCTs have been largely a mystery for years. The hypothesis that iGCTs represent the neoplastic offspring of primordial germ cells was proposed and has been discussed (1, 9). Isochromosome 12p and gain of chromosome X have been the features of GCTs. Recent developments in molecular genetics elucidated whole-genome characteristics of many brain tumours such as medulloblastoma and ependymoma, and iGCTs (10, 11).

Clinical presentation

The three major locations of iGCTs are the pineal region, neurohypophysis, and basal ganglia. Tumours of the pineal region often obstruct the aqueduct, resulting in obstructive hydrocephalus with intracranial hypertension. When lesions compress the tectal plate, a characteristic paralysis of upward gaze and convergence known as Parinaud syndrome occurs. Neurohypophyseal GCTs typically impinge on the optic chiasm causing bitemporal hemianopsia. They also damage the hypothalamo–hypophyseal axis as evidenced by the occurrence of diabetes insipidus that sometimes precedes the finding of tumours by years. These tumours used to be called suprasellar GCTs. Careful observation of their magnetic resonance imaging (MRI) features revealed those tumours would be better described as neurohypophyseal GCTs (12). Basal ganglia GCTs typically show an enhanced mass in and around the basal ganglia causing hemiparesis. However, their early feature is atrophy of the basal ganglia that is recognizable before development of hemiparesis (13).

Imaging, biomarkers, and endoscopic biopsies

Magnetic resonance imaging is of diagnostic importance. However, MRI does not distinguish histological subtypes of iGCT in the pineal region (14). Human chorionic gonadotropin (HCG) or HCG-beta would be a marker for choriocarcinoma. If serum HCG is higher than 2000 mIU/mL, the histology of the tumour is most likely choriocarcinoma (2). If serum alpha-fetoprotein (AFP) is higher than 2000 ng/mL, the histology of the tumour is most likely yolk sac tumour (2). However, moderately elevated HCG would not distinguish highly malignant choriocarcinomas that require maximum strength of treatment including whole neuroaxis irradiation and intermediate prognostic mixed tumours of immature teratoma and choriocarinoma that would not need whole neuroaxis irradiation but whole ventricle + local boost radiotherapy (details will be discussed later). Furthermore, most germinomas secrete HCG that is detectable by mRNA analyses (15). Therefore biomarkers would not be definitely diagnostic.

Recent surgical innovations, especially endoscopic techniques, have been integrated into the surgical treatment of iGCTs. The major advantage is performing tumour biopsy and third ventriculostomy, and CSF sampling for biomarkers if necessary, as a one-time procedure with minimum morbidity (16). On the other hand, the possible disadvantage would be diagnostic accuracy with endoscopic tumour biopsy, which should be looked at retrospectively and prospectively.

Treatment

Surgery

It is widely accepted that biopsy is enough for germinoma. This notion is based on a small series of 29 germinomas; biopsy samples were obtained in 16 patients, partial resection was attained in 5, and gross total resection was achieved in 8. After postoperative radiotherapy with or without chemotherapy, complete remission was achieved in all 29 patients, and the overall tumour-free survival rate was 100% at a median follow-up period of 42 months (17). This is a reasonable strategy as the response rate of postoperative chemoradiotherapy is quite effective for germinomas. However, there would be a rationale for aggressive resection of germinoma for the purpose of increasing diagnostic accuracy. Many tumours classified as germinomas have been shown to contain non-germinomatous elements upon further evaluation. So, the question remains if a more aggressive resection of germinomas would improve outcome from the standpoint of more accurate diagnostic interpretation and/or reduced tumour burden.

Then, the next question would be if aggressive resection for the intermediate prognostic group of iGCTs, such as immature teratoma or mixed tumours of immature teratoma and germinoma, still needs to be performed. Aggressive resection would accompany certain surgical morbidity. The experience in systemic GCTs suggested that a mature teratoma that became evident after initial treatment with chemotherapy or radiotherapy would be a good candidate for delayed or second-look surgery. A number of published reports substantiate the approach of using second-look surgery (18–20). The role of resection in iGCTs warrants further investigation.

Radiotherapy

Children and young adults receive similar radiation treatment (RT) although series report mainly the paediatric age group. Recent and current studies include patients either until 21 years old (COG) or at all ages (International Society of Paediatric Oncology (SIOP)).

Localized, 'pure germinoma' with 'low' level of HCG (pineal, neurohypophyseal, and bifocal)

Radiation treatment-only early approaches, using craniospinal irradiation (CSI) at 36 Gy, with tumour bed (TB) boost at a total dose of 50 Gy, gave excellent results (relapse-free survival >90%), which emphasized the high radiosensitivity of CNS germinoma tumours. This treatment was recognized as the gold standard until the early 1990S (21, 22).

The potential for adverse late effects on neurocognition and health-related quality of life of CSI RT led to general attempts to lower RT weight, starting in the 1990. Radiation treatment dose de-escalation was evaluated in RT approaches using CSI and TB boost. The German MAKEI successive studies concluded that respectively 30 Gy CSI and 45 Gy to the TB were safe (23). Hardenbergh et al. reported in 1997 a low-dose RT group receiving 18.8–25.5 Gy CSI and 44.5–49.5 Gy to the TB (24), similar to Merchant et al. (25). De-escalation over time was also reported by Cho et al. (26) and 19.5 Gy CSI and 39.3 to the TB were recommended. Concomitantly, RT to reduced volumes was explored: to whole brain or to whole ventricle (WV), in mono- or multicentric studies although at relatively high doses, around 50 Gy (27–29).

In parallel, chemotherapy-only approaches were initiated. In a multi-institutional trial, including 45 patients, it proved to be inferior to RT-based approaches. Indeed unacceptably high recurrence rates were shown with event-free survival (EFS) at 6 years of 45.6%, assessing that CNS germinoma tumours were chemosensitive but not chemo-curable (30–32). This confirmed the essential role of RT for germinoma disease control.

In the 1990S, clinical research dedicated to CNS GCT was developed, and multicentre/international trials were launched, in histologically documented germinoma, potentially allowing for larger numbers to be analysed in this rare condition. The general tendency was to deliver primary chemotherapy aiming at reducing both RT volume and RT dose: the first multi-institutional clinical study in Japan was in 1995; the French SFOP (Société Française d'Oncologie Pédiatrique/French Pediatric Oncology Society) was in 1990, followed by the European SIOP study (1996); the first multimodality clinical trials in North America were POG 9530 (1999) followed by the Beth Israel consortium and COG ACNS 0232 (2002).

Results of the Japanese study with primary chemotherapy (CARE-VP) followed by focal TB RT initially and ventricular RT after 1999 for all germinoma and HCG germinoma, at 24 Gy, without boost to the primary site, were recently updated and showed a 10-year progression-free survival (PFS) and overall survival (OS) of 84.7% and 97.5% respectively, in 115 germinoma patients. Thirty-five additional cases with high HCG secretion resulted in a similar outcome (33).

The European SIOP-96 study results were published in 2013 (34). This trial compared in a prospective, non-randomized trial, CSI at 24 Gy followed by a TB boost up to 40 Gy (option A, 125 patients) and a combined approach with primary chemotherapy followed by focal TB RT at 40 Gy (option B, 65 patients). While OS was similar in the two treatment arms, PFS was decreased in option B: 88% versus 97%.

North American first trials were based on adaptation of RT dose and volume to response to chemotherapy. Results of the POG trial have been reported on 12 germinoma patients (35). The COG ACNS 0232 trial, that followed the Beth Israel Germinoma consortium, unfortunately had low accrual. This phase III study, in histologically confirmed germinoma, was aimed at comparing standard RT only (WV RT 24 Gy, with a boost up to 45 Gy to the primary tumour) to chemotherapy followed by a response-based, reduced RT. Patients with a complete response (CR) received only involved-field TB RT at 30 Gy (36).

Relapses were reviewed in the French SFOP (Société Française d'Oncologie Pédiatrique/French Pediatric Oncology Society) series first reported in 2002 and subsequent SIOP-96 study, as well as in the interim analysis of the Japanese study in 1999, that showed after combined approaches with RT volume limited to the TB, a relatively high rate of relapses at 10 years: 27% in Japan (in patients who did not received the planned ventricular RT), 17% in France, and for the SIOP-96 study 11% at 5 years. A characteristic, subependymal ventricular pattern of relapses was observed with no or very few recurrences away from the ventricular system (37, 38). These relapses occurred mainly out of RT fields or at margins. SIOP-96 analysis also underlined that those patients who did not have complete initial work-up (extension or markers) were more susceptible to recurrence when treated according to the combined option with RT volume limited to the TB. Consequently that led, in combined approaches, to enlargement of RT fields to encompass the ventricular system including the fourth ventricle (Europe) or not (Japan). Other groups confirmed this pattern and emphasized the very low incidence of relapses in the spinal compartment (39–47).

Single institutions also have adopted primary chemotherapy followed by ventricular RT, such as the Los Angeles Children's Hospital group in the germinoma series from 2003 to 2008 using chemotherapy followed by WV RT at 21.4–24 Gy and simultaneous integrated TB boost up to 30 Gy with at 7 years PFS of 91.5% and OS of 96.5% (48, 49).

After reduced RT dose/volume, relapses appear to be salvageable including a re-irradiation component (33, 37, 50). This has led to more convergence in the volume of choice for radiation treatment in the current generation of protocols used across the world, with CSI no longer being prescribed for localized germinoma provided that the initial work-up is complete, and the whole ventricular system is being recognized as the new reference for RT-target volume (second multi-institutional clinical study in Japan (33), SIOP CNS GCT 2 (49), COG ACNS 1123 (52)). Total dose to the ventricles and/or to the primary site vary according to studies and most frequently are adapted to the response of the tumour to primary chemotherapy; WV irradiation doses for good responders of 18 Gy (COG) or of 24 Gy (Japan, SIOP); and, in non-responders, of 24 Gy for all studies. Total dose to the TB: in good responders 24 Gy (Japan, SIOP) or 30 Gy (COG), and, in non-responders of 24 Gy (Japan), 36 Gy (COG), or 40 Gy (SIOP).

Of note, high radiosensitivity with rapid kinetics of response to ionizing radiation has allowed prescribing a lower dose per fraction (1.5 Gy/fraction COG, 1.6 Gy/fraction SIOP) with the aim of improving normal brain parenchyma tolerance (SIOP studies). Future analysis of the ongoing multicentre/international studies will help in determining the minimal necessary RT dose/volume in combination with chemotherapy.

Whether chemotherapy followed by focal TB RT only might still be an option in selected cases for younger patients remains to be addressed with the help of additional prognostic factors (53). Radiotherapy only might be a challenging option as discussed by Rogers et al. (43), and by Yen et al. (53), with the minimal relevant volume being the ventricles (including the primary sites areas) and minimal dose to be determined.

A specific pattern of relapse for a basal ganglia primary site, suggests a requirement for whole-brain irradiation in this peculiar site (33).

The radiation oncologist community currently investigates recent techniques that offer potential for optimization of the dose distribution with the aim of maximizing sparing of normal brain. These include both X-ray delivery techniques: intensity-modulated RT

(IMRT) (54, 55), tomotherapy, and volumetric modulated arc therapy (VMAT) (56); and proton beam delivery techniques (57): conformal PT, intensity-modulated PT (IMPT) (37, 49, communication at the 52nd Particle Therapy Cooperative Group meeting (PTCOG) and SIOP 2013). Indeed, WV represents a large and complex volume and normal brain sparing might be best optimized using the unique dose distribution of proton beams with finite range, resulting in no exposure of normal tissues down to the target volume.

Technical recommendations including delineation of target volume, dedicated workshops, and prospective RT-quality control as part of the trials are necessary in multicentre studies and will help to optimize/homogenize radiotherapy practice, and to minimize the risk of relapse in the distal parts of the horns of the ventricular system. Prospective evaluation of neurocognitive outcome and health-related quality of life is part of all new protocols and will help in determining the best possible approach for optimized therapeutic index.

'Disseminated' germinoma, 'low' level of HCG

Craniospinal irradiation is the common practice. Chemotherapy may not be necessary as documented in the SIOP-96 which showed similar excellent survival in the CSI + boost RT-only arm in comparison to the combined arm with additional chemotherapy (34). However, definition of dissemination varies among countries, and results in different RT volumes delivery. Indeed, ventricular dissemination at diagnosis will receive ventricular irradiation in Japan, but CSI in Europe. Classification is an area of further consensus to be possibly obtained.

Non-germinoma germ cell tumours

Non-germinoma germ cell tumours (NGGCTs) are less radiosensitive than germinoma. A radiotherapy-alone procedure offers a 5- and 10-year survival of 36% (58). Alternatively, chemotherapy alone is associated with poor outcome and hardly salvageable relapses (30, 59, 60). This implies that, in association with the best possible surgical resection, both chemotherapy and radiotherapy are required in the management of NGGCT. Multimodality treatment is the rule. This heterogeneous histological group, including embryonal carcinoma, endodermal sinus tumour (yolk sac tumour), choriocarcinoma, malignant teratoma and mixed tumours, with sometimes germinoma components, is presently treated according to the same approach.

For localized NGGCTs, radiation treatment modalities are discussed, with no clear conclusions in early studies which delivered either focal TB RT or CSI with a TB boost, with a total dose to the primary site of 55 Gy (59, 61). Indeed reported relapses occurred mostly inside focal RT fields, less frequently at distance, with some in the ventricles.

Several multicentre trials opened in the 1990s: the first multi-institutional clinical study for CNS GCT (1995) in Japan treated this poor-prognosis group with postoperative, post-chemotherapy CSI at 30 Gy followed by a boost to ventricles and primary site up to 60 Gy with additional post-RT chemotherapy. Analysis at 10 years showed a PFS of 62.7% and an OS of 58.8%. Early progressions led to a modified approach during the study with concomitant chemo-radiotherapy (33).

The European SIOP 96 study (1996) was used in a combined setting, for localized disease, focal RT fields, limited to the TB at 54 Gy. PFS of patients with localized disease was 69% ± 4% (median follow-up 53 months), OS: 78% ± 4%; (median follow-up

41 months). A total of 41/146 relapses were observed, local (24), distant (5), combined (8), and gave arguments for continuing the focal RT approach. The analysis of the trial identified prognosis factors allowing for new risk stratification in the next current protocol with intensified chemotherapy in high-risk patients but no modification of the RT volume. The prognostic role of pre-RT residual disease was also underlined. Disseminated disease received craniospinal RT at 30 Gy, followed by a TB boost up to 54 Gy. Results are similar to localized disease. CSI does not prevent distant relapses (34).

In the POG 9530 protocol (1996), RT doses were adapted to the response to chemotherapy with non-responders receiving CSI 36 Gy followed by a TB boost up to 54 Gy, while responders had decreased doses: CSI 30.6 Gy and boost to the primary site 50 Gy. Results showed 11/14 were progression-free at 58 months (35)

The following COG ACNS 0122 trial (2004) in localized disease evaluated a chemotherapy response-adapted procedure, with or without second-look surgery and intensified chemotherapy. CSI appeared a safe conservative approach, and was homogeneously applied, with CSI at 36 Gy and TB boost up to 54 Gy. Results were introduced during the third international CNS GCT symposium (2013), by S. Goldman, and showed good local control (EFS 84%) and OS (93%) with optimal results in responders (49). All cases with dissemination received CSI.

It must be kept in mind that the threshold for the HCG marker for classification as non-germinoma GCT is subject to debate. In the European and North America trials, cut-off was 50 IU/L. This might jeopardize conclusions of trials and might have contributed to over-treating some patients. In the Japanese experience, higher levels (up to 200 IU/L) have not been associated with adverse outcome provided that RT volume encompasses the third and the lateral ventricles together with the primary site (38, 40).

Other groups used multimodal approaches including CSI (62). Current Japanese and European multicentre approaches have not introduced modifications in the radiation treatment phase. The Japanese second multi-institutional clinical study for CNS GCT phase II emphasizes strict application of concurrent chemotherapy and CSI plus TB boost up to 60 Gy (33); the SIOP CNS GCT II study is a risk-adapted chemotherapy regimen, and stays with focal TB RT up to 54 Gy in localized NGGCT (51). The current COG protocol ACNS 1123 replaces previous CSI by WV irradiation at slightly reduced doses (30.6 Gy) but stays with total dose to the TB of 54 Gy (63).

In terms of radiotherapy technical evolutions, again, best possible conformity is provided in order to optimize the radiotherapeutic index. Three-dimensional conformal planning is necessary for all X-ray and proton beam delivery. Proton therapy, due to the unique dose distribution, reduces by a factor of two the exposure of non-target normal tissues in comparison to standard radiotherapy and is an option especially in younger patients (57).

Central nervous system teratoma

Documented outcomes for CNS teratoma, in respect to radiation treatment have been seldom reported. In Japanese studies, and SIOP studies, mature teratoma when associated with a germinoma component is part of the good prognostic group. In this mixed germinoma-teratoma tumour, surgery is the treatment of choice for the teratoma component, non-sensitive to chemotherapy. After complete removal, radiation treatment delivery is performed

similarly to pure germinoma. If there is incomplete resection, the SIOP protocol recommends higher doses to the primary site (54 Gy).

Immature teratoma and teratoma with malignant transformation are part of the intermediate group in Japanese studies and receive chemotherapy followed by 30 Gy to the ventricles including the primary tumour site, followed by a boost up to 50 Gy to the TB. In the current SIOP study those cases will be documented, and treatment recommendations will be given on an individual basis—no overall therapeutic strategy is outlined in the protocol. The goal for the future is to accrue sufficient data on teratoma, including the impact of radiotherapy, in order to develop standardized guidelines for diagnosis and treatment of this subgroup of patients.

Chemotherapy

Investigation protocols for localized and metastatic testicular GCTs employing a synergetic combination of cytotoxic agents succeeded in durable remission rates of 60–90% with the following surgery and radiotherapy (64, 65). These included vinblastine, actinomycin-D, bleomycin, doxorubicin, cyclophosphamide, and cisplatin. Cisplatin-based combination chemotherapy has significantly enhanced the survival rates among patients with bulky and/or metastatic disease (64, 65). Carboplatin was later shown to have comparable efficacy to cisplatin with less ototoxicity and nephrotoxicity. Vinblastine was largely replaced by etoposide for synergism with cisplatin. Ifosfamide was found to be the third most active agent and was investigated initially as salvage therapy in patients with refractory disease (66). The most common combination regimens are PEB (cisplatin, etoposide, and bleomycin), PVB (cisplatin, vinblastine, and bleomycin), and JEB (carboplatin, etoposide, and bleomycin). Most of the agents could be delivered systemically to achieve concentration sufficient to cross the blood–brain barrier and led to the significant improvement of survival in cases of brain metastases in testicular GCTs. This experience enhanced the incorporation of chemotherapy among CNS GCTs at relapse and then at diagnosis during the 1980s (64, 65).

Chemotherapy-only approaches

The treatment of CNS GCTs remains controversial for their pathological heterogeneity and rarity. Germinomas are extremely radiosensitive and 5-year survival rates exceed 90% with radiotherapy alone. In contrast, malignant NGGCTs are less radiosensitive and previous studies reported 20–76% 5-year survival rates following radiotherapy, with or without chemotherapy. Radiotherapy can lead to several significant long-term adverse sequelae including endocrinopathy, neurocognitive impairment, and second malignancy. In addition, morbidities in GCT and NGGCT in developing countries are higher, due to the paucity of modern radiotherapy techniques. These together led to the seeking of alternative chemotherapy-based regimens. A number of investigators examined the novel strategy of chemotherapy alone in the management of GCT to avoid radiotherapy because of the relative ineffectiveness of irradiation alone on MMGCT and the well-known sensitivity of systemic GCT to chemotherapy.

The SFOP group treated 18 patients with GCT secreting either AFP or β-HCG by six cycles of a chemotherapy-only regimen of vinblastine, bleomycin, carboplatin, and etoposide, and/or ifosfamide with surgical resection of residual tumour after chemotherapy. Focal external beam radiotherapy (EBRT) was reserved for cases with viable residual tumour. Thirteen (72%) patients were treated only with chemotherapy and two were additionally treated with radiation. Twelve of the cases (67%) without radiotherapy developed recurrent tumour. Of 18 patients, 12 survived, but required EBRT. The investigators acknowledged that AFP- or β-HCG-secreting GCTs were not curable with conventional chemotherapy only and recommended that focal irradiation should be added to the treatment (60).

The First International Germ Cell Tumor Study investigated a chemotherapy-only regimen of carboplatin, etoposide, and bleomycin to avoid radiotherapy. In this study, germinoma patients with a complete remission (CR) after four cycles of induction chemotherapy were treated with two additional cycles. Those with less than a CR were treated with a chemotherapy regimen intensified by cyclophosphamide and following EBRT. This study accessioned 45 patients with germinoma and 26 with NGGCT, of whom 68 were considered evaluable. Thirty-nine of 68 (57%) patients achieved a CR within four cycles. Of 29 patients less than a CR, 16 achieved a CR with intensified chemotherapy or second surgery. Overall, 55 of the 71 patients (78%) achieved a CR without irradiation. The CR rate was 84% for germinoma and 78% for NGGCT. Twenty-eight of 71 patients (39%) remained disease free with a median follow-up period of 31 months. Twenty-eight patients (39%) showed tumour recurrence and seven patients showed disease progression on treatment. Ninety-three per cent of the recurrent disease underwent successful salvage therapy. Seven patients (10%) died of chemotherapy related toxicity. In conclusion, 41% of surviving patients and 50% of all patients were treated successfully with chemotherapy only without radiotherapy. The 2-year OS was 84% for germinoma and 62% for NGGCT (30). The Second International CNS Germ Cell Study Group employed two cycles of intensive cisplatin, etoposide, cyclophosphamide, and bleomycin (regimen A) to access the response in a group of 20 patients with NGGCT. According to this protocol, patients achieving a CR were treated with two additional cycles of carboplatin, etoposide, and bleomycin (regimen B). Those in CR after four cycles of treatment received one additional courses of regimen A and regimen B. Those not in CR underwent second-look surgery and/or EBRT. Ninety-four per cent of evaluable patients (n = 17) achieved CR or partial response after two cycles of regimen A. The median EFS for patients with CR was 62 months compared with 23 months mean EFS for those with a partial response (PR). Sixty-nine per cent of the evaluable patients developed progressive disease during or following chemotherapy. The 5-year EFS and OS for all the patients were 36% and 75%, respectively (31).

The other report from this study showed the results among 19 patients with germinoma, treated with the same protocol. All 11 patients with postoperative residual disease assessable for response achieved a CR. However, only 8 of 19 patients (42%) remained in remission, with a median follow-up of 6.5 years. Regarding the toxicities, three patients died of treatment-related toxicities and one patient died from an uncharacterized leucoencephalopathy. A toxic-death rate resulted in 19%. The 5-year EFS and 5-year OS were 47% and 68%, respectively. The investigators concluded the ineffectiveness of this approach for maintaining long-term disease control even among germinoma patients and were critical of the treatment-related toxicities (67).

The Third International CNS Germ Cell Tumor Study aimed to examine the efficacy of a risk-tailored chemotherapy-only regimen. Regimen A consisted of four to six cycles of carboplatin–etoposide alternating with cyclophosphamide–etoposide for low-risk localized germinoma with normal CSF and serum tumour markers. Regimen B consisted of four to six cycles of carboplatin–cyclophosphamide–etoposide for intermediate-risk germinoma with positive β-HCG and/or CSF β-HCG less than 50 mU/mL and high-risk, biopsy-proven non-germinomatous malignant element (MMGCT) or elevated serum/CSF AFP and/or β-HCG serum/CSF greater than 50mU/mL. Eleven patients were classified as low risk, 2 as intermediate risk and 12 as high risk. Seventeen (68%) patients achieved a CR after two courses and 19 (76%) after four courses of chemotherapy. Eleven patients relapsed at a mean of 30.8 months. The 6-year EFS and OS for 25 patients were 45.6% and 75.3%, respectively. The investigators concluded that standard treatment for CNS GCT continues to include radiotherapy either alone or combined with chemotherapy for pure germinoma and with chemotherapy with MMGCT (32).

All other studies also show that a chemotherapy-only strategy is associated with a significantly inferior outcome to radiotherapy-only treatment in spite of chemosensitivity in germinoma. They also show that very intensive chemotherapy does not contribute to the improvement of survival in NGGCT, without EBRT.

Chemotherapy in combined modality treatment

The addition of neoadjuvant chemotherapy has been attempted in order to reduce the dose and/or volume of radiotherapy in germinoma and to intensify the treatment for NGGCT in the multimodal treatment. Combined modality therapy including both chemotherapy and radiotherapy is considered the current standard of care. Investigators from the Memorial Sloan-Kettering Cancer Center used two cycles of carboplatin for 11 patients with primary CNS germinoma without metastatic disease. Patients achieving a CR were treated with reduced-dose EBRT (30 Gy to the involved field with 21 Gy to the neuroaxis). Those with lesser responses underwent two additional course of chemotherapy followed by full-dose irradiation (50 Gy to the involved filed with 36 Gy to the neuroaxis). There were five patients (45%) with a CR after two cycles and an additional two (64%) after the fourth course. Two patients demonstrated over 50% tumour reduction after two cycles and one after a total of four cycles of chemotherapy. Ninety-one per cent of the patients remained in complete remission for a median of 25 months (68).

The SFOP investigators reported the results of neoadjuvant chemotherapy in 51 patients with biopsy proven, localized germinoma. Four alternating courses of etoposide–carboplatin and etoposide–ifosfamide were administered prior to EBRT. EBRT consisted of limited-field irradiation (40 Gy) for patients for localized disease (51 patients) and low-dose craniospinal EBRT for those with dissemination. With a median follow-up period of 42 months, the 3-year EFS and OS were 96.4% and 98%, respectively (69). They later reported the pattern of relapse and outcome of neoadjuvant chemotherapy studies. Neoadjuvant chemotherapy with involved-field radiation therapy resulted in an unacceptably high rate of relapse within ventricle outside the radiation field (37).

The practice at the University of Tokyo has been to stratified GCT patients by relative risk into three subgroups: (i) germinoma and mature teratoma, (ii) mixed GCT with predominance of germinoma or teratoma with some pure malignant tumour (embryonal carcinomas, endodermal sinus tumours, and choriocarcinomas), and (iii) mixed tumours with predominance of pure malignant tumour.

Surgery and EBRT produced 10-year OS rates of 91.7% among the germinoma patients. Combination chemotherapy (cisplatin–vinblastine–bleomycin, cisplatin–etoposide, or carboplatin–etoposide) and radiotherapy was shown to significantly reduce the risk of disease recurrence in the intermediate prognostic group when compared with irradiation alone (P = 0.049). Forty-one per cent of these patients experienced a CR following induction chemotherapy (2). Based upon these observations, the Japanese Pediatric Brain Tumor Study Group conducted a clinical trial for CNS GCT. Germinoma patients were treated with neoadjuvant chemotherapy with carboplatin–etoposide or cisplatin–etoposide and followed with EBRT. Among those with germinomas, 94% achieved a CR with induction chemotherapy. Over a median follow-up period of 2.9 years, recurrent disease developed in 12%. In the majority of these, relapse occurred outside the radiation portal in the ventricle (70).

The SIOP CNS GCT-96 trials conducted a non-randomized internal study for germinoma that compared chemotherapy followed by focal irradiation with reduced dose CSI alone. Patients with localized disease (n = 190) received two cycles of carboplatin–etoposide alternating with ifosfamide and etoposide followed with focal primary tumour site irradiation of 40 Gy (n = 65) or dose-reduced CSI alone (24 Gy CSI with 16 Gy boost to the primary tumour site) (n = 125). There was no difference in 5-year EFS or OS, but a difference in PFS between two groups. Four of the 125 patients with reduced dose CSI alone experienced relapse at the primary tumour site compared with 7 of the 65 patients with combination treatment. The six of the seven relapsed patients treated with chemotherapy and focal irradiation experienced ventricular recurrence outside the primary radiotherapy field. They recommend including the whole ventricle irradiation to focal irradiation in patients treated without CSI (34). Together with the results from other studies, the current standard care of the multimodal treatment of germinoma includes 21–24 Gy WV irradiation with or without a boost to the primary tumour site.

The Hokkaido University Group protocol combined induction chemotherapy with low-dose involved-field EBRT. Pure germinomas are initially treated with etoposide–cisplatin. The clinical treatment volume for EBRT includes the tumour site for germinomas and multifocal germinomas received irradiation (24 Gy) to the whole ventricle, which includes the second and lateral ventricles; for pineal region tumours the fourth ventricle is also treated. They reported their results with 16 germinoma patients, 11 with β-HCG secreting germinomas. Eight patients had multifocal origin and three suffered from metastatic disease. Every germinoma patient achieved a CR by the third course of chemotherapy. The presence of β-HCG did not affect the response to therapy. Relapse-free survival rates at 5 years were 90% for the germinoma, and 44% for those with β-HCG secreting germinomas (the difference between the last two being P = 0.0025) (71).

The University of Eppendorf group paid attention to the risk of iatrogenic dissemination following surgical biopsy and/or resection among biomarker-positive GCT of the pineal region. They employed one course of neoadjuvant bleomycin–etoposide–cisplatin to induce significant regression and better delineation of the tumour's margins. After attempt for gross total resection, vinblastine–ifosfamide–cisplatin chemotherapy and craniospinal EBRT (50 Gy to tumour boost with 30 Gy to the neuroaxis) followed. Three patients, two with elevated β-HCG and one with

AFP, were treated with this protocol. Following induction therapy, pathological analysis revealed benign, mature teratoma with derivatives from all three germinal layers. There was also haemorrhagic necrosis with granulomatous and lymphocytic inflammation. In one case, there was small admixture of immature teratoma with mitosis. None of them demonstrated malignant extraembyonal surgery (72). The investigators of Kumamoto University also proposed treating patients with NG-GCT with neoadjuvant chemotherapy employing cisplatin–etoposide, carboplatin–etoposide, or ifosfamide–cisplatin–etoposide and EBRT to cytoreduce the tumour as to allow gross total resection. In 11 patients (five with yolk sac tumour, one with embryonal carcinoma, one with immature teratoma, and four with mixed malignant GCT), induction treatment produced two CR, six PR, two SD and one progressive disease. Ten of the 11 patients are alive at a mean of 96 months (20). They confirmed the effectiveness of this strategy in their later report of the results of the treatment of 14 patients with NGGCT with the same neoadjuvant chemotherapy and EBRT. Residual tumour was confirmed in 11 of the 14 patients after chemotherapy. Total removal was successful in 10 of the 11 patients. The 5-year EFS and OS rates were 86% and 93%, respectively (73).

The recent Children's Oncology Group (COG) phase II trial (ACNS0122) evaluated the effect of neoadjuvant chemotherapy with or without second-look surgery before CSI on response rates and survival outcomes. Patients demonstrating less than complete response after induction chemotherapy were encouraged to undergo second-look surgery. Patients who did not achieve completely response or partial response with any treatments proceeded to high-dose chemotherapy with peripheral blood stem cell rescue before CSI. Patients with newly diagnosed NGGCT (n = 102) received six cycles of carboplatin–etoposide alternating with ifosfamide–etoposide. Sixty-nine percent of patients achieved complete response or partial response with this neoadjuvant chemotherapy. Two patients with residual disease underwent consolidation high-dose chemotherapy with thiotepa and etoposide. At 5 years, EFS was 84% ± 4% (SE) and OS was 93% ± 3%, with medial follow-up of 5.1 years. There were no treatment-related deaths. This study showed that a neoadjuvant chemotherapy regimen, together with or without second-look surgery, is feasible and well tolerated but also produces a high response rate contributing to excellent survival outcomes in NGGCT patients (74).

Combined modality therapy including both chemotherapy and EBRT is considered the current standard of care in NGGCT. As CSI or whole-brain irradiation are both associated with significant late effects, there have been some trials to minimize the RT by stratifying patients according to risk of disease progression (75).

In the Japanese Pediatric Brain Tumor Study Group, the NG-GCT patients received ifosfamide–cisplatin–etoposide for three courses followed with irradiation. The intermediate prognosis group consisted of 18 patients with malignant teratoma and mixed tumours. There were no CRs noted with chemotherapy. However, following the completion of radiotherapy, 56% were tumour free. Two patients relapsed during a median observation period of 3.7 years. The poor prognosis group was made up of nine patients, of whom two were still alive without recurrence more than 2 years after the treatment (70).

The later Japanese Germ Cell Tumor study group treated intermediate prognosis patients with five cycles of carboplatin–etoposide followed by whole ventricle to 30.6 Gy and IFR to 50 Gy. The 10-year PFS and OS rates of this group were 81.5% and 91.3%, respectively. Patients with predominantly malignant germ cell tumour elements, called the poor prognosis group, were treated with three cycles of ifosfamide–cisplatin–etoposide and EBRT (CSI 30.6 Gy with focal irradiation to primary tumour site of 50 Gy). Second-look surgery was recommended for removal of residual tumour after EBRT. Patients received an additional five cycles of the same regimen after CSI and/or surgery. The 10-year-PFS and OS rate were 58.5% and 62.7% respectively (75).

In spite of the modest improvement of survival from these studies, it is still difficult to identify the standard management of NGGCT because of the historical differences in diagnosis, classification or risk stratification, and role of surgery among the study groups in the world, as well as its rarity and insufficient findings of biology of this disease. We need to have consensus on these subjects to perform larger-scale multi-institutional clinical trials and collaborative biology research to improve outcome and quality of life in patients with this disease.

High-dose chemotherapy with autologous stem cell transplantation for recurrent or progressive disease on treatment

Patients with progressive disease on treatment and those with relapse following multimodal treatment suffered a dismal prognosis. Investigators from the Memorial Sloan-Kettering Cancer Center evaluated the efficacy of high-dose chemotherapy (HDCT) utilizing thiotepa with autologous stem cell transplantation (auto-SCT) in 21 patients with recurrent or progressive CNS GCT. EFS and OS rates for the entire group 4 years after HDCT were 52% and 57%, respectively. Seven of 9 (78%) patients with germinoma survived disease free after HDCT with a median survival of 48 months. Only 4 of 12 (33%) patients with NGGCT survived without evidence of disease, with a median survival of 35 months. Patients achieving a CR had significantly better outcome. There was no toxic death for HDCT (76).

The Korean Society of Pediatric Neuro-Oncology conducted the prospective study of HDCT with autologous stem cell transplantation. They enrolled 20 patients with recurrent or progressive disease (9 with germinoma and 11 with NGGCT). Patients received two to eight cycles of conventional chemotherapy prior to HDCT with auto SCT with or without radiotherapy. Sixteen patients proceeded to the first HDCT with auto SCT, and 9 proceeded to the second HDCT with auto SCT. A carboplatin–thiotepa–etoposide regimen was used for the first and cyclophosphamide–melphalan was used for the second HDCT. Twelve patients (four NGGCT and eight germinoma) remain alive with a median follow-up of 47 months after relapse or progression. The 3-year OS was 59.1% (36.4% for NGGCT and 88.9% for germinoma). There were no treatment-related deaths (77).

Together with the reported results from other groups, sustained tumour control can be achieved with HDCT with auto-SCT both in germinoma and NGGCT. The success rate is higher in patients with recurrent germinoma. The role of adjuvant radiotherapy remains unclear (78).

References

1. Rosenblum MK, Nakazato Y, Matsutani M. Germ cell tumours. In: Louis DN, Ohgaki H, Wiestler OD, et al. (eds) *WHO Classification of Tumours of the Central Nervous System.* Lyon: International Agency for Research on Cancer, 2007; 198–204.

2. Matsutani M, Sano K, Takakura K, et al. Primary intracranial germ cell tumors: a clinical analysis of 153 histologically verified cases. *J Neurosurg* 1997; 86:446–455.

3. Report of Brain Tumor Registry of Japan (2001-2004) 13th Edition. *Neurol Med Chir (Tokyo)* 2014; 54:9–102.

4. Suh YL, Koo H, Kim TS, et al. Tumors of the central nervous system in Korea: a multicenter study of 3221 cases. *J Neurooncol* 2002; 56:251–259.

5. CBTRUS Statistical Report: Primary brain and central nervous system tumors diagnosed in the United States, 2006-2010. *Neuro-Oncol* 2013; 15 (suppl 2).

6. Kuratsu J, Ushio Y. A population-based survey in Kumamoto prefecture, Japan. Epidemiological study of primary intracranial tumors in childhood. *Pediatr Neurosurg* 1996; 25:240–247.

7. McCarthy BJ, Shibui S, Kayama T, et al. Primary CNS germ cell tumors in Japan and the United States: an analysis of 4 tumor registries. *Neuro-Oncology* 2012; 14:1194–1200.

8. Nakamura H, Makino K, Yano S, et al. Epidemiological study of primary intracranial tumors: a regional survey in Kumamoto prefecture in southern Japan -20-year study. *Int J Clin Oncol* 2011; 16:314–321.

9. Sano K. Pathogenesis of intracranial germ cell tumors reconsidered. *J Neurosurg* 1999; 90:258–264.

10. Wang L, Yamaguchi S, Burstein MD, et al. Novel somatic and germline mutations in intracranial germ cell tumours. *Nature* 2014; 511:241–245.

11. Ichimura K, Fukushima S, Totaki Y, et al. Recurrent neomorphic mutations of MTOR in central nervous system and testicular germ cell tumors may be targeted for therapy. *Acta Neuropathol* 2016; 131:889–901.

12. Fujiwara I, Asato R, Okumura R, et al. Magnetic resonance imaging of neurohypophyseal germinomas. *Cancer* 1991; 68:1009–1014.

13. Mutoh K, Okuno T, Ito M, et al. Ipsilateral atrophy in children with hemispheric cerebral tumors: CT findings. *J Comput Assist Tomogr* 1988; 12:740–743.

14. Fujimaki T, Matsutani M, Funada N, et al. CT and MRI features of intracranial germ cell tumors. *J Neurooncol* 1994; 19:217–226.

15. Takami H, Fukushima S, Fukuoka K, et al. Human chorionic gonadotropin is expressed virtually in all intracranial germ cell tumors. *J Neurooncol* 2015; 123:23–32.

16. Souweidane MM, Krieger MD, Weiner HL, et al. Surgical management of primary central nervous system germ cell tumors. Proceedings from the Second International Symposium on Central Nervous System Germ Cell Tumors. A review. *J Neurosurg Pediatr* 2010; 6:125–130.

17. Sawamura Y, De Tribolet N, Ishii N, et al. Management of primary intracranial germinomas: diagnostic surgery or radical resection? *J Neurosurg* 1997; 87:262–266.

18. Weiner HL, Lichtenbaum RA, Wisoff JH, et al. Delayed surgical resection of central nervous system germ cell tumors. *Neurosurgery* 2002; 50:727–733.

19. Friedman JA, Lynch JJ, Buckner JC, et al. Management of malignant pineal germ cell tumors with residual mature teratoma. *Neurosurgery* 2001; 48:518–523.

20. Kochi M, Itoyama Y, Shiraishi S, et al. Successful treatment of intractanial nongerminomatous malignant germ cell tumors by administering neoadjuvant chemotherapy and radiotherapy before excision of residual tumors. *J Neurosurg* 2003; 99:106–114.

21. Jenkin D, Berry M, Chan H, et al. Pineal region germinomas in childhoof treatment considerations. *Int J Radiat Oncol Biol Phys* 1990; 18:541–545.

22. Maity A, Shu HK, Janss A, et al. Craniospinal radiation in the treatment of biopsy-proven intracranial germinoma: twenty-five years' experience in a single center. *Int J Radiat Oncol Biol Phys* 2004; 58:1165–1170.

23. Bamberg M, Kortmann RD, Calaminus G, et al. Radiation therapy for intracranial germinoma: results of the German cooperative prospective trials MAKEI 83/86/89. *J Clin Oncol* 1999; 17:2585–2592.

24. Hardenbergh PH, Golden J, Billet A, et al. Intracranial germinoma: the case for lower dose radiation therapy. *Int J Radiat Oncol Biol Phys* 1997; 39:419–426.

25. Merchant TE, Sherwood SH, Mulhem RK, et al. CNS germinoma: disease control and long-term functional outcome for 12 children treated with craniospinal irradiation. *Int J Radiat Oncol Biol Phys* 2000; 46:1171–1176.

26. Cho J, Choi JU, Kim DS, et al. Low-dose craniospinal irradiation as a definitive treatment for intracranial germinoma. *Radiother Oncol* 2009; 91:75–79.

27. Wolden SL, Wara WM, Larson DA, et al. Radiation therapy for primary intracranial germ-cell tumors. *Int J Radiat Oncol Biol Phys* 1995; 32:943–949.

28. Haas-Kogan DA, Missett BT, Wara WM, et al. Radiation therapy for intracranial germ cell tumors. *Int J Radiat Oncol Biol Phys* 2003; 56:511–518.

29. Ogawa K, Shikama N, Toita T, et al. Long-term results of radiotherapy for intracranial germinoma: a multi-institutional retrospective review of 126 patients. *Int J Radiat Oncol Biol Phys* 2004; 58:705–713.

30. Balmaceda C, Heller G, Rosenblum M, et al. Chemotherapy without irradiation—a novel approach for newly diagnosed CNS germ cell tumors: results of an international cooperative trial. The First International Central Nervous System Germ Cell Tumor Study. *J Clin Oncol* 1996; 14:2908–2915.

31. Kellie SJ, Boyce H, Dunkel IJ, et al. Primary chemotherapy for intracranial nongerminomatous germ cell tumors: results of the second international CNS germ cell study group protocol. *J Clin Oncol* 2004; 22:846–853.

32. Da Silva NS, Cappellano AM, Diez B, et al. Primary chemotherapy for intracranial germ cell tumors: results of the third international CNS germ cell tumor study. *Pediatr Blood Cancer* 2010; 54:377–383.

33. Matsutani M, et al. Presented at the 3rd International CNS GCT Symposium, Cambridge, 17–20 April, 2013.

34. Calaminus G, Kortmann R, Worch J, et al. SIOP CNS GCT 96: final report of outcome of a prospective, multinational nonrandomized trial for children and adults with intracranial germinoma, comparing craniospinal irradiation alone with chemotherapy followed by focal primary site irradiation for patients with localized disease. *Neuro Oncol* 2013; 15:786–796.

35. Kretschmar C, Kleinberg L, Greenberg M, et al. Pre-radiation chemotherapy with response-based radiation therapy in children with central nervous system germ cell tumors: a report from the Children's Oncology Group. *Pediatr Blood Cancer* 2007; 48:285–291.

36. Allen J, et al. Presented at the 2nd International CNS GCT Symposium, Los Angeles, 18–21 November, 2005.

37. Alapetite C, Brisse H, Patte C, et al. Pattern of relapse and outcome of non-metastatic germinoma patients treated with chemotherapy and limited field radiation: the SIOP experience. *Neuro Oncol* 2010; 12:1318–1325.

38. Matsutani M. Clinical management of primary central nervous system germ cell tumors. *Semin Oncol* 2004; 31:676–683.

39. Brada M, Rajan B. Spinal seeding in cranial germinoma. *Br J Cancer* 1990; 61:239–240.

40. Shirato H, Aoyama H, Ikeda J, et al. Impact of margin for target volulme in low-dose involved field radiotherapy after induction chemotherapy for intracranial germinoma. *Int J Radiat Oncol Biol Phys* 2004; 60:214–217.

41. Timmerman RD, Patel D, Boaz JC, et al. Pattern of failure after induction chemotherapy followed by consolidative radiation therapy

for children with central nervous system germinoma. *Med Pediatr Oncol* 2003; 41:564–566.

42. Shikama N, Ogawa K, Tanaka S, et al. Lack of benefit of spinal irradiation in the primary treatment of intracranial germinoma: a multiinstitutional, retrospective review of 180 patients. *Cancer* 2005; 104:126–134.

43. Rogers SJ, Mosleh-Shirazi MA, Saran FH. Radiotherapy of localized intracranial germinoma: time to sever historical ties? *Lancet Oncol* 2005; 6:509–519.

44. Douglas JG, Rockhill JK, Ilson JM, et al. Cisplatin-based chemotherapy followed by focal, reduced-dose irradiation for pediatric primary central nervous system germinomas. *J Pediatr Hematol Oncol* 2006; 28:36–39.

45. Nguyen QN, Chang EL, Allen PK, et al. Focal and craniospinal irradiation for patients with intracranial germinoma and patterns of failure. *Cancer* 2006; 107:2228–2236.

46. Eom KS, Kim IH, Park CI, et al. Upfront chemotherapy and involved-field radiotherapy results in more relapses than extended radiotherapy for intracranial germinomas: modification in radiotherapy volume might be needed. *Int J Radiat Oncol Biol Phys* 2008; 71:667–671.

47. Paximadis P, Hallock A, Bhambhani K, et al. Patterns of failure in patients with primary intracranial germinoma treated with neoadjuvant chemotherapy and radiotherapy. *Pediatr Neurol* 2012; 47:162–166.

48. Khatua S, Dhall G, O'Neill S, et al. Treatment of primary CNS germinomatous germ cell tumors with chemotherapy prior to reduced dose whole ventricular and local boost irradiation. *Pediatr Blood Cancer* 2010; 55:42–46.

49. Murray MJ, Horan G, Lowis S, et al. Highlights from the Third International Central Nervous System Germ Cell Tumour symposium: laying the foundations for future consensus. *Ecanermedicalscience* 2013; 7:333.

50. Hu YW, Huang PI, Wong TT, et al. Salvage treatment for recurrent intracranial germinoma after reduced-volume radiotherapy: a single-institution experience and review of the literature. *Int J Radiat Oncol Biol Phys* 2012; 84:639–647.

51. Calaminus G, et al. Presented at the 3rd International CNS GCT Symposium, Cambridge, 17–20 April, 2013.

52. Bartels U, et al. Presented at the 3rd International CNS GCT Symposium, Cambridge, 17–20 April, 2013.

53. Yen SH, Chen YW, Huang PI, et al. Optimal treatment for intracranial germinoma: can we lower radiation dose without chemotherapy? *Int J Radiat Oncol Biol Phys* 2010; 77:980–987.

54. Raggi E, Mosleh-Shirazi MA, Saran FH. An evaluation of conformal and intensity-modulated radiotherapy in whole ventricular radiotherapy for localized primary intracranial germinomas. *Clin Oncol (R Coll Radiol)* 2008; 20:253–260.

55. Sakanaka K, Mizowaki T, Hiraoka M. Dosimetric advantage of intensity-modulated radiotherapy for whole ventricles in the treatment of localized intracranial germionoma. *Int J Radiat Oncol Biol Phys* 2012; 82:e273–e280.

56. Qi XS, Stinauer M, Togers B, et al. Potential for improved intelligence quotient using volumetric modulated arc therapy compared with conventional 3-dimensional conformal radiation for whole-ventricular radiation in children. *Int J Raiat Oncol Biol Phys* 2012; 84:1206–1211.

57. MacDonald SM, Trofimov A, Safai S, et al. Proton radiotherapy for pediatric central nervous system germ cell tumors: early clinical outcomes. *Int J Radiat Oncol Biol Phys* 2011; 79:121–129.

58. Fuller BF, Kapp DS, Cox R. Radiation therapy of pineal region tumors: 25 new cases and a review of 208 previously reported cases. *Int J Radiat Oncol Biol Phys* 1994; 28:229–245.

59. Calaminus G, Bamberg M, Baranzelli MC, et al. *Neuropediatrics* 1994; 25:26–32.

60. Baranzelli MC, Patte C, Bouffet E, et al. An attempt to treat pediatric intracranial alphaFP and betaHCG secreting germ cell tumors with

chemotherapy alone. SFOP experience with 18 cases. Societe Francaise d'Oncologie Pediatrique. *J Neurooncol* 1998; 37:229–239.

61. Robertson PL, DaRosso RC, Allen JC. Improved prognosis of intracranial non-germinoma germ cell tumors with multimodality therapy. *J Neurooncol* 1997; 32:71–80.

62. Kim JW, Kim WC, Cho JH, et al. A multimodal approach including craniospinal irradiation improves the treatment outcome of high-risk intracranial nongerminomatous germ cell tumors. *Int J Radiat Oncol Biol Phys* 2012; 84:625–631.

63. Dhall G, Fungusaro J. Presented at the 3rd International CNS GCT Symposium, Cambridge, 17–20 April, 2013.

64. Jennings MT. Current therapeutic management strategies for primary intracranial germ cell tumors. In: Newton HB (ed.) *Handbook of Brain Tumor Chemotherapy*. New York: Academic Press, 2005; 448–462.

65. Pinkerton R. Malignant germ cell tumors. In: Pinkerton C, Shankar AG, Matthay K (eds) *Evidence-Based Pediatric Oncology*. Oxford: Wiley-Blackwell, 2013; 65–68.

66. Nicols CR. Ifosfamide in the treatment of germ cell tumors. *Semin Oncol* 1996; 23:65–73.

67. Kellie S, Boyce H, Dunkel IJ, et al. Intensive chemotherapy and cyclophosphamide-based chemotherapy without radiotherapy for intracranial germinomas: failure of a primary chemotherapy approach. *Pediatr Blood Cancer* 2004; 43:126–133.

68. Allen JC, DaRoss RC, Donahue B, et al. A phase II trial of preirradiation carboplatin in newly diagnosed germinoma of the central nervous system. *Cancer* 1994; 74:940–944.

69. Bouffet E, Branzelli MC, Patte C, et al. Combined treatment modality for intracranial germinomas: results of a multicenter SFOP experience. *Br J Cancer* 1999; 79:1199–1204.

70. Matsutani M, The Japanese Pediatric Brain Tumor Study Group. Combined chemotherapy and radiation therapy for CNS germ cell tumors- The Japanese experience. *J Neurooncol* 2001; 54:311–316.

71. Aoyama H, Shirato H, Ikeda J, et al. Induction-chemotherapy followed by low-dose involved field radiotherapy for intracranial germ cell tumors. *J Clin Oncol* 2002; 20:857–865.

72. Knappe UJ, Bentele K, Horstmann M, et al. Treatment and long-term outcome of pineal nongerminomatous germ cell tumor. *Pediatr Neurosurg* 1998; 28:241–245.

73. Nakamura H, Makino K, Kochi M, et al. Evaluation of neoadjuvant therapy in patients with nongerminomatous germ cell tumors. *J Neurosurg Pediatr* 2011; 7:431–438.

74. Goldman S, Bouffet E, Fisher PG, et al. Phase II trial assessing the ability of neoadjuvant chemotherapy with or without second-look surgery to eliminate measurable disease for nongerminomatous germ cell tumors: a Children's Oncology Group Study. *J Clin Oncol* 2015; 33:2464–2471.

75. Matsutani M. Treatment results of intracranial GCT: final results of the Japanese Group for CNS GCT (abstract). *Neuro-Oncology* 2008; 9:169–222.

76. Modak S, Gardner S, Dunkel IJ, et al. Thiotepa-based high-dose chemotherapy with autologous stem-cell rescue in patients with recurrent or progressive CNS germ cell tumors. *J Clin Oncol* 2004; 22:1934–1943.

77. Baek HJ, Park HJ, Sung KW, et al. Myeloablative chemotherapy and autologous transplantation in patients with relapsed or progressed central nervous system germ cell tumors: results of Korean Society of Pediatric Neuro-Oncology (KSPNO) S-053 study. *J Neurooncol* 2013; 114:329–338.

78. Bouffet E. The role of myeloablative chemotherapy with autologous hematopoietic cell rescue in central nervous system germ cell tumors. *Pediatr Blood Cancer* 2010; 54:644–646.

CHAPTER 15

Familial tumour syndromes: neurofibromatosis, schwannomatosis, rhabdoid tumour predisposition, Li–Fraumeni syndrome, Turcot syndrome, Gorlin syndrome, and Cowden syndrome

Scott R. Plotkin, Jaclyn A. Biegel, David Malkin, Robert L. Martuza, and D. Gareth Evans

Introduction

Several familial tumour syndromes are associated with an increased incidence of nervous system tumours. Recognition of these syndromes is necessary to provide optimal clinical care and to provide genetic counselling to affected patients and their families. The hereditary syndromes included in this chapter are limited to those associated with nervous system tumours. These include neurofibromatosis type 1 (NF1), neurofibromatosis type 2 (NF2), schwannomatosis, rhabdoid tumour predisposition, Li–Fraumeni syndrome (LFS), Turcot syndrome, Gorlin syndrome, and Cowden syndrome. The majority of these syndromes are inherited in an autosomal dominant fashion, and the genes involved function primarily as tumour suppressors (Table 15.1). Consistent with Knudson's 'two-hit hypothesis', germline mutations in these genes result in increased susceptibility to tumours, which develop following a secondary somatic mutation or loss of heterozygosity of the normal copy of the gene (1). Study of these tumour syndromes has provided critical insight into mechanisms of tumourigenesis and recent large-scale genetic studies have confirmed the importance of these tumour suppressor genes in the formation of common sporadic cancers such as glioblastoma, meningioma, lung cancer, breast cancer, and colon cancer.

General principles

Genetic counselling is an essential component of the care of the patient with tumour suppressor syndromes. Genetic testing is routinely used to confirm a diagnosis for some conditions but not usually for others (e.g. NF1). Genetic testing for single-gene disorders can be used for family planning (i.e. prenatal or pre-implantation genetic diagnosis) or for pre-symptomatic diagnosis of individuals at risk (especially in LFS, NF1, and NF2). If a causative mutation can be identified in the proband, molecular testing with 100% specificity will be available for that family.

Cancer screening is commonly recommended for patients with tumour suppressor syndromes. Screening presents both advantages and disadvantages which must be weighed. The goal of screening programmes is to promote detection of benign and malignant tumours at an early stage where treatment outcomes are improved. Screening can also improve patients' emotional well-being by providing a sense of expectation and control (2). However, false-positive results of imaging or laboratory studies can lead to unnecessary procedures and increased patient anxiety. In addition, the benefit of screening recommendations has not been established for most tumour suppressor syndromes.

Table 15.1 Clinical and genetic features of tumour suppressor syndromes that predispose to nervous system tumours

Disease	Gene	Hallmark tumour	Other tumours	Epidemiology
NF1	NF1	Neurofibroma	Optic pathway glioma, MPNST, GIST, phaeochromocytoma	Birth incidence: 1/2700–3300
NF2	NF2	Vestibular schwannoma	Meningioma, spinal ependymoma	Birth incidence: 1/25,000–40,000
Schwannomatosis	SMARCB1 LTZR1	Schwannoma	Meningiomas (rarely)	Birth incidence: 1/40,000–100,000
Rhabdoid tumour predisposition	SMARCB1 SMARCA4	Atypical teratoid/rhabdoid tumours	Renal rhabdoid tumours	Not defined
LFS	TP53	Sarcoma	Astrocytic brain tumours, adrenocortical carcinoma, breast cancer	Estimated incidence: 1/5000–20,000
Gorlin syndrome	PTCH	Multiple basal cell carcinomas	Medulloblastoma, meningioma	Estimated incidence 1/19,000
Turcot syndrome	APC and DNA-repair mismatch genes	Colorectal cancer	Medulloblastoma, astrocytoma, ependymoma, glioblastoma	Not defined
Cowden syndrome	PTEN	Cerebellar gangliocytoma (Lhermitte–Duclos syndrome)	Breast cancer, thyroid cancer, endometrial cancer	Incidence: not defined Prevalence: 1/200,000

Neurofibromatosis 1

Definition

Neurofibromatosis 1 (OMIM #162200) is a tumour suppressor syndrome characterized by a predisposition to develop neurofibromas, gliomas, pigmentary lesions, and bony abnormalities.

Epidemiology

Neurofibromatosis 1 is the most common neurogenetic disorder with a birth incidence between 1 in 2000 and 1 in 3300 (3–6). The disease affects all racial groups and genders equally. NF1 is an autosomal dominant disorder with full penetrance and phenotypic variability both within and between families. About 42% of patients have new mutations with clinically unaffected parents (5). Life expectancy of patients with NF1 is reduced compared with the local population in England (71.5 vs 80 years) (7) and even more in Finland (6).

Aetiology/genetics

A germline mutation in the *NF1* gene can be identified in more than 95–97% of classically affected individuals if a combined approach including RNA analysis is utilized (8, 9). Thus far, no particular mutational hot spot has been identified in the *NF1* gene and most unrelated patients carry distinct mutations, including nonsense (~37%), splice-site (~28%), frameshift (~18%), and missense mutations (~9%) (8, 9). Despite intense investigation, few discrete genotype–phenotype relationships have been described. Deletion of the entire gene is associated with a more severe phenotype with greater burden of cutaneous and internal neurofibromas but higher degrees of dysmorphism and increased rates of mental retardation and malignant peripheral nerve sheath tumours (MPNSTs) compared with NF1 patients in general (10, 11). It is not yet clear whether this phenotype is due to the deletion of flanking elements, although deletion of the 3 intronic genes which are reverse transcribed may well be the cause (12). In addition, absence of cutaneous

neurofibromas has been associated with a 3-bp in-frame deletion in exon 17 of the *NF1* gene (13). Recently, germline mutations in the *SPRED1* gene have been identified in patients with a mild NF1 phenotype who do not have a germline *NF1* mutation (14). This condition, termed Legius syndrome, is characterized by the presence of multiple cafe-au-lait macules, skinfold freckling, and macrocephaly. Patients with Legius syndrome represent approximately 1.9% of anonymous individuals that meet the National Institutes of Health (NIH) criteria for NF1 in a large mutational analysis database (15) and 8% of sporadic children with 6+ café-au-lait patches (9). Diagnosis of Legius syndromes in patients with clinical features of NF1 is important since these individuals do not appear to be at risk for nerve sheath tumours, optic pathway glioma, or malignancy and have a milder phenotype than NF1 patients (15).

Mosaic NF1 is caused by postzygotic mutation of the *NF1* gene (16). The clinical phenotype depends on the timing of the mutation and the cell types affected. Mutations occurring early in development will lead to a mild, generalized form of NF1, similar to patients with an inherited mutation. Mutations occurring at a later stage of development, in a more specialized cell type, lead to segmental disease localized to one region, quadrant, or occasionally half of the body (Fig. 15.1). Gonadal mosaicism occurs when gametes are affected but other tissues are unaffected. This situation is rare and is usually diagnosed when clinically unaffected parents have two or more affected offspring (17). It is important to be able to identify mosaic forms of the disease as the risk of transmitting the affected gene to offspring is usually much lower than in those with an inherited germline mutation.

Pathogenesis

Neurofibromin, the most common *NF1* gene product, is a 2818-amino acid protein with a GTPase-activating protein (GAP) domain which functions to inactivate RAS signalling. Loss-of-function mutations of the *NF1* gene are associated with increased RAS activity and with the occurrence of benign and malignant

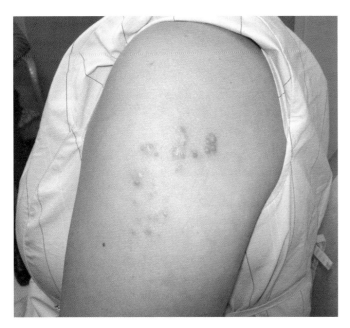

Fig. 15.1 Photograph of a patient with segmental NF1 manifested as a localized patch of cutaneous neurofibromas without other manifestations of NF1.

tumours, suggesting a tumour suppressor function for the gene (18, 19). The demonstration of *NF1* mutations or 'second hits' in NF1-related tumours has been complicated by the heterogeneous pathological composition of neurofibromas. The presence of Schwann cells, fibroblasts, vascular structures, and mast cells within these tumours suggests that *NF1* is lost in a single cell type, which then recruits other wild-type elements into the tumour. Supporting this hypothesis, loss of *NF1* in Schwann cells alone is sufficient to generate tumours in mice (20) and can be demonstrated in Schwann cells, but not in fibroblasts, from human tumours (21).

Genetically engineered mouse models of NF1 suggest that the microenvironment plays an important role in tumourigenesis. In these models, complete loss of neurofibromin is necessary but not sufficient for gliomagenesis. For example, neither $Nf1^{+/-}$ mice nor mice with targeted loss of *Nf1* in astroglial cells develop optic pathway gliomas (22, 23). In contrast, mice with *Nf1* loss in astroglial cells on a heterozygous background do develop optic pathway gliomas. Similarly, mice with *Nf1* loss in Schwann cells do not develop neurofibromas while mice with *Nf1* loss in Schwann cells on a heterozygous background develop neurofibromas (20).

Clinical presentation

Nearly all patients with NF1 present with clinical signs in the first decade of life. The most common presenting feature is café-au-lait macules which are typically present before the age of 1 year (24). Skinfold freckling and Lisch nodules (iris hamartomas) develop in childhood, and cutaneous neurofibromas often develop during adolescence. Optic pathway gliomas and plexiform neurofibromas are thought to be congenital lesions; when symptomatic, they often present in childhood. The lifetime risk of malignant MPNST is about 10–15% (25, 26); these tumours represent the primary cause of disease-specific mortality in NF1 patients (12, 23, 24, 26). The majority of MPNSTs occur by age 40 in most clinical series (22, 27). Non-nervous system tumours that may be seen in association with NF1 include gastrointestinal stromal tumours,

phaeochromocytomas, rhabdomyosarcoma, myeloid leukaemia, breast cancer, and carcinoid.

Diagnostic criteria

Diagnostic criteria were developed through the NIH Consensus Conference in 1987 and updated in 1997 (28). These criteria require the presence of at least two of the following clinical features: six or more café-au-lait macules, two or more neurofibromas or one plexiform neurofibroma, freckling in the axillary or inguinal regions, optic pathway glioma, two or more Lisch nodules, a distinctive bony lesion such as sphenoid dysplasia or thinning of the long bone cortex, and a first-degree relative with NF1. Reliance on just pigmentary criteria alone may misdiagnose NF1 in a third of cases (9), but the presence of at least one non-pigmentary criterion retains specificity.

Neurofibromas and MPNST

Neurofibromas are benign tumours derived from the nerve sheath which contain multiple cell types including Schwann cells, perineural cells, fibroblasts, and mast cells embedded in extracellular matrix and collagen (29). Neurofibromas grow within the nerve bundle and do not usually have a surrounding capsule. By puberty, more than 80% of NF1 patients develop neurofibromas (24), which can be cutaneous, subcutaneous, or deep in location. Radiographic evidence of spinal neurofibromas is common but symptomatic lesions are rare, representing less than 2% of patients in a large observational study (30). Intracranial neurofibromas are exceedingly rare; in contrast, neurofibromas of the head and neck are common.

Malignant peripheral nerve sheath tumours are sarcomas derived from the nerve sheath. In NF1 patients, these tumours typically develop within pre-existing plexiform neurofibromas (29) although some appear to develop *de novo*. The capacity for malignant transformation is not shared equally by all forms of neurofibroma: MPNSTs typically develop within plexiform and localized intraneural neurofibromas and never within cutaneous neurofibromas (29). The lifetime risk of MPNSTs in NF1 is about 10–15%; the prognosis of MPNSTs in patients with NF1 is worse compared with MPNSTs in the general population (25, 31, 32). At the present time, there is no effective screening protocol for MPNSTs although positron emission tomography scanning has excellent sensitivity and specificity to identify MPNSTs transformed from pre-existing neurofibromas (33).

Gliomas

Pilocytic astrocytomas are closely associated with NF1. These World Health Organization (WHO) grade I tumours have low cellularity and exhibit a biphasic histological pattern that includes compact areas with bipolar piloid cells and Rosenthal fibres, and loosely textured microcystic areas. Although these tumours may appear in any part of the brain, pilocytic astrocytomas in NF1 patients preferentially involve the optic nerve, chiasm, and tract, and the adjacent hypothalamus (i.e. optic pathway gliomas) (Fig. 15.2) (34). Optic pathway gliomas are identified in approximately 15% of patients with NF1; in most cases, such disease is limited to non-progressive enlargement of the optic pathway structures. Symptomatic optic gliomas occur in only 4% of patients (24) and typically present as proptosis, visual loss, or precocious puberty. Children less than 7 years old are at greatest risk for these neoplasms although older children and adults may rarely present with symptomatic tumours (35).

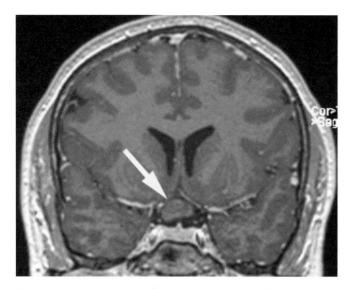

Fig. 15.2 Coronal MRI scan of the brain after administration of contrast demonstrating expansion of the optic chiasm consistent with an optic pathway glioma.

Non-optic gliomas also occur at increased frequency in NF1. The prevalence in patients less than 50 years of age is 100-fold greater than expected according to Surveillance, Epidemiology, and End Results (SEER) estimates for this age group (36). The most common sites include the brainstem (49%), cerebral hemispheres (21%), and basal ganglia (14%); histologies include both low-grade and high-grade tumours (34). The outcome of NF1 patients with glioblastoma is not well characterized due to the relative rarity of these tumours but small studies in children suggest that patients with NF1 fare better than their sporadic counterparts (37). Despite this advantage, gliomas are the second most common cause of death in NF1 patients (27).

Genetic testing

Genetic testing for *NF1* is not necessary to confirm a diagnosis in patients who meet clinical criteria, except if these are just pigmentary (freckling and café-au-lait) (9). The role of genetic testing in individuals with some features of NF1 but who do not meet criteria is controversial. Many clinicians recommend genetic testing for children with multiple café-au-lait macules and clinically unaffected parents while other clinicians monitor these patients clinically. Nonetheless, in childhood there should be suspicion for congenital mismatch repair deficiency that can mimic NF1. In contrast, genetic testing is certainly appropriate for affected individuals who wish to receive prenatal diagnosis or preimplantation genetic diagnosis.

Imaging and monitoring

Asymptomatic neurofibromas are common in patients with NF1 (38, 39). For many years, experts have questioned the utility of imaging asymptomatic patients. However, the introduction of whole-body magnetic resonance imaging (MRI) scanning has permitted the rapid assessment of whole-body tumour burden (40), introducing a new element into the ongoing debate regarding the role of imaging in these patients. Plexiform neurofibromas grow more rapidly in childhood, raising the question of whether early detection can be helpful.

Imaging studies of the brain and spine should be reserved for those NF1 patients with unexplained or progressive symptoms since identification of asymptomatic optic glioma in 10–15% of patients may lead to unnecessary procedures (41). In contrast, screening for symptomatic optic glioma is recommended and includes annual ophthalmological examinations between ages 2 and 7 years and review of growth and sexual development to identify hypothalamic dysfunction (41). Ophthalmological assessment should include measures of visual acuity and evaluation of the optic disc; visual-evoked potentials are not recommended (42). Routine laboratory investigations are not needed for patients with NF1.

Management

Neurofibroma

Surgery is the mainstay for treatment of neurofibroma although complete resection of plexiform neurofibromas is challenging given the invasive nature of these tumours (Fig. 15.3). Surgery may be considered for patients with symptomatic or progressive tumours but the benefit of treatment must be weighed carefully against the possibility of surgical morbidity. In patients with little or no neurological dysfunction related to their tumours, watchful waiting may allow patients to retain neurological function for many years. Radiation is typically deferred in patients with NF1 given the increased risk of malignant transformation (43). Chemotherapy trials for NF1-related plexiform neurofibroma have been performed but no drugs are currently approved for this indication (44). In a single-arm phase II study, administration of sirolimus to NF1 patients with progressive plexiform neurofibroma resulted in longer median time to progression (15.4 months) than historical control (11.9 months) (45). For NF1 patients with non-progressive plexiform neurofibroma, no patients experienced a radiographic response by 6 months and the stratum was closed by design (46).

Glioma

Patients with symptomatic optic gliomas should be followed closely, but therapy should be reserved for those lesions that are progressive. Surgery should be considered for patients with painful proptosis and blindness or those with hydrocephalus from chiasmal lesions. Similarly, radiation therapy is reserved for patients who progress through chemotherapy because of the risk of developing moyamoya syndrome (47), endocrinological dysfunction, and cognitive problems after treatment. In addition, radiation has been associated with an increased risk of malignant transformation of optic pathway gliomas (48). Current treatment options for progressive optic gliomas include chemotherapy such as carboplatin/vincristine, vinblastine, or temozolomide.

Asymptomatic, homogenously enhancing lesions outside the optic pathway can be followed serially by MRI without intervention. Tumour growth or new symptoms should prompt consideration of surgical sampling to establish tumour grade. Specific treatment guidelines for high-grade glioma are not defined for NF1 patients and these tumours are typically treated in a similar fashion to sporadic tumours. However, radiation therapy should be deferred in low-grade tumours, if possible, for the reasons outlined above. The recent finding that the mammalian target of rapamycin (mTOR) pathway is involved in the development of tumours in NF1 (49) has led to a clinical trial of everolimus for NF1-related glioma.

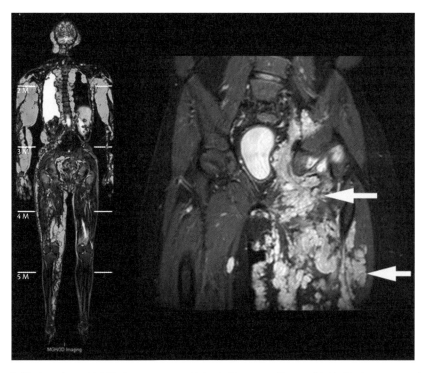

Fig. 15.3 Whole-body MRI scan (left) of a patient with NF1 demonstrates multiple plexiform neurofibromas (pink) affecting numerous body regions. Regional MRI scan (right) highlights the invasive nature of these tumours (arrows), a factor that limits the ability to achieve a complete resection.

Neurofibromatosis 2

Definition

Neurofibromatosis 2 (OMIM #101000) is characterized by the predisposition to develop multiple tumours including schwannomas, meningiomas, and spinal cord ependymomas.

Epidemiology

Neurofibromatosis 2 is significantly less common than NF1 with a birth incidence of 1 in 25,000–33,000 (50). NF2 is transmitted in autosomal dominant fashion with full penetrance. The proportion of cases due to *de novo* mutation is around 56% (5). There is no evidence for gender preference or racial imbalance. Life expectancy of patients with NF2 is reduced compared with the local population in England (69 vs 80 years) (7) but is improving in the modern era with specialist care (51).

Aetiology/genetics

A causative germline mutation in the *NF2* gene can be identified in 70–90% of affected individuals (52). Factors which prevent the identification of all mutations include the presence of large deletions, mutations in promoter or intronic regions, and somatic mosaicism. The introduction of improved detection methods has increased mutation detection rates. Currently, an *NF2* alteration is not identified in 33% of *de novo* patients presenting with bilateral vestibular schwannomas and in 60% of patients presenting with unilateral vestibular schwannomas, likely due to somatic mosaicism (53), but found in 95% of second-generation affected individuals.

Constitutional mutations of the *NF2* gene include nonsense (29–39%), splice-site (~25%), frameshift (25–27%), and missense mutations (5–7%) (54, 55). Mutation hot spots have been

identified at CpG dinucleotides that lead to TGA nonsense mutations, particularly in exons 2, 6, 8, and 11 (54). To date, genotype–phenotype correlations have been identified, with truncating mutations more common in severely affected patients (51, 56) and non-truncating mutations being more associated with milder disease (57). There is also a correlation between site of mutation and meningiomas, with 3′ mutations giving earlier diagnosis and more frequent disease. Constitutional truncating mutations in exons 2–13 are also associated with significantly poorer life expectancy (51).

Genetic mosaicism is a common cause of non-informative testing in sporadic NF2 patients. For these individuals, tumour specimens should be frozen for molecular analysis, if possible. If two genetic alterations (e.g. one mutation and one allele loss of the *NF2* gene) can be identified in a tumour, one is inferred to be the constitutional mutation. Haplotype analysis can then be used to screen at-risk individuals for the mutation(s) in constitutional DNA (58). In families with two or more affected individuals, linkage analysis using intragenic markers or markers flanking the *NF2* gene can be used for pre-symptomatic diagnosis with greater than 99% certainty of affected status.

Pathogenesis

The *NF2* gene was mapped to chromosome 22 in 1987 (59, 60) and then identified by two independent groups in 1993 (61, 62). The *NF2* gene is composed of 17 exons spanning 110 kb. There are three alternative messenger RNA species (7 kb, 4.4 kb, and 2.6 kb) due to variable length of the 3′ untranslated region. The predominant *NF2* gene product is a 595-amino acid protein and is a member of the 4.1 family of cytoskeletal proteins named Merlin (*m*oezin, *e*zrin, *r*adixin-like protein). The protein links membrane-associated proteins to the actin cytoskeleton, thereby acting as an interface with the extracellular environment (63).

The NF2 protein is a true tumour suppressor, as biallelic loss of the gene results in tumour growth. Inactivation of the *NF2* gene can be detected in the great majority of sporadic vestibular schwannomas (64) and in about 50–60% of sporadic meningiomas (65). Despite significant progress in understanding the role of the *NF2* gene product, the molecular mechanism by which loss of Merlin leads to tumourigenesis has not been fully elucidated. Multiple binding partners have been identified for Merlin with implications in a variety of signalling pathways involved in maintenance of contact-dependent inhibition of growth and proliferation, stabilization of adherens junctions, and the regulation of receptor tyrosine kinases at the cell surface (63). There is evidence implicating a novel nuclear function of Merlin to interact with an E3-ubiqiutin ligase (66).

Clinical presentation

The hallmark feature of NF2 is vestibular schwannomas which develop in more than 95% of patients with the disorder (Fig. 15.4). Non-vestibular schwannomas of cranial, spinal, and peripheral nerves are also common (Fig. 15.5). NF2-related schwannomas are histologically benign, and there does not appear to be an increased risk of spontaneous malignancy in this condition. However, MPNSTs may occur in patients who have received prior radiation therapy. Intradermal schwannomas help distinguish NF2 from schwannomatosis.

Meningiomas are common in NF2 patients. The cumulative incidence is approximately 80% by 70 years of age without a clear gender bias (67). Intracranial meningiomas most commonly arise along the cerebral falx and convexity (~70%), followed by the skull

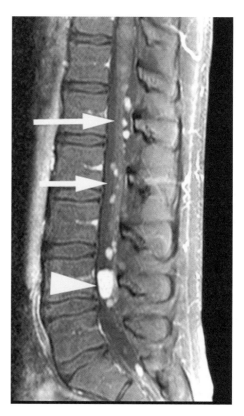

Fig. 15.5 Post-contrast sagittal MRI scan of the lumbar spine in a patient with NF2 demonstrating multiple schwannomas (arrows) in the lumbar spine and cauda equina with a larger lesion (arrowhead) that has enlarged over time. Patients with heavy tumour burden in this region can be asymptomatic.

base (~25%), and within the ventricles (~3%) (Fig. 15.4) (68). Optic sheath meningiomas occur in 4–8% of patients with NF2 and are a disproportionate cause of decreased visual acuity. The majority of meningiomas (>60%) show little or no growth over clinical follow-up times; a minority of tumours progress and require surgery (68). Among symptomatic meningiomas resected in a large case series, WHO grade II and III tumours were found in 29% and 6% of cases, respectively (68).

Spinal ependymomas in patients with NF2 present as intramedullary spinal cord lesions (Fig. 15.6) and occur in up to 50% of patients (69, 70). Two-thirds of patients with ependymomas have multiple tumours. The cervicomedullary junction or cervical spine is most commonly involved (63–82%) followed by the thoracic spine (36–44%) (69, 70). The brain and lumbar spine, common sites for sporadic ependymomas, are rarely involved. Radiographic evidence of tumour progression occurs in less than 10% of patients and progressive neurological dysfunction requiring ultimate surgical intervention occurs in only 12–20% of patients with ependymoma (69, 70).

The average age of onset of symptoms for NF2 is between 17 and 21 and typically precedes a formal diagnosis of NF2 by 5 to 8 years. Signs of eighth nerve dysfunction (deafness, tinnitus, or imbalance) are the most common presenting symptoms in adults, but occur in only a minority of paediatric patients (71). In younger patients, presenting signs include cranial nerve dysfunction, peripheral nerve dysfunction, myelopathy, seizures, skin tumours, café-au-lait macules, and juvenile cataracts (72).

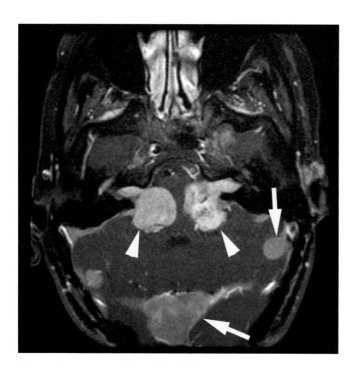

Fig. 15.4 Post-contrast axial MRI of the skull base in a patient with NF2 reveals bilateral vestibular schwannomas (arrowheads) extending out of the internal auditory canals to compress the brainstem. Multiple meningiomas are present in the posterior fossa (arrows).

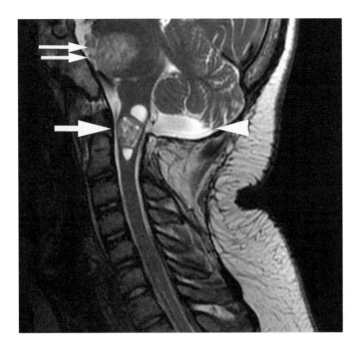

Fig. 15.6 Post-contrast sagittal MRI scan of the cervical spine in a patient with NF2 reveals an ependymoma (single arrow) at the cervicomedullary junction with cystic components superior and inferior to the solid tumour. The patient required suboccipital craniectomy for progressive symptoms (arrowhead). Note the presence of a large vestibular schwannoma (double arrows).

Diagnostic criteria

Clinical criteria for the diagnosis of NF2 were first formulated at the NIH Consensus Conference on NF1 and NF2 in 1987 and revised in 1991 (28, 73). By NIH criteria, a diagnosis of NF2 is based on either (i) the presence of bilateral vestibular schwannomas or (ii) a family history of NF2 and either a unilateral vestibular schwannoma or any two other tumours typically associated with NF2 (28, 73). Thus, only patients with bilateral vestibular schwannomas or a family history can qualify for a diagnosis under NIH criteria. Patients who do not fulfil these criteria but have multiple features associated with NF2 represent a diagnostic dilemma. For this reason, revised criteria were proposed by the Manchester group in 1992 and by the National Neurofibromatosis Foundation (NNFF) in 1997. The relative merits of these criteria continue to be debated by researchers and while all three diagnostic criteria identify the majority of patients with NF2, there remains difficulty in diagnosing some sporadic patients who present without bilateral vestibular schwannomas (74). There is also now some overlap with LZTR1 schwannomatosis which can present with unilateral vestibular schwannomas and other schwannomas fulfilling Manchester criteria (75). Indeed, even the presence of bilateral vestibular schwannoma in older patients with no other NF2 features may occur by chance alone (76).

Imaging and monitoring

Initial evaluation of patients who have or are at risk for NF2 should include testing to confirm a diagnosis and to identify potential problems such as hearing loss, visual loss, myelopathy, or gait problems. A medical history should include questions about auditory and vestibular function, focal neurological symptoms, skin tumours, seizures, headache, and visual symptoms. A family history should explore unexplained neurological and audiological symptoms in all first-degree relatives. MRI scanning of the brain should include contrast and axial and coronal thin cuts through the brainstem to identify vestibular schwannomas. A MRI scan of the spine with contrast should be performed given the predisposition to spinal ependymomas. Ophthalmological examination serves to identify characteristic lesions such as lens opacities, retinal hamartomas, or epiretinal membranes. A complete neurological examination serves as a baseline for future comparison and may assist in the selection of sites within the nervous system that require further imaging studies. Audiology (including pure tone threshold and word recognition) documents eighth cranial nerve dysfunction related to vestibular schwannomas and sets a baseline for future comparisons.

After initial diagnosis, patients should be evaluated relatively frequently (every 3–6 months) until the growth rate and biological behaviour of the tumour is determined. Consultation with an experienced surgeon after initial diagnosis is often helpful for pre-symptomatic patients (i.e. those with adequate hearing) to discuss the risks and benefits of hearing-sparing surgery. After the initial evaluation period most patients without acute problems can be followed on an annual basis. Evaluation at these visits should include a complete neurological examination, an MRI scan of the brain with contrast and thin cuts (≤3 mm) through the brainstem, MRI scans with contrast of symptomatic lesions outside the brain (if present), and audiology testing. Ophthalmological evaluation should be performed in selected patients with visual impairment or facial weakness. Yearly audiology exams serve to document changes in pure tone threshold and word recognition. This information can be helpful in planning early surgical intervention for vestibular schwannomas and for counselling patients regarding possible deafness. The frequency with which routine spinal imaging is obtained varies, but is clearly indicated in patients with new or progressive symptoms referable to the spinal cord. Patients with dysphonia or dysphagia should undergo evaluation of lower cranial nerve function with direct laryngoscopy and swallow evaluation. These evaluations are particularly important since lower cranial nerve dysfunction contributes to mortality in NF2 (7).

Management

The approach to management of NF2-associated tumours differs from that of sporadic tumours. The surgical removal of every lesion is not possible or advisable and the primary goal is to preserve function and maximize quality of life.

Vestibular schwannomas

Surgery is the mainstay of treatment of NF2-related tumours. Surgery is clearly indicated for patients with significant brainstem or spinal cord compression or with obstructive hydrocephalus. In patients with little or no neurological dysfunction related to their tumours, watchful waiting may allow patients to retain neurological function for many years (77). Facial weakness and laryngeal weakness are common complications of surgery for vestibular schwannomas. Treatment of these complications with facial reanimation and laryngoplasty can significantly improve quality of life for these patients.

Indications for surgical resection of other tumours are less defined. In general, schwannomas of other cranial nerves are slow growing and produce few symptoms. Surgical resection in these patients should be reserved for those with unacceptable neurological symptoms or rapid tumour growth. With demonstrated tumour growth, surgery may be indicated to prevent neurological deficit rather than delaying surgery until deficit occurs.

Radiation is often used as adjuvant therapy for treatment of sporadic brain tumours, but treatment outcomes for patients with NF2-related vestibular schwannomas are worse than for patients with sporadic tumours (78). Most clinicians prefer surgical extirpation of tumours when possible and reserve radiation treatment for tumours that are not surgically accessible or for those that progress after surgery. This practice is based on the experience that radiation therapy makes subsequent resection of vestibular schwannomas and function of auditory brainstem implants more difficult (79). In addition, there are reports of malignant transformation of NF2-associated schwannomas after radiation treatment and indirect evidence of increased numbers of malignancy in NF2 patients who have received radiation (80, 81). More recently, fractionated stereotactic radiotherapy has been advocated to minimize the risk of hearing loss after radiation. The actuarial 5-year local control rate using this technique is 93% with a hearing-preservation rate of 64% (82).

More recently, a number of targeted agents have been studied in patients with NF2 and progressive vestibular schwannoma. Despite preclinical evidence suggesting that the EGFR and ERBB2 pathways are important for schwannoma formation, clinical studies with erlotinib (an EGFR inhibitor) and lapatinib (an EGFR/ERBB2 inhibitor) have been disappointing (83, 84). Similarly, a small study of everolimus, an mTOR inhibitor, did not reveal any radiographic responses in NF2 patients with progressive vestibular schwannoma (85). However, there is mounting evidence that treatment with bevacizumab, an anti-vascular endothelial growth factor (VEGF) antibody, can produce durable hearing and radiographic responses in these patients (86). In a prospective, multi-institutional phase II study of NF2 patients with progressive vestibular schwannomas, 36% of patients experienced confirmed hearing improvement and no patients experienced hearing decline (87). A radiographic response was noted in 43% of target vestibular schwannomas.

Meningiomas

NF2 patients may have multiple meningiomas, and resection of all lesions in these patients is often not advisable. The benefit of surgery must be carefully weighed against potential complications. As a general rule, indications for resection include rapid tumour growth and worsening neurological symptoms or signs. Intervention for spinal cord tumours is necessary in a minority of patients (69). Surgery is more often required in patients with extramedullary tumours like meningiomas or schwannomas (59%) than for intramedullary tumours (12%) (70). The role of adjuvant radiation in other tumours such as meningiomas and ependymomas is not established but the majority of these tumours demonstrate benign histology and can be controlled surgically. No case series have been published on radiation therapy for NF2-related meningiomas.

Schwannomatosis and rhabdoid tumour predisposition

Definition

Schwannomatosis (OMIM #162091) and rhabdoid tumour predisposition (OMIM #609322) are discussed together since there is genetic and phenotypic overlap between these conditions. Schwannomatosis is characterized by the predisposition to develop multiple schwannomas and, less commonly, meningiomas. This is clinically distinguished from the predisposition to renal and extra-renal rhabdoid tumours, including atypical teratoid/rhabdoid tumours (AT/RTs) of the central nervous system (CNS) that develop in childhood (88, 89).

Epidemiology

Schwannomatosis was observed to be as be as prevalent as NF2 in a small Finnish study, but was only one-third of the NF2 incidence (1 in 33,000) in a larger UK-based study (90). The true prevalence of schwannomatosis is likely higher given the difficulty in case ascertainment. Unlike patients with NF1 who have characteristic dermatological findings and patients with NF2 who have eighth cranial nerve dysfunction at a young age, patients with schwannomatosis have non-specific symptoms that may not lead to medical evaluation. Familial schwannomatosis accounts for 15% of cases and is transmitted in autosomal dominant fashion with incomplete penetrance. Sporadic schwannomatosis accounts for the remaining 85% of patients, who have clinically unaffected parents.

Rhabdoid tumours account for approximately 1–2% of paediatric brain tumours. Twenty-five to thirty-five per cent of patients with rhabdoid tumours have a germline alteration of a rhabdoid tumour-associated gene that predisposes them to the development of AT/RTs, renal rhabdoid tumours, and less frequently, extra-renal rhabdoid tumours. The overall survival of patients with AT/RTs has increased from 16% to 40% in limited institution studies with the use of very aggressive therapeutic strategies (91).

Aetiology/genetics

Germline mutations or deletions in *SMARCB1* are identified in 40–50% of kindreds affected by familial schwannomatosis, in 10% of sporadic schwannomatosis patients, in one-third of patients with rhabdoid tumours, and in virtually all patients with multiple primary rhabdoid tumours, or rhabdoid tumour with a family history of schwannomatosis or rhabdoid tumour (92, 93). Germline alterations in rhabdoid tumour patients tend to be truncating (frameshift/nonsense) mutations in the central exons, or deletions or duplications of one or more exons, leading to complete knockout of the *SMARCB1* gene (94, 95). In tumours, this is coupled with a somatic loss of the second allele, leading to biallelic inactivation of *SMARCB1*. In contrast, inherited mutations found in familial schwannomatosis are more likely to be non-truncating (missense or splice-site) mutations which predominate at either end of the gene (96, 97), which might account for the milder phenotype as compared to rhabdoid tumour cases, as these mutations are potentially hypomorphic. However, sporadic schwannomatosis patients may carry truncating (frameshift or nonsense) or non-truncating (missense/splice-site) mutations (98, 99), which are predicted to knock out the protein product. Schwannomatosis-associated *SMARCB1* mutations are more frequent at either end of the gene whereas mutations associated with the inherited predisposition to rhabdoid tumours are more centrally located. It is possible that the specific combination of resulting somatic mutations, including the frequent co-mutation of the *NF2* gene in tumours from schwannomatosis patients (96, 97), may regulate the severity of the resulting phenotype.

In 2013, a second schwannomatosis gene, *LZTR1*, was found to be the cause of a high proportion of *SMARCB1*-negative schwannomatosis cases with NF2 loss in their tumours (100). LZTR1-related schwannomatosis has more overlap with NF2 with a likely 10–15% risk of developing vestibular schwannoma (75). Mutations in a second rhabdoid tumour locus, *SMARCA4* (*BRG1*) (101), also a component of the SWI/SNF complex, has been reported in a small number of patients.

Clinical testing for *SMARCB1* mutations is now recommended as standard of care for patients with rhabdoid tumours. For schwannomatosis patients, clinical testing for *SMARCB1* and *LZTR1* mutations is available.

Pathogenesis

SMARCB1 (also called *hSNF5, INI1*, and *BAF47*) and *SMARCA4* are subunits of the SWI/SNF complex, an ATP-dependent chromatin remodelling complex (101–105). SMARCB1 exerts its tumour suppressor function by regulating the cell cycle and inducing senescence (106, 107). In addition to regulating cell cycle, SMARCB1 and the SWI/SNF components regulate lineage specific gene expression and embryonic stem cell programming. SMARCB1 and SWI/SNF complexes have been shown to be involved in the control of neurogenesis, myogenesis, adipogenesis, osteogenesis, and haematopoiesis (108–113). *LZTR1* mutations have been identified in several cancers, and the gene functions as a tumour suppressor in glioblastoma where biallelic mutations have been reported (100). The LZTR1 protein belongs to the BTB/POZ superfamily and is involved in multiple cellular processes including regulation of chromatin conformation and the cell cycle (100).

Clinical presentation

Patients with schwannomatosis most commonly develop symptoms in the second or third decade of life but a formal diagnosis is usually delayed by approximately 10 years (114). Patients typically come to medical attention with complaints of pain (46%), a mass (27%), or both (11%). Indeed, pain is the most frequent symptom reported by patients, with 68% of patients experiencing chronic pain. Schwannomas commonly affect the spine (74%) and peripheral nerves (89%) but cranial nerve schwannomas (mostly trigeminal) are uncommon (8%). Neurological dysfunction related to schwannomas is uncommon and, when present, is often a complication of surgery. Anatomically limited disease, presumably due to genetic mosaicism, is seen in about 30% of patients.

In contrast to patients with NF2, vestibular schwannomas are rare particularly in *SMARCB1* schwannomatosis and the presence of a vestibular schwannoma in a patient with schwannomatosis should raise concern for an alternative diagnosis (e.g. mosaic NF2) (92). Until recently, the presence of a vestibular schwannoma excluded a diagnosis of schwannomatosis but a patient with a germline *SMARCB1* mutation has been described (115) and five with *LZTR1* mutations met NF2 criteria (75). Meningiomas occur in approximately 5% of schwannomatosis patients (114) and have a predilection for the cerebral falx (116). Families with multigenerational meningiomas and *SMARCB1* germline mutations have been reported (116, 117).

Patients with a genetic predisposition to rhabdoid tumour typically come to clinical attention by their initial diagnosis of a CNS, renal, or extra-renal malignancy, confirmed by the identification of a germline *SMARCB1* or *SMARCA4* mutation or deletion.

Patients with a chromosome 22q11.2 deletion syndrome that includes *SMARCB1* are also at increased risk for rhabdoid tumours (118, 119).

Diagnostic criteria

The diagnostic criteria for schwannomatosis were revised in 2013 (92) and incorporate both molecular and clinical features. A *molecular diagnosis* of schwannomatosis is confirmed by either (i) two or more pathologically proven schwannomas or meningiomas *and* genetic studies of at least two tumours with loss of heterozygosity (LOH) for chromosome 22 and two different *NF2* mutations—if there is a common *SMARCB1* mutation, this defines *SMARCB1*-associated schwannomatosis; or (ii) one pathologically proven schwannoma or meningioma *and* a germline *SMARCB1* pathogenic mutation. A *clinical diagnosis* of schwannomatosis is confirmed by either (i) two or more non-intradermal schwannomas, one with pathological confirmation, including no bilateral vestibular schwannoma on brain MRI (detailed, contrast-enhanced study of the internal auditory canals with slices no more than 3 mm thick); or (ii) one pathologically confirmed schwannoma or intracranial meningioma *and* an affected first-degree relative. Clinicians should consider schwannomatosis as a possible diagnosis if a patient has two or more non-intradermal nerve sheath tumours but none pathologically proven to be a schwannoma; the occurrence of chronic pain in association with the tumour(s) increases the likelihood of schwannomatosis. Patients cannot fulfil the diagnosis for schwannomatosis if they have a germline pathogenic *NF2* mutation, fulfil diagnostic criteria for NF2, have a first-degree relative with NF2, or have schwannomas limited to a previous radiation field. Despite the detailed formulation of these criteria, some mosaic NF2 patients will be misdiagnosed with schwannomatosis at a young age, and some schwannomatosis patients will be misdiagnosed as having unilateral vestibular schwannomas (rarely) or multiple meningiomas. Mosaic NF2 can be excluded by identifying different *NF2* mutations in separate schwannomas from the same patient.

The genetic predisposition to rhabdoid tumour is a molecular diagnosis based on the identification of a germline mutation or deletion of *SMARCB1* or *SMARCA4* in the context of an affected individual or family member with a primary rhabdoid tumour. It should be noted that other types of brain tumours may also be observed in association with *SMARCB1* mutations, but the incidence of germline *SMARCB1* mutations is unknown based on the small number of cases reported to date.

Imaging and monitoring

Initial evaluation of patients who have or are at risk for schwannomatosis should include testing to confirm a diagnosis (usually by excluding NF1 and NF2) and to identify potential problems such as weakness, pain, or myelopathy. A medical history should include questions about auditory and vestibular function, focal neurological symptoms, skin tumours or hyperpigmented lesions, seizures, headache, and visual symptoms. A family history should explore unexplained neurological, dermatological, and audiological symptoms in all first-degree relatives. A contrast-enhanced MRI scan of the brain with attention to the internal auditory canals (with slices no more than 3 mm thick) should be performed to exclude vestibular schwannomas. MRI scans of other body parts should be obtained based on the history and clinical exam. A combination of

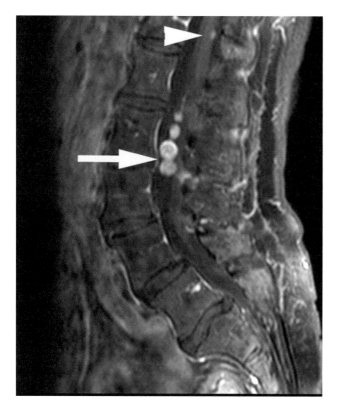

Fig. 15.7 Axial FLAIR MRI sequence demonstrating multiple peripheral schwannomas in a patient with schwannomatosis.

MRI scanning and pathological analysis is used to establish a diagnosis of schwannomatosis.

The radiographic appearance of schwannomatosis is characterized by multiple, discrete lesions along peripheral or spinal nerves (Fig. 15.7). Pathologically, schwannomas in patients with schwannomatosis resemble those from patients with NF2 and sporadic lesions. Although no single feature can reliably distinguish schwannomatosis-associated schwannomas, they tend to have more peritumoural oedema in the adjacent nerve, intratumoural myxoid changes, and intraneural growth patterns versus other schwannomas (120).

Patients at risk for rhabdoid tumour should have baseline contrast-enhanced brain and spine MRI scans and abdominal ultrasound to rule out the presence of a renal rhabdoid tumour. While frequent scans are recommended during the first several years of life for an infant with a germline *SMARCB1* alteration, the recommended intervals are not yet established. The tumours have an extremely rapid growth rate, and may cause clinical symptoms over the course of months.

Management

Schwannomas
Management of patients with schwannomatosis is primarily symptom oriented. As noted earlier, pain is the hallmark of this disorder. Surgery should be reserved for patients with symptomatic tumours or rapidly expanding lesions in the spinal cord. Surgery is the treatment of choice for symptomatic schwannomas and, in many patients, can relieve local pain or symptoms arising from compression of neighbouring tissues. The major risk of surgery is secondary

nerve injury and hence, surgeons experienced with nerve-sparing surgery should be involved when considering a schwannoma resection.

Experience with radiation therapy for management of schwannomatosis-related schwannomas is limited. Over the past two decades, there has been increasing experience with stereotactic radiation for sporadic vestibular schwannomas and spinal schwannomas (121, 122). Early results suggest that this modality is safe and effective for individuals without an underlying tumour suppressor syndrome. However, there is a theoretical possibility that radiation treatment could increase the risk for malignant transformation in patients with schwannomatosis, as has been reported for NF1 and NF2 (123). To date, there are no available data on the risk of secondary malignant transformation of tumours in schwannomatosis patients. At this time, most experts reserve the use of radiation for patients who require treatment for enlarging schwannomas that cannot be treated with surgery. The role of chemotherapy for symptomatic (i.e. painful) schwannomas remains unclear, although bevacizumab may be effective in some individuals.

Most patients require pain medication; these patients may benefit from referral to a comprehensive pain clinic with experience in managing neuropathic pain. Chronic pain is common in patients with schwannomatosis (114). The aetiology of pain in schwannomatosis is unclear: there is no clear relationship between tumour number, size, location, and the intensity of pain, and the pain has both neuropathic and nociceptive features. Perhaps for this reason, there is no consensus approach for treating pain in these patients.

CNS atypical teratoid/rhabdoid tumours
Currently, there are no National Comprehensive Cancer Network (NCCN) guidelines for treatment of AT/RTs, but therapy typically involves maximal safe surgical resection followed by chemotherapy with or without stem cell rescue and radiation. The prognosis is generally poor. In a registry review of 42 patients, the median overall survival was 16.75 months (124). A subset of patients (~25%) had prolonged survival; many of these patients were treated with radiation therapy, chemotherapy, and stem cell rescue (124). For this reason, prospective studies using intensive, multimodality therapy are under way. One study demonstrated 40% overall survival with intensive chemotherapy, although the morbidity associated with this treatment was high.

Li–Fraumeni syndrome

Definition
Li–Fraumeni syndrome is an autosomal dominant tumour disorder that predisposes to early onset of multiple specific neurological and non-neurological cancers and very high lifetime cumulative cancer risk.

Epidemiology
The true incidence of LFS is difficult to ascertain but it is thought to affect about 1 in 5000–20,000 individuals (125). The occurrence of multiple cancers, especially in a young person, should prompt consideration of LFS. *De novo* mutations in *TP53* are uncommon (<20% of cases), and a high index of suspicion is necessary to diagnose LFS in patients with little or no family history of cancer (126).

The penetrance of cancer is high in LFS patients. The cumulative risk of cancer in patients with a germline *TP53* may be up to

40% before the age of 20, and is greater than 80% by age 70 (127, 128). The mean age at diagnosis of first tumour is 24.9 years (128). Cancer penetrance is also more pronounced in women than in men, where the lifetime risk is 90% versus 70% (125). The excess number of cancers in *TP53*-positive females is primarily due to the sex-specific breast cancers in this group. Women also have an earlier average age of onset of cancer than men (29 vs 40 years, respectively) (129), with many breast cancers occurring age less than 30 years where mutations are as common as with the *BRCA2* gene (125).

Aetiology/genetics

Li–Fraumeni syndrome 1 (LFS1, OMIM #151623) is caused by germline mutations in the *TP53* tumour suppressor gene, which accounts for 56–83% of individuals with LFS (125, 130). The majority of gene alterations correspond to point mutations or small deletions or insertions which are widely distributed between exons 3–11; a small percentage represent genomic rearrangements (131). Missense mutations, particularly in the DNA core binding domain, are associated with an earlier age at tumour onset (131) but no strong genotype–phenotype correlations exist.

Germline mutations in the checkpoint kinase gene, *CHEK2*, have been identified in a small percentage of *TP53*-negative families (132, 133). The CHEK2 protein causes cell cycle arrest in response to DNA damage. However, several subsequent analyses of LFS families have not confirmed an underlying role for *CHEK2* (134).

Pathogenesis

The encoded protein of the *TP53* gene (p53) is one of the major proteins that control genome integrity in the context of DNA damage, hypoxia, and other stressors. *TP53* activation results in cell cycle arrest, senescence, and apoptosis.

Clinical presentation

Sarcomas and premenopausal breast cancer are the most frequent cancers associated with LFS, although approximately 13% of LFS kindreds with *TP53* mutations develop CNS tumours (128, 135). In a study of 738 evaluable cancers in 185 affected patients or kindreds, 70 were brain tumours making it the fourth most common cancer in these patients (136). Of brain tumours with reported histology, about 44–70% are of astrocytic origin, 30% are choroid plexus carcinomas, and 17% are medulloblastomas or primitive neuroectodermal tumours (128, 137). The age distribution of patients with brain tumours is bimodal, with a peak during childhood and a smaller peak in the third to fourth decade of life (137). The majority of brain tumours occur in children with a mean age of diagnosis of 16 years (138). Choroid plexus carcinoma is uncommon in LFS but patients with this tumour should be referred for genetic counselling regardless of family cancer history since choroid plexus carcinoma is strongly associated with germline *TP53* mutations (125).

Diagnostic criteria

Multiple diagnostic criteria exist for LFS including classic LFS criteria, Li–Fraumeni-like syndrome criteria (LFL), and Chompret criteria (138). In the 'classic' definition, LFS is confirmed when all three criteria are fulfilled: (i) a proband diagnosed with sarcoma before 45 years of age, (ii) a first-degree relative with cancer before 45 years of age, and (iii) another first- or second-degree relative

with any cancer diagnosed under 45 years of age or with sarcoma at any age (125). The sensitivity and specificity for germline *TP53* mutations vary among the criteria, and *TP53* mutation detection rates among families meeting classic LFS, LFL, and Chompret criteria are 56–83%, 30–40%, and 30% respectively (131, 138–140).

Imaging and monitoring

Surveillance protocols for LFS patients have been proposed to detect asymptomatic cancers at an early stage. Preliminary results from a small, non-randomized study suggest that active surveillance using non-invasive biochemical screening and imaging may reduce mortality through early detection and therapeutic intervention (141). The patients with the greatest benefit from this protocol appear to be children with malignant brain tumours who benefit from early detection followed by resection.

Treatment

Treatment of brain tumours associated with LFS is similar to that for sporadic tumours, although LFS patients should also be monitored for the development of secondary malignancies following administration of DNA-damaging treatments such as ionizing radiation or most chemotherapeutics (43).

Gorlin syndrome (nevoid/basal cell carcinoma syndrome)

Definition

Gorlin syndrome (GS), also called nevoid basal cell carcinoma syndrome (NBCCS), is an autosomal dominant disorder that predisposes to multiple basal cell carcinomas, jaw cysts, partial absence of the stratum corneum on the hands and feet (palmar/plantar pits), dural calcifications, rib abnormalities, medulloblastoma, and meningioma.

Epidemiology

The estimated prevalence of Gorlin syndrome is 1 in 30,000–164,000 (5, 142, 143) and the estimated birth incidence is 1 in 15,000 (5). The frequency of new mutations in the absence of a family history is about 50%. Life expectancy of patients with Gorlin syndrome is slightly reduced compared with the local population in England (73.4 vs 80 years) (7).

Genetics

Gorlin syndrome is linked to germline mutations of the human homolog of the *Drosophila melanogaster Patched* gene (*PTCH*) on chromosome 9q (144). Exon scanning of the *PTCH* gene of 106 unrelated pedigrees submitted to a DNA diagnostics laboratory identified mutations in 47 kindreds (44%). Pedigrees with only a single feature of GS, including patients with multiple basal cell carcinomas, did not have mutations in *PTCH*.

Pathogenesis

The protein product of *PTCH* is a transmembrane receptor for the secreted ligand sonic hedgehog (SHH) which is essential for cerebellar development. In the absence of SHH, PTCH exists as an inactive form in association with the transmembrane receptor smoothened (SMO). Binding of SHH to PTCH releases the inhibition of SMO and allows it to transduce freely within the SHH signalling pathway. The majority of *PTCH* mutations result in a truncated protein product with resultant unregulated activation of this pathway (145).

Clinical features

Most patients with GS are diagnosed on the basis of compatible clinical findings, including two major or one major and two minor criteria (146). The lifetime risk for developing medulloblastomas in GS is about 3–5%; conversely, GS is identified in 1–2% of patients with medulloblastomas (147). However, in reality the risks are about 1–2% for medulloblastoma in PTCH-related GS and up to 30% in SUFU-related GS (148). Gorlin syndrome-related medulloblastomas tend to occur at an earlier age than their sporadic counterparts, and medulloblastomas may often represent the initial tumour manifestation of GS (147). Medulloblastomas in GS patients are most commonly classified as desmoplastic (149), particularly in infants. Dural calcifications and meningioma are found in up to 70% and 5% of patients with GS, respectively (150). Less commonly, astrocytoma, oligodendroglioma, and craniopharyngioma are diagnosed in patients with GS.

Diagnostic criteria

A diagnosis of GS is confirmed when two major or one major and two minor criteria are fulfilled (149). The major criteria include: (i) more than two or one basal cell carcinoma diagnosed in patients younger than 20 years; (ii) odontogenic keratocyst of the jaw proven by histology; (iii) three or more palmar or plantar pits; (iv) bilamellar calcification of the falx cerebri; (v) bifid, fused, or markedly splayed ribs; or (vi) first-degree relative with NBCCS. The minor criteria include: (i) macrocephaly determined after adjustment for height; (ii) congenital malformations: cleft lip or palate, frontal bossing, 'coarse face', moderate or severe hypertelorism; (iii) other skeletal abnormalities: Sprengel deformity, marked pectus deformity, marked syndactyly of the digits; (iv) radiological abnormalities: bridging of the sella turcica, vertebral anomalies such as hemivertebrae, fusion, or elongation of the vertebral bodies, modelling defects of the hands and feet, and flame-shaped lucencies of the hands or feet; (v) ovarian fibroma; and (vi) medulloblastoma.

Imaging and monitoring

Consensus guidelines for surveillance of patients with GS have not been established. However, some authorities recommend a neurological examination every 6 months in order to detect deficits related to a medulloblastoma (146). At 3 years of age, the frequency of examinations may be reduced to once a year until 7 years of age, after which a medulloblastoma is very unlikely. Routine MRI screening of asymptomatic individuals has not been studied but is not considered routine for all individuals with GS, except perhaps those with *SUFU* mutations (149).

Management

Management of patients with GS-associated medulloblastomas is similar to that for sporadic tumours. However, careful consideration should be given to radiation planning due to the predisposition for radiation-induced tumours (151). Some experts recommend deferral of radiation for patients with desmoplastic medulloblastoma given the increased risk of secondary tumours. Some, but not all

reports, suggest GS-associated medulloblastomas are associated with a better prognosis than sporadic medulloblastomas (152).

Future treatment of both sporadic medulloblastomas as well as those associated with GS may include the use of small molecule inhibitors of the SHH pathway. These molecules have been tested in preclinical murine models (153) and vismodegib has been approved for treatment of advanced basal cell carcinoma (154).

Turcot syndrome

Definition

Turcot syndrome refers to the rare association of brain tumours and colorectal polyposis/adenocarcinoma. Two forms of hereditary colorectal cancer have been established, including familial adenomatous polyposis (FAP) and hereditary nonpolyposis colorectal cancer (HNPCC), now known as Lynch syndrome (LS). As such, the syndrome may represent an extreme form of the risk spectrum in these dominantly inherited conditions and not a family-specific diagnosis. More recently described recessive forms of LS with congenital mismatch repair deficiency may be a better fit for the originally described family with a very high risk of CNS malignancy and polyps/colorectal cancer.

Epidemiology

The estimated prevalence of FAP in the Danish population is 1 in 31,260, and the estimated birth incidence is 1 in 7021 (155). The frequency of new mutations in the absence of a family history is about 20–25% (156). The prevalence of HNPCC is more difficult to estimate but the proportion of all colorectal cancers due to this condition is around 2.2%. In the Danish HNPCC Registry, primary CNS tumours were identified in 14% of families (157). The median age of diagnosis was 42 years; the most common tumour type was glioblastoma (56%) followed by astrocytoma (22%) and oligodendroglioma (9%). The cumulative risk of brain tumour by age 70 was 2.5% for *MSH2* carriers, 0.8% for *MSH6* carriers, and 0.5% for *MLH1* carriers (157).

Aetiology/genetics

The complex molecular basis for Turcot syndrome was first reported in 1995 (158). Tumours in patients with FAP result from mutations in the *APC* gene on chromosome 5 while HNPCC-related tumours result from mutations in a series of DNA-mismatch repair (MMR) genes. The majority of affected HNPCC families have mutations in the *MSH2* and *MLH1* genes, but additional mutations have also been described in other MMR genes including *PMS1*, *PMS2*, and *MSH6* (158).

Rarely, patients with biallelic inactivation of MMR genes have been reported. This autosomal recessive tumour syndrome is termed brain tumour-polyposis syndrome 1 and is characterized by early-onset malignancies, including glioblastoma. Interestingly, these patients may demonstrate an NF1-type phenotype with multiple cafe-au-lait macules and skinfold freckling.

Pathogenesis

The primary mechanism by which mutations in the *APC* gene are believed to result in tumourigenesis is through disruption of the WNT signalling pathway, a pathway that is also commonly disrupted in sporadic colorectal cancers and medulloblastomas.

Germline mutations in MMR genes result in the characteristic finding of microsatellite instability, a consequence of failure to repair mismatched nucleotides during DNA replication and subsequent misalignment of DNA strands (158). Such mutations have been identified as a cause of sporadic high-grade gliomas in young individuals (159).

Clinical presentation

FAP is characterized by the development of hundreds to thousands of polyps in the colon and rectum during adolescence. Although these polyps are benign, progression to malignancy typically occurs by the age of 35–40 years. The absolute risk of an individual with FAP developing a brain tumour is low, but the relative risk is significantly elevated compared to the general population (158, 160). Pooled data on families with FAP indicate that medulloblastomas are the most common type of brain tumour (60%), followed by astrocytomas (14%), and ependymoma (10%). In contrast, patients with HNPCC usually develop fewer adenomatous polyps, but they are typically larger and more likely to represent adenocarcinomas. Affected patients have an increased incidence of extra-colonic malignancies, including glioblastoma.

Diagnostic criteria

Turcot syndrome is typically diagnosed clinically in patients with a primary CNS tumour and evidence of colorectal polyposis. In practice, genetic studies are recommended to differentiate mutations in MMR genes (Turcot syndrome type 1) from *APC* mutations (Turcot syndrome, type 2), a distinction that is most relevant in affected patients with attenuated forms of FAP and fewer adenomatous polyps.

Imaging and monitoring

Although Turcot syndrome is a rare disorder, patients with either FAP or HNPCC who develop neurological symptoms must be thoroughly evaluated for the presence of an underlying CNS tumour, including contrast-enhanced brain MRI scanning.

Treatment

No NCCN guidelines exist for treating CNS tumours related to Turcot syndrome. Treatment of brain tumours in this population is similar to that for sporadic tumours; however, treatment with DNA-damaging agents such as ionizing radiation should be used with caution due to the increased risk of secondary malignancies.

Cowden syndrome

Definition

Cowden syndrome (CS) is an autosomal dominant disorder characterized by the presence of hamartomas in multiple organ systems, including the CNS, as well as an increased predisposition for cancers of the breast, thyroid, and endometrium. Within the CNS, the pathognomonic feature is the presence of Lhermitte–Duclos disease (LDD), although other associations include megencephaly, heterotopias, seizures, vascular abnormalities, and mental retardation.

Epidemiology

While the incidence of the disorder has been estimated at 1 in 200,000 (161), this likely represents an underestimate given the variable expression of CS and often subtle cutaneous signs.

Genetics

In 1996, the genetic basis for CS was identified as a germline mutation in the *PTEN* gene on chromosome 10 (161). Diagnostic criteria for Cowden disease were proposed by an international consortium of researchers in 1996 before identification of the CS gene (162). In early studies, *PTEN* mutations were identified in approximately 80% of patients fulfilling these criteria (163). More recent data suggests that the detection rate of *PTEN* mutations using these criteria is around 60% and that germline mutations can be identified in about 40% of patients who do not fulfil these criteria (164). For this reason, updated criteria have been suggested that increase the specificity of the diagnosis (164).

Pathogenesis

The product of the *PTEN* gene is a phosphatase that inhibits signal transduction within the PI3K/AKT pathway that regulates important processes including cellular growth, migration, differentiation, and apoptosis. Mutations in *PTEN* also lead to increased activation of the downstream target mTOR, and increased activation of AKT and mTOR have been demonstrated in immunohistochemical analyses from the majority of adult-onset LDD patients. Conversely, samples from patients with childhood LDD reveal normal levels of PTEN activity and germline *PTEN* mutations are not observed, and childhood LDD is not considered a manifestation of CS (165, 166).

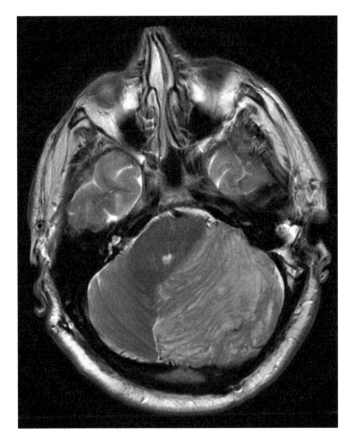

Fig. 15.8 Axial T2-weighted MRI of the cerebellum of a patient with Cowden syndrome showing Lhermitte–Duclos syndrome (cerebellar gangliocytoma).

Clinical presentation

The primary neuro-oncological manifestation of Cowden disease is LDD—a space-occupying lesion of the cerebellar cortex that most commonly presents as headaches, nausea, vomiting, and ataxia. Secondary obstructive hydrocephalus may result in obstruction of the fourth ventricle. Histologically, LDD is characterized by the replacement and expansion of the internal granular layer of the cerebellum with hypertrophic neurons, as well as loss of Purkinje cells and increased myelination within the molecular layer (166). The hamartomatous nature of LDD is suggested by the absence of mitoses, atypia, or proliferation within pathological specimens from affected patients.

LDD is typically identified in the third or fourth decade of life. The prevalence of LDD in Cowden disease is difficult to estimate since most asymptomatic patients are not imaged. Estimates of the prevalence range from 2% to 15% in clinical and research series (167–169). Adult-onset LDD appears to have a stronger association with germline PTEN mutations than does paediatric-onset LDD, and adult-onset LDD is no longer considered pathognomonic for Cowden disease (164).

Imaging and monitoring

Although the definitive diagnosis of LDD is made histopathologically, the unique features of LDD allow for an accurate diagnosis to be made by radiographic imaging. MRI reveals a well-circumscribed, non-enhancing lesion resulting in enlargement of the cerebellar folia (Fig. 15.8). T2-hyperintensity is typically present and the involved cerebellar cortex has a striated, laminated appearance often described as 'tiger-striped' (170).

Consensus guidelines for surveillance of patients with CS have not been published. Routine neurological examination should be performed in order to detect any deficit related to LDD. Routine MRI screening of asymptomatic individuals has not been studied but is not considered standard for all individuals with CS.

Management

Although LDD represents a benign lesion, it frequently demonstrates progressive enlargement and resection is considered the only effective method of treatment. Recurrences are not uncommon, most likely due to difficulty in identifying distinct borders between the normal and affected cerebellum during surgery (166). Symptoms from LDD result from hypertrophy of individual cells rather than cellular proliferation, and concordantly, radiation therapy has not been effective in achieving regression of these lesions. Demonstration of increased mTOR activity within LDD samples suggests that inhibitors of the mTOR pathway may be effective.

References

1. Knudson AG, Jr. Mutation and cancer: statistical study of retinoblastoma. *Proc Natl Acad Sci U S A* 1971; 68(4):820–823.

2. Teplick A, Kowalski M, Biegel JA, et al. Educational paper: screening in cancer predisposition syndromes: guidelines for the general pediatrician. *Eur J Pediatr* 2011; 170(3):285–294.

3. Friedman JM. Epidemiology of neurofibromatosis type 1. *Am J Med Genet* 1999; 89(1):1–6.

4. Lammert M, Friedman JM, Kluwe L, et al. Prevalence of neurofibromatosis 1 in German children at elementary school enrollment. *Arch Dermatol* 2005; 141(1):71–74.

5. Evans DG, Howard E, Giblin C, et al. Birth incidence and prevalence of tumor-prone syndromes: estimates from a UK family genetic register service. *Am J Med Genet A* 2010; 152A(2):327–332.

6. Uusitalo E, Leppävirta J, Koffert A, Suominen S, Vahtera J, Vahlberg T, Pöyhönen M, Peltonen J, Peltonen S. Incidence and mortality of neurofibromatosis: a total population study in Finland. *J Invest Dermatol* 2015; 135(3):904–906.

7. Wilding A, Ingham SL, Lalloo F, et al. Life expectancy in hereditary cancer predisposing diseases: an observational study. *J Med Genet* 2012; 49(4):264–269.

8. Messiaen LM, Callens T, Mortier G, et al. Exhaustive mutation analysis of the NF1 gene allows identification of 95% of mutations and reveals a high frequency of unusual splicing defects. *Hum Mutat* 2000; 15(6):541–555.

9. Evans DG, Bowers N, Burkitt-Wright E, et al. Comprehensive RNA analysis of the NF1 gene in classically affected NF1 affected individuals meeting NIH criteria has high sensitivity and mutation negative testing is reassuring in isolated cases with pigmentary features only. *eBioMedicine* 2016;7:212–220.

10. Cnossen MH, van der Est MN, Breuning MH, et al. Deletions spanning the neurofibromatosis type 1 gene: implications for genotype-phenotype correlations in neurofibromatosis type 1? *Hum Mutat* 1997; 9(5):458–464.

11. Kehrer-Sawatzki H, Kluwe L, Funsterer C, et al. Extensively high load of internal tumors determined by whole body MRI scanning in a patient with neurofibromatosis type 1 and a non-LCR-mediated 2-Mb deletion in 17q11.2. *Hum Genet* 2005; 116(6):466–475.

12. Douglas J, Cilliers D, Coleman K, et al. Mutations in RNF135, a gene within the NF1 microdeletion region, cause phenotypic abnormalities including overgrowth. *Nat Genet* 2007; 39(8):963–965.

13. Upadhyaya M, Huson SM, Davies M, et al. An absence of cutaneous neurofibromas associated with a 3-bp inframe deletion in exon 17 of the NF1 gene (c.2970-2972 delAAT): evidence of a clinically significant NF1 genotype-phenotype correlation. *Am J Hum Genet* 2007; 80(1):140–151.

14. Brems H, Chmara M, Sahbatou M, et al. Germline loss-of-function mutations in SPRED1 cause a neurofibromatosis 1-like phenotype. *Nat Genet* 2007; 39(9):1120–1126.

15. Messiaen L, Yao S, Brems H, et al. Clinical and mutational spectrum of neurofibromatosis type 1-like syndrome. *JAMA* 2009; 302(19):2111–2118.

16. Maertens O, De SS, Vandesompele J, et al. Molecular dissection of isolated disease features in mosaic neurofibromatosis type 1. *Am J Hum Genet* 2007; 81(2):243–251.

17. Ruggieri M, Huson SM. The clinical and diagnostic implications of mosaicism in the neurofibromatoses. *Neurology* 2001; 56(11):1433–1443.

18. Serra E, Puig S, Otero D, et al. Confirmation of a double-hit model for the NF1 gene in benign neurofibromas. *Am J Hum Genet* 1997; 61(3):512–519.

19. Gutmann DH, Donahoe J, Brown T, et al. Loss of neurofibromatosis 1 (NF1) gene expression in NF1-associated pilocytic astrocytomas. *Neuropathol Appl Neurobiol* 2000; 26(4):361–367.

20. Zhu Y, Ghosh P, Charnay P, et al. Neurofibromas in NF1: Schwann cell origin and role of tumor environment. *Science* 2002; 296(5569):920–922.

21. Serra E, Rosenbaum T, Winner U, et al. Schwann cells harbor the somatic NF1 mutation in neurofibromas: evidence of two different Schwann cell subpopulations. *Hum Mol Genet* 2000; 9(20):3055–3064.

22. Bajenaru ML, Zhu Y, Hedrick NM, et al. Astrocyte-specific inactivation of the neurofibromatosis 1 gene (NF1) is insufficient for astrocytoma formation. *Mol Cell Biol* 2002; 22(14):5100–5113.

23. Jacks T, Shih TS, Schmitt EM, et al. Tumour predisposition in mice heterozygous for a targeted mutation in Nf1. *Nat Genet* 1994; 7(3):353–361.

24. DeBella K, Szudek J, Friedman JM. Use of the national institutes of health criteria for diagnosis of neurofibromatosis 1 in children. *Pediatrics* 2000; 105(3 Pt 1):608–614.

25. Evans DG, Baser ME, McGaughran J, et al. Malignant peripheral nerve sheath tumours in neurofibromatosis 1. *J Med Genet* 2002; 39(5):311–314.

26. Duong TA, Sbidian E, Valeyrie-Allanore L, et al. Mortality associated with neurofibromatosis 1: a cohort study of 1895 patients in 1980-2006 in France. *Orphanet J Rare Dis* 2011; 6:18.

27. Evans DG, O'Hara C, Wilding A, et al. Mortality in neurofibromatosis 1: in North West England: an assessment of actuarial survival in a region of the UK since 1989. *Eur J Hum Genet* 2011; 19(11):1187–1191.

28. NIH Consensus Conference. Neurofibromatosis. Conference statement. National Institutes of Health Consensus Development Conference. *Arch Neurol* 1988; 45(5):575–578.

29. Woodruff JM. Pathology of tumors of the peripheral nerve sheath in type 1 neurofibromatosis. *Am J Med Genet* 1999; 89(1):23–30.

30. Thakkar SD, Feigen U, Mautner VF. Spinal tumours in neurofibromatosis type 1: an MRI study of frequency, multiplicity and variety. *Neuroradiology* 1999; 41(9):625–629.

31. Carli M, Ferrari A, Mattke A, et al. Pediatric malignant peripheral nerve sheath tumor: the Italian and German soft tissue sarcoma cooperative group. *J Clin Oncol* 2005; 23(33):8422–8430.

32. Uusitalo E, Rantanen M, Kallionpää RA, et al. Distinctive cancer associations in patients with neurofibromatosis type 1. *J Clin Oncol* 2016; 34(17):1978–1986.

33. Ferner RE, Golding JF, Smith M, et al. [18F]2-fluoro-2-deoxy-D-glucose positron emission tomography (FDG PET) as a diagnostic tool for neurofibromatosis 1 (NF1) associated malignant peripheral nerve sheath tumours (MPNSTs): a long-term clinical study. *Ann Oncol* 2008; 19(2):390–394.

34. Guillamo JS, Creange A, Kalifa C, et al. Prognostic factors of CNS tumours in Neurofibromatosis 1 (NF1): a retrospective study of 104 patients. *Brain* 2003; 126(Pt 1):152–160.

35. Listernick R, Ferner RE, Liu GT, et al. Optic pathway gliomas in neurofibromatosis-1: Controversies and recommendations. *Ann Neurol* 2007; 61(3):189–198.

36. Gutmann DH, Rasmussen SA, Wolkenstein P, et al. Gliomas presenting after age 10 in individuals with neurofibromatosis type 1 (NF1). *Neurology* 2002; 59(5):759–761.

37. Huttner AJ, Kieran MW, Yao X, et al. Clinicopathologic study of glioblastoma in children with neurofibromatosis type 1. *Pediatr Blood Cancer* 2010; 54(7):890–896.

38. Tonsgard JH, Kwak SM, Short MP, et al. CT imaging in adults with neurofibromatosis-1: frequent asymptomatic plexiform lesions. *Neurology* 1998; 50(6):1755–1760.

39. Plotkin SR, Bredella MA, Cai W, et al. Quantitative assessment of whole-body tumor burden in adult patients with neurofibromatosis. *PLoS One* 2012; 7(4):e35711.

40. Cai W, Kassarjian A, Bredella MA, et al. Tumor burden in patients with neurofibromatosis types 1 and 2 and schwannomatosis: determination on whole-body MR images. *Radiology* 2009; 250(3):665–673.

41. Listernick R, Louis DN, Packer RJ, et al. Optic pathway gliomas in children with neurofibromatosis 1: consensus statement from the NF1 Optic Pathway Glioma Task Force. *Ann Neurol* 1997; 41(2):143–149.

42. Fisher MJ, Avery RA, Allen JC, et al. Functional outcome measures for NF1-associated optic pathway glioma clinical trials. *Neurology* 2013; 81(21 Suppl 1):S15–S24.

43. Evans DGR, Birch JM, Ramsden RT, et al. Malignant transformation and new primary tumours after therapeutic radiation for benign disease: substantial risks in certain tumour prone syndromes. *J Med Genet* 2006; 43(4):289–294.

44. Plotkin SR, Blakeley JO, Dombi E, et al. Achieving consensus for clinical trials: the REiNS International Collaboration. *Neurology* 2013; 81(21 Suppl 1):S1–S5.

45. Weiss B, Widemann BC, Wolters P, et al. Sirolimus for progressive neurofibromatosis type 1-associated plexiform neurofibromas: a neurofibromatosis Clinical Trials Consortium phase II study. *Neuro Oncol* 2015; 17(4):596–603.

46. Weiss B, Widemann BC, Wolters P, et al. Sirolimus for non-progressive NF1-associated plexiform neurofibromas: an NF clinical trials consortium phase II study. *Pediatr Blood Cancer* 2014; 61(6):982–986.

47. Ullrich NJ, Robertson R, Kinnamon DD, et al. Moyamoya following cranial irradiation for primary brain tumors in children. *Neurology* 2007; 68(12):932–938.

48. Sharif S, Ferner R, Birch JM, et al. Second primary tumors in neurofibromatosis 1 patients treated for optic glioma: substantial risks after radiotherapy. *J Clin Oncol* 2006; 24(16):2570–2575.

49. Dasgupta B, Yi Y, Chen DY, et al. Proteomic analysis reveals hyperactivation of the mammalian target of rapamycin pathway in neurofibromatosis 1-associated human and mouse brain tumors. *Cancer Res* 2005; 65(7):2755–2760.

50. Evans DG, Moran A, King A, et al. Incidence of vestibular schwannoma and neurofibromatosis 2 in the North West of England over a 10-year period: higher incidence than previously thought. *Otol Neurotol* 2005; 26(1):93–97.

51. Hexter A, Jones A, Joe H, et al. Clinical and molecular predictors of mortality in neurofibromatosis 2: a UK national analysis of 1192 patients. *J Med Genet* 2015; 52(10):699–705.

52. Wallace AJ, Watson CJ, Oward E, et al. Mutation scanning of the NF2 gene: an improved service based on meta-PCR/sequencing, dosage analysis, and loss of heterozygosity analysis. *Genet Test* 2004; 8(4):368–380.

53. Evans DG, Ramsden RT, Shenton A, et al. Mosaicism in neurofibromatosis type 2: an update of risk based on uni/bilaterality of vestibular schwannoma at presentation and sensitive mutation analysis including multiple ligation-dependent probe amplification. *J Med Genet* 2007; 44(7):424–428.

54. Ahronowitz I, Xin W, Kiely R, et al. Mutational spectrum of the NF2 gene: a meta-analysis of 12 years of research and diagnostic laboratory findings. *Hum Mutat* 2007; 28(1):1–12.

55. Baser ME, Kuramoto L, Woods R, et al. The location of constitutional neurofibromatosis 2 (NF2) splice site mutations is associated with the severity of NF2. *J Med Genet* 2005; 42(7):540–546.

56. MacCollin M, Braverman N, Viskochil D, et al. A point mutation associated with a severe phenotype of neurofibromatosis 2. *Ann Neurol* 1996; 40(3):440–445.

57. Ruttledge MH, Andermann AA, Phelan CM, et al. Type of mutation in the neurofibromatosis type 2 gene (NF2) frequently determines severity of disease. *Am J Hum Genet* 1996; 59(2):331–342.

58. Kluwe L, Friedrich RE, Tatagiba M, et al. Presymptomatic diagnosis for children of sporadic neurofibromatosis 2 patients: a method based on tumor analysis. *Genet Med* 2002; 4(1):27–30.

59. Rouleau GA, Wertelecki W, Haines JL, et al. Genetic linkage of bilateral acoustic neurofibromatosis to a DNA marker on chromosome 22. *Nature* 1987; 329(6136):246–248.

60. Wertelecki W, Rouleau GA, Superneau DW, et al. Neurofibromatosis 2: clinical and DNA linkage studies of a large kindred. *N Engl J Med* 1988; 319(5):278–283.

61. Trofatter JA, MacCollin MM, Rutter JL, et al. A novel moesin-, ezrin-, radixin-like gene is a candidate for the neurofibromatosis 2 tumor suppressor. *Cell* 1993; 75(4):826.

62. Rouleau GA, Merel P, Lutchman M, et al. Alteration in a new gene encoding a putative membrane-organizing protein causes neuro-fibromatosis type 2. *Nature* 1993; 363(6429):515–521.

63. McClatchey AI, Giovannini M. Membrane organization and tumorigenesis--the NF2 tumor suppressor, Merlin. *Genes Dev* 2005; 19(19):2265–2277.

64. Jacoby LB, MacCollin M, Barone R, et al. Frequency and distribution of NF2 mutations in schwannomas. *Genes Chromosomes Cancer* 1996; 17(1):45–55.

65. Wellenreuther R, Kraus JA, Lenartz D, et al. Analysis of the neurofibromatosis 2 gene reveals molecular variants of meningioma. *Am J Pathol* 1995; 146(4):827–832.

66. Li W, You L, Cooper J, et al. Merlin/NF2 suppresses tumorigenesis by inhibiting the E3 ubiquitin ligase CRL4(DCAF1) in the nucleus. *Cell* 2010; 140(4):477–490.

67. Smith MJ, Higgs JE, Bowers NL, et al. Cranial meningiomas in 411 neurofibromatosis type 2 (NF2) patients with proven gene mutations: clear positional effect of mutations, but absence of female severity effect on age at onset. *J Med Genet* 2011; 48(4):261–265.

68. Goutagny S, Bah AB, Henin D, et al. Long-term follow-up of 287 meningiomas in neurofibromatosis type 2 patients: clinical, radiological, and molecular features. *Neuro Oncol* 2012; 14(8):1090–1096.

69. Mautner VF, Tatagiba M, Lindenau M, et al. Spinal tumors in patients with neurofibromatosis type 2: MR imaging study of frequency, multiplicity, and variety. *AJR Am J Roentgenol* 1995; 165(4):951–955.

70. Patronas NJ, Courcoutsakis N, Bromley CM, et al. Intramedullary and spinal canal tumors in patients with neurofibromatosis 2: MR imaging findings and correlation with genotype. *Radiology* 2001; 218(2):434–442.

71. Nunes F, MacCollin M. Neurofibromatosis 2 in the pediatric population. *J Child Neurol* 2003; 18(10):718–724.

72. Ruggieri M, Iannetti P, Polizzi A, et al. Earliest clinical manifestations and natural history of neurofibromatosis type 2 (NF2) in childhood: a study of 24 patients. *Neuropediatrics* 2005; 36(1):21–34.

73. Mulvihill JJ, Parry DM, Sherman JL, et al. NIH conference. Neurofibromatosis 1 (Recklinghausen disease) and neurofibromatosis 2 (bilateral acoustic neurofibromatosis). An update. *Ann Intern Med* 1990; 113(1):39–52.

74. Baser ME, Friedman JM, Wallace AJ, et al. Evaluation of clinical diagnostic criteria for neurofibromatosis 2. *Neurology* 2002; 59(11):1759–1765.

75. Smith MJ, Bulman M, Gokhale C, et al. Revisiting neurofibromatosis type 2 diagnostic criteria to exclude LZTR1 related schwannomatosis. *Neurology* 2017; 88(1):87–92.

76. Evans DG, Freeman S, Gokhale C, et al. Bilateral vestibular schwannomas in older patients: NF2 or chance? *J Med Genet* 2015; 52:422–425.

77. Liu R, Fagan P. Facial nerve schwannoma: surgical excision versus conservative management. *Ann Otol Rhinol Laryngol* 2001; 110(11):1025–1029.

78. Fuss M, Debus J, Lohr F, et al. Conventionally fractionated stereotactic radiotherapy (FSRT) for acoustic neuromas. *Int J Radiat Oncol Biol Phys* 2000; 48(5):1381–1387.

79. Slattery WH, III, Brackmann DE. Results of surgery following stereotactic irradiation for acoustic neuromas. *Am J Otol* 1995; 16(3):315–319.

80. Baser ME, Evans DG, Jackler RK, et al. Neurofibromatosis 2, radiosurgery and malignant nervous system tumours. *Br J Cancer* 2000; 82(4):998.

81. Thomsen J, Mirz F, Wetke R, et al. Intracranial sarcoma in a patient with neurofibromatosis type 2 treated with gamma knife radiosurgery for vestibular schwannoma. *Am J Otol* 2000; 21(3):364–370.

82. Combs SE, Volk S, Schulz-Ertner D, et al. Management of acoustic neuromas with fractionated stereotactic radiotherapy (FSRT): long-term results in 106 patients treated in a single institution. *Int J Radiat Oncol Biol Phys* 2005; 63(1):75–81.

83. Plotkin SR, Halpin C, McKenna MJ, et al. Treatment of progressive neurofibromatosis type 2-related vestibular schwannoma with erlotinib. *J Clin Oncol* 2008; 15(Suppl pt I):100s.

84. Karajannis MA, Legault G, Hagiwara M, et al. Phase II trial of lapatinib in adult and pediatric patients with neurofibromatosis type 2 and progressive vestibular schwannomas. *Neuro Oncol* 2012; 14(9):1163–1170.

85. Karajannis MA, Legault G, Hagiwara M, et al. Phase II study of everolimus in children and adults with neurofibromatosis type 2 and progressive vestibular schwannomas. *Neuro Oncol* 2014; 16(2):292–297.

86. Plotkin SR, Merker VL, Halpin C, et al. Bevacizumab for progressive vestibular schwannoma in neurofibromatosis type 2: a retrospective review of 31 patients. *Otol Neurotol* 2012; 33(6):1046–1052.

87. Blakeley JO, Ye X, Duda DG, et al. Efficacy and biomarker study of bevacizumab for hearing loss resulting from neurofibromatosis type 2-associated vestibular schwannomas. *J Clin Oncol* 2016; 34(14):1669–1675.

88. Hulsebos TJ, Plomp AS, Wolterman RA, et al. Germline mutation of INI1/SMARCB1 in familial schwannomatosis. *Am J Hum Genet* 2007; 80(4):805–810.

89. Versteege I, Sevenet N, Lange J, et al. Truncating mutations of hSNF5/INI1 in aggressive paediatric cancer. *Nature* 1998; 394(6689):203–206.

90. Antinheimo J, Sankila R, Carpen O, et al. Population-based analysis of sporadic and type 2 neurofibromatosis-associated meningiomas and schwannomas. *Neurology* 2000; 54(1):71–76.

91. Chi SN, Zimmerman MA, Yao X, et al. Intensive multimodality treatment for children with newly diagnosed CNS atypical teratoid rhabdoid tumor 3. *J Clin Oncol* 2009; 27(3):385–389.

92. Plotkin SR, Blakeley JO, Evans DG, et al. Update from the 2011 International Schwannomatosis Workshop: From genetics to diagnostic criteria. *Am J Med Genet A* 2013; 161A(3):405–416.

93. Bruggers CS, Bleyl SB, Pysher T, et al. Clinicopathologic comparison of familial versus sporadic atypical teratoid/rhabdoid tumors (AT/RT) of the central nervous system 1. *Pediatr Blood Cancer* 2011; 56(7):1026–1031.

94. Bourdeaut F, Lequin D, Brugieres L, et al. Frequent hSNF5/INI1 Germline mutations in patients with rhabdoid tumor. *Clin Cancer Res* 2011; 17(1):31–38.

95. Eaton KW, Tooke LS, Wainwright LM, et al. Spectrum of SMARCB1/INI1 Mutations in Familial and Sporadic Rhabdoid Tumors. *Pediatr Blood Cancer* 2011; 56:7–15.

96. Boyd C, Smith MJ, Kluwe L, et al. Alterations in the SMARCB1 (INI1) tumor suppressor gene in familial schwannomatosis. *Clin Genet* 2008; 74(4):358–366.

97. Hadfield KD, Newman WG, Bowers NL, et al. Molecular characterisation of SMARCB1 and NF2 in familial and sporadic schwannomatosis. *J Med Genet* 2008; 45(6):332–339.

98. Rousseau G, Noguchi T, Bourdon V, et al. SMARCB1/INI1 germline mutations contribute to 10% of sporadic schwannomatosis. *BMC Neurol* 2011; 11:9.

99. Smith MJ, Wallace AJ, Bowers NL, et al. Frequency of SMARCB1 mutations in familial and sporadic schwannomatosis. *Neurogenetics* 2012; 13(2):141–145.

100. Piotrowski A, Xie J, Liu YF, et al. Germline loss-of-function mutations in LZTR1 predispose to an inherited disorder of multiple schwannomas 1. *Nat Genet* 2014; 46(2):182–187.

101. Schneppenheim R, Fruhwald MC, Gesk S, et al. Germline nonsense mutation and somatic inactivation of SMARCA4/BRG1 in a family with rhabdoid tumor predisposition syndrome 1. *Am J Hum Genet* 2010; 86(2):279–284.

102. Martens JA, Winston F. Recent advances in understanding chromatin remodeling by Swi/Snf complexes. *Curr Opin Genet Dev* 2003; 13(2):136–142.

103. Narlikar GJ, Fan HY, Kingston RE. Cooperation between complexes that regulate chromatin structure and transcription. *Cell* 2002; 108(4):475–487.

104. Wang W, Cote J, Xue Y, et al. Purification and biochemical heterogeneity of the mammalian SWI-SNF complex. *EMBO J* 1996; 15:5370–5382.

105. Wang W, Xue Y, Zhou S, et al. Diversity and specialization of mammalian SWI/SNF complexes. *Genes Dev* 1996; 10:2117–2130.

106. Kalpana GV, Smith ME. Development of targeted therapies for rhabdoid tumors based on the functions of INI1/hSNF5 tumor suppressor. In: Arceci B, Houghton P (eds) *Molecularly Targeted Therapies for Pediatric Tumors*. Springer Verlag, 2009; 305–330.

107. Wilson BG, Roberts CW. SWI/SNF nucleosome remodellers and cancer. *Nat Rev Cancer* 2011; 11(7):481–492.

108. Krosl J, Mamo A, Chagraoui J, et al. A mutant allele of the Swi/Snf member BAF250a determines the pool size of fetal liver hemopoietic stem cell populations. *Blood* 2010; 116(10):1678–1684.

109. Yoo AS, Crabtree GR. ATP-dependent chromatin remodeling in neural development. *Curr Opin Neurobiol* 2009; 19(2):120–126.

110. Albini S, Puri PL. SWI/SNF complexes, chromatin remodeling and skeletal myogenesis: it's time to exchange! *Exp Cell Res* 2010; 316(18):3073–3080.

111. Caramel J, Medjkane S, Quignon F, et al. The requirement for SNF5/INI1 in adipocyte differentiation highlights new features of malignant rhabdoid tumors. *Oncogene* 2008; 27(14):2035–2044.

112. Nowak SJ, Aihara H, Gonzalez K, et al. Akirin links twist-regulated transcription with the Brahma chromatin remodeling complex during embryogenesis. *PLoS Genet* 2012; 2012:e1002547.

113. Young DW, Pratap J, Javed A, et al. SWI/SNF chromatin remodeling complex is obligatory for BMP2-induced, Runx2-dependent skeletal gene expression that controls osteoblast differentiation. *J Cell Biochem* 2005; 94(4):720–730.

114. Merker VL, Esparza S, Smith MJ, et al. Clinical features of schwannomatosis: a retrospective analysis of 87 patients. *Oncologist* 2012; 17(10):1317–1322.

115. Smith MJ, Kulkarni A, Rustad C, et al. Vestibular schwannomas occur in schwannomatosis and should not be considered an exclusion criterion for clinical diagnosis. *Am J Med Genet A* 2012; 158A(1):215–219.

116. van den Munckhof P, Christiaans I, Kenter SB, et al. Germline SMARCB1 mutation predisposes to multiple meningiomas and schwannomas with preferential location of cranial meningiomas at the falx cerebri. *Neurogenetics* 2012; 13(1):1–7.

117. Bacci C, Sestini R, Provenzano A, et al. Schwannomatosis associated with multiple meningiomas due to a familial SMARCB1 mutation. *Neurogenetics* 2010; 11(1):73–80.

118. Eaton KW, Tooke LS, Wainwright LM, et al. Spectrum of SMARCB1/INI1 mutations in familial and sporadic rhabdoid tumors. *Pediatr Blood Cancer* 2011; 56(1):7–15.

119. Jackson EM, Shaikh TH, Gururangan S, et al. High-density single nucleotide polymorphism array analysis in patients with germline deletions of 22q11.2 and malignant rhabdoid tumor 1. *Hum Genet* 2007; 122(2):117–127.

120. MacCollin M, Chiocca EA, Evans DG, et al. Diagnostic criteria for schwannomatosis. *Neurology* 2005; 64(11):1838–1845.

121. Gerszten PC, Quader M, Novotny J, et al. Radiosurgery for benign tumors of the spine: clinical experience and current trends. *Technol Cancer Res Treat* 2012; 11(2):133–139.

122. Niranjan A, Mathieu D, Flickinger JC, et al. Hearing preservation after intracanalicular vestibular schwannoma radiosurgery. *Neurosurgery* 2008; 63(6):1054–1062.

123. Evans DG, Birch JM, Ramsden RT, et al. Malignant transformation and new primary tumours after therapeutic radiation for benign disease: substantial risks in certain tumour prone syndromes. *J Med Genet* 2006; 43(4):289–294.

124. Hilden JM, Meerbaum S, Burger P, et al. Central nervous system atypical teratoid/rhabdoid tumor: results of therapy in children enrolled in a registry. *J Clin Oncol* 2004; 22(14):2877–2884.

125. Gonzalez KD, Noltner KA, Buzin CH, et al. Beyond Li Fraumeni syndrome: clinical characteristics of families with p53 germline mutations. *J Clin Oncol* 2009; 27(8):1250–1256.

126. Gonzalez KD, Buzin CH, Noltner KA, et al. High frequency of de novo mutations in Li-Fraumeni syndrome. *J Med Genet* 2009; 46(10):689–693.

127. Wu CC, Strong LC, Shete S. Effects of measured susceptibility genes on cancer risk in family studies. *Hum Genet* 2010; 127(3):349–357.

128. Bougeard G, Renaux-Petel M, Flaman JM, et al. Revisiting Li-Fraumeni syndrome from TP53 mutation carriers. *J Clin Oncol* 2015; 33(21):2345–2352.

129. Hwang SJ, Lozano G, Amos CI, et al. Germline p53 mutations in a cohort with childhood sarcoma: sex differences in cancer risk. *Am J Hum Genet* 2003; 72(4):975–983.

130. Varley JM, McGown G, Thorncroft M, et al. Germ-line mutations of TP53 in Li-Fraumeni families: an extended study of 39 families. *Cancer Res* 1997; 57(15):3245–3252.

131. Bougeard G, Sesboue R, Baert-Desurmont S, et al. Molecular basis of the Li-Fraumeni syndrome: an update from the French LFS families. *J Med Genet* 2008; 45(8):535–538.

132. Bell DW, Varley JM, Szydlo TE, et al. Heterozygous germ line hCHK2 mutations in Li-Fraumeni syndrome. *Science* 1999; 286(5449):2528–2531.

133. Vahteristo P, Tamminen A, Karvinen P, et al. p53, CHK2, and CHK1 genes in Finnish families with Li-Fraumeni syndrome: further evidence of CHK2 in inherited cancer predisposition. *Cancer Res* 2001; 61(15):5718–5722.

134. Sodha N, Houlston RS, Bullock S, et al. Increasing evidence that germline mutations in CHEK2 do not cause Li-Fraumeni syndrome. *Hum Mutat* 2002; 20(6):460–462.

135. Olivier M, Goldgar DE, Sodha N, et al. Li-Fraumeni and related syndromes: correlation between tumor type, family structure, and TP53 genotype. *Cancer Res* 2003; 63(20):6643–6650.

136. Nichols KE, Malkin D, Garber JE, et al. Germ-line p53 mutations predispose to a wide spectrum of early-onset cancers. *Cancer Epidemiol Biomarkers Prev* 2001; 10(2):83–87.

137. Kleihues P, Schauble B, zur Hausen A, et al. Tumors associated with p53 germline mutations: a synopsis of 91 families. *Am J Pathol* 1997; 150(1):1–13.

138. Mai PL, Malkin D, Garber JE, et al. Li-Fraumeni syndrome: report of a clinical research workshop and creation of a research consortium. *Cancer Genet* 2012; 205(10):479–487.

139. Varley JM. Germline TP53 mutations and Li-Fraumeni syndrome. *Hum Mutat* 2003; 21(3):313–320.

140. Birch JM, Hartley AL, Tricker KJ, et al. Prevalence and diversity of constitutional mutations in the p53 gene among 21 Li-Fraumeni families. *Cancer Res* 1994; 54(5):1298–1304.

141. Villani A, Shore A, Wasserman JD, et al. Biochemical and imaging surveillance in TP53 mutation carriers with Li-Fraumeni syndrome: 11 year followup of a prospective observational study. *Lancet Oncology* 2016; 17(9):1295–1305.

142. Farndon PA, Del Mastro RG, Evans DG, et al. Location of gene for Gorlin syndrome. *Lancet* 1992; 339(8793):581–582.

143. Shanley S, Ratcliffe J, Hockey A, et al. Nevoid basal cell carcinoma syndrome: review of 118 affected individuals. *Am J Med Genet* 1994; 50(3):282–290.

144. Hahn H, Wicking C, Zaphiropoulous PG, et al. Mutations of the human homolog of Drosophila patched in the nevoid basal cell carcinoma syndrome. *Cell* 1996; 85(6):841–851.

145. Wicking C, Shanley S, Smyth I, et al. Most germ-line mutations in the nevoid basal cell carcinoma syndrome lead to a premature termination of the PATCHED protein, and no genotype-phenotype correlations are evident. *Am J Hum Genet* 1997; 60(1):21–26.

146. Evans DG, Ladusans EJ, Rimmer S, et al. Complications of the naevoid basal cell carcinoma syndrome: results of a population based study. *J Med Genet* 1993; 30(6):460–464.

147. Evans DG, Farndon PA, Burnell LD, et al. The incidence of Gorlin syndrome in 173 consecutive cases of medulloblastoma. *Br J Cancer* 1991; 64(5):959–961.

148. Smith MJ, Beetz C, Williams SG, et al. Germline mutations in SUFU cause Gorlin syndrome-associated childhood medulloblastoma and redefine the risk associated with PTCH1 mutations. *J Clin Oncol* 2014; 32(36):4155–4161.

149. Amlashi SF, Riffaud L, Brassier G, et al. Nevoid basal cell carcinoma syndrome: relation with desmoplastic medulloblastoma in infancy. A population-based study and review of the literature. *Cancer* 2003; 98(3):618–624.

150. Kimonis VE, Goldstein AM, Pastakia B, et al. Clinical manifestations in 105 persons with nevoid basal cell carcinoma syndrome. *Am J Med Genet* 1997; 69(3):299–308.

151. Choudry Q, Patel HC, Gurusinghe NT, et al. Radiation-induced brain tumours in nevoid basal cell carcinoma syndrome: implications for treatment and surveillance. *Childs Nerv Syst* 2007; 23(1):133–136.

152. Lacombe D, Chateil JF, Fontan D, et al. Medulloblastoma in the nevoid basal-cell carcinoma syndrome: case reports and review of the literature. *Genet Couns* 1990; 1(3–4):273–277.

153. Romer JT, Kimura H, Magdaleno S, et al. Suppression of the Shh pathway using a small molecule inhibitor eliminates medulloblastoma in Ptc1(+/-)p53(-/-) mice. *Cancer Cell* 2004; 6(3):229–240.

154. Tang JY, Mackay-Wiggan JM, Aszterbaum M, et al. Inhibiting the hedgehog pathway in patients with the basal-cell nevus syndrome 1. *N Engl J Med* 2012; 366(23):2180–2188.

155. Bulow S, Faurschou NT, Bulow C, et al. The incidence rate of familial adenomatous polyposis. Results from the Danish Polyposis Register 2. *Int J Colorectal Dis* 1996; 11(2):88–91.

156. Bisgaard ML, Fenger K, Bulow S, et al. Familial adenomatous polyposis (FAP): frequency, penetrance, and mutation rate 1. *Hum Mutat* 1994; 3(2):121–125.

157. Therkildsen C, Ladelund S, Rambech E, et al. Glioblastomas, astrocytomas and oligodendrogliomas linked to Lynch syndrome. *Eur J Neurol* 2015; 22(4):717–724.

158. Hamilton SR, Liu B, Parsons RE, et al. The molecular basis of Turcot's syndrome. *N Engl J Med* 1995; 332(13):839–847.

159. Leung SY, Chan TL, Chung LP, et al. Microsatellite instability and mutation of DNA mismatch repair genes in gliomas. *Am J Pathol* 1998; 153(4):1181–1188.

160. Attard TM, Giglio P, Koppula S, et al. Brain tumors in individuals with familial adenomatous polyposis: a cancer registry experience and pooled case report analysis. *Cancer* 2007; 109(4):761–766.

161. Nelen MR, Kremer H, Konings IB, et al. Novel PTEN mutations in patients with Cowden disease: absence of clear genotype-phenotype correlations. *Eur J Hum Genet* 1999; 7(3):267–273.

162. Nelen MR, Padberg GW, Peeters EA, et al. Localization of the gene for Cowden disease to chromosome 10q22–23. *Nat Genet* 1996; 13(1):114–116.

163. Marsh DJ, Coulon V, Lunetta KL, et al. Mutation spectrum and genotype-phenotype analyses in Cowden disease and Bannayan-Zonana syndrome, two hamartoma syndromes with germline PTEN mutation. *Hum Mol Genet* 1998; 7(3):507–515.

164. Pilarski R, Burt R, Kohlman W, et al. Cowden syndrome and the PTEN hamartoma tumor syndrome: systematic review and revised diagnostic criteria. *J Natl Cancer Inst* 2013; 105(21):1607–1616.

165. Zhou XP, Marsh DJ, Morrison CD, et al. Germline inactivation of PTEN and dysregulation of the phosphoinositol-3-kinase/Akt pathway cause human Lhermitte-Duclos disease in adults. *Am J Hum Genet* 2003; 73(5):1191–1198.

166. Abel TW, Baker SJ, Fraser MM, et al. Lhermitte-Duclos disease: a report of 31 cases with immunohistochemical analysis of the PTEN/AKT/mTOR pathway. *J Neuropathol Exp Neurol* 2005; 64(4):341–349.

167. Pilarski R, Stephens JA, Noss R, et al. Predicting PTEN mutations: an evaluation of Cowden syndrome and Bannayan-Riley-Ruvalcaba syndrome clinical features. *J Med Genet* 2011; 48(8):505–512.

168. Tan MH, Mester J, Peterson C, et al. A clinical scoring system for selection of patients for PTEN mutation testing is proposed on the basis of a prospective study of 3042 probands. *Am J Hum Genet* 2011; 88(1):42–56.

169. Riegert-Johnson DL, Gleeson FC, Roberts M, et al. Cancer and Lhermitte-Duclos disease are common in Cowden syndrome patients. *Hered Cancer Clin Pract* 2010; 8(1):6.

170. Kulkantrakorn K, Awwad EE, Levy B, et al. MRI in Lhermitte-Duclos disease. *Neurology* 1997; 48(3):725–731.

CHAPTER 16

Familial tumour syndromes: von Hippel–Lindau disease

Hiroshi Kanno and Joachim P. Steinbach

Definition

This chapter addresses von Hippel–Lindau (VHL) disease with haemangioblastoma as the primary manifestation affecting the nervous system as well as sporadic haemangioblastomas. Sporadic haemangioblastomas and those arising in association with von Hippel–Lindau disease are graded as grade I by the World Health Organization (WHO) classification (1).

Epidemiology

The incidence of VHL is estimated to be 1 in 36,000–43,000 live births and the prevalence to be 1 in 53,000–91,000 (2, 3). VHL is an autosomal dominant disorder with full penetrance and phenotypic variability within molecular subtypes of the condition (4, 5). The proportion of cases due to *de novo* mutation is around 20% (6). Life expectancy of patients with VHL is substantially reduced compared with the local population in England (52.5 vs 80 years) (7).

Pathology

Haemangioblastomas appear as circumscribed, highly vascularized tumours commonly associated with large cysts (1). Histologically, they are characterized by two distinct components: large and vacuolated stromal cells and abundant endothelial cells forming vascular structures. The stromal cells have been regarded to constitute the neoplastic component of the tumour and may display some degree of atypia, but usually show little proliferative activity (8). Recent data suggests that an embryological, developmentally arrested haemangioblast is the tumour cell of origin for VHL-associated haemangioblastomas (9). Intratumoural haemorrhage as well as reactive changes in the surrounding brain tissue such as gliosis and Rosenthal fibres are frequently observed (WHO classification, haemangioblastoma section). Stromal cells are negative for glial fibrillary acidic protein and endothelial cell markers. They commonly express vimentin, neuron-specific enolase, neural cell adhesion molecule, S-100, and other markers. In addition, they express high levels of vascular endothelial growth factor (VEGF), which is complemented by expression of vascular endothelial growth factor receptor (VEGFR)-2 and other receptors for angiogenic growth factors on the endothelial cell fraction. This loop is considered the key driver of vessel formation. VEGF secretion is also considered to contribute to peritumoural oedema.

Pathogenesis

Research into the pathogenesis of VHL has been instrumental for the definition of the canonical and widely conserved oxygen-sensing hypoxia-inducible factor (HIF) system. In summary, in the presence of oxygen, VHL protein serves to prevent the accumulation of HIF protein by targeting it to the proteasomal pathway. The mechanism includes hydroxylation of proline residues of the HIF protein by oxygen-dependent prolyl hydroxylase domain factors. These hydroxylated residues are necessary for the interaction with the beta-domain of VHL protein, which is part of an ubiquitin E3 ligase complex that targets HIF-alpha subunits to the ubiquitin–proteasome pathway. Biallelic inactivation of VHL thus blocks oxygen-dependent degradation of HIF-alpha and leads to constitutive activation of the HIF pathway although oxygen is present (10, 11). This may be referred to as pseudohypoxia and causes many biological changes that are normally observed in cells exposed to hypoxia and include prominent metabolic and proangiogenic responses. HIF then acts as a transcription factor promoting expression of several hundred target genes that are involved in angiogenesis, proliferation and survival, metabolism, and other processes enabling neoplastic growth. These include VEGF, platelet-derived growth factor, erythropoietin, and many others. The proangiogenic signals mediated mainly via VEGF and VEGFR have been considered the most important oncogenic capacities of VHL inactivation and are consistent with the angiogenic appearance of many tumour types in VHL syndrome. However, the metabolic reprogramming resulting from disinhibition of HIF signalling may be equally important, with altered metabolism recently having been recognized as one additional hallmark of cancer (12). It would appear that the uniform activation of HIF should result in true pathway addiction which may be exploited by therapies targeting VEGF/VEGFR. This has been moderately successful in renal cell cancer, but results in haemangioblastomas and other tumour of the VHL spectrum have been disappointing (see 'Clinical features'). One explanation for this is the HIF-independent effects of VHL deficiency which have more recently been recognized and which include effects on the regulation of extracellular matrix assembly and apoptosis (13, 14).

Clinical features

Central nervous system manifestation of VHL is haemangioblastoma, which is the most common manifestation of all VHL-associated lesions, found in 70–80% of VHL patients.

Haemangioblastoma is a WHO grade I benign tumour of uncertain cytogenesis that does not metastasize to remote organs, but it is associated with significant neurological morbidity and mortality based on its location and multiplicity. Since the management of VHL is complex, a deep understanding of the natural course of haemangioblastoma in VHL is needed (1). A diagnostic and therapeutic flowchart for this tumour is shown in Fig. 16.1 (15).

Approximately 25% of CNS haemangioblastomas are associated with VHL, with approximately 75% of them being sporadic. In VHL patients, 50–60% of haemangioblastomas are located in the cerebellum, 40–50% in the spinal cord, 10–20% in the brainstem, and 2–4% in the pituitary stalk. In the spinal cord, 30–50% are located in the thoracic segments, 40–50% in the cervical segments, and 10–20% in the lumbar segments (16, 17). CNS haemangioblastoma is the earliest or the second earliest manifestation of VHL patients, and the onset age of CNS haemangioblastoma ranges from 7 to 73 years, with the mean age being 29 years (17, 18). Signs and symptoms vary based on the anatomical tumour location, associated oedema and cyst, and tumour size. Usually, tumours that become symptomatic and require resection grow faster than asymptomatic ones (1). Patients with cerebellar haemangioblastomas can present with symptoms as a result of cerebellar impairment, and with those symptoms due to increased intracranial pressure. Those symptoms are mainly attributed not to the solid tumours themselves but to cyst enlargement. Patients with spinal haemangioblastomas can present with symptoms stemming from radiculopathy and with those owing to myelopathy. In addition, patients with brainstem haemangioblastomas can display symptoms mainly due to both lower cranial nerve impairment and high intracranial pressure. As mentioned previously, most symptoms caused by haemangioblastomas do not arise from the solid tumour itself but from the associated rapidly growing cyst or syrinx (16). Therefore, symptoms can occasionally develop rapidly, though usually they develop slowly. Previous large-scale studies on VHL patients have shown that haemangioblastomas have a sporadic growth pattern with periods of growth followed by growth arrest, that is, a saltatory growth pattern (16, 20–23). Patterns of growth vary and are categorized as saltatory (70–75% of growing tumours), linear (5–7%), or exponential (20–25%). Many tumours will remain the same size for several years (16). In one study, VHL patients were found to have a mean of 8.5 tumours/

patient (range, 1–33 tumours/patient) at initial evaluation. Mean tumour development was 0.4 new tumours/year and was correlated with age, with more frequent development in the younger patients (23). If located close to the ventricular system, these tumours can cause cerebrospinal fluid obstructions, which may be lethal. In rare cases, haemangioblastomas present by intraparenchymal or subarachnoid haemorrhage (1). Approximately 5% of patients develop polyglobulia, which can be cured by removing the solid tumour mass (1, 23). Performance status (PS) of VHL patients with CNS haemangioblastomas has been assessed according to the Eastern Cooperative Oncology Group performance status (ECOG PS).

This study result revealed that most patients have a low ECOG PS score (PS = 0, 1). The mean ECOG PS of patients with a single CNS haemangioblastoma was significantly lower than that of patients with multiple CNS haemangioblastomas (17).

Diagnostic strategy

Central nervous system haemangioblastoma in VHL disease is diagnosed according to symptoms and signs, past and family histories, neurological assessment, laboratory data, neuroradiological findings, pathological findings, and genetic testing.

Symptoms of patients with CNS haemangioblastomas, which vary based on the anatomical location, are shown in Table 16.1 (1). VHL-related past and/or family histories support the diagnosis of

Table 16.1 Symptoms based on anatomical location of tumours

Location	Percentage
Cerebellum	
Headache	77.0%
Gait ataxia	57.0%
Nausea/vomiting	19.0%
Vertigo	18.0%
Speech difficulties	15.0%
Dysmetria	11.0%
Spinal cord	
Paresthesia	75.7%
Pain	64.9%
Gait ataxia	35.1%
Dysesthesias	24.3%
Urinary/bowel abnormalities	18.9%
Brainstem	
Headache	83.3%
Singultus	66.6%
Nausea/vomiting	50.0%
Dysphagia	41.7%
Cough	25.0%
Paresthesia	25.0%

Reproduced from *J Transl Med Epidemiol.*, 2(1), Huntoon K, Lonser RR, Nervous system manifestations of von Hippel-Lindau disease, pp. 1015, Copyright (2014), JSciMed Central, reproduced under the Creative Commons License 4.0.

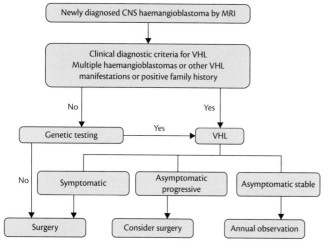

Fig. 16.1 Diagnostic and therapeutic flowchart for CNS haemangioblastoma.

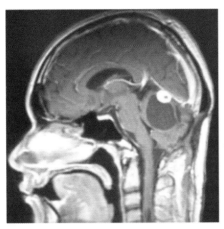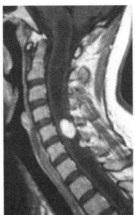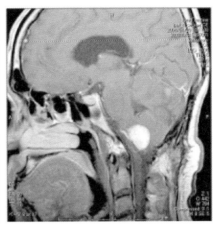

Fig. 16.2 Contrast-enhanced T1-weighed MRIs of CNS haemangioblastomas in VHL patients. Left, cerebellar haemangioblastoma associated with a cyst. Centre, multiple spinal cord haemangioblastomas. Right, brainstem haemangioblastoma.

CNS haemangioblastoma in VHL patients. Neurological assessment suggesting cerebellar, spinal, or brainstem lesions leads to a diagnosis of their lesions. In terms of laboratory data, patients bearing haemangioblastomas often show polycythemia as a result of erythropoietin secreted from haemangioblastoma cells, suggesting the presence of haemangioblastoma.

Regarding neuroradiological findings, haemangioblastomas are most often visualized by contrast-enhanced T1-weighted magnetic resonance imaging (MRI) (Fig. 16.2) or contrast enhanced computed tomography (CT). In post-contrast images, the tumour tissue appears as a homogenous, bright contrast-enhanced mass that clearly stands out from the surrounding tissue. T2-weighted or FLAIR MRI allows excellent quantification of oedema and peritumoural cysts, which appear as high-signal areas. Cyst walls of haemangioblastomas are not usually enhanced on MRI or CT. Angiography can be used to highlight the tumour staining, arteriovenous shunting, and early draining veins associated with these tumours prior to resection. Angiography is also performed for intended preoperative embolization in the case of large solid haemangioblastomas (15).

The pathohistological diagnosis of tumour tissue is the final diagnosis of haemangioblastoma. A haemangioblastoma is mainly composed of two different constituents, that is, stromal cells and vascular cells, of which the stromal cells represent the neoplastic component (24, 25). It has been suggested that these stromal cells are derived from haemangioblast progenitor cells (26, 27) and that the vascular cells represent reactive angiogenesis (28). Markers commonly positive in the stromal cells are commonly positive for various markers, including neuron-specific enolase, neural cell-adhesion molecule (CD56), and vimentin (27; whereas the vascular cells are commonly positive for CD34 and CD31 (2). Haemangioblastoma histologically mimics the clear cell type of renal cell carcinoma (RCC), but a differential diagnosis can be made.

Genetic testing to detect *VHL* gene mutations can be performed using a VHL patient's peripheral blood or tumour tissue. This testing can reveal *VHL* gene mutations in both peripheral blood (29) and tumour tissue in VHL patients, whereas it can detect such mutations in tumour tissue only in the case of sporadic haemangioblastoma (31). Germline *VHL* gene mutations,

spread diversely and producing three distinct cancer phenotypes, have been identified: (i) type 1, renal carcinoma without phaeochromocytoma; (ii) type 2A, renal carcinoma with phaeochromocytoma; and (iii) type 2B, phaeochromocytoma alone (30; Fig. 16.3).

In addition, VHL is diagnosed according to clinical diagnostic criteria (20). In the presence of a positive family history, VHL can be diagnosed clinically in a patient with at least one typical VHL tumour, such as retinal or CNS haemangioblastoma, RCC, phaeochromocytoma, or pancreatic tumour. Endolymphatic sac tumours and multiple pancreatic cysts suggest a positive carrier. In contrast, in patients with a negative family history of VHL-associated tumours, diagnosis of VHL can be made when such patients exhibit two or more CNS haemangioblastomas or a single haemangioblastoma in association with a visceral tumour such as RCC, phaeochromocytoma, or pancreatic tumour (19).

Therapeutic strategy

Using well-defined microsurgical techniques, the vast majority of haemangioblastomas in the CNS can be resected safely (21, 22). Because of the inability to accurately predict which tumours will become symptomatic and the sporadic growth patterns of tumours, surgical resection principally is better postponed until the tumours become symptomatic. This surgical management paradigm avoids unnecessary surgery and can be used to maintain neurological function in most patients (20, 22).

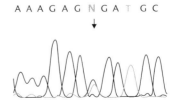

Fig. 16.3 Genetic testing of the *VHL* gene from blood of a VHL patient bearing a CNS haemangioblastoma. A germline mutation (Cys161Thr) is shown (arrow).

Surgical indication

In VHL patients, the therapeutic strategy of each haemangioblastoma has to be discussed individually with respect to the tumour location, tumour size or associated cysts, as well as symptoms and general condition of the patient, because most VHL patients will develop numerous haemangioblastomas growing at different rates and at several locations. Although the appropriate treatment strategies for haemangioblastomas are still a matter of debate, there is a general consensus that the symptomatic tumours should be treated (16, 31). Since these haemangioblastomas do not grow continuously at the same rate but with intermittent quiescent and rapid-growth phases, therapeutic strategies for asymptomatic tumours in VHL patients are controversial. Although asymptomatic tumours, which are stable in MRI screening, are recommended to be followed radiographically, those which imminently cause obstruction of the cerebrospinal fluid should be treated promptly. In the case of asymptomatic but progressive tumours, treatment strategies slightly differ in the literature. However, the majority of reports recommend early surgery (31, 32), since preoperative neurological symptoms are usually not reversible, and surgical resection can usually be performed with low morbidity.

Preoperative embolization

Preoperative embolization can be helpful in the case of large solid tumours to prevent intraoperative haemorrhage. Since this procedure is, however, occasionally associated with side effects such as swelling, haemorrhage, and infarction, preoperative embolization is controversial. The time span between embolization and an operation should not exceed 3 days, since perifocal swelling can cause enhanced unnecessary risks (15).

Surgical treatment

Surgical treatment is usually the most recommended therapy for CNS haemangioblastomas, and its final goal is the complete resection of all tumour components. Since most VHL patients bear multiple haemangioblastomas and undergo multiple surgeries causing deterioration of PS (17), during removal of symptomatic tumours any small asymptomatic tumours in the same anatomical location should be removed simultaneously if they can be found. The cystic wall, not contrast-enhanced, may be left untreated, since the cyst fluid is solely caused by the tumour cells (32). But cysts associated with tumours will refill again in the case of incomplete resection of the solid tumour (33). The cystic wall consists of reactive gliosis without an epithelial lining (32). Since haemangioblastomas are highly vascular tumours, it is not recommended to cut the tumour into pieces, and debulking of the tumour should be avoided since it can cause extensive bleeding. Resection must be carried out with careful visualization, and cutting and coagulation of each feeding vessel must be done. It is therefore necessary to consequently dissect the area between the tumour capsule and the surrounding tissue. In many cases the cyst has grown much bigger than the solid part and is causative of progressive neurological symptoms. Upon removal of the solid part of the tumour, the cyst has usually opened and become reduced in size (34, 35). The solid tumour itself can be distinguished from the surrounding brain tissue due to its reddish or orange colour and can usually be removed completely. However, distinction from the surrounding vessels is occasionally difficult.

In this case, indocyanine green video-angiography and fluorescent visualization with 5-ALA are useful (36, 37). Doppler flow sonography can also be useful, since it is a sensitive intraoperative tool to guide the surgical approach and resection (36–39). Intraoperative monitoring including motor-evoked potentials for spinal cord haemangioblastomas and an additional D-wave for those located in the vicinity of motor tracts should be applied in the case of surgery of spinal cord haemangioblastomas (35). If the spinal haemangioblastoma is not visible on the surface of the spinal cord, enlarged arterialized veins can be helpful for finding the tumour. Enhanced-power Doppler ultrasonography can also be of help in this case. These enlarged arterialized veins except for those penetrating the tumour should be preserved to avoid swelling and haemorrhage from the tumour. Even if a dorsal fascicle is involved in the tumour, it can usually be removed with no neurological deficit or only slight disturbance of deep sensation (32, 35).

Radiotherapy

It has been demonstrated that stereotactic radiosurgery for haemangioblastomas has an acceptable risk for adverse radiation effects, but results in partial diminishment of tumour control over long-term follow-up (40). Principally, stereotactic radiosurgery can be used for surgically inaccessible or multiple cranial and spinal tumours (41). More recently, fractionated external beam radiotherapy (42) and infratentorial craniospinal radiation therapy (43) have been investigated for use against haemangioblastomas, and favourable outcomes were reported for VHL-associated haemangioblastomas.

Pharmacological treatment

Despite their highly vascular nature and the presence of VEGF, inhibition of the VEGF/VEGFR system, in contrast to RCC, has not demonstrated substantial benefit in haemangioblastomas. Smaller series of patients treated with SU5416/semaxanib, a first-generation inhibitor of VEGFR-2 (44), and bevacizumab, an anti-VEGF-A antibody (45), have primarily shown disease stabilization in some cases, which may have been mainly due to anti-oedema effects. A single-arm phase II trial with the multi-tyrosine kinase inhibitor sunitinib, now the standard therapy for VHL RCC patients, has confirmed that haemangioblastomas respond worse to VEGF/VEGFR-based therapies. From fifteen patients treated, 18 RCC and 21 haemangioblastoma lesions were evaluable. Six of the RCCs (33%) responded partially, but none of the haemangioblastomas did (46). A larger study with bevacizumab as well as studies with vatalanib and pazopanib, two multi-tyrosine kinase inhibitors, are ongoing.

Follow-up of central nervous system haemangioblastomas in VHL patients

Patients with VHL and CNS haemangioblastomas should undergo MRIs of the brain and spinal cord at least once a year. VHL patients above 10 years old, who do not display CNS haemangioblastomas, should undergo MRI screening of their whole neuroaxis every 2 years. Ophthalmological examination should be performed to screen for retinal haemangioblastomas. In addition, MRI of the abdomen is performed to screen for RCC, pancreatic lesions, and phaeochromocytoma (15, 20, 27).

Current research topics

In contrast to renal cell cancer, research and clinical trials into hae-mangioblastomas have been underpowered. One major challenge will be to exploit VHL pathway addiction beyond VEGF/VEGFR inhibition, which appears to be less efficient in haemangioblas-tomas (46). This may be accomplished by inhibitors of the more upstream HIF protein, or more specific downstream interventions targeting other HIF effectors. Interestingly, a synthetic lethality screen identified a HIF-dependent essential requirement for the glucose transporter Glut-1 in VHL mutant renal cell cancer (47). Fibroblast growth factor signalling may also be a relevant target in haemangioblastomas, since it is expressed there in higher levels compared to RCC (46). HIF-independent effects of VHL deficiency should also be exploited. It has also been suggested that immuno-therapy has particular prospects in VHL-mutated tumours, because decreased expression of HLA-I molecules in mutated VHL renal tumour cells sensitizes them to NK-mediated lysis (48).

In general, specifically for haemangioblastomas, more trans-lational research on tumour tissue is necessary in order to define specific driver alterations there, to determine target modulation in trials with candidate drugs, and to explore alternative targets. Based on the recognition of the embryological, developmentally arrested haemangioblast as the tumour cell of origin for VHL-associated hae-mangioblastomas, therapies that exploit the differentiation poten-tial of the haemangioblast may offer such an alternative treatment paradigm for CNS haemangioblastoma (9). In missense mutation VHL disease, the rapid degradation of a malformed protein within the tumours causes VHL pathway deficiency. Treatment with the histone deacetylase inhibitor vorinostat appears to increase VHL protein levels (49) and a clinical trial is ongoing.

References

1. Huntoon K, Lonser RR. Nervous system manifestations of von Hippel-Lindau disease. *J Transl Med Epidemiol* 2014; 2(1):1015.

2. Evans DG, Howard E, Giblin C, et al. Birth incidence and prevalence of tumor-prone syndromes: estimates from a UK family genetic register service. *Am J Med Genet A* 2010; 152A(2):327–332.

3. Maher ER, Iselius L, Yates JR, et al. Von Hippel-Lindau disease: a genetic study. *J Med Genet* 1991; 28(7):443–447.

4. Maher ER, Webster AR, Richards FM, et al. Phenotypic expression in von Hippel-Lindau disease: correlations with germline VHL gene mutations. *J Med Genet* 1996; 33(4):328–332.

5. Stolle C, Glenn G, Zbar B, et al. Improved detection of germline mutations in the von Hippel-Lindau disease tumor suppressor gene. *Hum Mutat* 1998; 12(6):417–423.

6. Sgambati MT, Stolle C, Choyke PL, et al. Mosaicism in von Hippel-Lindau disease: lessons from kindreds with germline mutations identified in offspring with mosaic parents. *Am J Hum Genet* 2000; 66(1):84–91.

7. Wilding A, Ingham SL, Lalloo F, et al. Life expectancy in hereditary cancer predisposing diseases: an observational study. *J Med Genet* 2012; 49(4):264–269.

8. Miyagami M, Katayama Y, Nakamura S. Clinicopathological study of vascular endothelial growth factor (VEGF), p53, and proliferative potential in familial von Hippel-Lindau disease and sporadic hemangioblastomas. *Brain Tumor Pathol* 2000; 17:111–120.

9. Zhuang Z, Frerich JM, Huntoon K, et al. Tumor derived vasculogenesis in von Hippel-Lindau disease-associated tumors. *Sci Rep* 2014; 4:4102.

10. Kaelin WG Jr, Ratcliffe PJ. Oxygen sensing by metazoans: the central role of the HIF hydroxylase pathway. *Mol Cell* 2008; 30:393–402.

11. Richard S, Gardie B, Couvé S, et al. Von Hippel-Lindau: how a rare disease illuminates cancer biology. *Semin Cancer Biol* 2013; 23:26–37.

12. Hanahan D, Weinberg RA. Hallmarks of cancer: the next generation. *Cell* 2011; 144:646–674.

13. Ohh M, Yauch RL, Lonergan KM, et al. The von Hippel-Lindau tumor suppressor protein is required for proper assembly of an extracellular fibronectin matrix. *Mol Cell* 1998; 1:959–968.

14. Esteban-Barragán M, Avila P, Alvarez-Tejado M, et al. Role of the von Hippel-Lindau tumor suppressor gene in the formation of beta1-integrin fibrillar adhesions. *Cancer Res* 2002; 62:2929–2936.

15. Krüger MT, Klingler JH, Steiert C, et al. Current diagnostic and therapeutic strategies in treatment of CNS hemangioblastomas in patients with VHL. *J Trans Med Epidemiol* 2014; 2(1):1016.

16. Wanebo JE, Lonser RR, Glenn GM, et al. The natural history of hemangioblastomas of the central nervous system in patients with von Hippel-Lindau disease. *J Neurosurg* 2003; 98:82–94.

17. Kanno H, Kuratsu J, Nishikawa R, et al. Clinical features of patients bearing central nervous system hemangioblastoma in von Hippel-Lindau disease. *Acta Neurochir (Wien)* 2013; 155:1–7.

18. Maher ER, Yates JR, Ferguson-Smith MA. Statistical analysis of the two stage mutation model in von Hippel-Lindau disease, and in sporadic cerebellar haemangioblastoma and renal cell carcinoma. *J Med Genet* 1990; 27:311–314.

19. Lonser, RR, Glenn GM, Walther M, et al. von Hippel-Lindau disease. *Lancet* 2003; 361:2059–2067.

20. Lonser RR, Weil RJ, Wanebo JE, et al. Surgical management of spinal cord hemangioblastomas in patients with von Hippel-Lindau disease. *J Neurosurg* 2003; 98:106–116.

21. Weil RJ, Lonser RR, DeVroom HL, et al. Surgical management of brainstem hemangioblastomas in patients with von Hippel-Lindau disease. *J Neurosurg* 2003; 98:95–105.

22. Lonser RB, Butman JA, Huntoon K, et al. Prospective natural history study of central nervous system hemangioblastomas in von Hippel-Lindau disease. *J Neurosurg* 2014; 120:1055–1062.

23. Gläsker S, Van Velthoven V. Risk of hemorrhage in hemangioblastomas of the central nervous system. *Neurosurgery* 2005; 57:71–76.

24. Vortmeyer AO, Gnarra JR, Emmert-Buck MR, et al. von Hippel-Lindau gene deletion detected in the stromal cell component of a cerebellar hemangioblastoma associated with von Hippel-Lindau disease. *Hum Pathol* 1997; 28:540–543.

25. Vortmeyer AO, Frank S, Jeong SY, et al. Developmental arrest of angioblastic lineage initiates tumorigenesis in von Hippel-Lindau disease. *Cancer Res* 2003; 63:7051–7055.

26. Glasker S, Li J, Xia JB, et al. Hemangioblastomas share protein expression with embryonal hemangioblast progenitor cell. *Cancer Res* 2006; 66:4167–4172.

27. Hasselblatt M, Jeibmann A, Gerss J, et al. Cellular and reticular variants of haemangioblastoma revisited: a clinicopathologic study of 88 cases. *Neuropathol Appl Neurobiol* 2005; 31:618–622.

28. Zbar B, Kishida T, Chen F, et al. Germline mutations in the Von Hippel-Lindau disease (VHL) gene in families from North America, Europe, and Japan. *Hum Mutat* 1996; 8:348–357.

29. Kanno H, Kondo K, Ito S, et al. Somatic mutations of the von Hippel-Lindau tumor suppressor gene in sporadic central nervous system hemangioblastomas. *Cancer Res* 1994; 54:4845–4847.

30. Van Velthoven V, Reinacher PC, Klisch J, et al. Treatment of intramedullary hemangioblastomas, with special attention to von Hippel-Lindau disease. *Neurosurgery* 2003; 53:1306–1313.

31. Kanno H, Yamamoto I, Nishikawa R, et al. Spinal cord hemangioblastomas in von Hippel–Lindau disease. *Spinal Cord* 2009; 47:447–452.

32. Lonser RR, Vortmeyer AO, Butman JA, et al. Edema is a precursor to central nervous system peritumoral cyst formation. *Ann Neurol* 2005; 58:392–399.

33. Gläsker S, Vortmeyer AO, Lonser RR, et al. Proteomic analysis of hemangioblastoma cyst fluid. *Cancer Biol Ther* 2006; 5:549–553.

34. Lonser RR, Oldfield EH. Microsurgical resection of spinal cord hemangioblastomas. *Neurosurgery* 2005; 57:372–376.

35. Gläsker S, Klingler JH, Muller K, et al. Essentials and pitfalls in the treatment of CNS hemangioblastomas and von Hippel-Lindau disease. *Cent Eur Neurosurg* 2010; 71:80–87.

36. Utsuki S, Oka H, Sato K, et al. Fluorescence diagnosis of tumor cells in hemangioblastoma cysts with 5-aminolevulinic acid. *J Neurosurg* 2010; 112:130–132.

37. Murai Y, Adachi K, Matano F, et al. Indocyanine green videoangiography study of hemangioblastomas. *Can J Neurol Sci* 2011; 38:41–47.

38. Kanno H, Ozawa Y, Sakata K, et al. Intraoperative power Doppler ultrasonography with a contrast-enhancing agent for intracranial tumors. *J Neurosurg* 2005; 102:295–301.

39. Gläsker S, Shah MJ, Hippchen B, et al. Doppler-sonographically guided resection of central nervous system hemangioblastomas. *Neurosurgery* 2011; 68:267–275.

40. Asthagiri AR, Mehta GU, Zach L, et al. Prospective evaluation of radiosurgery for hemangioblastomas in von Hippel-Lindau disease. *Neuro Oncol* 2010; 12:80–86.

41. Moss JM, Choi CY, Adler JR Jr, et al. Stereotactic radiosurgical treatment of cranial and spinal hemangioblastomas. *Neurosurgery* 2009; 65:79–85.

42. Koh ES, Nichol A, Millar BA, et al. Role of fractionated external beam radiotherapy in hemangioblastoma of the central nervous system. *Int J Radiat Oncol Biol Phys* 2007; 69:1521–1526.

43. Simone CB 2nd, Lonser RR, Ondos J, et al. Infratentorial craniospinal irradiation for von Hippel-Lindau: a retrospective study supporting a new treatment for patients with CNS hemangioblastomas. *Neuro Oncol* 2011; 13:1030–1036.

44. Schuch G, de Wit M, Höltje J, et al. Case 2. Hemangioblastomas: diagnosis of von Hippel-Lindau disease and antiangiogenic treatment with SU5416. *J Clin Oncol* 2005; 23:3624–3626.

45. Seystahl K, Weller M, Bozinov O, et al. Neuropathological characteristics of progression after prolonged response to bevacizumab in multifocal hemangioblastoma. *Oncol Res Treat* 2014; 37(4):209–212.

46. Jonasch E, McCutcheon IE, Waguespack SG, et al. Pilot trial of sunitinib therapy in patients with von Hippel-Lindau disease. *Ann Oncol* 2011; 22:2661–2666.

47. Chan DA, Sutphin PD, Nguyen P, et al. Targeting GLUT1 and the Warburg effect in renal cell carcinoma by chemical synthetic lethality. *Sci Transl Med* 2011; 3:94ra70.

48. Perier A, Fregni G, Wittnebel S, et al. Mutations of the von Hippel-Lindau gene confer increased susceptibility to natural killer cells of clear-cell renal cell carcinoma. *Oncogene* 2011; 30:2622–2632.

49. Yang C, Huntoon K, Ksendzovsky A, et al. Proteostasis modulators prolong missense VHL protein activity and halt tumor progression. *Cell Rep* 201; 3:52–59.

CHAPTER 17

Familial tumour syndromes: tuberous sclerosis complex

Howard Weiner and Peter B. Crino

Definition

The tuberous sclerosis complex (TSC) was first described in 1880 by Bourneville who reported a young woman with severe epilepsy who died following status epilepticus, and who was found to have lesions in the heart and kidneys. Over the past century, numerous clinical reports have described the protean clinical manifestations of TSC and in the 1990s, the identification of mutations in two distinct TSC genes (*TSC1* and *TSC2*) ushered in the modern era of molecular and cellular pathogenesis of TSC (see reference 1). Mutations in TSC genes lead to tissue hamartomas (lesions exhibiting abnormal growth) that disrupt or interfere with normal organ functioning. TSC is a multisystem disorder that can affect virtually any organ system in varying severity but exhibits a proclivity for the brain, lung, heart, skin, and kidney (1–3). The manifestations of TSC in each organ system lead to an often complicated set of clinical features including epilepsy, cognitive disability, autism, hydrocephalus, renal dysfunction, retroperitoneal haemorrhage, progressive pulmonary failure, and often cosmetically disfiguring skin lesions. Thus, the multiple manifestations of TSC require ongoing surveillance and care, usually by a multidisciplinary team.

Epidemiology

An autosomal dominant disorder, TSC has an estimated annual incidence of 1 in 6000–10,000 live births (4) and currently affects an estimated 1 million individuals worldwide. There seems to be no ethnic or racial predisposition and males and females are affected to approximately equal extents. Patients can develop TSC by an inherited mode of transmission from affected parents or by a spontaneous *de novo* mutation in either *TSC1* or *TSC2*. As an autosomal dominant disease, there is no carrier state for TSC. However, the clinical severity can be highly variable with a spectrum and bimodal distribution of severely and mildly affected individuals.

Aetiology and genetics

TSC results from mutations in the *TSC1* (9q34) (5) or *TSC2* (16p13.3) (6) gene. *TSC1* is a 23-exon gene encoding an 8.6 kb transcript, and a 30 kDa protein, TSC1 (hamartin). *TSC2* encodes a 5.5 kb transcript and a 180 kDa protein, TSC2 (tuberin). These proteins are ubiquitously expressed in most organ systems and cell types. There is high interspecies sequence conservation of these genes

and proteins, from *Drosophila* to man. Approximately 80% of TSC cases result from sporadic *TSC1* or *TSC2* mutations, while approximately 20% of affected TSC patients exhibit a dominant inheritance pattern (7, 8). There are over 2000 unique *TSC1* and *TSC2* allelic variants encompassing missense, nonsense, insertion, and deletion mutations, distributed within nearly all exons of *TSC1* and *TSC2* (see http://chromium.liacs.nl/LOVD2/TSC/home.php?select_db=TSC1 or =TSC2). *TSC2* mutations account for 60% of TSC, and *TSC1* mutations account for 30% of cases (9, 10). While *TSC1* or *TSC2* mutations are identified in 70–90% of TSC patients, approximately 10–15% of clinically defined TSC patients have no mutation identified ('NMI') (11), perhaps reflecting low-level somatic mosaicism or perhaps an unidentified *TSC3* gene. A sequencing analysis of TBC1 domain family member 7 (*TBC1D7*), whose encoded protein binds to TSC1, failed to identify pathogenic mutations suggesting a *TSC3* gene locus (12). Patients with NMI pose a particular diagnostic challenge as subjects with major diagnostic features on clinical examination may have NMI following genotype screening.

Interestingly, there are few specific genotype–phenotype correlations in TSC in which a particular genotype reliably predicts the clinical features or course of any one TSC patient (13–15). Broadly, studies suggest that patients with a sporadic *TSC1* gene mutation generally have milder disease manifestations, in particular neurological manifestations, than patients of similar age with *TSC2* mutations. However, this is not a uniform finding and many patients with identified *TSC1* mutations have severe neurological features. Additionally, patients with NMI can have clinically severe TSC but may also have less severe disease than patients with identified *TSC1* or *TSC2* mutations. Modifier genes have been proposed as one mechanism to account for phenotypic variability of TSC, although to date, none have been identified for neurological features.

Pathogenesis

The TSC1 and TSC2 proteins form a heterodimeric complex that serves as an upstream regulator of the mammalian target of rapamycin (sirolimus) (mTOR) signalling pathway (Fig. 17.1).

The effects, regulators, and targets of mTOR have been recently reviewed (see reference 16). mTOR is a ubiquitous serine/threonine kinase that integrates signals from growth factors (e.g. IGF-1), nutrients, energy, and cellular stressors (e.g. hypoxia) (17, 18) to regulate multiple cellular processes such as cell growth and proliferation, gene transcription, protein translation, and cell

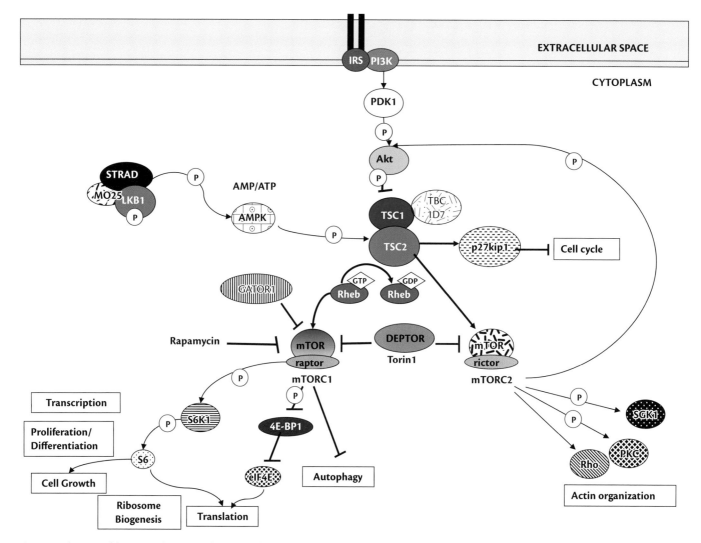

Fig. 17.1 Schematic of the mammalian target of rapamycin (mTOR) signalling cascade. Upstream signalling of cell surface molecules, e.g. IGF-1, through PI3K, PDK1, and Akt. TSC1 and TSC2 (and TBC1D7) proteins form a heterodimeric complex that modulates the mTOR signalling pathway via Rheb. mTOR forms two distinct complexes with other proteins, e.g. raptor, specific to mTOR complex 1 (mTORC1), and rictor, specific to mTORC2, to regulate protein translation, gene transcription, cell proliferation, differentiation, and autophagy. mTORC1 signals downstream to numerous target proteins including p70S6K1 and STAT3 while mTORC2 modulates signalling through SGK1 and PKC.

death and autophagy. mTOR binds with other proteins to form two structurally and functionally distinct protein complexes: mTOR complex 1 (mTORC1), comprised of mTOR, raptor (regulatory-associated protein of mTOR) and PRAS40, and mTORC2, comprised of mTOR, rictor (rapamycin-insensitive component of mTOR), mSin1, and Protor1/2 (19). DEPTOR interacts with and inhibits both mTORC1 and mTORC2 (20). The stress response gene *REDD1* is a novel mTOR inhibitor that regulates mTOR signalling through the TSC1/TSC2 complex as a function of cellular oxygen tension (21). REDD1 is induced in response both to hypoxia and energy stress, and cells that lack REDD1 exhibit defective mTOR regulation in response to either of these stress signals. TSC1 protein stabilizes TSC2 by direct binding, preventing its ubiquitination and when bound to TSC1, TSC2 acts as a GTPase-activating protein towards the signalling protein Ras homologue enriched in brain (Rheb), which then constitutively activates mTOR signalling. A third component of the complex, TBC1D7 (12), has been shown to bind to TSC1 and to play an important

role in modulating the GAP activity exerted by TSC2 on Rheb. In experimental studies, TBC1D7 knockdown diminishes the association between TSC1 and TSC2, decreases the Rheb-GAP activity, and increases mTORC1 signalling.

mTORC1 governs a variety of cellular processes including pyrimidine synthesis, amino acid utilization, gene transcription, ribosome biogenesis, mRNA translation, and autophagy, via phosphorylation of substrate proteins including p70S6K, ribosomal S6, and 4E-BP1 (22–24). In virtually all organ systems assessed in TSC patients, loss-of-function mutations in *TSC1* or *TSC2* lead to enhanced activation of mTOR signalling, evidenced by increased phosphorylation of p70S6K1, S6, and 4E-BP1. Phosphoproteomic analyses have shown that in addition to its well-defined substrates (e.g. p70S6K), mTORC1 may modulate phosphorylation of several hundred downstream proteins thus positing TSC1:TSC2:mTOR as a pivotal signalling node in many cell types (25, 26). The macrolide antibiotic sirolimus (rapamycin) is a highly specific mTORC1 inhibitor that has been used successfully in several TSC clinical trials (see 'Management'). Sirolimus inhibits mTORC1 through association with another mTOR binding protein, FKBP12.

In contrast to mTORC1, mTORC2 signals through Akt, PIK3, and serum and glucocorticoid-inducible kinase 1 (SGK1) (27, 28). mTORC2 regulates actin cytoskeletal organization and hyperactivated mTORC2 signalling results in altered cell motility in endothelial cells and glioma cell lines. mTORC2 is relatively insensitive to sirolimus inhibition although long-term treatment in mammalian cells can prevent *de novo* mTORC2 assembly. Torin1 is a recently defined compound that inhibits both mTORC1 and mTORC2 signalling *in vitro*. While the TSC1:TSC2 complex serves an inhibitory role on mTORC1 signalling, some studies have reported opposite effects on mTORC2, suggesting that TSC1:TSC2 is required for its proper activation. In renal angiomyolipomas (AMLs) and $Tsc2^{+/-}$ mouse kidney tumours, mTORC1 biomarkers are increased while mTORC2 effectors are attenuated (29). Conversely, following knockdown of *Tsc2* in mouse neural progenitor cells, mTORC2 signalling is activated (30). Thus, there may be temporal, regional, and cellular specificity to how mTOR signalling is regulated within each of its complexes.

TSC1:TSC2:mTOR complex signalling contributes to numerous functions in the developing and mature brain. For example, in the brain, neuronal and glial size is regulated by mTOR activity and loss of either *Tsc1* or *Tsc2 in vitro* or *in vivo* leads to enhanced cell soma size. For example, Cre-mediated deletion of exons 17 and 18 of *Tsc1* in cultured mouse hippocampal neurons results in enhanced S6 phosphorylation and increased neuronal soma size (31). Conditional knockout of *Tsc1* or *Tsc2* under synapsin- (32), Emx- (33), GFAP- (34), or nestin-specific promoters (35) leads to enhanced cell size and mTORC1 activation. *Tsc2* knockdown with shRNA *in vitro* and *in vivo* causes a two-fold increase in cell size (30). In all systems tested, increased cell size by reduced Tsc1 or Tsc2 can be reversed with sirolimus suggesting that regulation of cell size is mTORC1 dependent.

Clinical presentation

The diagnosis of TSC is made according to a set of clinical criteria in which individual manifestations of TSC are identified in single or multiple organ systems (36). Thus, a combination of a detailed physical examination and select radiographic studies are necessary to assemble a comprehensive clinical evaluation of each patient. Surveillance criteria have been published to guide long-term follow-up in TSC patients (37). The features of TSC have been divided into major and minor diagnostic criteria that are used to yield either definite or possible TSC. For example, major diagnostic criteria include cortical dysplasias (cortical tubers and white matter radial migration lines), subependymal nodules (SENs), and subependymal giant cell astrocytomas (SEGAs), retinal hamartomas, pulmonary lymphangioleiomyomatosis (LAM; occurs almost exclusively in females with TSC), AMLs in the kidney or liver, cardiac rhabdomyomas, ungual fibromas, facial angiofibromas, hypomelanotic macules ('ash leaf spots'), the Shagreen patch, and the detection of clearly deleterious mutations in *TSC1* or *TSC2* (Table 17.1) (36, 37). Detection of a clearly pathogenic mutation in either *TSC1* or *TSC2*, can serve as an independent diagnostic criterion that is sufficient for the diagnosis of TSC regardless of the individual clinical findings (36). Minor diagnostic criteria include intraoral hamartomas, 'confetti lesions' on the skin (e.g. multiple, small, and scattered hypomelanotic areas),

Table 17.1 Revised diagnostic criteria for TSC. Definite diagnosis: two major features or one major feature with at least two minor features. Possible diagnosis: either one major feature or at least two minor features

Major	Minor
Cortical dysplasias	Intraoral fibromas
Subependymal giant cell astrocytoma	Retinal achromic patch
Subependymal nodules	Non-renal hamartomas
Retinal hamartomas	'Confetti' skin lesions
Angiofibromas	Renal cysts
Ungual fibromas	Dental enamel pits
Shagreen patch	
Hypomelanotic macules	
Angiomyolipomas	
Cardiac rhabdomyoma	
Lymphangioleiomyomatosis	
TSC1 or *TSC2* pathogenic mutation	

Adapted from *Pediatr Neurol.*, 49(4), Northrup H, Krueger DA, International Tuberous Sclerosis Complex Consensus Group. Tuberous sclerosis complex diagnostic criteria update: recommendations of the 2012 international tuberous sclerosis complex consensus conference, pp. 243–54, Copyright (2013), with permission from Elsevier; *Pediatr Neurol.*, 49(4), Krueger DA, Northrup H, International Tuberous Sclerosis Complex Consensus Group. Tuberous sclerosis complex surveillance and management: recommendations of the 2012 international tuberous sclerosis complex consensus conference, pp. 255–65, Copyright (2013), with permission from Elsevier.

and renal cysts. The identification of two or more major diagnostic criteria, or one major feature with at least two minor features confirms a clinical diagnosis of 'definite' TSC, whereas one major feature, or two or more minor features suggests 'possible' TSC.

The diagnosis for many TSC patients is straightforward with easy identification of major features in the skin, brain, or kidney. However, in some individuals, ascertaining the clinical diagnosis can be more challenging, especially if a pathogenic mutation is not identified. For example, clinicians may be faced with patients exhibiting minimal skin abnormalities and normal renal imaging but who exhibit a single brain lesion. Alternatively, there are some individuals with renal cysts (a minor criterion) and a single skin lesion. The numerous possible combinations of features require a detailed physical examination including Wood's lamp examination for hypomelanotic lesions, coupled with imaging of kidney, brain, and, in female patients, lungs to assess LAM to fully evaluate the presence of major and minor diagnostic features.

The classic neuropathological manifestations of TSC include cortical tubers (Fig. 17.2), SENs, and SEGAs in variable percentages of TSC patients (38). The revised diagnostic criteria include cortical tubers and radial migration lines seen radiographically under the heading of cortical dysplasias. The incidence of each varies across the TSC population with tubers found in over 80% of TSC patients and SENs in 50%. SEGAS are found in 10–20% of TSC patients. While tubers and SEGAs are associated with neurological features, SENs are believed to be asymptomatic. Each can typically be visualized by brain computerized tomography (CT) and magnetic resonance imaging (MRI) and serve as useful diagnostic signposts.

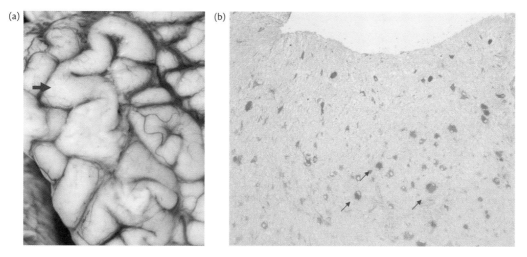

Fig. 17.2 (a) A brain specimen depicting a tuber (arrow) as a focal thickening in cortical gyration. (b) Note complete loss of normal hexalaminar cortical structure and the presence of numerous giant cells (arrows) immunoreactive for the p70S6 kinase substrate phosphorylated ribosomal S6 protein, a biomarker of mTORC1 activation. Adapted from *N Engl J Med*, 355(13), Crino PB, Nathanson KL, Henske EP, Medical Progress: The tuberous sclerosis complex, pp. 1345–1356, Copyright (2006), with permission from Massachusetts Medical Society.

Tuber and SEGA number and size are closely tied to overall patient morbidity and mortality in TSC.

Imaging

There is evidence that distinct tuber subtypes can be defined by brain MRI based on signal intensity (39). For example, 'type A' tubers appear isointense on T1 images but may exhibit subtle hyperintensity on T2-weighted and FLAIR sequences. 'Type B' tubers are hypointense on T1, and hyperintense on T2 and FLAIR sequences (Fig. 17.3). Finally, 'type C' tubers are hypointense on T1, hyperintense on T2, and heterogeneous on FLAIR sequences. In this study, patients with type A tubers had a milder neurological phenotype, whereas patients with type C tubers tended to have additional MRI findings in addition to tubers (e.g. SEGAs), and a higher probability of having intractable epilepsy, a history of infantile spasms, and autism spectrum disorder, compared to patients with type A or type B tubers.

Management

Epilepsy

More than 80% of TSC patients suffer from epilepsy and for many patients seizures will be intractable to medical therapies. The mechanisms by which seizures are generated in TSC remain to be fully defined. Seizures of all types, for example, simple partial, complex partial, generalized tonic–clonic, and atonic, may be observed. There is commonly an association between the localization of a tuber and onset zone for seizures in most TSC patients with the

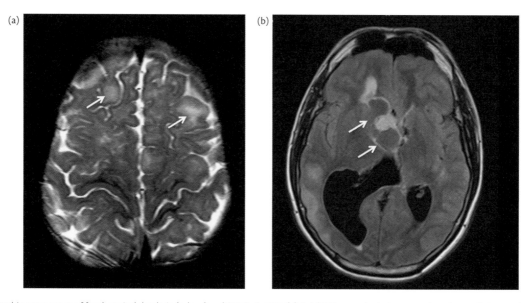

Fig. 17.3 Radiographic appearance of focal cortical dysplasia (tubers) and SEGAs in TSC. (a) Axial T2 image depicting two tubers (arrows) that are hyperintense (type B). (b) Axial FLAIR image depicting a SEGA (arrows) causing obstructive hydrocephalus.

presumption being that tubers serve as the epileptogenic substrate for seizures in TSC. Because tubers can be multiple, TSC patients may suffer from multifocal seizure onset or a more pervasive epilepsy syndrome such as infantile spasms or Lennox–Gastaut syndrome. The development of recurrent seizures in TSC likely results from multifactorial contributions of *TSC1* or *TSC2* gene mutations, abnormal cortical cytoarchitecture, altered synaptic connections, changes in neurotransmitter receptor or ion channel expression, aberrant expression of growth or trophic factors, and a robust pro-inflammatory response. Surgical resection of tubers is associated with seizure reduction, although the ictal onset zone may not lie within the tuber itself but at the interface between the tuber and the surrounding perituberal cortex (see 'Treatment of epilepsy').

Several mouse models of TSC exhibit spontaneous seizures, suggesting that effects of TSC gene mutations on brain development can cause robust changes in excitability. For example, there are changes in astrocyte regulation of extracellular glutamate homeostasis leading to impaired glutamate transport by astrocytes, elevated extracellular glutamate concentrations, neuronal hyperexcitability, excitotoxic cell death, and seizures (40). In addition to regulation of glutamate homeostasis, a defect in potassium buffering by inward-rectifying potassium (Kir) channels on astrocytes could lead to neuronal hyperexcitability and seizures. The expression and function of specific Kir channels are significantly reduced in astrocytes from *Tsc1*^{GFAP}CKO mice. There are limited data on the electrophysiological properties of dysplastic neurons (DNs) and giant cells (GCs) in tubers obtained from slice recordings in surgically resected tubers (41). For example, analysis of tuber acute slice specimens revealed that passive membrane properties of normal-appearing pyramidal neurons (e.g. cell capacitance, input resistance, time constant, resting membrane potentials, firing properties, or current–voltage relationships) did not differ from that of normal pyramidal neurons. Cytomegalic DNs exhibit a larger membrane capacitance, time constant, and input resistance than normal-appearing pyramidal neurons. DNs display repetitive calcium oscillations, a sign of hyperexcitability. GCs do not display inward currents and in current clamp mode, they do not fire action potentials.

Analysis of human tuber specimens resected at the time of epilepsy surgery reveals significant changes in the expression of mRNAs and proteins encoding NMDA, AMPA, and GABA$_A$ receptor subunits and uptake sites (42, 43). Subsequent studies demonstrated alterations in expression and cell-specific distribution of group I (mGluR1, mGluR5), group II (mGluR2/3), and group III (mGluR4 and mGluR8) mGluR subtypes in cortical tubers using immunocytochemistry (44). Robust group I mGluR immunoreactivity, in particular mGluR5, was observed in a large majority of TSC specimens in DNs and GCs within cortical tubers. mGluR1 was detected in a subpopulation of neurons and giant cells. Group II and particularly group III mGluR immunoreactivity was less frequently observed than group I mGluRs in dysplastic neurons and giant cells of tubers.

Treatment of epilepsy

Research in TSC has provided a highly successful and progressive model to study both rare and common disorders using a paradigmatic 'bedside-to-bench-to-bedside' approach. Beginning with TSC patient samples, both TSC genes were defined and then a compelling link to a cell signalling pathway (mTOR) was defined.

Fortuitously, sirolimus (rapamycin) was found to be a potent inhibitor of this cascade and thus rapid progress to pre-clinical studies, and ultimately human clinical trials was made. In virtually all *in vitro* and whole animal TSC models, sirolimus or other mTOR inhibitory compounds, can rescue phenotypic abnormalities induced by loss of either Tsc1 or Tsc2 including enhanced cell size, impaired migration, altered dendrite or axon outgrowth, abnormal cognitive behaviour, or recurrent seizures.

Clinical treatment of TSC is largely focused on symptomatic management of specific features of TSC. Recurrent seizures are a particular clinical challenge for many TSC patients. While antiepileptic drugs (AEDs) remain the mainstay of epilepsy therapy, many TSC patients will suffer from medically refractory seizures despite multiple AEDs. One recent and promising study showed that the mTOR inhibitor everolimus can reduce seizure frequency in children and adults with TSC associated epilepsy (45). Cortical tubers visualized on brain MRI are thought to be epileptogenic and have been the traditional target of resective epilepsy surgery in those TSC patients with intractable seizures not responsive to medications. However, there remains debate regarding the relationship between tubers and seizures in TSC, because some TSC patients have no visible tubers on MRI yet have severe epilepsy, and animal models of TSC with a seizure phenotype exist without obvious tubers.

Seizures can be severe and frequent in TSC. In more than half of TSC patients, seizures may be refractory to medical therapy with AEDs. This often will lead to repeated visits to the neurologist as well as multiple trips to the emergency room. Families can be thrown into crisis very quickly in these situations. While seizures may develop in a patient with known TSC, sometimes the new onset of seizures in children may be the initial presentation of the child's TSC, and the diagnosis is made by brain MRI, which typically shows tubers. If seizures are difficult to control in children with TSC, then the treating physician should consider additional treatment options, including epilepsy surgery. It is now well recognized that uncontrolled frequent seizures are detrimental to the developing brain and, therefore, an aggressive approach towards controlling these are in the child's best interest. As in other cases of childhood epilepsy, the first line of therapy is medical management with AEDs. Children with TSC will often require more than one medication because their seizures may be very difficult to control. Because uncontrolled chronic seizures are detrimental to the child's neurological and cognitive development, each case should be referred to a centre with expertise in the evaluation of these children for epilepsy surgery.

The main diagnostic modalities used in the evaluation of children with TSC and medically refractory epilepsy include the scalp electroencephalogram (EEG) and MRI scan of the brain. Of course, the clinical semiology of the seizures is critical, as is the neurological examination, in further developing a surgical hypothesis about where the primary seizure onset zone may localize to in the brain. This critical localization is essential for surgery to be a consideration, and the precise localization of the ictal onset will often determine how successful epilepsy surgery can be. As part of the pre-surgical evaluation, children will often be admitted to an epilepsy monitoring unit for video EEG monitoring. In TSC, the ability to easily pinpoint the child's seizures to a single tuber or location in the brain is the exception rather than the rule. Rather, more often, the presence of multiple cortical tubers is associated with what appears to be multifocal epilepsy, rendering the situation more complicated. In the past, these children were uniformly dismissed as potential surgical candidates. However, increasing evidence supports the notion that, despite multiple potentially epileptogenic areas in the TSC brain, a detailed diagnostic evaluation can unmask one or more surgical targets, providing hope for children previously excluded from surgical consideration. The medical literature contains data supporting a number of non-invasive functional imaging approaches which can help determine the major epileptogenic zone(s) in TSC patients, including positron emission tomography, single-photon emission tomography, magnetoencephalography, diffusion transfer imaging, and functional MRI. TSC children often have multiple seizure types, each associated with a different tuber location. Surgery may only target one of these seizure types, depending on the clinical scenario. Of course, in order to proceed with surgery, the potential benefits of surgery must clearly outweigh the potential risks. All of this is discussed in great detail with the child's parents, including the possibility that surgery might not help the seizures despite this exhaustive evaluation.

The goal of surgery is to target and remove the main seizure focus thought to be responsible for the onset of the targeted seizures, if this can be done safely. Epilepsy surgery therefore involves resection of the epileptogenic tuber(s) and any surrounding epileptic non-tuber brain tissue. If the non-invasive pre-surgical testing, including the brain MRI, clearly demonstrates the area to be removed, then surgery can be accomplished in a single operation. Intraoperative electrocorticography can provide real-time EEG data in the operating room, to aide in determining the tissue that needs to be resected. More often, because of the complexity of the epilepsy in TSC, invasive EEG monitoring will be necessary to refine the ictal localization in order to optimize the benefit of surgery. A combination of grid, strip, and depth electrodes are typically implanted surgically to create a volumetric assessment of the electrophysiology *in vivo*. After this initial operation, children are monitored in the paediatric intensive care unit, during which time they undergo video EEG invasive monitoring. The epileptologists may reduce the patient's medication during this time, to enhance the recording of seizures. This entire process requires a multidisciplinary team of specialists dedicated to the expert care of these children. After an ictal and interictal 'map' are created from the data gathered during this inpatient monitoring phase, the second surgery is performed, during which the seizure focus/tuber(s) is resected. Occasionally, to determine if another unresected tuber will then give rise to surgical failure, an additional phase of invasive monitoring is done. This 'third stage' of surgery, involves re-implanting an EEG electrode array intracranially at the second operation after the seizure focus has been resected. Several international centres have shown that epilepsy surgery can significantly benefit more than half of severely affected patients, at acceptable risk comparable to other types of neurosurgery.

Treatment of SEGA and other TS-related conditions

The advent of the mTOR inhibitors, sirolimus (rapamycin) and everolimus, has changed the landscape of clinical TSC care. An initial clinical trial revealed the efficacy of sirolimus in reducing the volume of renal AMLs and improving pulmonary function tests in LAM (46). While AMLs showed reduced overall volume after 12 months of sirolimus, in the ensuing 12 months in which sirolimus was discontinued, there was re-growth of AMLs in many

patients. A subsequent trial demonstrated that patients treated with sirolimus for 52 weeks had regression of renal and hepatic AMLs and SEGAs (47). The mTOR inhibitor everolimus was shown to reduce SEGA volume after 6 months of treatment (48). In this cohort, there was modest reduction in seizure frequency in 9 out of 16 TSC patients with seizures; however, seizure frequency did not change in 6 individuals, and worsened in 1 patient. Everolimus is the first mTOR inhibitor to be approved by the US Food and Drug Administration (FDA) for the treatment of SEGAs and AMLs associated with TSC. A trial of 20 TSC patients treated with everolimus revealed that seizure frequency was reduced by 50% or more in 12 of 20 subjects, suggesting a possible role for mTOR inhibitors in the treatment of medically refractory epilepsy in TSC (49). These clinical studies show that modulation of the mTOR pathway in TSC could provide benefit to a subset of TSC patients and suggests the possibility of 'syndrome-specific' therapy in TSC.

Appropriate management of SEGA remains a clinical challenge in TSC since aggressive SEGA growth leads to mortality in TSC. There are several questions regarding the definition of a SEGA that are relevant to clinical management. For example, what minimum size defines a SEGA? Are SEGAs really SENs that achieve a certain size and enhance with gadolinium? Is serial growth on MRI scanning necessary for a small (<5 mm) enhancing lesion at the foramen of Monro to be considered a SEGA? What about a larger (>1 cm) enhancing lesion that does not grow on serial MRI imaging? In general, most clinicians would agree that an enlarging lesion, in this typical location, would be considered a SEGA, even if it were small. Similarly, most would agree that a large enhancing lesion at the foramen of Monro is a SEGA, even in the absence of radiographic growth. Finally, it is even less obvious what proportion of TSC patients will become clinically symptomatic from a SEGA.

Natural history studies have shown that SEGAs have variable biological behaviour in TSC patients. A proportion of SEGAs will grow, as demonstrated by radiographic progression on serial MRI scans. Those tumours that do grow tend to do so at a very slow rate, with only a small fraction presenting with acute, significant tumour enlargement and, on occasion, obstructive hydrocephalus. Most patients will not have any symptoms despite a noted change on imaging. Only a subgroup of the SEGAs that show radiographic enlargement will give rise to neurological symptoms such as headache, nausea, vomiting, seizure exacerbation, visual changes, or behavioural and cognitive deterioration. Because the growth rate is unknown and cannot be reliably predicted in individual patients, it is advisable to repeat MRI scanning approximately 3–4 months after the initial MRI in newly diagnosed TSC patients. If one or two such serial scans show no significant change, then the interval between scans can be increased to 6 months and then to annually or every 2 years, in stable situations.

Options for enlarging or symptomatic SEGAs include surgical intervention or medical therapy. Radiation does not have an established role in the management of this type of neoplasm. It is noteworthy that TSC patients are referred for neurosurgical care of either an enlarging or symptomatic SEGA or for epilepsy surgery in the setting of medically intractable seizures, but only rarely for surgical intervention for both problems in the same patient. In fact, a significant number of SEGA patients do not have seizures and may not be taking AEDs at all, despite having numerous tubers on MRI scanning. Similarly, TSC patients who undergo epilepsy surgery will often have SEGAs noted on MRI scanning, but these may not grow over time and may never require treatment. The genetic factors that influence the clinical phenotype in TSC patients have not been fully defined. Indeed, another analysis of MRI scans in a large group of TSC patients revealed an association between SEGAs and the presence of cerebellar tubers, the latter of which had a greater tendency to change over time when compared with supratentorial cortical tubers, which remained stable over time (50).

It is clear that TSC patients experiencing acute neurological symptoms from a SEGA and/or associated hydrocephalus require neurosurgical intervention. Moreover, asymptomatic tumours that progressively enlarge on serial MRI scanning should be treated prior to the development of symptoms or hydrocephalus, which may not necessarily be reversible once it has already occurred. Certainly, if ventricular enlargement develops in the absence of symptoms, treatment should be strongly considered. In contrast, patients harbouring larger SEGAs (≥2 cm), in the absence of symptoms or of raised intracranial pressure, that remain unchanged on serial MRI scans can be closely monitored without neurosurgical intervention, assuming reliable follow-up can be assured.

In the current setting of an FDA-approved medical treatment for SEGAs with mTOR inhibitors, a question of relevance to patient care presently is whether medical or surgical treatment should be selected when the situation is not one of acute clinical urgency. The most obvious scenario in which this choice presents itself is when a SEGA has demonstrated radiographic enlargement, in the absence of symptoms. Proponents of both the medical and the surgical interventions exist, and arguments in favour of both have been proposed. Surgery has a generally well-defined set of infrequent risks, in experienced neurosurgical hands, which are taken upfront, all at once, with the goal of achieving the potential surgical cure of a pathologically low-grade brain tumour. In contrast, medical therapy obviates the surgical risks, but entails drug treatment of indefinite duration, with its own risk of potential side effects and unknown long-term effects for the patient.

The microsurgical approach for removing a SEGA is generally either transcallosal or transcortical, with most neurosurgeons favouring the transcallosal, interhemispheric approach (51). Some surgeons have utilized a transcortical approach to the tumour in the lateral ventricle in the setting of hydrocephalus. Recent experience with minimally invasive, endoscopic, stereotactic, neurosurgical SEGA resection has been reported (52, 53). The goal of surgery should always be complete tumour resection. When this is not possible, unfortunately, residual tumour tends to grow over time. With the increasing number of treatment options for SEGAs in TSC patients, one could potentially envision a strategy that incorporates a multimodality therapeutic paradigm. For example, is there a possible role for initial mTOR inhibition medical therapy to shrink a SEGA, followed by planned endoscopic, minimally invasive resection? Could mTOR inhibitors be used for a residual mass when complete tumour resection could not be achieved surgically?

Current research topics

Despite major advance in the diagnosis, surveillance, clinical assessment, animal modelling, and molecular genetics of TSC, there remain numerous unanswered questions and issues that are directly relevant to clinical care. Unresolved issues include understanding the high clinical variability of TSC, defining the lack of clear genotype–phenotype correlations, and identifying biomarkers for prognosis and stratification. A primary question is whether any more definitive genotype–phenotype correlations can be established so that particular mutations or classes of mutations could, for example, be used to predict the prognosis of any one TSC patient. This would have obvious importance in defining the clinical course of patients and the need for prophylactic therapy. A second issue is to better understand the disparity between tuber burden and neurological disability in TSC. While many individuals with numerous tubers will exhibit a severe neurological phenotype, often a patient with multiple tubers will have no or very mild neurological involvement. Conversely, there are patients with only a single tuber with severe intractable epilepsy and autism. Are these differences due to brain micropathology in TSC, the type of germline mutation, or perhaps other genetic modifiers? A third issue is whether credible predictive biomarkers for infantile spasms, seizures, cognitive disabilities, SEGA growth, response to AEDs, or autism can be identified so that prophylactic therapy with an mTOR inhibitor can be initiated. Identification of a blood, cerebrospinal fluid, or genetic marker that could be obtained in fetal or early neonatal life could provide life-altering information for TSC patients. As a corollary to this issue, the possibility of fetal therapy must be addressed. New strategies to devise mTOR cascade inhibitors that are not harmful to fetal development are warranted. Finally, while the advent of everolimus therapy heralds a new era for some aspects of TSC patient care, it remains unknown whether mTOR inhibitors will be effective for infantile spasms, cognitive disability, or autism in TSC. In addition, there is as of yet, no clear guideline for duration of therapy with mTOR inhibitors (e.g. weeks, months, years, or lifetime). Further studies will be required to define a definitive treatment algorithm for TSC patients.

Acknowledgements

This work was supported by NS045021, a Department of Defense-CDMRP-TSC Program grant, and the TS Alliance (PBC).

References

1. Crino PB, Nathanson KL, Henske EP. The tuberous sclerosis complex. *N Engl J Med* 2006; 355:1345–1356.
2. Curatolo P, Bombardieri R, Jozwiak S. Tuberous sclerosis. *Lancet* 2008; 372(9639):657–668.
3. Napolioni V, Moavero R, Curatolo P. Recent advances in neurobiology of tuberous sclerosis complex. *Brain Dev* 2009; 31:104–113.
4. Osborne JP, Fryer A, Webb D. Epidemiology of tuberous sclerosis. *Ann N Y Acad Sci* 1991; 615:125–127.
5. van Slegtenhorst M, de Hoogt R, Hermans C, et al. Identification of the tuberous sclerosis gene TSC1 on chromosome 9q34. *Science* 1997; 277:805–808.
6. European Tuberous Sclerosis Consortium. Identification and characterization of the tuberous sclerosis gene on chromosome 16. *Cell* 1993; 75:1305–1315.
7. Au KS, Williams AT, Roach ES, et al. Genotype/phenotype correlation in 325 individuals referred for a diagnosis of tuberous sclerosis complex in the United States. *Genet Med* 2007; 9:88–100.
8. Dabora SL, Jozwiak S, Franz DN, et al. Mutational analysis in a cohort of 224 tuberous sclerosis patients indicates increased severity of TSC2, compared with TSC1, disease in multiple organs. *Am J Hum Genet* 2001; 68:64–80.
9. Jones AC, Daniells CE, Snell RG, et al. Molecular genetic and phenotypic analysis reveals differences between TSC1 and TSC2 associated familial and sporadic tuberous sclerosis. *Hum Mol Genet* 1997; 6:2155–2161.
10. Jones AC, Shyamsundar MM, Thomas MW, et al. Comprehensive mutation analysis of TSC1 and TSC2-and phenotypic correlations in 150 families with tuberous sclerosis. *Am J Hum Genet* 1999; 64:1305–1315.
11. Sancak O, Nellist M, Goedbloed M, et al. Mutational analysis of the TSC1 and TSC2 genes in a diagnostic setting: genotype–phenotype correlations and comparison of diagnostic DNA techniques in Tuberous Sclerosis Complex. *Eur J Hum Genet* 2005; 13:731–741.
12. Dibble CC, Elis W, Menon S, et al. TBC1D7 is a third subunit of the TSC1-TSC2 complex upstream of mTORC1. *Mol Cell* 2012; 47:535–546.
13. van Slegtenhorst M, Verhoef S, Tempelaars A, et al. Mutational spectrum of the TSC1 gene in a cohort of 225 tuberous sclerosis complex patients: no evidence for genotype-phenotype correlation. *J Med Genet* 1999; 36:285–289.
14. Au KS, Williams AT, Roach ES, et al. Genotype/phenotype correlation in 325 individuals referred for a diagnosis of tuberous sclerosis complex in the United States. *Genet Med* 2007; 9(2):88–100.
15. Sancak O, Nellist M, Goedbloed M, et al. Mutational analysis of the TSC1 and TSC2 genes in a diagnostic setting: genotype–phenotype correlations and comparison of diagnostic DNA techniques in tuberous sclerosis complex. *Eur J Hum Genet* 2005; 13(6):731–741.
16. Maiese K, Chong ZZ, Shang YC, et al. mTOR: on target for novel therapeutic strategies in the nervous system. *Trends Mol Med* 2013; 19(1):51–60.
17. Huang J, Manning BD. The TSC1-TSC2 complex: a molecular switchboard controlling cell growth. *Biochem J* 2008; 412:179–190.
18. Wullschleger S, Loewith R, Hall MN. TOR signaling in growth and metabolism. *Cell* 2006; 124:471–484.
19. Oh WJ, Jacinto E. mTOR complex 2 signaling and functions. *Cell Cycle* 2011; 10:2305–2316.
20. Peterson TR, Laplante M, Thoreen CC, et al. DEPTOR is an mTOR inhibitor frequently overexpressed in multiple myeloma cells and required for their survival. *Cell* 2009; 137:873–886.
21. Ellisen LW. Growth control under stress: mTOR regulation through the REDD1-TSC pathway. *Cell Cycle* 2005; 4:1500–1502.
22. Tee AR, Manning BD, Roux PP, et al. Tuberous sclerosis complex gene products, Tuberin and Hamartin, control mTOR signaling by acting as a GTPase-activating protein complex toward Rheb. *Curr Biol* 2003; 13:1259–1268.
23. Ben-Sahra I, Howell JJ, Asara JM, et al. Stimulation of de novo pyrimidine synthesis by growth signaling through mTOR and S6K1. *Science* 2013; 339(6125):1323–1328.
24. Efeyan A, Zoncu R, Sabatini DM. Amino acids and mTORC1: from lysosomes to disease. *Trends Mol Med* 2012; 18(9):524–533.
25. Hsu PP, Kang SA, Rameseder J, et al. The mTOR-regulated phosphoproteome reveals a mechanism of mTORC1-mediated inhibition of growth factor signaling. *Science* 2011; 332:1317–1322.
26. Yu Y, Yoon SO, Poulogiannis G, et al. Phosphoproteomic analysis identifies Grb10 as an mTORC1 substrate that negatively regulates insulin signaling. *Science* 2011; 332:1322–1326.
27. Jacinto E, Loewith R, Schmidt A, et al. Mammalian TOR complex 2 controls the actin cytoskeleton and is rapamycin insensitive. *Nat Cell Biol* 2004 6:1122–1128.
28. Huang J, Wu S, Wu CL, et al. Signaling events downstream of mammalian target of rapamycin complex 2 are attenuated in cells and tumors deficient for the tuberous sclerosis complex tumor suppressors. *Cancer Res* 2009; 69:6107–6114.
29. Zeng Z, Sarbassov dos D, Samudio IJ, et al. Rapamycin derivatives reduce mTORC2 signaling and inhibit AKT activation in AML. *Blood* 2007; 109:3509–3512.
30. Tsai V, Parker WE, Orlova KA, et al. Fetal brain mTOR signaling activation in tuberous sclerosis complex. *Cereb Cortex* 2014; 24:315–327.
31. Tavazoie SF, Alvarez VA, Ridenour DA, et al. Regulation of neuronal morphology and function by the tumor suppressors Tsc1 and Tsc2. *Nat Neurosci* 2005; 8:1727–1734.
32. Meikle L, Talos DM, Onda H, et al. A mouse model of tuberous sclerosis: neuronal loss of Tsc1 causes dysplastic and ectopic neurons, reduced myelination, seizure activity, and limited survival. *J Neurosci* 2007; 27:5546–5558.
33. Carson RP, Van Nielen DL, Winzenburger PA, et al. Neuronal and glia abnormalities in Tsc1-deficient forebrain and partial rescue by rapamycin. *Neurobiol Dis* 2012; 45:369–380.
34. Uhlmann EJ, Wong M, Baldwin RL, et al. Astrocyte-specific TSC1 conditional knockout mice exhibit abnormal neuronal organization and seizures. *Ann Neurol* 2002; 52:285–296.
35. Anderl S, Freeland M, Kwiatkowski DJ, et al. Therapeutic value of prenatal rapamycin treatment in a mouse brain model of Tuberous Sclerosis Complex. *Hum Mol Genet* 2011; 20:4597–4604.
36. Northrup H, Krueger DA; International Tuberous Sclerosis Complex Consensus Group. Tuberous sclerosis complex diagnostic criteria update: recommendations of the 2012 international tuberous sclerosis complex consensus conference. *Pediatr Neurol* 2013; 49(4):243–254.
37. Krueger DA, Northrup H; International Tuberous Sclerosis Complex Consensus Group. Tuberous sclerosis complex surveillance and management: recommendations of the 2012 international tuberous sclerosis complex consensus conference. *Pediatr Neurol* 2013; 49(4):255–265.
38. Mizuguchi M, Takashima S. Neuropathology of tuberous sclerosis. *Brain Dev* 2001; 23(7):508–515.
39. Gallagher A, Grant EP, Madan N, et al. MRI findings reveal three different types of tubers in patients with tuberous sclerosis complex. *J Neurol* 2010; 257:1373–1381.
40. Wong M, Crino PB. Tuberous sclerosis and epilepsy: role of astrocytes. *Glia* 2012; 60:1244–1250.
41. Cepeda C, André VM, Yamazaki I, et al. Comparative study of cellular and synaptic abnormalities in brain tissue samples from pediatric tuberous sclerosis complex and cortical dysplasia type II. *Epilepsia* 2010; 51(Suppl 3):160–165.
42. White R, Hua Y, Lynch DR, et al. Differential transcription of neurotransmitter receptor subunits and uptake sites in giant cells and dysplastic neurons in cortical tubers. *Ann Neurol* 2001; 49:67–78.
43. Talos DM, Kwiatkowski DJ, Cordero K, et al. Cell-specific alterations of glutamate receptor expression in tuberous sclerosis complex cortical tubers. *Ann Neurol* 2008; 63:454–465.

44. Boer K, Troost D, Timmermans W, et al. Cellular localization of metabotropic glutamate receptors in cortical tubers and subependymal giant cell tumors of tuberous sclerosis complex. *Neuroscience* 2008; 156:203–215.

45. French JA, Lawson JA, Yapici Z, et al. Adjunctive everolimus therapy for treatment-resistant focal-onset seizures associated with tuberous sclerosis (EXIST-3): a phase 3, randomised, double-blind, placebo-controlled study. *Lancet* 2016; 388(10056):2153–2163.

46. Bissler JJ, McCormack FX, Young LR, et al. Sirolimus for angiomyolipoma in tuberous sclerosis complex or lymphangioleiomyomatosis. *N Engl J Med* 2008; 358:140–151.

47. Dabora SL, Franz DN, Ashwal S, et al. Multicenter phase 2 trial of sirolimus for tuberous sclerosis: kidney angiomyolipomas and other tumors regress and VEGF-D levels decrease. *PLoS One* 2011; 6:e23379.

48. Krueger DA, Care MM, Holland K, et al. Everolimus for subependymal giant-cell astrocytomas in tuberous sclerosis. *N Engl J Med* 2010; 363:1801–1811.

49. Krueger DA, Wilfong AA, Holland-Bouley K, et al. Everolimus treatment of refractory epilepsy in tuberous sclerosis complex. *Ann Neurol* 2013; 74(5):679–687.

50. Vaughn J, Hagiwara M, Katz J, et al. MRI characterization and longitudinal study of focal cerebellar lesions in a young tuberous sclerosis cohort. *AJNR Am J Neuroradiol* 2013; 34(3):655–659.

51. Harter DH, Bassani L, Rodgers SD, et al. A management strategy for intraventricular subependymal giant cell astrocytomas in tuberous sclerosis complex. *J Neurosurg Pediatr* 2014; 13:21–8.

52. Morita A, Kelly PJ. Resection of intraventricular tumors via computer-assisted volumetric stereotactic resection. *Neurosurgery* 1993; 32:920–926.

53. Rodgers SD, Bassani L, Weiner HL, et al. Stereotactic endoscopic resection and surgical management of a subependymal giant cell astrocytoma: case report. *J Neurosurg Pediatr* 2012; 9:417–420.

CHAPTER 18

Pituitary tumours

Edward R. Laws, Jr, Whitney W. Woodmansee,
and Jay S. Loeffler

Introduction

Disorders of the pituitary gland and the region of the sella turcica present a wide spectrum of clinical problems. A variety of lesions in this area tend to present with similar problems, namely headache, hormonal disorders, and loss of vision. The lesions involve a variety of tumours, cerebrovascular problems, infections, and inflammatory diseases. Benign adenomas of the pituitary gland are by far the most common disorder, along with craniopharyngiomas, Rathke cleft cysts, and meningiomas (Table 18.1) (1,2). These entities are the primary focus of this chapter.

Pituitary adenomas are in fact the second most common primary brain tumour. Depending on the specific tumour type, they range in incidence from 7 to 92 cases per 100,000 people per year, and in prevalence to approximately 1020 per 100,000 (2). Meningiomas are fairly frequent benign tumours of the sellar region. These include meningiomas of the tuberculum sellae, the planum sphenoidale, the clinoid processes, and the optic canals. Often they are grouped together as meningiomas of the anterior skull base. Craniopharyngiomas are the most common tumour of the sellar region in children, and most of these congenital tumours are thought to arise from the pituitary stalk. They can affect adults as well as children, are frequently cystic, and often contain areas of calcification.

The goals of therapy for tumours in the sellar region include relief of mass effect, maintenance or restoration of visual function, normalization of hormonal hypersecretion, preservation or restoration of pituitary hormonal function, prevention of recurrence, and the obtaining of pathological tissue for diagnosis (Box 18.1) (2).

Pituitary adenomas

In considering pituitary adenomas, the major distinction is between hyperfunctioning tumours presenting with typical hormonal syndromes, and clinically non-functioning tumours which usually present as relatively silent masses, causing headache, hypopituitarism, and compression of the optic chiasm, often producing the classical bitemporal hemianopia. They are classified by functional subtype, size, and invasiveness (3). The functional subtype is often obvious from the clinical presentation, as we see with prolactinomas, acromegaly, and Cushing's disease. A classification scheme related to size and regional extension was developed by Jules Hardy and has been widely accepted (4). The most commonly used size distinction

is between a microadenoma, 10 mm or less in diameter, and a macroadenoma, greater than 10 mm in diameter.

In addition to extending into the parasellar region, some pituitary adenomas are invasive regionally, and a scheme for classification of invasiveness has been developed by Knosp and colleagues, and is widely utilized (5). Magnetic resonance imaging (MRI) demonstrates the anatomical aspects of pituitary adenomas, and MRI is the basis not only for diagnosis, but for surgical planning (Figs 18.1 and 18.2).

When one considers the goals of therapy, the physiology and the anatomy of lesions, and the methods available for treatment, it is evident that each patient treatment plan must be individualized, and in most cases a multidisciplinary approach and a programme of therapy should be developed (6). Once the clinical and anatomical diagnoses have been made, one must consider a spectrum of therapies and combinations of therapies that may be recommended. In some cases this will involve simple observation and careful follow-up. In others, medical therapy may be indicated, and can be highly effective. For some patients, and some lesions, surgical excision may be the initial treatment of choice. For others, several forms of radiation therapy, including radiosurgery, are available as adjunctive treatments. Often, a programme of management involving several of these modalities is necessary for long-term control.

Medical management of pituitary adenomas

Medical management, of varying degrees of efficacy, is available for all of the hyperfunctioning pituitary adenomas.

Prolactinomas

Prolactinomas are the most common type of hyperfunctioning pituitary adenoma (7, 8). The population prevalence varies by study and gender with a 2010 publication reporting a prevalence of 44 per 100,000 (8). Most prolactinomas are effectively controlled by the use of dopamine agonists, such as cabergoline or bromocriptine, and medical therapy is generally the initial treatment of choice. Prolactin secretion is under inhibitory control by dopaminergic neurons in the hypothalamus and thus dopamine agonists have been useful for treatment of hyperprolactinemia.

These agents inhibit cellular proliferation and prolactin secretion from prolactin-producing cells. The goal of medical therapy is to reduce or normalize prolactin levels and to control tumour

Table 18.1 Differential diagnosis of pituitary lesions

Pituitary adenoma	Meningioma
Rathke cleft cyst	Germ cell tumour
Craniopharyngioma	Pituicytoma
Arachnoid cyst	Ganglioglioma
Lymphocytic hypophysitis	Metastatic lesion
Carcinoma	

growth. With normalization of prolactin levels, many of the clinical symptoms associated with hyperprolactinemia, such as amenorrhea, galactorrhoea, sexual dysfunction, and infertility, often reverse. Dopamine agonist therapy for prolactinomas has been associated with tumour shrinkage, and normalization of prolactin levels, as well as improvement in many of the clinical sequelae. Numerous studies have examined the effects of dopamine agonists on clinical outcomes and although the results vary by study, duration of treatment, agent used, and tumour type, the majority of patients do respond to therapy (9). Reported median response rates are as follows: tumour shrinkage (62%), resumption of menses (78%), resolution of galactorrhoea (86%), and normalization of prolactin levels (68%) (9). Cabergoline is currently the preferred drug because of its increased efficacy and tolerability. Cabergoline therapy is associated with a high rate of normalization of prolactin levels and tumour shrinkage, even in macroprolactinomas (10). Patients generally tolerate dopamine agonists with few side effects, particularly if they are started at low doses which are titrated slowly. In recent years, there has been concern regarding the development of cardiac valvulopathy in patients on high-dose ergot-derivative dopamine agonists as used in Parkinson's disease (11–13). The risk of valvular disease has been less clear in hyperprolactinemia/prolactinoma patients who are typically treated with lower doses of dopamine agonists (13). However, two meta-analyses of cabergoline use in hyperprolactinemia/prolactinomas have demonstrated an increased risk of tricuspid regurgitation in these patients as well (14, 15). Therefore, caution is advised, especially in patients on long-term, high-dose cabergoline, and echocardiography should be considered on an individualized basis. Duration of dopamine agonist therapy for prolactinomas should be individualized as well, and the most recent Endocrine Society guidelines (9) on this topic suggest that patients who have been treated for 2 or more years and show normal prolactin levels and tumour resolution on MRI may be considered for a trial of discontinuation of therapy. Approximately 20% of patients withdrawn from dopamine agonist therapy can maintain normal prolactin levels and success is

---

Box 18.1 Goals of therapy of pituitary adenomas

1. Relief of compressive mass effect—optic chiasm, cavernous sinus, brain
2. Normalization of excessive hormone secretion—GH, PRL, ACTH, TSH
3. Preservation/restoration of normal pituitary function
4. Prevention of recurrent disease.

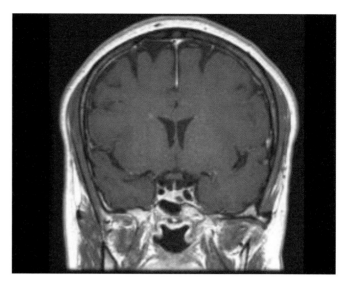

Fig. 18.1 Coronal, T1-weigted MRI of a patient with a pituitary microadenoma.

highest in patients treated with cabergoline for greater than 2 years (16). Long-term monitoring is required. Surgery for prolactinoma removal is certainly considered in patients intolerant of or resistant to dopamine agonist therapy.

Acromegaly

As with prolactinomas, medical therapy is available for patients with growth hormone (GH)-producing pituitary tumours. Generally, surgery is recommended as the initial treatment of choice, but in some patients primary medical therapy may be considered. The most commonly used medications are the somatostatin (SST) analogues. The SST analogues bind with variable affinity to the five different SST receptor subtypes (SST1–5) which are expressed on somatotroph cells, and, with ligand binding, inhibit GH secretion and cellular proliferation (17). The long-acting formulations, such as octreotide LAR and lanreotide, bind with highest affinity to SST receptor subtypes 2 and 5. In addition to controlling tumour growth

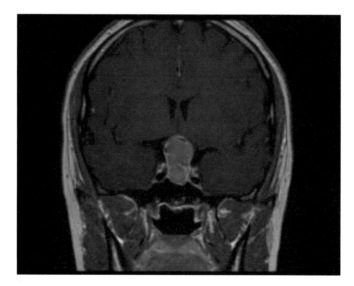

Fig. 18.2 Coronal, T1-weigted MRI of a patient with a contrast-enhancing, pituitary macroadenoma.

and managing the co-morbidities associated with GH excess, the goal of medical therapy in acromegaly is to induce a biochemical remission. Optimal hormonal control is associated with reduced mortality and improved co-morbidity associated with active acromegaly (18, 19). Biochemical remission, or optimal disease control, has been defined as a normal age-appropriate insulin-like growth factor (IGF)-1 level in a reliable assay, and a random GH level less than 1 mcg/L (ultrasensitive assay) or a nadir GH level less than 0.4 mcg/L in an oral glucose tolerance test (20). Both octreotide LAR and lanreotide have been shown to be efficacious in controlling biochemical parameters and causing tumour shrinkage (17) and appear to have comparable effectiveness (21). In one study of primary medical therapy of acromegalic patients, approximately 75% of patients had 25% or more reduction in tumour size and 42.5% had biochemical control (GH ≤2.5mcg/L and normal IGF-1) (22). A phase II clinical trial with the newest SST analogue, pasireotide, has shown efficacy in the treatment of acromegalic patients (23, 24). Pasireotide has a broader affinity for the SST receptor and binds SST1, SST2, SST3, and SST5, and thus has the potential to have greater efficacy. Unfortunately, this newer agent has been associated with increased risk of hyperglycaemia (25). Pegvisomant is another agent that may be used to control acromegaly and is typically considered when patients are inadequately controlled with SST analogues (26). Pegvisomant is a GH receptor antagonist given as a subcutaneous injection either as monotherapy, or may be combined with SST analogues. GH levels are not used to monitor therapy and typically they increase during treatment. IGF-1 normalization and improvement in clinical parameters are the main outcomes followed on pegvisomant therapy. Safety concerns include liver function abnormalities and pituitary tumour growth. Cabergoline may also be useful in some patients, particularly those with mild elevations in IGF-1 or those who have tumours that co-secrete prolactin (27). Finally, these medications may be used in combination to allow biochemical remission for those patients not controlled on one agent alone (28). For many patients, biochemical remission or disease control can be achieved using one or more of the medication options outlined above.

Cushing's disease

Currently, medical therapy for Cushing's disease remains in evolution. Medical therapy has more frequently been considered as an interim treatment modality while either contemplating additional surgery (pituitary or adrenalectomy) or waiting for radiation to be effective. Previously, agents that block the synthesis of cortisol were the major medications used to ameliorate the symptoms and signs of this devastating disease in patients not in biochemical remission following pituitary surgery. Metyrapone ketoconazole and mitotane (also adrenolytic) have been used for some time with moderate success, but side effects often limit their utility (29). Although clinical experience is somewhat limited, cabergoline has been shown to improve hypercortisolism in some patients with persistent disease after surgery (30, 31). Two additional agents have been approved by the US Food and Drug Administration for use to control hypercortisolism in Cushing's disease, mifepristone and pasireotide. Mifepristone is a progesterone antagonist that at high concentrations acts also as a cortisol antagonist. In a small trial of patients with Cushing's syndrome (N = 50, the majority due to pituitary disease) with type 2 diabetes mellitus, 87% demonstrated improvement in clinical status as measured by the area under the curve for glucose

on a 2-hour oral glucose tolerance test and by diastolic blood pressure (32). Side effects included fatigue, hypokalaemia, nausea, vomiting, arthralgias, oedema, and endometrial thickening in women. Importantly, urinary cortisol excretion cannot be used as a biochemical marker to assess efficacy of this medication. The SST analogue pasireotide has also been approved for medical therapy of Cushing's disease. The pivotal phase III clinical trial, published by Colao and colleagues (25), studied 162 patients with Cushing's disease and persistent hypercortisolism. Patients were randomized to either 600 or 900 mcg subcutaneously twice daily for 6 months, and the effects on urinary free cortisol, as well as other secondary endpoints, were assessed. The primary endpoint was urinary free cortisol in the normal range at the 6-month time point without a pasireotide dose escalation. Fifteen and twenty-six per cent of the low- and high-dose pasireotide groups, respectively, met the primary endpoint. Pasireotide treatment was associated with the expected side effects of SST analogues (gastrointestinal symptoms), but demonstrated a high rate of hyperglycaemia-related adverse events (25). Although this medication is currently approved for use in Cushing's disease patients for whom surgery is not indicated or has not been curative, its exact role has not been thoroughly determined. The availability of these new medications for Cushing's disease certainly introduces new treatment options for patients, but their long-term safety and efficacy remain under investigation.

Thyrotropin-stimulating hormone-producing pituitary adenomas

Thyrotropin-stimulating hormone (TSH)-producing pituitary adenomas are relatively rare and account for less than 1% of pituitary adenomas. Patients present with the typical signs and symptoms of hyperthyroidism, and diagnosis rests on demonstrating a normal or elevated TSH in the setting of hyperthyroxinaemia (33, 34). Surgery is the treatment of choice, but many of these tumours can be large and invasive, and are not always cured with surgery alone. The thyrotrope expresses SST receptors and TSH-producing pituitary tumours are responsive to SST analogues. Tumour shrinkage and TSH reduction have been demonstrated in patients who have been treated with SST analogues (35–39).

Non-functioning pituitary adenomas

Clinically non-functioning pituitary tumours, which usually present as macroadenomas, do not currently have any effective form of medical therapy to reduce the size of the tumour, and are primarily treated surgically (40, 41). Because many of these tumours are associated with hypopituitarism and pituitary insufficiency, active and effective hormone replacement therapy is essential. Fortunately, appropriate hormonal replacement therapy is available.

Surgical management of pituitary adenomas

Indications for surgery vary among the differing types of pituitary adenomas. For clinically non-functioning adenomas, usual indications are progressive visual loss from chiasmal compression, progressive hypopituitarism from the tumour compressing the normal pituitary, clinical manifestations of cavernous sinus compression (ptosis, diplopia, facial numbness, or pain), and intractable incapacitating headache. Results with regard to reversal of these symptoms are generally favourable (Table 18.2) (1).

Table 18.2 Outcomes of surgery for pituitary adenomas

Adenoma subtype	Remission criteria	Remission (%)	% Recurrence (10 yrs)
Non-functioning— Null cell/ Gonadotrope	Visual improvement	87	16
Acromegaly—GH	Normal IGF-1	Micro-87 Macro-50	8
Prolactin	Normal PRL	Micro-87 Macro-45	14
Cushing's disease—ACTH	Normal or subnormal Cortisol	Micro-89 Macro-55	12

ACTH, adrenocorticotropin-releasing hormone; GH, growth hormone; PRL, prolactin.

Reproduced from *J Am Coll Surg*, 193(6), Jane JA Jr, Laws ER Jr, The surgical management of pituitary adenomas in a series of 3,093 patients, pp. 651–59, Copyright (2001), with permission from Elsevier.

For the hyperfunctioning adenomas (prolactin, GH, adrenocorticotropin-releasing hormone (ACTH), TSH), the indications for surgery vary considerably. Prolactin-secreting adenomas are ordinarily very responsive to medical therapy. About 6% of patients will be intolerant of the rare but important side effects of dopamine agonist therapy, and some will be concerned about the very small risk of cardiac valvular disease provoked by these agents. These patients may become candidates for surgery. Other patients may have tumours that are hyporesponsive to dopamine agonist therapy, in that the prolactin levels may not normalize, or the tumour may not decrease in size in response to therapy (42). Cystic variants of prolactinomas are particularly prone to lack of medication-induced shrinkage. It is important to remember that in most patients medical therapy is suppressive and likely will not produce a lasting remission when discontinued. Although initial surgical results are good, especially for microadenomas (Table 18.2), it is important to note that the postsurgical recurrence rate for these tumours is high, and often requires subsequent medical management (1, 2).

For GH-secreting pituitary adenomas that ordinarily are associated with acromegaly, surgical management is currently first-line therapy for most of these lesions. Medical management has become increasingly more sophisticated and effective, and often is used to augment surgery in achieving remission and control of the co-morbidities associated with acromegaly. As with other pituitary adenomas, surgical results vary with the size and stage of the tumour, and whether or not there is invasion of the parasellar structures, particularly the cavernous sinus. The level of GH at the time of surgery is also an effective predictor of biochemical remission, with the best results in patients with immediate postoperative GH levels of less than 5 mcg/L (43).

In Cushing's disease resulting from an ACTH-secreting pituitary adenoma, surgery currently is first-line management for the majority of patients (44). Medical therapy includes some new strategies that have been tested in clinical trials; these agents, as with other medical therapies, are primarily suppressive in action, and those used for Cushing's disease have significant side effects. The majority of patients with Cushing's disease have ACTH-secreting pituitary microadenomas, and they have good initial responses to surgical management (Table 18.2) (1). As with prolactinomas, however, the recurrence rates at 10 and 20 years are high, and may necessitate

adjunctive therapy (45). Some patients with Cushing's disease are so fragile and ill from the co-morbidities associated with the disease that they are candidates for bilateral adrenalectomy (46). With current endoscopic techniques, this procedure can provide immediate lowering of circulating cortisol. The major concern with adrenalectomy is the possible subsequent development of Nelson's syndrome, associated with aggressive pituitary tumours secreting ACTH, uncontrolled by the loss of negative feedback from circulating cortisol.

TSH-secreting pituitary adenomas are uncommon, but can ordinarily be managed by medical therapy with SST analogues, or by surgery, or a combination of these modalities (34, 39).

Clinically non-functioning tumours are usually classified as null cell or gonadotrophic tumours based on immunocytochemistry. The gonadotrophic tumours may stain for follicle stimulating hormone, luteinizing hormone, or the alpha subunit of glycoprotein hormones, but rarely do they have clinical expression. There are so-called silent types of other pituitary tumours that stain for ACTH, GH, prolactin, or even multiple hormones that are clinically non-functioning. These tumours often present with visual loss. Outcomes are measured by return of vision, remission of headache, or lack of recurrence over time (47). Postoperative improvement in vision occurs in more than 87% of surgically treated tumours.

When surgical therapy is indicated, most tumours can be approached using a minimally invasive transnasal, transsphenoidal route, using the operating microscope, or more recently, the operating endoscope (48). Only 4–5% of pituitary adenomas currently are treated by craniotomy and these are usually 'giant' tumours, which often have eccentric suprasellar projection. The transsphenoidal approach is highly effective in most cases, and provides excellent outcomes and low levels of complications in experienced hands and in a multidisciplinary setting.

When surgery fails to achieve remission, or when tumours recur, adjunctive medical therapy and radiation therapy can be used to control the manifestations of this common disease.

Radiation therapy/radiosurgery

The advent of modern radiation delivery techniques allows radiation oncologists to deliver radiation that conforms the full dose distribution to the pituitary target volume while reducing the dose to surrounding critical structures. If the dose to the pituitary tumour is given in one to five fractions, the term stereotactic radiosurgery (SRS) is applied. If more than five fractions are used, fractionated radiation (FR) is the appropriate term (49). If possible, SRS is preferred, based upon equivalence in treatment efficacy and patient convenience. If the target volume is too close (<3 mm) to the optic system, SRS is not feasible and fractionated treatment is required (50). Fractionated treatment ranges from 25 to 30 fractions delivered over 5–6 weeks. Although it is potentially less damaging to surrounding structures, there are increasing data that suggest that biochemical response is slower with FR than what is seen after SRS (51). Types of conformal delivery systems in the United States and throughout the world include Gamma Knife® (Elekta, Stockholm), linear accelerators, CyberKnife® (Accuray, Sunnyvale, CA), and proton beam (52).

FR or SRS is used for surgically recurrent non-functioning adenomas if further surgery is felt not to be curative (e.g. invasion into the clivus or cavernous sinus). Radiation alone is essentially not performed in modern medical practice except for the very rare case of surgically inoperable patients. In a review of over 1000 patients treated for surgically recurrent non-functioning adenoma with FR or SRS, control rates were typically over 90% (53). The endpoint of success for FR or SRS is lack of progression, not extent of tumour reduction; however, two-thirds of patients treated will demonstrate tumour reduction on follow-up imaging. Typical doses used for FR were 45–50 Gy and with SRS 14–18 Gy. Tumours that show radiographic evidence of invasion, or have histological evidence of high proliferation, probably require FR because of the need to include more tissue in the irradiated volume.

For patients with secretory adenomas, there are a few important caveats for the radiation oncologist to be aware of in patient selection, treatment techniques, dose, and timing of irradiation. For these patients, higher biological equivalent doses lead to more rapid biochemical response. In our practice, it is not uncommon for patients to undergo reoperations to reduce remaining volume, so that higher doses of radiation can be applied. Patients with GH-secreting adenomas should not take long-acting SST analogues for at least 4 weeks prior to radiation, though they may begin as soon as the radiation is completed. In the rare patient irradiated for an aggressive prolactin-secreting tumour, cabergoline or bromocriptine should be discontinued for the month leading up to treatment, but they may resume as the radiation is concluded (54). Although the exact biological effects of these hormonal medical therapies are not understood, it is thought that they interfere with the cell cycle, making the adenomas less responsive to radiation. This results in decreased control rates as well as prolonged intervals to biochemical response and possibly increased rates of radiation-induced pituitary dysfunction. Although tumour arrest rates in secretory patients are as high as those for patients with non-functioning tumours, time to biochemical cure can be quite prolonged, and ranges from 9 months to several years (53). Patients must remain on suppressive medical therapy until there is clear evidence of radiation response based on biochemical testing. For patients with Cushing's disease, defining the target volume is quite challenging. In the last 200 Cushing's disease patients treated with radiation at the Massachusetts General Hospital, only a minority had visible tumour present on the radiation planning MRI and computed tomography. The target volume in these patients includes the dura

of the sella turcica and the medial wall of both the left and right cavernous sinus. These are areas where ACTH tumour is found at reoperation or at postmortem examinations (55). Biochemical remission rates for Cushing's disease and acromegaly are about 50% at 4 years. With longer observation periods, most patients will eventually be controlled if the data are analysed in an actuarial fashion (56).

In summary, it is generally agreed that radiation therapy is indicated for non-functioning adenomas in the following circumstances: (i) non-surgical candidate, (ii) recurrence of tumour after surgery, and (iii) surgically inaccessible tumour (e.g. cavernous sinus). For functioning adenomas radiation therapy is indicated for the following patients: (i) hormonally uncontrolled after maximal surgical and medical therapy, (ii) intolerance of medical therapy, and (iii) tumour expansion into non-operable sites.

The type of radiation to be used remains controversial. We believe SRS should be the treatment of choice for tumours greater than 3 mm distant from the optic nerves and chiasm, and for tumours with an average diameter of less than 3 cm. FR should be the treatment of choice for the remaining patients. For SRS patients, we recommend 15–18 Gy for non-functioning lesions and 20 Gy or more for secretory tumours. For FR patients, doses between 45–54 Gy in 25–30 fractions delivered over 5–5.5 weeks at 1.8 Gy/fraction are advised.

Late effects of pituitary radiation

The most common late effect of pituitary radiation is hypopituitarism. At least 20% of patients will require at least one hormonal axis needing replacement by 5 years and approximately 70% by 10 years. GH appears to be the most common hormone affected, followed by thyroid, female and male sex hormones, and cortisol. Mild, asymptomatic increase in prolactin levels is a common late finding. Diabetes insipidus is not a result of pituitary radiation and if seen, should suggest tumour recurrence. It is imperative that an endocrinologist follows these patients monitoring for early biochemical evidence of gonadal dysfunction, hypothyroidism, and subtle abnormalities in adrenal function (57). Although for decades it was recommended that the patient not be replaced with GH after pituitary irradiation (because of concern about stimulating tumour growth), it has now become the standard of care, producing substantial improvement in quality of life for long-term survivors of pituitary adenoma radiation (58).

There are no long-term data regarding the risk of radiation-associated brain tumours after pituitary radiation using modern techniques. The cumulative risk of second brain tumours was 2% at 10 years and 2.4% at 20 years measured from the date of large-field, low-energy, FR completion. These tumours included meningioma, sarcoma, high-grade glioma, and primitive neuroectodermal tumour (59). It has been estimated that with modern techniques, secondary tumour risks from FR will be lower than these numbers. It is clear that the risk of secondary tumours following SRS is extremely low, and has been estimated to be 1/1000–10,000 (60).

The incidence of cerebrovascular accidents (CVAs) in patients following pituitary radiation has always been a concern, since the majority of the vessels in the circle of Willis receive a full dose. In the only study with long-term observation, the actuarial incidence of CVA was 4% at 5 years, 11% at 10 years, and 21% at 20 years measured from the date of completion of radiation. The relative risk of CVA compared to the general population in the United Kingdom was 4.1. Patients treated with more modern radiation techniques had a significantly lower risk (61)

Pituitary Carcinoma

Pituitary carcinomas account for approximately 0.1% of all pituitary adenomas. They occur in the presence of a previous benign adenoma. By definition, pituitary carcinomas are lesions not in continuity with the previous adenoma within the intracranial space and/or have disseminated to extracranial sites (e.g. bone, lung, liver). Pituitary carcinomas should be separated from aggressive and invasive pituitary adenomas which are classified as aggressive adenoma. The mean latency period from adenoma to carcinoma is approximately 6 years but has been reported as late as 18 years. The most common histologies associated with carcinoma are ACTH "silent" tumors and prolactin secreting adenomas (62). Historically, re-irradiation and surgery have been the mainstay of treatment. Many chemotherapeutic agents have been used with little or no success. However, recently, the alkylating drug temozolomide has been employed with response rates as high as 60%. However, the duration of response has generally been 12 months or less though some patients continue to respond for up to 2 years (63). There is interest in targeted therapy based on whole genome sequencing of the carcinoma, but to date few "targetable" mutations have been identified.

In summary, numerous types of structural lesions can be found in the sellar and suprasellar region. The most common lesions identified are the benign pituitary adenomas, which typically can be treated successfully with medical therapy, surgical resection, and radiation, or a combination of modalities depending on the tumour type and response to the original treatment. These patients are best treated with a multidisciplinary approach that combines the expertise of endocrinology, neurosurgery, and radiation oncology specialists (6).

References

1. Jane JA Jr, Laws ER Jr. The surgical management of pituitary adenomas in a series of 3,093 patients. *J Am Coll Surg* 2001; 193(6):651–659.

2. Laws ER, Sheehan JP. *Sellar and Parasellar Tumors: Diagnosis, Treatments, and Outcomes.* New York: Thieme, 2012.

3. DeLellis RA, Lloyd RV, Heitz PU, et al. (eds). *World Health Organization Classification of Tumours: Pathology and Genetics of Tumours of Endocrine Organs.* Lyon: IARC Press, 2004.

4. Hardy J. Transsphenoidal surgery of the normal and pathological pituitary. *Clin Neurosurg* 1969; 16:185–217.

5. Knosp E, Steiner E, Kitz K, et al. Pituitary tumors with invasion of the cavernous sinus space: a magnetic resonance imaging classification compared with clinical findings. *J Neurosurg* 1993; 33:610–617.

6. Laws ER, McLaughlin N, Oyesiku NM, et al. Pituitary centers of excellence. *Neurosurgery* 2012; 71:916–923.

7. Daly AF, Rixhon M, Adam C, et al. High prevalence of pituitary adenomas: a cross-sectional study in the province of Liege, Belgium. *J Clin Endocrinol Metab* 2006; 91:4769–4775.

8. Fernandez A, Karavitaki N, Wass JA. Prevalence of pituitary adenomas: a community-based, cross-sectional study in Banbury (Oxfordshire, UK). *Clin Endocrinol (Oxf)* 2010; 72:377–382.

9. Melmed S, Casanueva FF, Hoffman AR, et al. Diagnosis and treatment of hyperprolactinemia: an Endocrine Society clinical practice guideline. *J Clin Endocrinol Metab* 2011; 96(2):273–288.

10. Colao A, DiSarno A, Landi ML, et al. Macroprolactinoma shrinkage during cabergoline treatment is greater in naive patients than in patients pretreated with other dopamine agonists: a prospective study in 110 patients. *J Clin Endocrinol Metab* 2000; 85:2247–2252.

11. Zanettini R, Antonini A, Gatto G, et al. Valvular heart disease and the use of dopamine agonists for Parkinson's disease. *N Engl J Med* 2007; 356:39–46.

12. Schade R, Andersohn F, Suissa S, et al. Dopamine agonists and the risk of cardiac-valve regurgitation. *N Engl J Med* 2007; 356:29–38.

13. Valassi E, Klibanski A, Biller BM. Clinical review: Potential cardiac valve effects of dopamine agonists in hyperprolactinemia. *J Clin Endocrinol Metab* 2010; 95(3):1025–1033.

14. Bogazzi F, Manetti L, Raffaelli V, et al. Cabergoline therapy and the risk of cardiac valve regurgitation in patients with hyperprolactinemia: a meta-analysis from clinical studies. *J Endocrinol Invest* 2008; 31(12):1119–1123.

15. De Vecchis R, Esposito C, Ariano C. Cabergoline use and risk of fibrosis and insufficiency of cardiac valves: meta-analysis of observational studies. *Herz* 2013; 38(8):868–880.

16. Dekkers OM, Largo J, Burman P, et al. Recurrence of hyperprolactinemia after withdrawal of dopamine agonists: systematic review of the literature and meta-analysis. *J Clin Endocrinol Metab* 2010; 95:43–51.

17. Freda PU. Somatostatin analogs in acromegaly. *J Clin Endocrinol Metab* 2002; 87(7):3013–3018.

18. Melmed S, Colao A, Barkan A, et al. Guidelines for acromegaly management: an update. *J Clin Endocrinol Metab* 2009; 94(5):1509–1517.

19. Swearingen B, Barker FG, 2nd, Katznelson L, et al. Long-term mortality after transsphenoidal surgery and adjunctive therapy for acromegaly. *J Clin Endocrinol Metab* 1998; 83(10):3419–3426.

20. Guistina A, Chanson P, Bronstein MD, et al. A consensus on criteria for cure of acromegaly. *J Clin Endocrinol Metab* 2010; 95:3141–3148.

21. Murray RD, Melmed S. A critical analysis of clinically available somatostatin analog formulations for therapy of acromegaly. *J Clin Endocrinol Metab* 2008; 93:2957–2968.

22. Colao A, Pivonello R, Auriemma RS, et al. Predictors of tumor shrinkage after primary therapy with somatostatin analogs in acromegaly: a prospective study in 99 patients. *J Clin Endocrinol Metab* 2006; 91(6):2112–2118.

23. Petersenn S, Schopohl J, Barkan A, et al. Pasireotide (SOM230) demonstrates efficacy and safety in patients with acromegaly: a randomized, multicenter, Phase II trial. *J Clin Endocrinol Metab* 2010; 95:2781–2789.

24. Petersenn S, Farrall AJ, Block C, et al. Long-term efficacy and safety of subcutaneous pasireotide in acromegaly: results from an open-ended, multicenter, Phase II extension study. *Pituitary* 2014; 17(2):132–40.

25. Colao A, Petersenn S, Newell-Price J, et al. A 12-month phase 3 study of pasireotide in Cushing's disease. *N Engl J Med* 2012; 366:914–924.

26. Trainer PJ, Drake WM, Katznelson L, et al. Treatment of acromegaly with the growth hormone-receptor antagonist pegvisomant. *N Engl J Med* 2000; 342(16): 1171–1177.

27. Abs R, Verhelst J, Maiter D, et al. Cabergoline in the treatment of acromegaly: a study in 64 patients. *J Clin Endocrinol Metab* 1998; 83(2):374–378.

28. Fleseriu M. The role of combination medical therapy in acromegaly: hope for the nonresponsive patient. *Curr Opin Endocrinol Diabetes Obes* 2013; 20(4):321–329.

29. Tritos NA, Biller BM, Swearingen B. Management of Cushing disease. *Nat Rev Endocrinol* 2011; 7(5):279–289.

30. Pivonello R, De Martino MC, Cappabianca P, et al. The medical treatment of Cushing's disease: effectiveness of chronic treatment with the dopamine agonist cabergoline in patients unsuccessfully treated by surgery. *J Clin Endocrinol Metab* 2009; 94(1):223–230.

31. Godbout A, Manavela M, Danilowicz K, et al. Cabergoline monotherapy in the long-term treatment of Cushing's disease. *Eur J Endocrinol* 2010; 163(5):709–716.

32. Fleseriu M, Biller BM, Findling JW, et al. Mifepristone, a glucocorticoid receptor antagonist, produces clinical and metabolic benefits in patients with Cushing's syndrome. *J Clin Endocrinol Metab* 2012; 97(6):2039–2049.

33. McDermott MT, Ridgway EC. Central hyperthyroidism. *Endocrinol Metab Clin North Am* 1998; 27(1):187–203.

34. Laws ER, Vance ML, Jane JA, Jr. TSH adenomas. *Pituitary* 2006; 9(4): 313–315.

35. Comi RJ, Gesundheit N, Murray L, et al. Response of thyrotropin-secreting pituitary adenomas to a long-acting somatostatin analogue. *N Engl J Med* 1987; 317:12–17.

36. Chanson P, Warnet A. Treatment of thyroid-stimulating hormone secreting adenomas with octreotide. *Metabolism* 1992; 4:62–65.

37. Chanson P, Weintraub BD, Harris AG. Treatment of TSH-secreting pituitary adenomas with octreotide: a follow-up of 52 patients. *Ann Intern Med* 1993; 119:236–240.

38. Caron P, Arlot S, Bauters C, et al. Efficacy of the long-acting octreotide formulation (octreotide-LAR) in patients with thyrotropin-secreting pituitary adenomas. *J Clin Endocrinol Metab* 2001; 86(6):2849–2853.

39. Beck-Peccoz P, Persani L. Medical management of thyrotropin-secreting pituitary adenomas. *Pituitary* 2002; 5(2):83–88

40. Young WF, Jr, Scheithauer BW, Kovacs KT, et al. Gonadotroph adenoma of the pituitary gland: a clinicopathologic analysis of 100 cases. *Mayo Clin Proc* 1996; 71(7):649–656.

41. Molitch ME. Management of incidentally found nonfunctional pituitary tumors. *Neurosurg Clin N Am* 2012; 23(4):543–553.

42. Molitch ME. Pharmacologic resistance in prolactinoma patients. *Pituitary* 2005; 8:43–52.

43. Kreutzer J, Vance ML, Lopes MB, et al. Surgical management of GH-secreting pituitary adenomas: an outcome study using modern remission criteria. *J Clin Endocrinol Metab* 2001; 86(9):4072–4077.

44. Prevedello DM, Pouratian N, Sherman J, et al. Management of Cushing's disease: outcome in patients with microadenoma detected on pituitary magnetic resonance imaging. *J Neurosurg* 2008; 109(4):751–759.

45. Patil CG, Prevedello DM, Lad SP, et al. Late recurrences of Cushing's disease after initial successful transsphenoidal surgery. *J Clin Endocrinol Metab* 2008; 93(2):358–362.

46. Smith PW, Turza KC, Carter, CO, et al. Bilateral adrenalectomy for refractory Cushing disease: a safe and definitive therapy. *J Am Coll Surg* 2009; 208(6):1059–1064.

47. Laws ER, Jr, Trautmann JC, Hollenhorst RW, Jr. Transsphenoidal decompression of the optic nerve and chiasm. Visual results in 62 patients. *J Neurosurg* 1977; 46(6):717–722.

48. Jane JA, Jr, Thapar K, Kaptain GJ, et al. Pituitary surgery: transsphenoidal approach. *Neurosurgery* 2002; 51(2):435–442.

49. Konziolka D, Lunsford LD, Loeffler JS, et al. Radiosurgery and radiotherapy: observations and clarifications *J Neurosurg* 2004; 4:585–589.

50. Tishler RB, Loeffler JS, Lunsford LD, et al. Tolerance of the cranial nerves of the cavernous sinus to radiosurgery. *Int J Radiat Oncol Biol Phys* 1993; 27:215–221.

51. Landolt AM, Haller D, Lomax N, et al. Stereotactic radiosurgery for surgically treated acromegaly: comparison with fractionated radiotherapy, *J Neurosurg* 1998; 88:1002–1008.

52. Loeffler JS, Durante M. Charged particle therapy—optimization, challenges and future directions. *Nat Rev Clin Oncol* 2013; 10:411–424.

53. Loeffler JS, Shih HA. Radiation therapy in the management of pituitary adenomas. *J Clin Endocrinol Metab* 2011; 96:1992–2003.

54. Sheehan JP, Pouratian N, Steiner L, et al. Gamma knife surgery for pituitary adenomas: factors related to radiographic and endocrine outcomes. *J Neurosurg* 2011; 114:303–309.

55. Petit JH, Biller BM, Yock TI, et al. Proton stereotactic radiotherapy for persistent adrenocorticotropin-producing adenomas *J Clin Endocrinol Metab* 2008; 93:393–399.

56. Estrada J, Boronat M, Mielgo M, et al. The long-term outcome of pituitary irradiation after unsuccessful transphenoidal surgery in Cushing's disease. *N Engl J Med* 1997; 336:172–177.

57. Constine LS, Woolf PD, Cann D, et al. Hypothalamic-pituitary dysfunction after radiation for brain tumors. *N Engl J Med* 1993; 328:87–94.

58. Wexler T, Gunnell L, Omer Z, et al. Growth hormone deficiency is associated with decreased quality of life in patients with prior acromegaly. *J Clin Endocrinol Metab* 2009; 94: 2471–2477.

59. Minniti G, Traish D, Ashley S, et al. Risk of second brain tumor after conservative surgery and radiotherapy for pituitary adenoma: update after an additional 10 years. *J Clin Endocrinol Metab* 2004; 90:800–804.

60. Loeffler JS, Niemierko A, Chapman PH. Second tumors after radiosurgery: tip of the iceberg or a bump in the road. *Neurosurgery* 2003; 52:1436–1440.

61. Brada M, Burchell L, Ashley S, et al. The incidence of cerebrovascular accidents in patients with pituitary adenomas. *Int J Radiat Oncolo Biol Phys* 1999; 45:693–698.

62. Hearney AP. Pituitary carcinoma: difficult diagnosis and treatment. J Clin Endocrinol Metab. 2011; 96:3649–3660.

63. Jordan JT, Miller JJ, Cushing T, et al. Temozolomide therapy for aggressive functioning pituitary adenomas refractory to surgery and radiation: a case series. *Neurooncol Pract* 2017.

CHAPTER 19

Metastatic brain tumours

Matthias Preusser, Gabriele Schackert,
and Brigitta G. Baumert

Definition

Brain metastases are secondary brain tumours that result from spread of cancers originating outside of the central nervous system (CNS). Thus, brain metastases are not a separate disease entity but a clinically and pathobiologically heterogeneous group of disease manifestations of systemic cancers (1).

Epidemiology

Central nervous system metastases are the most frequent malignant brain tumours and have been estimated to be up to ten times more common than gliomas. Up to 40% of cancer patients will develop brain metastases (2). However, the exact incidence of brain metastases remains unclear due to a lack of epidemiological studies on this subject, underdiagnosis, and inaccurate reporting in the literature. Incidence rates of up to 11 per 100,000 population per year have been reported, but the true incidence may in fact be considerably higher (2).

The relative incidence of brain metastases is highly variable among primary tumour types with lung cancer, breast cancer, melanoma, and kidney cancer showing the highest risk for metastatic CNS involvement in adults (2–7). Other common primary tumours such as prostate cancer and colorectal cancer are underrepresented among brain metastases, probably due to as yet undefined pathobiological/molecular differences in the propensity for brain invasion. In up to 15% of brain metastases no primary tumour is found at diagnosis (2). In children, germ cell tumours, sarcomas (osteosarcoma, rhabdomyosarcoma, and Ewing's sarcoma), and neuroblastomas are the most common primary tumours causing brain metastases (2, 8).

The incidence of brain metastases seems to be increasing over time. Probable reasons for this are the increasing incidence of smoking-associated lung cancer, higher availability and more intensive use of cranial magnetic resonance imaging (MRI) in cancer patients, and longer survival of cancer patients due to increased availability of effective therapy options (thus allowing greater opportunity for brain metastases to become clinically evident) (9). Moreover, some drugs used for the therapy of extracerebral neoplasms do not or only poorly cross the blood–brain barrier which may give tumour cells that invaded the CNS a survival benefit. This concern has been raised in particular with regard to monoclonal antibodies such as trastuzumab, which do not penetrate the intact blood–brain barrier due to their high molecular weight (11).

The prognosis of brain metastasis patients is in general poor with median overall survival times of only a few months for most patient populations. However, some patients do experience long-term survival of several years. Several prognostic scores based on clinical parameters, such as patient age, Karnofsky performance score, status of extracranial disease, and number of brain metastases, have been developed. The most commonly used ones are the recursive partitioning analysis score, the graded prognostic assessment (GPA) score, and the diagnosis-specific GPA (DS-GPA) (12–14). The GPA prognostic classification system takes into account Karnofsky performance status, age, number of brain metastases, and the status of extracranial disease. The DS-GPA includes the parameters of age, Karnofsky performance score, number of brain metastases, and status of extracranial disease depending on the primary tumour histology and may be preferable to other more generic prognostic scores. However, despite the use of prognostic scoring systems, prediction of individual patient outcome is difficult and prone to error (15). Incorporation of tissue-based or imaging characteristics may improve prognostic evaluation of brain metastasis patients, pending validation in large and ideally prospectively collected patient populations (16–18).

Aetiology and pathogenesis

So far, it is unclear what determines the difference in risk of histological tumour types and molecular subtypes causing brain colonization. Most probably, this can be explained by molecular parameters that influence the affinity of tumour cells to the milieu of the brain ('seed and soil theory') (19). The formation of brain metastases commonly necessitates haematogenous dissemination of tumour cells from the primary tumour or other non-CNS metastases. Exceptional routes may include direct spread from bone or venous sinuses or cerebrospinal fluid whereas lymphatic spread is highly unlikely given the paucity of lymphatic drainage of the brain. Successful CNS invasion requires attachment of tumour cells to brain microvessels and breaching of the blood–brain barrier and invasion into the brain parenchyma via upregulation of selectins, integrins, chemokines, heparanases, matrix metalloproteases, and other molecules (20). Within the brain parenchyma, tumour cells may be able to stay senescent or dormant in the perivascular area for prolonged periods of time. Outgrowth to micro- and then macrometastases involves tumour cell proliferation and induction of vascular endothelial growth factor (VEGF)-dependent angiogenesis (21). Brain metastases have been shown to invade the brain parenchyma in different ways. About half of brain metastases present with a well-demarcated border to the surrounding brain parenchyma and grow in an expansive manner, approximately 20% of cases show brain invasion by vascular co-option (tumour cell growth alongside pre-existing vascular structures), and around 30% of cases show single-cell invasion (22). Metastatic brain tumours elicit a variably intense reaction in the brain microenvironment with astrogliosis, recruitment of microglia and tumour-associated macrophages, collagenous fibrosis, and mixed lymphocytic infiltration (19, 23).

Clinical presentation

There is a high variability in clinical presentation of brain metastases. Symptoms depend on the localization of the cerebral lesions and may include focal neurological deficits, aphasia, epileptic seizures, signs of increased intracranial pressure (headache, nausea), personality changes, and others (24). Brain metastases may, however, also remain asymptomatic over long periods of time.

Imaging

Brain metastases are usually detected by neuroimaging in symptomatic patients or during staging investigations. Neuroimaging during initial disease staging is recommended for patients with small cell lung cancer, while screening in patients with non-small cell lung cancer (NSCLC) is currently under discussion and recommendations differ between clinical practice guidelines (25). In any case, patients with neurological symptoms should be referred for neuroimaging. Contrast-enhanced MRI with gadolinium is the preferred imaging technique for visualization of brain metastases and has been shown to have higher sensitivity than computed tomography or 18-fluorodeoxyglucose positron emission tomography (26). However, there are no guidelines that define many important imaging variables such as gadolinium dose and technical scanning parameters (MRI field strength, slice thickness, slice gap, etc.). Moreover, no generally accepted response criteria for brain metastases are available. The response criteria commonly used in neuro-oncology trials on primary brain tumours such as MacDonald criteria or Response Assessment in Neuro-Oncology (RANO) criteria are not directly applicable to brain metastases, because they do not consider the extracranial disease status (26). Brain metastases-specific RANO criteria are under development and recommend volumetric measurements using contrast-enhanced MRI as well as the inclusion of neurological functioning, neurological symptoms, functional independence, and health-related quality of life for response assessment in brain metastases trials (26, 27). However, these criteria need validation in appropriate studies before they can be applied in the clinical setting. Response Evaluation Criteria in Solid Tumors (RECIST) criteria that are used for extracranial cancers, on the other hand, do not take important brain-specific parameters such as neurological symptoms or corticosteroid use into account.

Advanced neuroimaging techniques such as dynamic contrast-enhanced MRI, magnetic resonance spectroscopy, perfusion-weighted imaging, susceptibility-weighted imaging, and diffusion-weighted imaging may aid differential diagnosis or be of prognostic value, or both, but more studies are needed to develop concrete recommendations for their incorporation into routine clinical use (28). Preliminary studies suggest the potential ability of dynamic susceptibility contrast MRI and diffusion-weighted imaging to differentiate between often observed radionecrosis after stereotactic radiosurgery (SRS) or high-dose radiotherapy and potential progression or recurrence (29, 30). Usually regular MRI is used for follow-up of brain metastases, although there is a lack of data to provide evidence-based recommendations on the use of neuroimaging in the follow-up of brain metastasis patients. One study indicated that routine brain surveillance using MRI in brain metastasis patients treated with SRS rather than symptom-prompted imaging may improve outcome and reduce the cost of care (31).

Treatment in adults

The principal treatment options in brain metastasis patients include local therapies like neurosurgical resection, radiotherapy (including SRS and stereotactic radiotherapy (SRT), whole-brain radiotherapy (WBRT), and new radiation techniques), and medical antineoplastic therapy (including cytotoxic chemotherapy and targeted agents) as well as supportive care measures. However, for many clinical situations there is a lack of high-level evidence to guide treatment decisions and lack of agreement on common clinical management issues (32). The choice of the therapeutic approach should ideally be discussed in a multidisciplinary tumour board and needs to take into account several important parameters such as the number of brain metastases, the status of the extracranial tumour burden, the patient's performance status, primary tumour type, molecular alterations, co-morbidities, and prior therapies.

Surgery

Neurosurgical resection is primarily considered in patients with surgically accessible single brain metastases, no or controlled extracranial tumour burden, and good performance status (9). In patients with significant mass effect from one or more brain metastases, surgical resection may be necessary for acute decompression. In patients with an unknown primary tumour, surgical resection offers the possibility to obtain tissue for histopathological and molecular tumour (sub-)typing. In patients with more than one brain metastasis, cerebral metastasectomy is sometimes performed in cases in which more than one lesion are accessible through the same craniotomy approach, although this approach is not backed by data from clinical trials (9).

Several studies have investigated the combination of surgical resection with WBRT (33). It has been reported that in patients with a single metastasis, surgical resection alone is associated with a higher recurrence rate when radiotherapy does not follow resection and that WBRT alone is associated with a lower survival rate compared to radiation plus surgical resection (34, 35). Kocher et al. reported that adjuvant WBRT after SRS or surgery of one to three brain metastases reduces intracranial relapses and neurological deaths but fails to improve the duration of functional independence and overall survival (36). These data have been used as an argument to withhold adjuvant WBRT in well-performing patients with otherwise stable systemic disease and a limited number (one to three) of brain metastases, who have been initially treated with either radiosurgery or surgery, as long as serial imaging for follow-up is performed. However, it must be noted that all of the mentioned studies are limited by imperfections in study design that limit their generalizability (1). For example, neuroimaging protocols were poorly standardized across studies and patients with highly heterogeneous primary tumour histologies (with NSCLC being the largest group) were enrolled. An unresolved question is also whether local postoperative irradiation of the tumour bed is a useful alternative to WBRT (37, 38). Adjuvant irradiation of the operation cavity substantially reduces the risk of recurrence in the tumour bed (39). Initial single-centre studies report high local control of about 80%; however, prospective evidence is lacking (40–42).

Radiotherapy

Stereotactic radiosurgery/radiotherapy

Stereotactic radiosurgery, a single-dose, high-precision focused radiotherapy, utilizes convergent beams or arcs to irradiate in a single fraction circumscribed lesions with a high dose in the planning target volume and a steep dose gradient at the margin (Fig. 19.1).

Brain metastases have long been considered a prototypic indication for SRS, especially when they are small (maximal diameter of up to 3 cm) and of limited number (less than three to four). Recently, hypofractionated SRT with few fractions for metastases larger than 2.5–3 cm in diameter metastases is also increasingly applied. An advantage of SRS/SRT over WBRT is the better preservation of neurocognitive function due to sparing of non-affected brain areas (1). On the other hand, SRS/SRT will not be able to treat microscopic tumour manifestations that escape detection by neuroimaging. Another advantage is that SRS is delivered in a single fraction in an outpatient setting and may thus be more convenient for many patients in this palliative disease setting than WBRT, which is typically delivered in 2–3-week courses. SRS and neurosurgical resection are often considered complementary approaches in patients with single or few (less than four) brain metastases and careful consideration between these two options needs to be undertaken on an individual case-to-case basis. Compared to neurosurgery, SRS has the advantages of being a non-invasive treatment that can be delivered in an outpatient setting, of being feasible also in lesions not amenable to resection due to sensitive localization in the CNS (e.g. brainstem, eloquent area), and also of being achievable

in patients who cannot be operated on due to co-morbidities (9). However, SRS does not provide the possibility of providing tissue collection for histology or determination of molecular markers and may induce significant radiation necrosis with brain oedema.

In general, drawing of evidence-based conclusions on the optimal use of SRS is limited by the lack of well-performed and adequately designed clinical trials. Most of the available clinical trials included heterogeneous patient populations and focused on subpopulations with relatively good prognosis. Still, based on the available evidence, SRS needs to be regarded as a main treatment option for brain metastases and should be considered for patients with single or few (up to three to four) brain metastases with a maximal diameter of 2.5–3 cm, especially if the metastases are not amenable to surgery (e.g. localization in eloquent brain areas or brainstem) and have no significant mass effect (43–45). A prospective, multiinstitutional, observational study investigated the use of SRS in 1194 patients with one, two to four, or five to ten brain metastases and found similar overall survival and treatment-related toxicity rates between the groups with two to four and five to ten metastases (46). Further research is needed to address the question of whether WBRT with hippocampal sparing or SRS/SRT should be preferred in patients with five to ten brain metastases and can only be answered by a prospective randomized study with inclusion of high-quality neurocognitive function testing and neurocognitive endpoints.

Newer radiation techniques make the combination of localized high-precision radiotherapy and the delivery of WBRT at the same time possible (Fig. 19.2) (47, 48). This new treatment strategy targets areas of known disease and microscopic disease simultaneously and carries the potential to enhance the therapeutic ratio. Randomized trials are required to evaluate this novel treatment.

Whole-brain radiotherapy

Whole-brain radiotherapy is a cornerstone in the treatment of brain metastases and is typically applied in patients with multiple brain metastases. WBRT may induce partial remission or disease stabilization; however, median overall survival times in patients treated

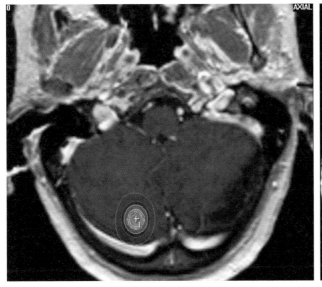
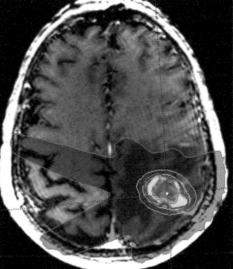

Fig. 19.1 (See colour plate section) Example of stereotactic radiosurgery (left) with an arc technique applied, and stereotactic radiotherapy (right) for a larger metastasis with multiple fixed convergent beams. Light blue colour: high-dose area, purple colour: low-dose area.

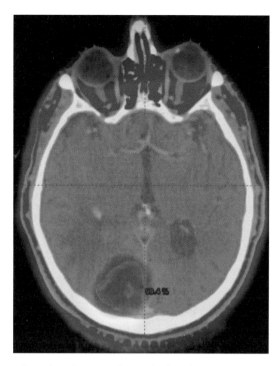

Fig. 19.2 (See colour plate section) Example of simultaneous integrated boost technique with whole-brain radiotherapy (WBRT). Green colour: dose for WBRT, red colour: a higher dose delivered at the same time as WBRT during the same daily radiotherapy session, for example, a total dose of 30 Gy for the whole brain and 60 Gy to the metastases.

with WBRT for multiple brain metastases are only a few months in most patient series. WBRT is associated with a significant risk for neurocognitive decline due to damage to the brain parenchyma or induction of intracerebral vascular changes and the benefits and expected adverse effects need to be carefully considered (1). A meta-analysis of 39 trials involving 10,835 patients concluded that altered WBRT dose-fractionation schemes are not superior in terms of overall survival, neurological function, or symptom control as compared to standard fractionation (3000 cGy in ten daily fractions or 2000 cGy in four or five daily fractions) (49). Adjuvant WBRT after SRS of up to four brain metastases improves intracranial control but does not seem to improve overall survival and carries a high risk of neurocognitive decline; it is therefore not unequivocally recommended (36, 43, 50–52).

Small cell lung cancer has a high risk for brain metastases and prophylactic cranial irradiation has been shown to prolong survival and decrease the incidence of cerebral metastases (53). Prophylactic cranial irradiation is recommended for patients with extensive disease achieving a complete or partial response to first-line chemotherapy and for patients with localized and stable disease (54).

Open issues that need to be addressed further in clinical trials include the definition of patient groups (e.g. patients with oligo- or asymptomatic brain metastases of tumour subtypes with sensitivity to specific inhibitors) that may benefit from a primary systemic therapy or a combination of WBRT with a targeted agent or a radiosensitizer, identification of approaches that preserve neurocognitive function in patients treated with WBRT (hippocampal-sparing WBRT), and the selection of patients that will not benefit from

WBRT or any other antineoplastic therapy and are best managed with 'best supportive care'.

Acute side effects such as fatigue, nausea, headache, and cognitive decline are transient, whereas adverse effects like memory dysfunction after WBRT are persistent. A significant decline in hippocampus-related memory function following WBRT has been reported. Several studies have shown that WBRT is related to neurocognitive decline. However, it has also been noted that neurocognitive decline recovered over time and then paralleled neurocognitive functioning of patients who had not received WBRT (55, 56). A study with 208 patients with brain metastases receiving WBRT, who underwent prospective evaluation of neurocognitive functioning, showed that the median time to neurocognitive decline was longer in those responding to the WBRT than those who did not (57). This means that brain metastases themselves probably contribute to cognitive decline to some extent.

Several strategies for prevention of neurocognitive toxicity in patients treated with WBRT are under investigation. In a randomized, double-blind, placebo-controlled phase II trial, patients treated with memantine (a *N*-methyl-D-aspartate receptor antagonist) in addition to WBRT had better cognitive function over time with a reduced rate of decline in memory, executive function, and processing speed (58). Sparing of the hippocampal region during brain irradiation may prevent damage to neural progenitor cells located in the subgranular zone of the hippocampus and may thus preserve short-term memory and recall (59). It has been shown that neural stem cells in the hippocampus are very sensitive to injury from radiotherapy. A lower radiation dose to the hippocampus might therefore spare some memory function. New radiation techniques like intensity-modulated radiotherapy or volumetric modulated arc therapy can reduce the radiation dose to the hippocampus while obtaining sufficient dose coverage of the brain to control brain metastases. The single-arm phase II Radiation Therapy Oncology Group (RTOG) 0933 study using hippocampal-avoidance WBRT techniques suggested that minimal adverse cognitive effects appeared when the hippocampus was spared (60). Performance on a standardized memory test declined 7% from baseline to 4 months, as compared with 30% in a historical control group. However, these effects appeared to dissipate over time as the decline versus baseline averaged 2% at 6 months. Quality of life seems to be connected to neurocognitive functioning as assessments also showed a more favourable profile for patients treated by hippocampal-avoidance WBRT.

Another feasible approach to sparing brain parenchyma could be the application of radiosurgery for multiple brain metastases (46). However, comparative trials with a WBRT control arm are missing so far.

Medical antineoplastic therapy
Chemotherapy
The role of cytotoxic chemotherapy in brain metastasis patients is poorly defined due to the lack of adequate clinical trials (61). Only a few trials have been performed and the available trials have pooled various tumour types and have used poorly standardized trial endpoints, thus considerably limiting their conclusiveness. None of the studies have demonstrated a proven survival benefit of chemotherapy for brain metastases, although intracranial responses have been observed. It must be noted that brain metastases of germ

cell tumours have to be recognized as chemosensitive and may be successfully treated with chemotherapy (62). The conduct of well-designed clinical trials to define the role of chemotherapy for the treatment of brain metastases is strongly encouraged. Such trials should focus on specific histological tumour types and should be performed in a randomized fashion to ensure informative results.

Targeted agents

A number of targeted agents with activity in brain metastasis patients have emerged and may be considered in selected patients. Clinical decision-making is complicated in many cases by the lack of clinical trials evaluating the optimal combination and sequencing of these novel therapeutic approaches with established therapies such as surgery, SRS, and WBRT. Therefore, novel agents should preferably be administered to brain metastasis patients within the context of clinical trials. Outside of clinical trials, treatment decisions should be made by a multidisciplinary tumour board (26).

Non-small cell lung cancer

Presently, three approved targeted agents with potential activity against brain metastases are available, namely the epidermal growth factor receptor (EGFR) tyrosine kinase inhibitors gefitinib and erlotinib and the anaplastic lymphoma kinase (ALK) tyrosine kinase inhibitor crizotinib.

EGFR inhibitors

Activating mutations of the *EGFR* gene are found in primary NSCLC specimens in up to 40% of Asian and up to 15% of Caucasians. The exact incidence of *EGFR* mutations in brain metastases and the relation of *EGFR* gene status between primary tumours and cerebral metastases have not been defined. The presence of *EGFR* mutations has been suggested to be associated with multiple brain metastases rather than with oligometastatic CNS involvement. Radiological responses of brain metastases to both erlotinib and gefitinib, given as single agents or in combination with radiotherapy, have been documented in a number of case reports, retrospective surveys, and some relatively small prospective studies (63, 64). However, the results of a phase III study implies that the addition of erlotinib to WBRT and SRS in patients with one to three brain metastases of NSCLC does not confer a survival benefit over radiation alone, although the study was closed prematurely due to poor accrual (65). Taken together, the current data do not define a specific role of EGFR inhibitors for the treatment of NSCLC brain metastases (66). Also, the role of next-generation EGFR inhibitors such as afatinib in brain metastases needs to be clarified in future studies.

ALK inhibitors

ALK gene rearrangements, most commonly *EML4-ALK* translocations occur in 2–5% of NSCLC. The *ALK* gene status seems to be constant between primary tumours and brain metastases (67). *ALK* rearrangement leads to upregulation of pro-neoplastic signalling cascades such as RAS/ERK and PI3K/AKT, and therapy with the oral ALK inhibitor crizotinib has shown compelling activity in ALK-positive NSCLC patients. Prospectively collected data on the efficacy of crizotinib in patients with brain metastases of *ALK*-rearranged NSCLC are missing, but intracranial response has been documented in case reports. According to single case studies, high-dose crizotinib application schedules seem to be able to induce responses in brain metastases refractory to standard dosing (68, 69). Next-generation ALK inhibitors (e.g. alectinib) may also be active in brain metastases (70).

Breast cancer

Human epidermal growth factor receptor 2 antagonists

The human epidermal growth factor receptor 2 (HER2)-positive breast cancer subtype has a high propensity for metastatic brain involvement, as up to 40% of patients will be diagnosed with brain metastases during their disease course. Therefore, the role of HER2-targeting agents for brain metastases is of interest.

Trastuzumab, a humanized monoclonal antibody directed against HER2, is active and clinically indicated in metastatic HER2-positive breast cancer. However, it is thought not to penetrate the intact blood–brain barrier due to its large molecular size. Of note, however, trastuzumab has been detected in the cerebrospinal fluid after intravenous infusion in situations associated with increased blood–brain barrier permeability (radiotherapy, carcinomatous meningitis) (71). Although prospective trials are lacking, some case series imply some benefit of trastuzumab in patients with brain metastases, although it is unclear whether this is related to control of extracranial or intracranial disease (72–74).

Lapatinib is a dual EGFR and HER2 tyrosine kinase inhibitor and is approved in patients progressing on trastuzumab. Lapatinib may be able to penetrate the blood–brain barrier, as it has a molecular weight of 943.5 Da. Indeed, several studies indicate that lapatinib may induce responses of brain metastases and may be a reasonable treatment option in selected cases. Two prospective phase II trials documented intracranial responses of progressive brain metastases after WBRT and prior trastuzumab exposure to lapatinib-containing therapy (75, 76). The LANDSCAPE trial, a single-arm prospective study, explored the role of primary systemic therapy with a combination of capecitabine and lapatinib in patients with HER2-positive breast cancer and previously untreated brain metastases (77). Objective CNS responses were seen in 29/44 (65.9%) of evaluable patients and the median time to radiotherapy was 8.3 months. Yet, a randomized trial comparing the effects of lapatinib/capecitabine and WBRT on overall survival and neurocognitive outcome is lacking.

Future studies should explore the relevance of novel HER2-targeting agents such as pertuzumab and trastuzumab-emtansine (T-DM1) for the treatment of patients with brain metastases (78).

Melanoma

For decades, no truly active treatments had been available for metastatic melanoma. Cytotoxic chemotherapy and interferons were routinely used, but showed only very limited, if any, benefit in most patients. However, in recent years, tyrosine kinase inhibitors of v-Raf murine sarcoma viral oncogene homologue B1 (BRAF) and the monoclonal antibody ipilimumab, an immune checkpoint inhibitor, have shown compelling activity against metastatic melanoma and have been approved for clinical use. Interestingly, for these agents clinically relevant activity against brain metastases has been documented, too.

BRAF inhibitors

Activating mutations of *BRAF* are found in approximately half of metastatic melanomas and affect other tumour types in varying frequencies (e.g. papillary thyroid cancer, ovarian cancer, hairy cell leukaemia, and others). *BRAF* mutations lead to constitutive kinase activity of the mutant gene product, which enhances the metastatic and proliferative tumour cell capacity by activation of the mitogen-activated protein kinase (MAPK) pathway. The most common mutation affecting more than 95% of mutation-bearing cases is characterized by a substitution of valine by glutamic acid in the kinase domain of BRAF (*BRAF* V600E point mutation). Two tyrosine kinase inhibitors of BRAF, vemurafenib and dabrafenib, have shown clinically meaningful activity and are both approved for therapeutic use in patients with *BRAF* V600 mutated metastatic melanoma. There is no clear superiority in efficacy of one of the two agents over the other, however they differ in their adverse effect profiles. Vemurafenib has more pronounced skin toxicity, while dabrafenib is associated with more severe fever episodes. BRAF inhibitors may lead to rapid regression of tumours and this effect may be particularly relevant for brain metastasis patients, as it may help to quickly alleviate symptoms caused by intracranial masses. However, BRAF inhibition leads to upregulation of secondary resistance mechanisms such as MEK activation and subsequently to tumour regrowth within a few months. Current trials are investigating whether the combination of BRAF inhibitors with MEK inhibitors (e.g. trametinib) may prolong the therapeutic activity.

Concerning brain metastases, several case reports, patient series, and clinical trials have indicated that BRAF inhibitors cross the blood–tumour barrier and can induce rapid and significant responses in brain metastases (10, 79–81). A phase I/II study showed confirmed responses of *BRAF* V600E mutated brain metastases to dabrafenib in 56% of patients with 47% of patients staying on treatment for more than 6 months (81). In a prospective open-label study, vemurafenib achieved greater than 30% intracranial tumour regression in 37% of patients. Median progression-free survival was 3.9 months and median overall survival was 5.3 months. Other signs of clinical improvement included reduced corticosteroid requirements and improvements in performance status (10). Importantly, the *BRAF* mutation status is consistent between primary tumours, extracranial metastases, and brain metastases (82). Open issues concern the optimal combination and sequencing of BRAF inhibitors with established treatment options such as SRS and WBRT, but also with ipilimumab. Retrospective investigations seem to suggest that ipilimumab therapy prior to treatment with a BRAF inhibitor may lead to more favourable outcome than the opposite sequence (83, 84).

Ipilimumab

Ipilimumab is a fully humanized immunoglobulin G1 monoclonal antibody against the extracellular domain of cytotoxic T-lymphocyte antigen 4 (CTLA4), a regulatory receptor that inhibits T cells. Blocking of CTLA4 by ipilimumab enhances the T-cell response against tumour cells, thus facilitating immunological antitumour activity. Ipilimumab has shown durable antitumour activity in trials of metastatic melanoma and is approved in this indication in many countries. A pooled analysis of three completed phase II studies on ipilimumab in advanced melanoma showed 4-year survival rates of 13.8–50%, with the highest rates achieved in treatment-naïve patients (85). Of note, ipilimumab is associated with grade 3 or 4 immune-related adverse events such as autoimmune colitis, hepatitis, and hypophysitis in up to 15% of patients.

Ipilimumab has been reported to show durable clinical benefits in some melanoma patients with brain metastases. A phase II trial enrolling 72 patients found intracranial disease control in 24% of patients with asymptomatic brain metastases and 5% of patients with symptomatic brain metastases (86). In a single-arm phase II trial, disease control was achieved in 10/20 (50%) patients with asymptomatic brain metastases by combined therapy with

ipilimumab and fotemustine (87). In a retrospective analysis of an Expanded Access Program in Italy, the global disease control rate in 146 patients with asymptomatic melanoma brain metastases was 27%, including 4 patients with complete responses and 13 with partial responses. Median progression-free survival and overall survival were 2.8 and 4.3 months, respectively and approximately 20% of patients were alive 1 year after initiation of ipilimumab treatment (88). Thus, ipilimumab seems to be a valid treatment option, particularly for asymptomatic melanoma brain metastases. Of particular interest for brain metastasis patients may be the finding that irradiation of tumours during ipilimumab therapy may induce shrinking of distant, non-irradiated tumours, possibly through enhanced activation of the immune system through release of tumour antigens (89, 90).

A number of next-generation inhibitors of additional immune checkpoint molecules, for example, of programmed death 1 (PD-1) and programmed death 1 ligand (PD-L1), are under clinical development and have shown relatively high rates of sustained tumour responses and favourable safety data in early clinical trials (91). Concurrent therapy with the PD-1 inhibitor nivolumab and ipilimumab has a manageable toxicity profile and induced tumour regressions in a significant fraction of patients (92). Future studies need to evaluate their activity in brain metastasis patients.

Best supportive care

A considerable proportion of patients with brain metastases present in a poor clinical state with low Karnofsky performance score and unfavourable prognostic parameters. Frequent symptoms and clinical complaints include pain, fatigue, dyspnoea, altered mental status, headache, cranial nerve palsy, epilepsy, nausea, and vomiting (93). For such patients, best supportive care measures including treatment with corticosteroids, anticonvulsants, analgesics and professional management by a palliative care team need to be considered. However, referrals to palliative care services usually are considered too late in the disease course (94, 95). Unfortunately, there are few studies on the optimal application of supportive and palliative care measures in the brain metastasis population. The Medical Research Council conducted a randomized, non-inferiority, phase III trial comparing best supportive care plus WBRT versus best supportive care in patients with inoperable NSCLC brain metastases (Quartz trial) (96). The trial was not completed owing to poor accrual and funding issues. The interim analysis after 151 enrolled patients (median age 67 years; 50% had a Karnofsky index below 70%, the planned accrual target was 534 patients), however, showed no evidence for a negative effect of withholding WBRT on quality of life, overall survival, or quality-adjusted life years. The median overall survival was 49 days in the WBRT-containing arm and 51 days in the best supportive care-only arm. A major unresolved issue remains the definition of optimal criteria for selection of patients who should be treated by optimal supportive care alone or who may derive a significant benefit from antineoplastic therapies.

Commentary on National Comprehensive Cancer Network and any other treatment guidelines

No comprehensive guidelines are available for the management of patients with brain metastases. Few and relatively non-specific recommendations are found in the National Comprehensive Cancer Network guidelines on central nervous system cancers, however they are limited by lack of high-level evidence for most clinically relevant situations (44). Furthermore, they do not consider the primary tumour histology or molecular tumour subtypes and are thus too generic for meaningful application in everyday practice.

Surveillance recommendations

For radiological follow-up of patients with brain metastases, cranial MRI is recommended every 2–3 months for 1 year and thereafter as clinically indicated (44).

Treatment in children

Brain metastases of solid cancers are rare in children and are most commonly derived from germ cell tumours, sarcomas (osteosarcoma, rhabdomyosarcoma, and Ewing's sarcoma) and neuroblastomas (2, 8). Treatment strategies are ill defined but rely mainly on neurosurgery, radiotherapy, and cytotoxic chemotherapy. In brain metastases of extracranial germ cell tumours, intensive chemotherapy regimens may be the preferred treatment option (97).

Current research topics

Clinical research

Patients with brain metastases have systematically been excluded from many clinical trials, especially from those investigating novel therapeutics. However, recent examples of trials focusing on brain metastases (e.g. on ipilimumab and BRAF inhibitors in melanoma patients), have been successfully conducted. In NSCLC, ongoing trial initiatives specifically include brain metastasis patients to study the intracranial response to novel ALK or EGFR inhibitors with improved blood–brain barrier penetration. 'Window of opportunity' studies, in which patients scheduled for neurosurgical resection of brain metastases are treated with drugs of interest and tissue sampling is performed during operation, may help to clarify the ability of novel drugs to reach therapeutic concentrations within CNS tumours. Prophylactic trials with the intent of inhibiting outgrowth of brain metastases in high-risk populations (e.g. through antiangiogenic treatment in stage III NSCLC) are being designed based on preclinical data (21, 98, 99).

An important issue for the meaningful conduct of clinical studies is the definition of universally acceptable endpoints. The RANO group is developing criteria for the standardized evaluation of radiological, neurocognitive, and quality-of-life measures in brain metastasis patients enrolled in clinical trials (26, 27).

Laboratory research

For decades, comparatively little laboratory-based research has been performed on brain metastases. However, recently more research groups are beginning to work on secondary CNS malignancies with the ultimate goal of identifying targets for prophylaxis and treatment of brain metastases.

Several research groups are applying high-throughput methods for characterization of (epi-)genetic aberrations in brain metastases and corresponding primary tumours and extracranial metastases (100). There are attempts to interrogate the evolution of brain metastases based on next-generation sequencing. Furthermore, ongoing studies are investigating methylation profiles of brain metastases and matched primary tumours.

Another important field of laboratory research is the investigation of the interaction of brain-metastatic tumour cells with elements of the CNS microenvironment. For example, microglial cells and astrocytes may play an important role in brain invasion and growth of brain metastases, as tumour cells seem to be able to exploit these resident cells of the brain parenchyma (101–104). Given the emerging role of immunotherapeutics such as immune checkpoint inhibitors in several cancer types typically manifesting with brain metastases (melanoma, NSCLC), a detailed characterization of the adaptive immune response to secondary CNS malignancies will also be critical.

References

1. Kondziolka D, Kalkanis SN, Mehta MP, et al. It is time to re-evaluate the management of patients with brain metastases. *Neurosurgery* 2014; 75(1):1–9.

2. Nayak L, Lee EQ, Wen PY. Epidemiology of brain metastases. *Curr Oncol Rep* 2012; 14(1):48–54.

3. Barnholtz-Sloan JS, Sloan AE, Davis FG, et al. Incidence proportions of brain metastases in patients diagnosed (1973 to 2001) in the Metropolitan Detroit Cancer Surveillance System. *J Clin Oncol* 2004; 22(14):2865–2872.

4. Gavrilovic IT, Posner JB. Brain metastases: epidemiology and pathophysiology. *J Neurooncol* 2005; 75(1):5–14.

5. Pestalozzi BC, Zahrieh D, Price KN, et al. Identifying breast cancer patients at risk for central nervous system (CNS) metastases in trials of the International Breast Cancer Study Group (IBCSG). *Ann Oncol* 2006; 17(6):935–944.

6. Schouten LJ, Rutten J, Huveneers HA, et al. Incidence of brain metastases in a cohort of patients with carcinoma of the breast, colon, kidney, and lung and melanoma. *Cancer* 2002; 94(10):2698–2705.

7. Tabouret E, Chinot O, Metellus P, et al. Recent trends in epidemiology of brain metastases: an overview. *Anticancer Res* 2012; 32(11):4655–4662.

8. Stefanowicz J, Iżycka-Świeszewska E, Szurowska E, et al. Brain metastases in paediatric patients: characteristics of a patient series and review of the literature. *Folia Neuropathol* 2011; 49(4):271–281.

9. Owonikoko TK, Arbiser J, Zelnak A, et al. Current approaches to the treatment of metastatic brain tumours. *Nat Rev Clin Oncol* 2014; 11(4):203–222.

10. Dummer R, Goldinger SM, Turtschi CP, et al. Vemurafenib in patients with BRAF(V600) mutation-positive melanoma with symptomatic brain metastases: final results of an open-label pilot study. *Eur J Cancer* 2014; 50(3):611–621.

11. Lin NU, Winer EP. Brain metastases: the HER2 paradigm. *Clin Cancer Res* 2007; 13(6):1648–1655.

12. Gaspar L, Scott C, Rotman M, et al. Recursive partitioning analysis (RPA) of prognostic factors in three Radiation Therapy Oncology Group (RTOG) brain metastases trials. *Int J Radiat Oncol Biol Phys* 1997; 37(4):745–751.

13. Sperduto PW, Berkey B, Gaspar LE, et al. A new prognostic index and comparison to three other indices for patients with brain metastases: an analysis of 1,960 patients in the RTOG database. *Int J Radiat Oncol Biol Phys* 2008; 70(2):510–514.

14. Sperduto PW, Kased N, Roberge D, et al. Summary report on the graded prognostic assessment: an accurate and facile diagnosis-specific tool to estimate survival for patients with brain metastases. *J Clin Oncol* 2012; 30(4):419–425.

15. Kondziolka D, Parry PV, Lunsford LD, et al. The accuracy of predicting survival in individual patients with cancer. *J Neurosurg* 2014; 120(1):24–30.

16. Berghoff A, Sax C, Klein M, et al. Alleviation of brain edema and restoration of functional independence by bevacizumab in brain-metastatic breast cancer: a case report. *Breast Care* 2014; 9(2):134–136.

17. Berghoff A, Spanberger T, Ilhan-Mutlu A, et al. Preoperative diffusion-weighted imaging of single brain metastases correlates with patient survival times. *PLoS One* 2013; 8(2):e55464.

18. Berghoff AS, Ilhan-Mutlu A, Wöhrer A, et al. Prognostic significance of Ki67 proliferation index, HIF1 alpha index and microvascular density in patients with non-small cell lung cancer brain metastases. *Strahlenther Onkol* 2014; 190(7):676–685.

19. Fidler IJ. The role of the organ microenvironment in brain metastasis. *Semin Cancer Biol* 2011; 21(2):107–112.

20. Preusser M, Capper D, Ilhan-Mutlu A, et al. Brain metastases: pathobiology and emerging targeted therapies. *Acta Neuropathol* 2012; 123(2):205–222.

21. Kienast Y, von Baumgarten L, Fuhrmann M, et al. Real-time imaging reveals the single steps of brain metastasis formation. *Nat Med* 2010; 16(1):116–122.

22. Berghoff AS, Rajky O, Winkler F, et al. Invasion patterns in brain metastases of solid cancers. *Neuro Oncol* 2013; 15(12):1664–1672.

23. Berghoff AS, Lassmann H, Preusser M, et al. Characterization of the inflammatory response to solid cancer metastases in the human brain. *Clin Exp Metastasis* 2013; 30(1):69–81.

24. Nieder C, Thamm R, Astner ST, et al. Disease presentation and treatment outcome in very young patients with brain metastases from lung cancer. *Onkologie* 2008; 31(6):305–308.

25. National Comprehensive Cancer Network. *NCCN Guidelines: Non-Small Cell Lung Cancer*. http://www.nccn.org/professionals/physician_gls/pdf/nscl.pdf.

26. Lin NU, Lee EQ, Aoyama H, et al. Challenges relating to solid tumour brain metastases in clinical trials, part 1: patient population, response, and progression. A report from the RANO group. *Lancet Oncol* 2013; 14(10):e396–e406.

27. Lin NU, Wefel JS, Lee EQ, et al. Challenges relating to solid tumour brain metastases in clinical trials, part 2: neurocognitive, neurological, and quality-of-life outcomes. A report from the RANO group. *Lancet Oncol* 2013; 14(10):e407–e416.

28. Lee EK, Lee EJ, Kim MS, et al. Intracranial metastases: spectrum of MR imaging findings. *Acta Radiol* 2012; 53(10):1173–1185.

29. Hoefnagels FW, Lagerwaard FJ, Sanchez E, et al. Radiological progression of cerebral metastases after radiosurgery: assessment of perfusion MRI for differentiating between necrosis and recurrence. *J Neurol* 2009; 256(6):878–887.

30. Huang J, Wang AM, Shetty A, et al. Differentiation between intra-axial metastatic tumor progression and radiation injury following fractionated radiation therapy or stereotactic radiosurgery using MR spectroscopy, perfusion MR imaging or volume progression modeling. *Magn Reson Imaging* 2011; 29(7):993–1001.

31. Lester SC, Taksler GB, Kuremsky JG, et al. Clinical and economic outcomes of patients with brain metastases based on symptoms: an argument for routine brain screening of those treated with upfront radiosurgery. *Cancer* 2014; 120(3):433–441.

32. Tsao MN, Rades D, Wirth A, et al. International practice survey on the management of brain metastases: Third International Consensus Workshop on Palliative Radiotherapy and Symptom Control. *Clin Oncol* 2012; 24(6):e81–e92.

33. Kalkanis SN, Kondziolka D, Gaspar LE, et al. The role of surgical resection in the management of newly diagnosed brain metastases: a systematic review and evidence-based clinical practice guideline. *J Neurooncol* 2010; 96(1):33–43.

34. Patchell RA, Tibbs PA, Regine WF, et al. Postoperative radiotherapy in the treatment of single metastases to the brain: a randomized trial. *JAMA* 1998; 280(17):1485–1489.

35. Patchell RA, Tibbs PA, Walsh JW, et al. A randomized trial of surgery in the treatment of single metastases to the brain. *N Engl J Med* 1990; 322(8):494–500.

36. Kocher M, Soffietti R, Abacioglu U, et al. Adjuvant whole-brain radiotherapy versus observation after radiosurgery or surgical resection of one to three cerebral metastases: results of the EORTC 22952-26001 study. *J Clin Oncol* 2011; 29(2):134–141.

37. Ueki K, Matsutani M, Nakamura O, et al. Comparison of whole brain radiation therapy and locally limited radiation therapy in the treatment of solitary brain metastases from non-small cell lung cancer. *Neurol Med Chir (Tokyo)* 1996; 36(6):364–369.

38. Soltys SG, Adler JR, Lipani JD, et al. Stereotactic radiosurgery of the postoperative resection cavity for brain metastases. *Int J Radiat Oncol Biol Phys* 2008; 70(1):187–193.

39. Kocher M, Soffietti R, Abacioglu U, et al. Adjuvant whole-brain radiotherapy versus observation after radiosurgery or surgical resection of one to three cerebral metastases: results of the EORTC 22952-26001 study. *J Clin Oncol* 2011; 29(2):134–141.

40. Do L, Pezner R, Radany E, et al. Resection followed by stereotactic radiosurgery to resection cavity for intracranial metastases. *Int J Radiat Oncol Biol Phys* 2009; 73(2):486–491.

41. Kelly PJ, Lin YB, Yu AY, et al. Stereotactic irradiation of the postoperative resection cavity for brain metastasis: a frameless linear accelerator-based case series and review of the technique. *Int J Radiat Oncol Biol Phys* 2012; 82(1):95–101.

42. Jensen CA, Chan MD, McCoy TP, et al. Cavity-directed radiosurgery as adjuvant therapy after resection of a brain metastasis. *J Neurosurg* 2011; 114(6):1585–1591.

43. Tsao MN, Rades D, Wirth A, et al. Radiotherapeutic and surgical management for newly diagnosed brain metastasis(es): an American Society for Radiation Oncology evidence-based guideline. *Pract Radiat Oncol* 2012; 2(3):210–225.

44. Nabors LB, Ammirati M, Bierman PJ, et al. Central nervous system cancers. *J Natl Compr Canc Netw* 2013; 11(9):1114–1151.

45. Kocher M, Wittig A, Piroth MD, et al. Stereotactic radiosurgery for treatment of brain metastases: a report of the DEGRO Working Group on Stereotactic Radiotherapy. *Strahlenther Onkol* 2014; 190(6):521–32.

46. Yamamoto M, Serizawa T, Shuto T, et al. Stereotactic radiosurgery for patients with multiple brain metastases (JLGK0901): a multi-institutional prospective observational study. *Lancet Oncol* 2014; 15(4):387–395.

47. Lagerwaard FJ, van der Hoorn EA, Verbakel WF, et al. Whole-brain radiotherapy with simultaneous integrated boost to multiple brain metastases using volumetric modulated arc therapy. *Int J Radiat Oncol Biol Phys* 2009; 75(1):253–259.

48. Rodrigues G, Yartsev S, Yaremko B, et al. Phase I trial of simultaneous in-field boost with helical tomotherapy for patients with one to three brain metastases. *Int J Radiat Oncol Biol Phys* 2011; 80(4):1128–1133.

49. Tsao MN, Lloyd N, Wong RK, et al. Whole brain radiotherapy for the treatment of newly diagnosed multiple brain metastases. *Cochrane Database Syst Rev* 2012; 4:CD003869.

50. Soon YY, Tham IW, Lim KH, et al. Surgery or radiosurgery plus whole brain radiotherapy versus surgery or radiosurgery alone for brain metastases. *Cochrane Database Syst Rev* 2014; 3:CD009454.

51. Chang EL, Wefel JS, Hess KR, et al. Neurocognition in patients with brain metastases treated with radiosurgery or radiosurgery plus whole-brain irradiation: a randomised controlled trial. *Lancet Oncol* 2009; 10(11):1037–1044.

52. Aoyama H, Shirato H, Tago M, et al. Stereotactic radiosurgery plus whole-brain radiation therapy vs stereotactic radiosurgery alone for treatment of brain metastases: a randomized controlled trial. *JAMA* 2006; 295(21):2483–2491.

53. Slotman B, Mauer ME, Bottomley A, et al. Prophylactic cranial irradiation in extensive small-cell lung cancer. *N Engl J Med* 2007; 357(7):664–672.

54. Früh M, De Ruysscher D, Popat S, et al. Small-cell lung cancer (SCLC): ESMO Clinical Practice Guidelines for diagnosis, treatment and follow-up. *Ann Oncol* 2013; 24(Suppl 6):vi99–105.

55. Le Péchoux C, Laplanche A, Faivre-Finn C, et al. Clinical neurological outcome and quality of life among patients with limited small-cell cancer treated with two different doses of prophylactic cranial irradiation in the intergroup phase III trial (PCI99-01, EORTC 22003-08004, RTOG 0212 and IFCT 99-01). *Ann Oncol* 2011; 22(5):1154–1163.

56. Sun A, Bae K, Gore EM, et al. Phase III trial of prophylactic cranial irradiation compared with observation in patients with locally advanced non-small-cell lung cancer: neurocognitive and quality-of-life analysis. *J Clin Oncol* 2011; 29(3):279–286.

57. Li J, Bentzen SM, Renschler M, et al. Regression after whole-brain radiation therapy for brain metastases correlates with survival and improved neurocognitive function. *J Clin Oncol* 2007; 25(10):1260–1266.

58. Brown PD, Pugh S, Laack NN, et al. Memantine for the prevention of cognitive dysfunction in patients receiving whole-brain radiotherapy: a randomized, double-blind, placebo-controlled trial. *Neuro Oncol* 2013; 15(10):1429–1437.

59. Gondi V, Tome WA, Mehta MP. Why avoid the hippocampus? A comprehensive review. *Radiother Oncol* 2010; 97(3):370–376.

60. Gondi V, Mehta MP, Pugh S, et al. Memory preservation with conformal avoidance of the hippocampus during whole-brain radiotherapy for patients with brain metastases: Primary endpoint results of RTOG 0933. *American Society for Radiation Oncology 55th Annual Meeting.* Abstract LBA1. Presented September 23, 2013.

61. Mehta MP, Paleologos NA, Mikkelsen T, et al. The role of chemotherapy in the management of newly diagnosed brain metastases: a systematic review and evidence-based clinical practice guideline. *J Neurooncol* 2010; 96(1):71–83.

62. Hardt A, Krell J, Wilson PD, et al. Brain metastases associated with germ cell tumors may be treated with chemotherapy alone. *Cancer* 2014; 120(11):1639–1646.

63. Welsh JW, Komaki R, Amini A, et al. Phase II trial of erlotinib plus concurrent whole-brain radiation therapy for patients with brain metastases from non-small-cell lung cancer. *J Clin Oncol* 2013; 31(7):895–902.

64. Burel-Vandenbos F, Ambrosetti D, Coutts M, et al. EGFR mutation status in brain metastases of non-small cell lung carcinoma. *J Neurooncol* 2013; 111(1):1–10.

65. Sperduto PW, Wang M, Robins HI, et al. A phase 3 trial of whole brain radiation therapy and stereotactic radiosurgery alone versus WBRT and SRS with temozolomide or erlotinib for non-small cell lung cancer and 1 to 3 brain metastases: Radiation Therapy Oncology Group 0320. *Int J Radiat Oncol Biol Phys* 2013; 85(5):1312–1318.

66. Chamberlain MC. Should erlotinib be coadministered with whole-brain radiotherapy in patients with brain metastases and non-small-cell lung cancer? *J Clin Oncol* 2013; 31(25):3164–3165.

67. Preusser M, Berghoff AS, Ilhan-Mutlu A, et al. ALK gene translocations and amplifications in brain metastases of non-small cell lung cancer. *Lung Cancer* 2013; 80(3):278–283.

68. Kim YH, Ozasa H, Nagai H, et al. High-dose crizotinib for brain metastases refractory to standard-dose crizotinib. *J Thorac Oncol* 2013; 8(9):e85–e86.

69. Peled N, Zach L, Liran O, et al. Effective crizotinib schedule for brain metastases in ALK rearrangement metastatic non-small-cell lung cancer. *J Thorac Oncol* 2013; 8(12):e112–e113.

70. Perez CA, Velez M, Raez LE, et al. Overcoming the resistance to crizotinib in patients with non-small cell lung cancer harboring EML4/ALK translocation. *Lung Cancer* 2014; 84(2):110–115.

71. Stemmler HJ, Schmitt M, Willems A, et al. Ratio of trastuzumab levels in serum and cerebrospinal fluid is altered in HER2-positive breast cancer patients with brain metastases and impairment of blood-brain barrier. *Anticancer Drugs* 2007; 18(1):23–28.

72. Bartsch R, Berghoff AS, Preusser M. Optimal management of brain metastases from breast cancer. Issues and considerations. *CNS Drugs* 2013; 27(2):121–134.

73. Bartsch R, Rottenfusser A, Wenzel C, et al. Trastuzumab prolongs overall survival in patients with brain metastases from Her2 positive breast cancer. *J Neurooncol* 2007; 85(3):311–317.

74. Metro G, Foglietta J, Russillo M, et al. Clinical outcome of patients with brain metastases from HER2-positive breast cancer treated with lapatinib and capecitabine. *Ann Oncol* 2011; 22(3):625–630.

75. Lin NU, Diéras V, Paul D, et al. Multicenter phase II study of lapatinib in patients with brain metastases from HER2-positive breast cancer. *Clin Cancer Res* 2009; 15(4):1452–1459.

76. Lin NU, Eierman W, Greil R, et al. Randomized phase II study of lapatinib plus capecitabine or lapatinib plus topotecan for patients with HER2-positive breast cancer brain metastases. *J Neurooncol* 2011; 105(3):613–620.

77. Bachelot T, Romieu G, Campone M, et al. Lapatinib plus capecitabine in patients with previously untreated brain metastases from HER2-positive metastatic breast cancer (LANDSCAPE): a single-group phase 2 study. *Lancet Oncol* 2013; 14(1):64–71.

78. Bartsch R, Berghoff AS, Preusser M. Breast cancer brain metastases responding to primary systemic therapy with T-DM1. *J Neurooncol* 2014; 116(1):205–206.

79. Rochet NM, Kottschade LA, Markovic SN. Vemurafenib for melanoma metastases to the brain. *N Engl J Med* 2011; 365(25):2439–2441.

80. Dzienis MR, Atkinson VG. Response rate to vemurafenib in patients with B-RAF-positive melanoma brain metastases: a retrospective review. *Melanoma Res* 2014; 24(4):349–353.

81. Falchook GS, Long GV, Kurzrock R, et al. Dabrafenib in patients with melanoma, untreated brain metastases, and other solid tumours: a phase 1 dose-escalation trial. *Lancet* 2012; 379(9829):1893–1901.

82. Capper D, Berghoff AS, Magerle M, et al. Immunohistochemical testing of BRAF V600E status in 1,120 tumor tissue samples of patients with brain metastases. *Acta Neuropathol* 2012; 123(2):223–233.

83. Ascierto PA, Simeone E, Sileni VC, et al. Sequential treatment with ipilimumab and BRAF inhibitors in patients with metastatic melanoma: data from the Italian cohort of the Ipilimumab Expanded Access Program. *Cancer Invest* 2014; 32(4):144–149.

84. Ackerman A, Klein O, McDermott DF, et al. Outcomes of patients with metastatic melanoma treated with immunotherapy prior to or after BRAF inhibitors. *Cancer* 2014; 120(11):1695–1701.

85. Wolchok JD, Weber JS, Maio M, et al. Four-year survival rates for patients with metastatic melanoma who received ipilimumab in phase II clinical trials. *Ann Oncol* 2013; 24(8):2174–2180.

86. Margolin K, Ernstoff MS, Hamid O, et al. Ipilimumab in patients with melanoma and brain metastases: an open-label, phase 2 trial. *Lancet Oncol* 2012; 13(5):459–465.

87. Di Giacomo AM, Ascierto PA, Pilla L, et al. Ipilimumab and fotemustine in patients with advanced melanoma (NIBIT-M1): an open-label, single-arm phase 2 trial. *Lancet Oncol* 2012; 13(9):879–886.

88. Queirolo P, Spagnolo F, Ascierto PA, et al. Efficacy and safety of ipilimumab in patients with advanced melanoma and brain metastases. *J Neurooncol* 2014; 118(1):109–116.

89. Silk AW, Bassetti MF, West BT, et al. Ipilimumab and radiation therapy for melanoma brain metastases. *Cancer Med* 2013; 2(6):899–906.

90. Stamell EF, Wolchok JD, Gnjatic S, et al. The abscopal effect associated with a systemic anti-melanoma immune response. *Int J Radiat Oncol Biol Phys* 2013; 85(2):293–295.

91. Hamid O, Robert C, Daud A, et al. Safety and tumor responses with lambrolizumab (anti-PD-1) in melanoma. *N Engl J Med* 2013; 369(2):134–144.

92. Wolchok JD, Kluger H, Callahan MK, et al. Nivolumab plus ipilimumab in advanced melanoma. *N Engl J Med* 2013; 369(2):122–133.

93. Yamanaka R, Koga H, Yamamoto Y, et al. Characteristics of patients with brain metastases from lung cancer in a palliative care center. *Support Care Cancer* 2011; 19(4):467–473.

94. Stavas M, Arneson K, Friedman J, et al. From whole brain to hospice: patterns of care in radiation oncology. *J Palliat Med* 2014; 17(6):662–666.

95. Gofton TE, Graber J, Carver A. Identifying the palliative care needs of patients living with cerebral tumors and metastases: a retrospective analysis. *J Neurooncol* 2012; 108(3):527–534.

96. Langley RE, Stephens RJ, Nankivell M, et al. Interim data from the Medical Research Council QUARTZ Trial: does whole brain radiotherapy affect the survival and quality of life of patients with brain metastases from non-small cell lung cancer? *Clin Oncol* 2013; 25(3):e23–e30.

97. Göbel U, von Kries R, Teske C, et al. Brain metastases during follow-up of children and adolescents with extracranial malignant germ cell tumors: risk adapted management decision tree analysis based on data of the MAHO/MAKEI-registry. *Pediatr Blood Cancer* 2013; 60(2):217–223.

98. Steeg PS. Perspective: the right trials. *Nature* 2012; 485(7400): S58–S59.

99. Preusser M, Winkler F, Collette L, et al. Trial design on prophylaxis and treatment of brain metastases: lessons learned from the EORTC Brain Metastases Strategic Meeting 2012. *Eur J Cancer* 2012; 48(18):3439–3447.

100. Bos PD, Zhang XH, Nadal C, et al. Genes that mediate breast cancer metastasis to the brain. *Nature* 2009; 459(7249):1005–1009.

101. Lin Q, Balasubramanian K, Fan D, et al. Reactive astrocytes protect melanoma cells from chemotherapy by sequestering intracellular calcium through gap junction communication channels. *Neoplasia* 2010; 12(9):748–754.

102. Pukrop T, Dehghani F, Chuang HN, et al. Microglia promote colonization of brain tissue by breast cancer cells in a Wnt-dependent way. *Glia* 2010; 58(12):1477–1489.

103. Rietkotter E, Menck K, Bleckmann A, et al. Zoledronic acid inhibits macrophage/microglia-assisted breast cancer cell invasion. *Oncotarget* 2013; 4(9):1449–1460.

104. Xing F, Kobayashi A, Okuda H, et al. Reactive astrocytes promote the metastatic growth of breast cancer stem-like cells by activating Notch signalling in brain. *EMBO Mol Med* 2013; 5(3):384–396.

CHAPTER 20

Metastatic tumours: spinal cord, plexus, and peripheral nerve

David Schiff, Jonathan Sherman, and Paul D. Brown

Epidural metastasis

Definition

Epidural neoplasms threaten normal neurological function via their potential to compress the spinal cord, cauda equina, or nerve roots exiting through the neuroforamina. Most such tumours are malignant, and many arise from bone metastases although some develop from direct contiguous spread from a primary bone or paraspinal tumour. This condition is broadly referred to as 'epidural spinal cord compression' (ESCC).

Epidemiology

Several factors make the precise incidence of ESCC elusive. The definition itself is not precise, since epidural tumours vary in the extent of thecal sac and spinal cord/cauda equina deformation they produce. ESCC is often a late-stage complication of cancer, and in such circumstances back pain may be treated empirically without definitive diagnostic tests. Moreover, patients with no or mild neurological dysfunction may be treated as outpatients, hampering some epidemiological search strategies. A population-based study in Ontario, Canada, that captured principally ESCC diagnoses requiring hospitalization found that 2.5% of patients with cancer experienced ESCC within 5 years of their death (1), with the incidence varying from as low as 0.2% of patients with pancreatic cancer to 8% of patients with multiple myeloma. More recently, a US-based study of inpatient diagnoses reported that the average annual incidence of ESCC was 3.4% of patients dying from cancer, with myeloma, lymphoma, and prostate cancer having the highest cancer-specific incidence (2). Overall, lung cancer (25%), prostate cancer (16%), myeloma (11%), non-Hodgkin's lymphoma (8%), and breast cancer (7%) were the most common causes of ESCC.

Clinical presentation: symptoms

The first symptom to raise consideration of ESCC is typically localized back pain. Back pain is the initial symptom in 95% of patients and on average precedes other symptoms by 7 weeks (3). Since bone metastases without epidural extension, as well as compression fractures from any cause, may manifest as localized back pain, many cases of ESCC are not investigated early. Pain typically worsens over time and is often increased with recumbency. Over time, the pain may develop radicular features: the patient with thoracic ESCC may note a gripping, girdle-like pain. Pain may develop or worsen substantially with vertebral collapse, and pain with movement raises the possibility of spinal instability.

Motor involvement is the most feared consequence of ESCC and unfortunately is present in a majority of patients at the time of diagnosis. Depending on the affected level of the neuraxis, weakness may reflect myelopathy or cauda equina compression. As weakness increases, the ability to ambulate may be lost. Sensory loss is almost as common as weakness, but patients may be unaware, mandating a careful examination for a spinal sensory level or radicular sensory loss. Urinary and faecal incontinence tend to be late findings in ESCC, paralleling the degree of weakness; rarely, these may occur early when the conus medullaris is compressed.

Physical examination

The physical examination may heighten a clinician's suspicion of ESCC, but a normal physical examination does not exclude the diagnosis. Spinal tenderness to percussion and spinal deformity should be sought. The clinician should examine carefully for radicular and myelopathic weakness and sensory loss. Gait must be tested, with an attempt to differentiate between an inability to ambulate due to pain versus weakness or sensory loss. Rectal examination including assessment of anal wink is valuable for determining conus or cauda dysfunction.

Differential diagnosis

In the cancer patient with isolated back pain, the differential diagnosis of ESCC necessarily includes vertebral metastasis without epidural compression. Benign causes of back pain most commonly affect the lumbosacral or cervical spine, whereas 60% of ESCC arises in the thoracic spine. Epidural abscess, intramedullary metastasis, leptomeningeal metastasis, malignant plexopathy, benign intradural-extramedullary tumours, and radiation myelopathy are also considerations. The medical history and imaging studies will generally separate out these entities.

Imaging

Advances in neuroimaging have transformed the ability to diagnosis ESCC in the last 25–30 years. Up until that time, definitive diagnosis of an epidural mass generally required a myelogram, often combined with a computed tomography (CT) scan. This test was invasive, uncomfortable, and sometimes contraindicated due to coagulopathy, thrombocytopenia, or other reasons. Consequently, plain radiographs, radionuclide bone scanning, CT scanning, and clinical features were sometimes incorporated into algorithms to spare low-risk patients invasive testing. At present, the widespread availability of magnetic resonance imaging (MRI) has relegated these other imaging studies to ancillary status.

MRI is a highly sensitive and specific test for the diagnosis of ESCC; it has the secondary virtue of assisting in the diagnosis of ESCC mimics such as leptomeningeal and intramedullary metastases, as well as bone metastases without epidural extension among others. MRI demonstrates the extent of tumour burden, assesses vertebral integrity, detects clinically silent lesions, and is critical for treatment planning. The entire spinal cord/cauda equina should be screened with at least sagittal sequences since 30% of patients with ESCC will have multiple sites (4); areas of suspected disease are further imaged in the cross-sectional and parasagittal planes.

Supportive therapies

Supportive therapies are an important part of ESCC management, with the goals of preserving neurological function, ameliorating pain, and preventing other complications while definitive antineoplastic treatment is undertaken. The supportive intervention that has received the most attention is corticosteroids. Corticosteroids decrease vasogenic oedema in the spinal cord (5), and have beneficial analgesic effects (6, 7) as well as potential oncolytic effects. A randomized clinical trial confirmed the favourable impact of corticosteroids in preserving ambulation in patients with ESCC undergoing fractionated radiotherapy (8). The optimal dose of steroids remains debatable; high doses of corticosteroids can lead to disabling complications in as little as 2 weeks. It is clear that regimens starting at 96 mg of dexamethasone daily are associated with substantially more side effects than with a daily starting dose of 16 mg (9). One reasonable approach is to reserve the high doses (100 mg bolus followed by 24 mg four times daily) for patients with severe neurological dysfunction, and to utilize 16 mg daily in divided doses for patients with relatively mild neurological dysfunction. When the higher doses are employed, they should be tapered fairly rapidly; one approach is to halve the dose every 3 days. Patients with small epidural lesions without compression of the spinal cord and a normal neurological examination may safely forgo the use of corticosteroids (10).

While pain often responds nicely to corticosteroids, pain with ESCC may be severe and refractory. In such instances, there should be a low threshold to utilize opioids, bearing in mind the tendency towards constipation from these agents is exacerbated in the setting of diminished mobility and neurological dysfunction. Immobilization and paresis also predispose to venous thromboembolism, and strong consideration should be given to deep vein thrombosis prophylaxis with heparin/low-molecular-weight heparinoids or pneumatic venous compression devices.

Surgery in epidural metastases

The role of surgery in the management of epidural metastases has changed as diagnosis and management has improved in this patient population. The primary goal of treatment is maximizing quality of life while minimizing morbidity. Consequently, the multidisciplinary treatment team must have a complete understanding of how each treatment modality can impact the patient not only in length of survival, but more importantly in the quality of that patient's remaining life.

Tomita et al. attempted to generate a decision framework for surgical treatment goals. The authors correlated the growth rate of the tumour based on histology, the presence or absence of visceral metastases, and the presence of solitary or multiple bony metastases to a surgical strategy. This strategy included wide or marginal excision, marginal or intralesional excision, palliative surgery, or supportive care (11). In a subsequent randomized trial by Patchell et al., surgery plus standard fractionated radiation was compared to radiation alone for patients with high-grade epidural spinal cord compression with myelopathy. Patients treated with surgical decompression were found to have significant improvement in either maintained or recovered ambulation and continence, with a lower use of narcotics as compared to the radiation-alone group (12).

While these publications justify the role of surgery in a group of patients with epidural metastases, the analysis does not account for development of stereotactic body radiation therapy (SBRT). The use of SBRT (see 'Radiotherapy in epidural metastases') in this patient population has directly affected the role of surgery in these patients. Integrating this technology, Bilsky et al. developed a new decision framework entitled NOMS to allow for a multidisciplinary method of assessing these patients. This framework includes a Neurological assessment, Oncological assessment, assessment of Mechanical instability, and an assessment of Systemic disease burden and medical co-morbidity. Neurological assessment includes evidence of myelopathy, functional radiculopathy, and the degree of epidural compression. The latter includes tumour not adjacent to the thecal sac, tumour abutting the thecal sac, tumour compressing the thecal sac but not the spinal cord, and tumour compressing the spinal cord. Oncological assessment primarily evaluates the radiosensitivity of the tumour such that sensitive tumours include multiple myeloma and lymphoma while moderately sensitive tumours include breast and prostate carcinoma. Moderately resistant tumours include colon and non-small cell lung carcinoma, while highly radioresistant tumours include renal cell carcinoma, thyroid carcinoma, melanoma, and sarcoma (13).

Mechanical instability is best assessed by the Spine Instability Neoplastic Score (SINS). The Spinal Oncology Study Group created this scoring system with high inter- and intra-relater reliability. The scoring system analyses numerous components including tumour location, presence of pain, presence of a lytic or blastic tumour, presence of a new subluxation or de novo deformity, collapse of the vertebral body, and degree of posterolateral involvement. Location includes junctional segments, mobile segments, semirigid segments, and rigid segments. Each area generates a score such that a total score of 0–6 equates to stability, a total score of 7–12 equates to potentially unstable, and a total score of 13–18 equates to unstable (14, 15).

The final component of the NOMS framework is systemic disease burden and medical co-morbidities. The former requires an evaluation of extent of disease via positron emission tomography (PET)-CT with or without a bone scan and a MRI of the neuraxis. The latter is patient dependent and may require cardiac work-up, pulmonary function testing, and ultrasound of the lower extremities depending on the patient's ability to mobilize (13).

Having defined the NOMS framework, the multidisciplinary team must look at each patient individually and evaluate the best course of action. For instance, a patient with a predictably radio sensitive tumour regardless of degree of compression would best be treated with conventional radiation therapy barring a lesion associated with mechanical instability. Similarly, a patient with a radioresistant tumour without compression of the thecal sac can be treated with SBRT without the need for surgical intervention. However, a patient with a radioresistant tumour with compression of the thecal sac requires surgical decompression.

The need for instrumentation is highly dependent on the tumour location both with regard to dorsal or ventral location and spinal level. The primary location for epidural metastases is within the vertebral body, and laminectomy alone removes posterior support and can generate instability (16). In the cervical spine, an isolated tumour within the vertebral body requiring surgery can be treated with an anterior vertebrectomy and fusion alone with dissection through the neck musculature. However, the majority of vertebral vertebral body metastases are not in isolation. Furthermore, up to 70% of tumours are located within the thoracic spine, and, consequently if surgery is indicated, a posterior decompression and fusion operation is often required (Fig. 20.1). The tumour is often confined by the posterior longitudinal ligament. By stripping this ligament away from the dura, tumour is resected and the thecal sac is reconstituted. For pathological compression fractures resulting in instability, resection of tumour within the vertebral body can also be achieved through this posterior approach with stability added via intraoperative placement of polymethylmethacrylate (PMMA) (17). Following surgery and wound healing, SBRT is provided for treatment of the remaining ventral disease.

As an alternative to open surgical approaches, vertebral body lesions resulting in pathological fracture with minimal ventral compression of the thecal sac can be treated with percutaneous kyphoplasty or vertebroplasty. This treatment is possible only for mid-thoracic to lumbar lesions and PMMA is injected via a transcostovertebral approach in the former and a posterolateral transpedicular approach in the latter. The treatment is very effective in improving pain related to the fracture. Pain relief can occur within 24–48 hours after treatment; this control is maintained at the 2-year follow-up examination (18, 19).

Radiotherapy in epidural metastases

Selecting the best treatment modality in ESCC to maximize quality of life while minimizing morbidity is crucial. The majority of patients with epidural metastases will be treated with conventional external beam radiotherapy (EBRT) since most patients are not

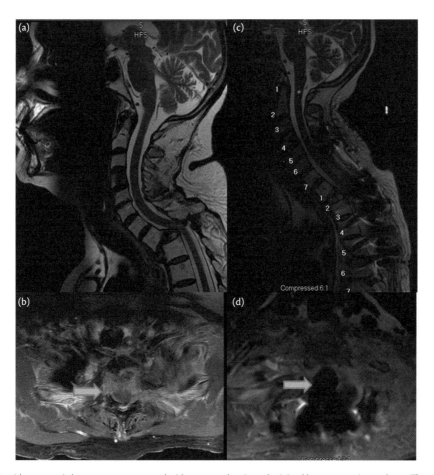

Fig. 20.1 A 59-year-old female with metastatic breast cancer presented with acute neck pain and minimal lower extremity weakness. There was stable systemic disease on recent PET-CT. (a) Preoperative sagittal T2 MRI scan displaying pathological fracture with subluxation. SINS scoring system = 18/18 confirming instability. (b) Preoperative axial T1 post-gadolinium MRI scan displaying significant epidural spinal cord compression in this patient. The patient underwent a C7–T2 decompression and tumour resection with a C3–T6 instrumentation and fusion. (c) Postoperative sagittal T2 MRI displaying improvement in alignment with decreased spinal cord compression. (d) Postoperative axial T1 post-gadolinium MRI displaying decompression of the spinal cord.

considered good surgical candidates. Spinal radiotherapy is generally well tolerated. Typically the radiotherapy portal covers the width of the vertebral body (and any paraspinal tumour extension if present) with margin and extends one to two vertebral bodies above and below the epidural metastasis (20). Approximately 70% of patients will experience an improvement in pain (21). Relief of tumour blockage has been noted in 80% of patients evaluated by pre- and post-treatment myelograms in a prospective trial (22). Neurological outcomes after radiotherapy are highly dependent on pretreatment neurological function. Typically 90% of treated patients will remain ambulatory after treatment, while approximately one-third of non-ambulatory patients will regain the ability to walk, and 0–5% of paraplegic patients will become ambulatory (21); however, higher response rates can be seen in radiosensitive neoplasms (23).

A variety of EBRT schedules have been used to treat epidural metastases. A retrospective analysis of over 1300 patients treated with five different treatment schedules, 8 Gy in 1 fraction, 20 Gy in 5 fractions, 30 Gy in 10 fractions, 37.5 Gy in 15 fractions, and 40 Gy in 20 fractions (24), demonstrated that motor function and post-treatment ambulatory rates were similar between the treatment regimens. However the more protracted schedules were associated with fewer recurrences within the radiation field. The authors recommended 8 Gy in 1 fraction for patients with poor predicted survival and 30 Gy in 10 fractions for better prognosis patients. Three randomized trials have evaluated fractionation schedules for patients with metastatic ESCC and short life expectancy. The first trial randomized 300 patients to short-course RT (8 Gy × 2 fractions with fractions a week apart) or to a split-course RT (5 Gy × 3 fractions, 4-day rest, and then 3 Gy × 5 fractions) (21). The median survival was 4 months. Both schedules were similarly effective and there were no differences in toxicity, ambulatory rate, or in-field recurrence rate. The second trial randomized 327 patients with ESCC to 8 Gy × 2 fractions (with fractions a week apart) or 8 Gy × 1 fraction and found no difference in response or overall survival (median 4 months) (25). A third trial randomized 203 poor to intermediate prognosis patients (median overall survival 3.2 months) to

4 Gy × 5 fractions or 3 Gy × 10 fractions (26). Again both schedules were similarly effective with no significant differences in toxicity, ambulatory rate, or in-field recurrence rate. Therefore, for patients with a relatively short life expectancy, a short course of EBRT (e.g. 1 fraction of 8 Gy or 5 fractions of 4 Gy) affords similar palliation, without the inconvenience of a more protracted treatment course; while for better prognosis patients a more protracted course (e.g. 30 Gy in 10 fractions) of radiotherapy is warranted.

Radiotherapy is often delivered after surgical resection of epidural metastases to improve the chance of durable local control. Timing of the radiotherapy is important as preoperative radiotherapy is associated with higher rates of wound complications. A retrospective review of 123 patients with metastatic ESCC found the major wound complication rate was 32% for patients treated with preoperative radiotherapy compared to 12% for those treated with postoperative radiotherapy (27). Therefore, it is recommended that radiotherapy be delivered postoperatively and delayed at least a week (typically radiotherapy is delayed 3–4 weeks) after surgery (28).

With advancements in technology, the role of radiotherapy in the management of epidural metastases has evolved. One of these advancements is stereotactic body radiotherapy (SBRT), also known as stereotactic spine radiosurgery (SSRS). SBRT utilizes image guidance to deliver precise, high-dose radiation, typically in 1–5 fractions (29). SBRT typically has a steep dose gradient between the tumour and primary dose-limiting structure, the spinal cord (Fig. 20.2). This steep dose gradient allows higher radiation doses to be delivered to the tumour than can be delivered with conventional techniques since SBRT is much better at limiting the dose to the spinal cord. For this reason, SBRT is often utilized in patients who have failed conventional radiotherapy and it has been found to be effective in this setting in phase I/II trials (30). In general, SBRT is utilized in patients with limited spine metastases (i.e. one to two metastases), disease limited to one or two contiguous vertebral bodies, non-mechanical pain, and because the anticipated benefit of SBRT is long-term tumour control, an estimated survival of greater than 6 months. SBRT is often used in patients deemed poor

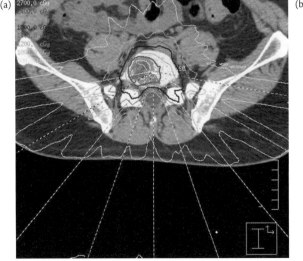
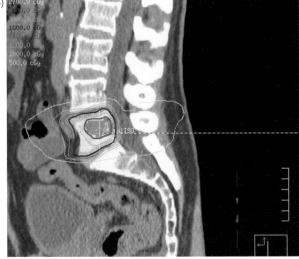

Fig. 20.2 (See colour plate section) Axial (a) and sagittal (b) MRI views of a L5 metastasis from renal cell carcinoma. The SBRT treatment plan is included. Note the rapid dose fall-off from the 24 Gy isodose line (red) to the 10 Gy isodose line (light blue) at the anterior edge of the spinal canal.

surgical candidates or in lieu of surgery since SBRT is an outpatient treatment, has quicker recovery time in a patient population with a relatively short survival, and causes less interference with ongoing systemic therapies than open surgery. However, SBRT and open surgery should not be considered competing treatment modalities but instead viewed as complementary treatment modalities; ideally treatment decisions will be made prospectively in a multidisciplinary tumour board, with orthopaedic surgeons, neurosurgeons, and radiation oncologists, with a strong clinical focus on cancers of the spine, selecting the best treatment based on multiple factors including quality of patient's pain, stability of spine, extent of disease, patient's co-morbidities and prognosis, tumour histology, and tumour location.

Promising results have been achieved with SBRT with long-term pain improvement and local control seen in 86% and 90% of patients, respectively (31). Garg et al. reported the results of a phase I/II trial of single-fraction SBRT 16–24 Gy (32). In this trial, 61 patients with 63 spinal metastases were enrolled and the 18-month local control rate was 88% with a median survival of 30 months. Only two patients experienced radiation adverse events (grade 3 or higher). A phase I/II trial of 149 patients with spinal metastases treated with 27–30 Gy in 3 fractions focused on quality of life and pain (33). The investigators found significant improvement in quality of life after SBRT and the number of patients reporting no pain from bone metastases increased from 26% at baseline to 54% at 6 months after SBRT. Toxicity was limited and there were no late spinal cord toxicities observed. In both of these trials, patients with acute ESCC were specifically excluded from enrolment. There are only a few SBRT studies focusing specifically on patients with epidural disease since SBRT is significantly limited by the interface of the tumour with the spinal cord. In a study of multiple myeloma, a radioresponsive neoplasm, 24 patients with 31 lesions causing ESCC were treated with single-fraction SBRT (median of 16 Gy) (34). Pain control was achieved in 86% of patients and complete radiographic response of the epidural tumour was observed in 81% of patients at 3 months after SBRT. Seven of these patients presented with neurological deficits and five neurologically improved or became normal after SBRT. A study of 62 patients with metastatic ESCC from many different tumour primaries (a large proportion were lung, prostate, or breast) and baseline muscle power 4 of 5 or better were treated with a single fraction of SBRT (median of 16 Gy) (35). Thecal sac patency significantly improved from 55% to 76% after SBRT and neurological function improved in 81%. Therefore, SBRT can achieve significant improvement in pain control, quality of life, and long-term local control. However due to inherent limitations in dose delivery, SBRT should be considered investigational in the treatment of ESCC, especially for those patients with radioresistant primary tumours. Exceptions would be patients who are not surgical candidates, although conventional radiotherapy is generally favoured in this clinical situation.

An alternative approach, often called separation surgery, is a more limited surgical approach, typically decompression by limited posterolateral tumour resection and posterior segmental instrumentation, followed by SBRT (36). The potential advantage of this approach is the surgery provides cord decompression and stabilization, while avoiding the risks of more extensive surgeries, and provides a small margin of 2–3 mm between the tumour and spinal cord that allows the delivery of tumouricidal radiation doses. A retrospective study of 187 patients treated with 'separation surgery' found 1-year local control rates greater than 90% for those treated with larger fraction size (8 Gy or larger) after operative radiosurgery.

Chemotherapy

Chemotherapy is a rational treatment for ESCC when the causative tumour is likely to be chemosensitive. Most common solid tumour causes of ESCC are not chemosensitive; however, for Hodgkin's lymphoma, germ cell tumours, and neuroblastoma, chemotherapy may effectively treat both the ESCC and other sites of disease (37–40). Hormonal manipulation has been documented to be beneficial in cases of ESCC from prostate and breast cancer.

Prognosis

A prospective study confirmed that radiation improved back pain in 60% of patients, with 70% of all patients able to ambulate and 90% continent (29). Several factors influence neurological outcome, with the most important being the pre-radiation neurological status. Other factors include the relative radiosensitivity of the underlying cancer, as well as the extent of anatomical compression of the thecal sac and deformation of the spinal cord or cauda equina. Finally, the tempo of onset of neurological deficits is pertinent, as a slower onset of dysfunction generally portends a better outcome (41).

Not surprisingly, survival following radiation therapy for ESCC depends on the presence and extent of visceral, brain, and other bone metastases. Additionally, a shorter interval between initial cancer diagnosis and ESCC onset predicts a shorter survival, as do radioresistant histologies, inability to walk, and rapidity of onset of ESCC-related neurological deficits (42). These factors have been combined into an ESCC prognostic scoring system to predict neurological outcome and overall survival to aid in decision-making (43, 44).

Intramedullary spinal cord metastases

Intramedullary spinal cord metastasis (ISCM) refers to metastases in the cord parenchyma. This complication of systemic cancer was rarely identified during the myelography era, since only masses producing substantial spinal cord swelling could be detected; diagnosis was more frequently made at autopsy (45). With the advent of MRI, ISCM has been more readily detected and has been the subject of several institutional case series (46, 47). Clinically, its incidence is approximately 1/16th that of ESCC (46). ISCM is recognized in about 2% of cancer autopsies (45). Prior to widespread MRI availability, physicians diagnosed only 5% of ISCM cases pre-mortem (48).

ISCM is typically a late complication of cancer, although up to 20% of cases arise as the initial manifestation of malignancy (46). A majority of patients with ISCM have brain metastases (65%), and one-quarter of patients have concomitant leptomeningeal metastases. Mean age of presentation is 55 and men are slightly more affected than women. ISCMs affect the cervical, thoracic, and lumbar cord equally (49). ISCMs are most often single.

Like spinal epidural metastases, ISCMs can produce myelopathy and back pain. Pain is less ubiquitous and severe than in patients with spinal epidural metastases, affecting about half of all patients. Another feature suggesting ISCM is Brown-Séquard syndrome, or a markedly asymmetric myelopathy. This feature is present in almost half of patients with ISCM but in only 3% of patients with ESCC (46). Rapid progression of symptoms distinguishes ISCM from primary intramedullary tumours such as ependymomas and other astrocytomas, which typically present with a slower progression of symptoms over months to years. In three-quarters of ISCM patients, the time from the onset of neurological symptoms to the development of the full neurological deficit is less than 1 month (50, 51).

Lung cancer (54%) accounts for a majority of ISCM cases, with small cell carcinoma disproportionally over-represented. Other common underlying aetiologies include breast carcinoma (13%), melanoma (9%), lymphoma (5%), and renal cell carcinoma (4%) (46, 52–54). When a spinal lesion is suspected in a patient with a history of systemic cancer, contrast-enhanced MRI should be performed to screen for ISCM as well as epidural compression. MRI scans readily differentiate ISCM from ESCC, revealing parenchymal circumscribed contrast enhancement with a larger surrounding area of T2 signal indicative of oedema (46).

Surgery in intramedullary spinal cord metastases

The role of surgical resection for intradural ISCMs is controversial. As stated previously, approximately 50% of ISCMs are secondary to lung carcinoma. The majority of these cases are small cell carcinoma, which is primarily treated via chemotherapy and radiation. Up to 12% of other cases are secondary to lymphoma, which is also treated via non-surgical adjuvant measures. The remainder of cases primarily metastasize from breast, renal cell, melanoma, or gastrointestinal carcinoma (50, 55–58). Consequently, a relatively small percentage of cases present with surgical resection as a viable treatment option.

As with every intervention, a risk/benefit analysis must be performed by the treating physicians. Approximately 75% of ISCMs display a 1-month time period from the time of initial symptoms to paraplegia (59). Consequently, prompt treatment is of primary importance. Patients with rapid progression of neurological deficits display improvement with early surgical management (56). However, there exist two distinct patterns of metastasis including (i) primary parenchymal involvement and (ii) parenchymal disease secondary to leptomeningeal involvement (45). As the goal of surgical resection is to maintain existing neurological function,

radiation is considered as adjuvant treatment if there is concern for residual disease (57, 60).

Patients who present with primary parenchymal involvement are also considered for surgical resection as the initial treatment option depending on the location of the tumour within the spinal cord. The primary surgical access point is the posterior median sulcus of the spinal cord. The relationship of the tumour to this sulcus must be taken into account when considering surgical resection. ISCMs are also typically well circumscribed, similar to intracerebral metastasis and are amenable to resection once accessed (Fig. 20.3) (56, 61, 62). Perhaps even more important is the size of the tumour. A multidisciplinary approach is critical in these patients; consideration should be given to the option of surgical debulking with radiation as an option for upfront or residual disease (63). As with any patient with metastatic disease in whom surgery is considered, the state of systemic disease must always be taken into account (59).

Radiotherapy in intramedullary spinal cord metastases

Conventional radiotherapy remains the primary treatment for ISCMs since a large percentage of the primary tumours are either small cell lung carcinoma or lymphoma and typically these histologies are very responsive to radiotherapy (57). Additionally, both surgical resection and SBRT are very difficult to perform with an intramedullary lesion. Although the prognosis for these patients is very poor (e.g. median survival 4 months), radiotherapy has been shown to extend survival and maintain ambulatory function in up to 90% of patients (57). A typical fractionation schedule is 30 Gy in 10 fractions.

Malignant plexopathy and peripheral nerve metastases

The brachial plexus is an anastomotic collection of nerves formed by the nerve roots of the fifth cervical through first thoracic spinal segments. Malignant involvement of the brachial plexus occurs by two mechanisms: compression by a mass or infiltration by cancer cells. The former arise by metastases to axillary lymph nodes or direct extension of an apical lung tumour, both of which lie in close proximity to the lower trunk of the brachial plexus. About 1% of patients with cancer develop a neoplastic brachial plexopathy;

(a)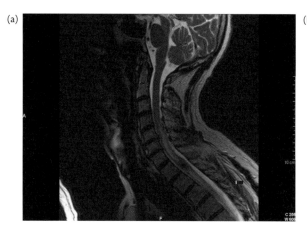

(b)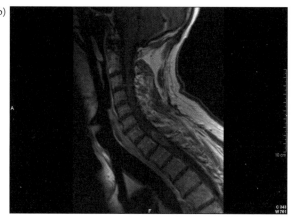

Fig. 20.3 A 74-year-old man with T3N0 bladder cancer developed subacute onset of left leg weakness over several days. Sagittal T2 (a) and post-gadolinium (b) MRI scans demonstrated an intramedullary spinal cord metastasis. Subtotal resection of the mass demonstrated metastatic carcinoma. Postoperative brain MRI revealed two small asymptomatic brain metastases.

the most common underlying malignancies are breast and lung cancers, accounting for approximately 70% of cases (64, 65). Both lesions tend preferentially to involve the lower trunk of the plexus derived primarily from the C8 and T1 roots. Lymphomas occasionally infiltrate the brachial plexi (66). Pain is the most common and significant symptom and may precede other symptoms by months. It commonly involves the shoulder region and radiates down the medial aspect of arm into the fourth and fifth digits. Muscle weakness and sensory loss may also be present. Horner's syndrome is present in approximately 50% of patients. Physical examination may reveal lymphoedema or an axillary mass.

The lumbar plexus derives from the ventral rami of the L1–L4 nerve roots, and the sacral plexus from the ventral roots of S1–S4. Colorectal tumours, genitourinary tumours, sarcomas, and lymphomas are the most common cancers to involve the lumbosacral plexus (67, 68). Tumours invade the plexus by direct extension from the primary tumour in a majority of cases, although metastases from extra-abdominal malignancies account for one-quarter of cases (67). As with neoplastic brachial plexopathy, pain is the predominant symptom in malignant lumbosacral plexopathy. Weakness and sensory abnormalities are common, the distribution dependent on the extent of plexus involvement. Symptoms are typically unilateral. Incontinence is rare and its presence suggests epidural extension of tumour. Leg oedema and the presence of an abdominopelvic mass should be sought on physical examination including rectal examination.

The differential diagnosis for malignant plexopathy in patients who have previously received radiation therapy is radiation plexopathy although this should be a diagnosis of exclusion as unnecessary delay in treatment of malignant plexopathy only prolongs a patient's suffering; non-malignant causes such as idiopathic brachial plexitis (Parsonage–Turner syndrome) and diabetic amyotrophy must also be considered. Radiation plexopathy is somewhat less likely to be extremely painful (64, 69). Electrophysiology may also be helpful, as the continuous, involuntary small muscle discharges that define myokymia are often present in radiation plexopathy and generally absent in malignant plexopathy (70).

Confirmation of the diagnosis of malignant plexopathy usually depends on imaging. CT scanning identifies abnormalities in 89% and 74% of patients with brachial and lumbosacral plexopathy, respectively (71). MRI provides much better anatomical detail and has become the imaging modality of choice. The most common finding with both CT and MRI scans is a mass either in or near the plexus (72, 73). Increased T2 signal adjacent to the brachial plexus is occasionally seen on MRI (11). Although imaging is usually sufficient to establish the diagnosis, 9% of MRI scans are normal; in such patients, surgical exploration is often necessary (64, 65, 72). More recently, PET has helped confirm metastases in patients with indeterminate MRI scans (74, 75). Spinal MRI may also be indicated, as coexistent epidural disease is present in approximately 50% of cases. Restaging with systemic imaging to evaluate for active disease outside of the plexus should be considered. Hydronephrosis should be sought in patients with lumbosacral plexopathy as it was detected in 44% of cases in one series (67).

The primary role of surgery in patients with brachial plexopathy is in differentiating between radiation-induced plexopathy and metastatic plexopathy. Either can present many years after initial treatment of underlying disease with a median of 5.5–6 years or

greater. The role of surgery in the setting of negative imaging of the brachial plexus remains controversial (76). The most common scenario is a breast carcinoma patient with a history of mastectomy and radiation. In a patient with previously diagnosed, widely metastatic disease, tumour as an aetiology is more likely. However, in patients with stable systemic disease, surgical exploration can be definitive, thereby preventing a delay in treatment if surgical exploration leads to a positive biopsy (64, 69, 72, 77, 78). Neurolymphomatosis, typically secondary to non-Hodgkin's lymphoma, can include multiple peripheral nerves including the brachial plexus and the diagnosis can be confirmed with open biopsy (79, 80).

Treatment of metastatic brachial plexopathy may include radiation, chemotherapy, or surgical resection. The latter is considered with a defined isolated lesion on imaging with consideration of systemic disease control, such as in isolated metastatic leiomyoma of the uterus (81, 82).

Similar to brachial plexus pathology, cancer patients can also present with signs of lumbosacral plexopathy. If the diagnosis is in question, surgical exploration and biopsy allows for definitive diagnosis (67, 83, 84). In addition to biopsy, surgical resection is considered for treatment of lesions with poor response to chemotherapy or radiation (67). With regard to peripheral nerve metastases, the primary role of surgery is in establishing the diagnosis in peripheral neuropathy after chemotherapy treatment for cancer. For example, lymphoma patients after chemotherapy treatment with apparent stable systemic disease can develop peripheral neuropathy with such diagnoses of progressive distal polyneuropathy or mononeuropathy multiplex. Peripheral nerve biopsy can confirm the presence of active tumour in order to establish the need for further treatment (85, 86). Perhaps less commonly, patients may present with metastatic peripheral neuropathy with otherwise negative surveillance imaging requiring nerve biopsy for initial diagnosis of cancer (87–89). This clinical scenario is most common in lymphoma and has been reported in neurolymphomatosis (88, 90). Surgical biopsy is second to MRI in establishing a diagnosis (66). However, despite diffuse metastatic disease, peripheral nerve biopsy may be negative (75, 91, 92).

Metastatic peripheral nerve disease can also present via direct extension from primary pathology. This clinical scenario is reported in a variety of carcinomas including prostate carcinoma metastatic to the sciatic nerve (93). These lesions require open surgical biopsy as an alternative to percutaneous biopsy. The former decreases the risk of neurological injury and increases the percentage of a positive biopsy (93, 94).

Radiation therapy is an important therapeutic modality for most patients with malignant plexopathy or peripheral nerve metastases. Unlike with bone metastases, in which a meta-analysis showed equivalence in complete and overall pain relief between single- and multi-fraction radiotherapy schedules (95), there is a suggestion that a more protracted course may be beneficial for those patients with neoplastic involvement of a nerve root causing neuropathic pain (96). While bone pain treated with radiation is relieved through molecular processes that are not completely understood and hence lower doses are sufficient (97), tumour compression of nerve roots requires higher doses of radiation to cause regression of the tumour. For these reasons, a typical schedule is 30 Gy in 10 fractions (or more protracted courses) for plexus and peripheral nerve metastases.

References

1. Loblaw DA, Laperriere NJ, Mackillop WJ. A population-based study of malignant spinal cord compression in Ontario. *Clin Oncol (R Coll Radiol)* 2003; 15(4):211–217.

2. Mak KS, Lee LK, Mak RH, et al. Incidence and treatment patterns in hospitalizations for malignant spinal cord compression in the United States, 1998-2006. *Int J Radiat Oncol Biol Phys* 2011; 80(3):824–831.

3. Helweg-Larsen S, Sorensen PS. Symptoms and signs in metastatic spinal cord compression: a study of progression from first symptom until diagnosis in 153 patients. *Eur J Cancer* 1994; 30A(3):396.

4. Schiff D, O'Neill BP, Wang CH, et al. Neuroimaging and treatment implications of patients with multiple epidural spinal metastases. *Cancer* 1998; 83(8):1593–1601.

5. Ushio Y, Posner R, Posner JB, et al. Experimental spinal cord compression by epidural neoplasm. *Neurology* 1977; 27(5):422–429.

6. Gilbert RW, Kim JH, Posner JB. Epidural spinal cord compression from metastatic tumor: diagnosis and treatment. *Ann Neurol* 1978; 3(1):40–51.

7. Greenberg HS, Kim JH, Posner JB. Epidural spinal cord compression from metastatic tumor: results with a new treatment protocol. *Ann Neurol* 1980; 8(4):361–366.

8. Sorensen PS, Helweg-Larsen S, Mouridsen H, et al. Effect of high-dose dexamethasone in carcinomatous metastatic spinal cord compression treated with radiotherapy: a randomised trial. *Eur J Cancer* 1994; 30A(1):22.

9. Heimdal K, Hirschberg H, Slettebo H, et al. High incidence of serious side effects of high-dose dexamethasone treatment in patients with epidural spinal cord compression. *J Neurooncol* 1992; 12(2):141–144.

10. Maranzano E, Latini P, Beneventi S, et al. Radiotherapy without steroids in selected metastatic spinal cord compression patients. A phase II trial. *Am J Clin Oncol* 1996; 19(2):179–183.

11. Tomita K, Kawahara N, Kobayashi T, et al. Surgical strategy for spinal metastases. *Spine* 2001; 26(3):298–306.

12. Patchell RA, Tibbs PA, Regine WF, et al. Direct decompressive surgical resection in the treatment of spinal cord compression caused by metastatic cancer: a randomised trial. *Lancet* 2005; 366(9486):643–648.

13. Bilsky M, Smith M. Surgical approach to epidural spinal cord compression. *Hematol Oncol Clin North Am* 2006; 20(6):1307–1317.

14. Fisher CG, DiPaola CP, Ryken TC, et al. A novel classification system for spinal instability in neoplastic disease: an evidence-based approach and expert consensus from the Spine Oncology Study Group. *Spine* 2010; 35(22):E1221–E1229.

15. Fourney DR, Frangou EM, Ryken TC, et al. Spinal instability neoplastic score: an analysis of reliability and validity from the spine oncology study group. *J Clin Oncol* 2011; 29(22):3072–3077.

16. Spinazze S, Caraceni A, Schrijvers D. Epidural spinal cord compression. *Crit Rev Oncol Hematol* 2005; 56(3):397–406.

17. Bilsky MH, Boland P, Lis E, et al. Single-stage posterolateral transpedicle approach for spondylectomy, epidural decompression, and circumferential fusion of spinal metastases. *Spine* 2000; 25(17):2240–2249.

18. Purkayastha S, Gupta AK, Kapilamoorthy TR, et al. Percutaneous vertebroplasty in the management of vertebral lesions. *Neurol India* 2005; 53(2):167–172.

19. Sabharwal T, Salter R, Adam A, et al. Image-guided therapies in orthopedic oncology. *Orthop Clin North Am* 2006; 37(1):105–112.

20. Brown PD, Stafford SL, Schild SE, et al. Metastatic spinal cord compression in patients with colorectal cancer. *J Neurooncology* 1999; 44(2):175–180.

21. Maranzano E, Bellavita R, Rossi R, et al. Short-course versus split-course radiotherapy in metastatic spinal cord compression: results of a phase III, randomized, multicenter trial. *J Clin Oncol* 2005; 23(15):3358–3365.

22. Helweg-Larsen S, Johnsen A, Boesen J, et al. Radiologic features compared to clinical findings in a prospective study of 153 patients with metastatic spinal cord compression treated by radiotherapy. *Acta Neurochir* 1997; 139(2):105.

23. Maranzano E, Latini P. Effectiveness of radiation therapy without surgery in metastatic spinal cord compression: final results from a prospective trial. *Int J Radiat Oncol Biol Phys* 1995; 32(4):959–967.

24. Rades D, Stalpers LJ, Veninga T, et al. Evaluation of five radiation schedules and prognostic factors for metastatic spinal cord compression. *J Clin Oncol* 2005; 23(15):3366–3375.

25. Maranzano E, Trippa F, Casale M, et al. 8Gy single-dose radiotherapy is effective in metastatic spinal cord compression: results of a phase III randomized multicentre Italian trial. *Radiother Oncol* 2009; 93(2):174–179.

26. Rades D, Segedin B, Conde-Moreno AJ, et al. Radiotherapy with 4 Gy x 5 versus 3 Gy x 10 for metastatic epidural spinal cord compression: final results of the SCORE-2 Trial (ARO 2009/01). *J Clin Oncol* 2016; 34(6):597–602.

27. Ghogawala Z, Mansfield FL, Borges LF. Spinal radiation before surgical decompression adversely affects outcomes of surgery for symptomatic metastatic spinal cord compression. *Spine* 2001; 26(7):818–824.

28. Itshayek E, Yamada J, Bilsky M, et al. Timing of surgery and radiotherapy in the management of metastatic spine disease: a systematic review. *Int J Oncol* 2010; 36(3):533–544.

29. Ahmed KA, Stauder MC, Miller RC, et al. Stereotactic body radiation therapy in spinal metastases. *Int J Radiat Oncol Biol Phys* 2012; 82(5):e803–e809.

30. Garg AK, Wang XS, Shiu AS, et al. Prospective evaluation of spinal reirradiation by using stereotactic body radiation therapy: The University of Texas MD Anderson Cancer Center experience. *Cancer* 2011; 117(15):3509–3516.

31. Gerszten PC, Burton SA, Ozhasoglu C, et al. Radiosurgery for spinal metastases: clinical experience in 500 cases from a single institution. *Spine* 2007; 32(2):193–199.

32. Garg AK, Shiu AS, Yang J, et al. Phase 1/2 trial of single-session stereotactic body radiotherapy for previously unirradiated spinal metastases. *Cancer* 2012; 118(20):5069–5077.

33. Wang XS, Rhines LD, Shiu AS, et al. Stereotactic body radiation therapy for management of spinal metastases in patients without spinal cord compression: a phase 1-2 trial. *Lancet Oncol* 2012; 13(4):395–402.

34. Jin R, Rock J, Jin JY, et al. Single fraction spine radiosurgery for myeloma epidural spinal cord compression. *J Exp Ther Oncol* 2009; 8(1):35–41.

35. Ryu S, Rock J, Jain R, et al. Radiosurgical decompression of metastatic epidural compression. *Cancer* 2010; 116(9):2250–2257.

36. Moulding HD, Elder JB, Lis E, et al. Local disease control after decompressive surgery and adjuvant high-dose single-fraction radiosurgery for spine metastases. *J Neurosurg Spine* 2010; 13(1):87–93.

37. Grommes C, Bosl GJ, DeAngelis LM. Treatment of epidural spinal cord involvement from germ cell tumors with chemotherapy. *Cancer* 117(9):1911–1916.

38. Matsubara H, Watanabe K, Sakai H, et al. Rapid improvement of paraplegia caused by epidural involvements of Burkitt's lymphoma with chemotherapy. *Spine (Phila Pa 1976)* 2004; 29(1):E4–E6.

39. Plantaz D, Rubie H, Michon J, et al. The treatment of neuroblastoma with intraspinal extension with chemotherapy followed by surgical removal of residual disease. A prospective study of 42 patients—results of the NBL 90 Study of the French Society of Pediatric Oncology. *Cancer* 1996; 78(2):311–319.

40. Wong ET, Portlock CS, O'Brien JP, et al. Chemosensitive epidural spinal cord disease in non-Hodgkins lymphoma. *Neurology* 1996; 46(6):1543–1547.

41. Rades D, Heidenreich F, Karstens JH. Final results of a prospective study of the prognostic value of the time to develop motor deficits before irradiation in metastatic spinal cord compression. *Int J Radiat Oncol Biol Phys* 2002; 53(4):975–979.

42. Rades D, Fehlauer F, Schulte R, et al. Prognostic factors for local control and survival after radiotherapy of metastatic spinal cord compression. *J Clin Oncol* 2006; 24(21):3388–3393.

43. Rades D, Douglas S, Veninga T, et al. Validation and simplification of a score predicting survival in patients irradiated for metastatic spinal cord compression. *Cancer* 2010; 116(15):3670–3673.

44. Rades D, Rudat V, Veninga T, et al. A score predicting posttreatment ambulatory status in patients irradiated for metastatic spinal cord compression. *Int J Radiat Oncol Biol Phys* 2008; 72(3):905–908.

45. Costigan DA, Winkelman MD. Intramedullary spinal cord metastasis. A clinicopathological study of 13 cases. *J Neurosurg* 1985; 62(2):227–233.

46. Schiff D, O'Neill BP. Intramedullary spinal cord metastases: clinical features and treatment outcome. *Neurology* 1996; 47:906–912.

47. Dam-Hieu P, Seizeur R, Mineo JF, et al. Retrospective study of 19 patients with intramedullary spinal cord metastasis. *Clin Neurol Neurosurg* 2009; 111(1):10–17.

48. Okamoto H, Shinkai T, Matsuno Y, et al. Intradural parenchymal involvement in the spinal subarachnoid space associated with primary lung cancer. *Cancer* 1993; 72(9):2583–2588.

49. Connolly ES, Jr, Winfree CJ, McCormick PC, et al. Intramedullary spinal cord metastasis: report of three cases and review of the literature. *Surg Neurol* 1996; 46(4):329–337.

50. Grem JL, Burgess J, Trump DL. Clinical features and natural history of intramedullary spinal cord metastasis. *Cancer* 1985; 56(9):2305–2314.

51. Jellinger K, Kothbauer P, Sunder-Plassmann E, et al. Intramedullary spinal cord metastases. *J Neurol* 1979; 220(1):31–41.

52. Fakih M, Schiff D, Erlich R, et al. Intramedullary spinal cord metastasis (ISCM) in renal cell carcinoma: a series of six cases. *Ann Oncol* 2001; 12(8):1173–1177.

53. Dunne JW, Harper CG, Pamphlett R. Intramedullary spinal cord metastases: a clinical and pathological study of nine cases. *Q J Med* 1986; 61(235):1003–1020.

54. Flanagan E, O'Neill B, Habermann T, et al. Secondary intramedullary spinal cord non-Hodgkin's lymphoma. *J Neurooncol* 107(3):575–580.

55. Edelson RN, Deck MD, Posner JB. Intramedullary spinal cord metastases. Clinical and radiographic findings in nine cases. *Neurology* 1972; 22(12):1222–1231.

56. Kalayci M, Cagavi F, Gul S, et al. Intramedullary spinal cord metastases: diagnosis and treatment—an illustrated review. *Acta Neurochir* 2004; 146(12):1347–1354.

57. Schiff D, O'Neill BP. Intramedullary spinal cord metastases: clinical features and treatment outcome. *Neurology* 1996; 47(4):906–912.

58. Villegas AE, Guthrie TH. Intramedullary spinal cord metastasis in breast cancer: clinical features, diagnosis, and therapeutic consideration. *Breast J* 2004; 10(6):532–535.

59. Sutter B, Arthur A, Laurent J, et al. Treatment options and time course for intramedullary spinal cord metastasis. Report of three cases and review of the literature. *Neurosurg Focus* 1998; 4(5):e3.

60. Conill C, Sanchez M, Puig S, et al. Intramedullary spinal cord metastases of melanoma. *Melanoma Res* 2004; 14(5):431–433.

61. Findlay JM, Bernstein M, Vanderlinden RG, et al. Microsurgical resection of solitary intramedullary spinal cord metastases. *Neurosurgery* 1987; 21(6):911–915.

62. Ogino M, Ueda R, Nakatsukasa M, et al. Successful removal of solitary intramedullary spinal cord metastasis from colon cancer. *Clin Neurol Neurosurg* 2002; 104(2):152–156.

63. Shin DA, Huh R, Chung SS, et al. Stereotactic spine radiosurgery for intradural and intramedullary metastasis. *Neurosurg Focus* 2009; 27(6):E10.

64. Kori SH, Foley KM, Posner JB. Brachial plexus lesions in patients with cancer: 100 cases. *Neurology* 1981; 31(1):45–50.

65. Wittenberg KH, Adkins MC. MR imaging of nontraumatic brachial plexopathies: frequency and spectrum of findings. *Radiographics* 2000; 20(4):1023–1032.

66. Baehring JM, Damek D, Martin EC, et al. Neurolymphomatosis. *Neuro Oncol* 2003; 5(2):104–115.

67. Jaeckle KA, Young DF, Foley KM. The natural history of lumbosacral plexopathy in cancer. *Neurology* 1985; 35(1):8–15.

68. Onufrey V, Mohiuddin M. Radiation therapy in the treatment of metastatic renal cell carcinoma. *Int J Radiat Oncol Biol Phys* 1985; 11(11):2007–2009.

69. Bagley FH, Walsh JW, Cady B, et al. Carcinomatous versus radiation-induced brachial plexus neuropathy in breast cancer. *Cancer* 1978; 41(6):2154–2157.

70. Krarup C, Crone C. Neurophysiological studies in malignant disease with particular reference to involvement of peripheral nerves. *J Neurol* 2002; 249(6):651–661.

71. Thomas JE, Cascino TL, Earle JD. Differential diagnosis between radiation and tumor plexopathy of the pelvis. *Neurology* 1985; 35(1):1–7.

72. Thyagarajan D, Cascino T, Harms G. Magnetic resonance imaging in brachial plexopathy of cancer. *Neurology* 1995; 45(3 Pt 1):421–427.

73. Cascino TL, Kori S, Krol G, et al. CT of the brachial plexus in patients with cancer. *Neurology* 1983; 33(12):1553–1557.

74. Hathaway PB, Mankoff DA, Maravilla KR, et al. Value of combined FDG PET and MR imaging in the evaluation of suspected recurrent local-regional breast cancer: preliminary experience. *Radiology* 1999; 210(3):807–814.

75. Trojan A, Jermann M, Taverna C, et al. Fusion PET-CT imaging of neurolymphomatosis. *Ann Oncol* 2002; 13(5):802–805.

76. Lingawi SS, Bilbey JH, Munk PL, et al. MR imaging of brachial plexopathy in breast cancer patients without palpable recurrence. *Skeletal Radiol* 1999; 28(6):318–323.

77. Thomas JE, Colby MY, Jr. Radiation-induced or metastatic brachial plexopathy? A diagnostic dilemma. *JAMA* 1972; 222(11):1392–1395.

78. Meller I, Alkalay D, Mozes M, et al. Isolated metastases to peripheral nerves. Report of five cases involving the brachial plexus. *Cancer* 1995; 76(10):1829–1832.

79. Bokstein F, Goor O, Shihman B, et al. Assessment of neurolymphomatosis by brachial plexus biopsy and PET/CT. Report of a case. *J Neurooncology* 2005; 72(2):163–167.

80. Giglio P, Gilbert MR. Neurologic complications of non-Hodgkin's lymphoma. *Curr Hematol Malig Rep* 2006; 1(4):214–219.

81. Fishman EK, Campbell JN, Kuhlman JE, et al. Multiplanar CT evaluation of brachial plexopathy in breast cancer. *J Comput Assist Tomogr* 1991; 15(5):790–795.

82. de Ruiter GC, Scheithauer BW, Amrami KK, et al. Benign metastasizing leiomyomatosis with massive brachial plexus involvement mimicking neurofibromatosis type 1. *Clin Neuropathol* 2006; 25(6):282–287.

83. Pettigrew LC, Glass JP, Maor M, et al. Diagnosis and treatment of lumbosacral plexopathies in patients with cancer. *Arch Neurol* 1984; 41(12):1282–1285.

84. Saphner T, Gallion HH, Van Nagell JR, et al. Neurologic complications of cervical cancer. A review of 2261 cases. *Cancer* 1989; 64(5):1147–1151.

85. Krendel DA, Stahl RL, Chan WC. Lymphomatous polyneuropathy. Biopsy of clinically involved nerve and successful treatment. *Arch Neurol* 1991; 48(3):330–332.

86. Glass J. Neurologic complications of lymphoma and leukemia. *Semin Oncol* 2006; 33(3):342–347.

87. Hughes RA, Britton T, Richards M. Effects of lymphoma on the peripheral nervous system. *J R Soc Med* 1994; 87(9):526–530.

88. Quinones-Hinojosa A, Friedlander RM, Boyer PJ, et al. Solitary sciatic nerve lymphoma as an initial manifestation of diffuse neurolymphomatosis. Case report and review of the literature. *J Neurosurg* 2000; 92(1):165–169.

89. Shibata-Hamaguchi A, Samuraki M, Furui E, et al. B-cell neurolymphomatosis confined to the peripheral nervous system. *J Neurol Sci* 2007; 260(1–2):249–252.

90. Kelly JJ, Karcher DS. Lymphoma and peripheral neuropathy: a clinical review. *Muscle Nerve* 2005; 31(3):301–313.

91. van den Bent MJ, de Bruin HG, Bos GM, et al. Negative sural nerve biopsy in neurolymphomatosis. *J Neurol* 1999; 246(12):1159–1163.

92. Ramchandren S, Dalmau J. Metastases to the peripheral nervous system. *J Neurooncol* 2005; 75(1):101–110.

93. Ladha SS, Spinner RJ, Suarez GA, et al. Neoplastic lumbosacral radiculoplexopathy in prostate cancer by direct perineural spread: an unusual entity. *Muscle Nerve* 2006; 34(5):659–665.

94. Gachiani J, Kim DH, Nelson A, et al. Management of metastatic tumors invading the peripheral nervous system. *Neurosurg Focus* 2007; 22(6):E14.

95. Wu JS, Wong R, Johnston M, et al. Meta-analysis of dose-fractionation radiotherapy trials for the palliation of painful bone metastases. *Int J Radiat Oncol Biol Phys* 2003; 55(3):594–605.

96. Roos DE, Turner SL, O'Brien PC, et al. Randomized trial of 8 Gy in 1 versus 20 Gy in 5 fractions of radiotherapy for neuropathic pain due to bone metastases (Trans-Tasman Radiation Oncology Group, TROG 96.05). *Radiother Oncol* 2005; 75(1):54–63.

97. Goblirsch M, Mathews W, Lynch C, et al. Radiation treatment decreases bone cancer pain, osteolysis and tumor size. *Radiat Res* 2004; 161(2):228–234.

CHAPTER 21

Neoplastic meningitis: metastases to the leptomeninges and cerebrospinal fluid

Marc C. Chamberlain, Stephanie E. Combs, and Soichiro Shibui

Definition

Carcinomatous meningitis or meningeal carcinomatosis is a term that defines leptomeningeal metastases arising as a result of metastases from systemic solid cancers (1, 2). Similarly, lymphomatous and leukaemic meningitis result from cerebrospinal fluid (CSF) dissemination of lymphoma or leukaemia. All three entities are commonly referred to as neoplastic meningitis (NM) or leptomeningeal metastases due to involvement of both the CSF compartment as well as the leptomeninges comprised of the pia and arachnoid.

Epidemiology

Though NM is the third most common metastatic complication of the central nervous system (CNS), NM is comparatively uncommon with 7000–9000 new cases diagnosed annually in the United States (1–5). The most common sources of systemic cancer metastatic to the leptomeninges are breast, lung, melanoma, aggressive non-Hodgkin's lymphoma, and acute leukaemia in that order.

Neoplastic meningitis is diagnosed in 1–5% of patients with solid tumours, 5–15% of patients with leukaemia and lymphoma, and 1–2% of patients with primary brain tumours (1–5). Autopsy studies show that 19% of patients with cancer and neurological signs and symptoms have evidence of leptomeningeal involvement (4). Adenocarcinoma is the most frequent histology and breast, lung, and melanoma are the most common primary sites to metastasize to the leptomeninges (1–5). Although small cell lung carcinoma and melanoma have the highest rates of spread to the leptomeninges (11% and 20% respectively), because of the higher incidence of breast cancer (with a 5% rate of spread), the latter accounts for most cases in large series of the disorder (1–5). Carcinomas of unknown primary constitute 1–7% of all cases of NM (1–5).

Aetiology

Neoplastic meningitis is a consequence of metastasis to the CNS and consequently has no known aetiology notwithstanding the observation that certain cancers, based upon incidence, have a predilection for metastasis to the leptomeninges such as breast, melanoma, acute lymphocytic leukaemia, and primitive neuroectodermal tumours such as medulloblastoma. Leptomeningeal metastasis does not appear to have a hereditary component nor are there environmental exposures that result in an increased risk of this metastatic complication. There has been controversy regarding the possible increased risk of CSF dissemination in patients undergoing resective surgery for parenchymal brain metastasis especially in surgery directed at cerebellar metastasis. At present, however, there is no compelling data to suggest that placement of a ventriculoperitoneal shunt in patients with NM increases the risk of dissemination to the peritoneum resulting in carcinomatosis peritonei.

Pathogenesis

Cancer cells reach the meninges by various routes: (i) haematogenous spread, either through the venous plexus of Batson or by arterial dissemination; (ii) direct extension from contiguous tumour deposits; and (iii) through centripetal migration from systemic tumours along perineural or perivascular spaces (1–5).

Once cancer cells have entered the subarachnoid space, they are transported by CSF flow resulting in disseminated and multifocal neuraxis seeding of the leptomeninges. Possible mechanisms of CSF dissemination are outlined in Box 21.1. Tumor infiltration is most prominent at the base of the brain, the dorsal surface of the spinal cord, and, in particular, the cauda equina (1–5). Hydrocephalus or impairment of CSF flow may occur at any level of the neuraxis and is due to ependymal nodules or tumour deposits obstructing CSF outflow. The pathophysiology of NM may involve up-regulation of vascular endothelial growth factor as measured by CSF analysis, up-regulation of interleukin-8 and proinflammatory cytokines, as well as constitutive activation of tumoural integrin promoting adhesion (6–8).

Clinical presentation

Neoplastic meningitis classically presents with pleomorphic clinical manifestations encompassing symptoms and signs in three

Box 21.1 Possible mechanisms of cerebrospinal fluid dissemination

- Decreased expression of adhesion molecules:
  1. VLA-4
  2. CD44
  3. P-selectin

- Downregulation of chemokine receptors:
  1. CCR1
  2. CCR2
  3. CXCR4

- Increased matrix metalloproteinase expression

- Angiogenesis:
  1. VEGF
  2. Angiopoietin-1

- Activation pathway:
  1. Mutation in alternative or classical NF-κB
  2. Mutation in Src
  3. EMT (epithelial–mesenchymal transition).

domains of neurological function: (i) the cerebral hemispheres (15% of all patients); (ii) the cranial nerves (35%); and (iii) the spinal cord and nerve roots (60%). Signs on examination generally exceed the symptoms reported by the patient (1–5).

The most common manifestations of cerebral hemisphere dysfunction are headache and mental status changes. Other signs include seizures and hemiparesis. Diplopia is the most common symptom of cranial nerve dysfunction with cranial nerve VI being the most frequently affected, followed by cranial nerves III and IV. Trigeminal sensory or motor loss, cochlear dysfunction, and optic neuropathy are also common findings. Spinal signs and symptoms include weakness (lower extremities more often than upper), dermatomal or segmental sensory loss, and pain in the neck, back, or following radicular patterns. Nuchal rigidity is only present in 15% of cases (1–5).

A high index of suspicion needs to be entertained in order to make the diagnosis of NM. The finding of multifocal neuraxis disease in a patient with known malignancy is strongly suggestive of NM, but it is also common for patients with NM to present with isolated syndromes such as symptoms of raised intracranial pressure, cauda equina syndrome, or cranial neuropathy.

New neurological signs and symptoms may represent progression of NM but must be distinguished from the manifestations of parenchymal disease (30–40% of patients with NM will have coexistent parenchymal brain metastases), from side effects of chemotherapy or radiation used for treatment, and rarely from paraneoplastic syndromes. At presentation, NM must also be differentiated from chronic meningitis due to tuberculosis, fungal infection, or sarcoidosis as well as from metabolic and toxic encephalopathies in the appropriate clinical setting (1–5).

Cerebrospinal fluid analysis

The most useful laboratory test in the diagnosis of NM is the CSF examination. Abnormalities include increased opening pressure (>200 mmH$_2$O), increased leucocytes (>4/mm^3), elevated protein (>50 mg/dL), or decreased glucose (<60 mg/dL), which though suggestive of NM are not diagnostic (1–5). The presence of malignant cells in the CSF is diagnostic of NM but in general, as is true for most cytological analysis, assignment to a particular tumour is not possible. Glass and colleagues demonstrated that up to 40% of patients with clinically suspected NM proven at time of autopsy are cytologically negative. This figure increased to greater than 50% in patients with focal NM (4).

A CSF examination is useful in all patients with suspected NM. Demonstrating positive CSF cytology or flow cytometry assist in managing patients with NM. Conversion from positive to negative cytology or flow cytometry is considered a response and would suggest continuation of therapy.

In patients with positive CSF cytology (see later in this section), up to 45% will be cytologically negative on initial examination (1–5). The yield is increased to 80% with a second CSF examination but little benefit is obtained from repeat lumbar punctures after two punctures (1–5). Of note, a series including lymphomatous and leukaemic meningitis observed the frequent dissociation between CSF cell count and malignant cytology (29% of cytologically positive CSF had concurrent CSF cell counts of less than 4/mm^3) (1–5). Another study showed that CSF levels of protein, glucose, and malignant cells vary at different levels of the neuraxis even if there is no obstruction of the CSF flow (1–5, 9). This finding reflects the multifocal nature of NM and explains that CSF obtained from a site distant to that of the pathologically involved meninges may yield a negative cytology.

The low sensitivity of CSF cytology makes it difficult not only to diagnose NM, but also to assess the response to treatment. Biochemical markers, immunohistochemistry, and molecular biology techniques applied to CSF have been explored in an attempt to find a reliable biological marker of disease (10). Numerous biochemical markers have been evaluated but, in general, their use has been limited by poor sensitivity and specificity. The use of biochemical markers can be helpful as adjunctive diagnostic tests and, when followed serially, to assess response to treatment. Occasionally, in patients with clinically suspected NM and negative CSF cytology, they may support the diagnosis of NM. Use of monoclonal antibodies for immunohistochemical analysis in NM does not significantly increase the sensitivity of cytology alone. However, in the case of leukaemia and lymphoma, antibodies against surface markers can be used to distinguish between reactive and neoplastic lymphocytes in the CSF. Cytogenetic studies have also been evaluated in an attempt to improve the diagnostic accuracy of NM. Flow cytometry and DNA single-cell cytometry, techniques that measure the chromosomal content of cells, and fluorescent *in situ* hybridization, that detects numerical and structural genetic aberrations as a sign of malignancy, can give additional diagnostic information and are especially useful in liquid tumours (leukaemia and lymphoma) and appear more sensitive than CSF cytology (11–13) (Table 21.1). Of greatest utility in patients with haematological cancers is the increased sensitivity of CSF flow cytometry as compared to CSF cytology in demonstrating NM, that in addition requires comparatively small volumes of CSF for analysis (approximately 2 mL) (11–13) (Table 21.1).

Table 21.1 Non-Hodgkin's lymphoma: comparison between cerebrospinal fluid (CSF) cytology versus flow cytometry

	Negative CSF cytology	Positive CSF cytology	Total
Negative flow cytometry	287 (72%)	21 (5%)	308 (76%)
Positive flow cytometry	63 (16%)	28 (7%)	91 (23%)
Total	350 (88%)	49 (12%)	399 (100%)

Source data from *Neurology*, 50(4), Chamberlain MC, Cytologically negative carcinomatous meningitis: usefulness of CSF biochemical markers, pp. 1173–1175, Copyright (1998), Wolters Kluwer Health, Inc.; *J Clin Oncol*, 27(9), Quijano S, Lopez A, Sanchos JM, et al, Identification of leptomeningeal disease in aggressive B-cell non-Hodgkin's lymphoma: improved sensitivity of flow cytometry, pp. 1462–1469, Copyright (2009), American Society of Clinical Oncology; *Neurology*, 66, Bromberg JEC, Breems DA, Kraan J, et al., CSF flow cytometry greatly improves diagnostic accuracy in CNS hematologic malignancies, pp. 1674–1679, Copyright (2007), Wolters Kluwer Health, Inc.

Imaging

Magnetic resonance imaging (MRI) with gadolinium enhancement is the technique of choice to evaluate patients with suspected NM (1–5, 14, 15). Because NM involves the entire neuraxis, imaging of the entire CNS is required in patients considered for further treatment. T1-weighted sequences, with and without contrast, combined with fat suppression T2-weighted sequences constitute the standard examination (1–5, 16). MRI has been shown to have a higher sensitivity than cranial contrast-enhanced computed tomography in several series, and is similar to computed tomographic myelography for the evaluation of the spine, but significantly better tolerated (1–5). Neuroradiographic imaging (i.e. MRI of brain or relevant spine) may suggest NM based upon focal or diffuse leptomeningeal enhancement, subarachnoid or ventricular tumour nodules, and the frequent (30–40%) coexistence of brain parenchymal metastases in instances of non-haematological cancers (14, 15). The reported rates of negative CSF imaging in patients with NM range from 30% to 70% suggesting normal CNS imaging does not exclude a diagnosis of NM.

Radionuclide studies using either ^{111}In-diethylenetriamine pentaacetic acid or ^{99}Tc macro-aggregated albumin constitute the technique of choice to evaluate CSF flow dynamics (1–5, 16). Abnormal CSF circulation has been demonstrated in 30–70% of patients with NM, with blocks commonly occurring at the skull base, the spinal canal, and over the cerebral convexities (16–19). Patients with interruption of CSF flow demonstrated by radionuclide ventriculography have been shown in three clinical series to have decreased survival when compared to those with normal CSF flow (16–19). Involved-field radiotherapy to the site of CSF flow obstruction restores flow in 30% of patients with spinal disease and 50% of patients with intracranial disease (16–19). Re-establishment of CSF flow with involved-field radiotherapy followed by intrathecal chemotherapy led to longer survival, lower rates of treatment-related morbidity, and lower rate of death from progressive NM, compared to the group that had persistent CSF blocks (17–19).

Treatment

Adults and children

Surgery

The requirement for surgery in NM is infrequent and when performed is for limited indications. These include placement of a ventricular access device (VAD) such as an Ommaya reservoir to permit intra-CSF chemotherapy administration, instillation of a ventriculoperitoneal shunt (VPS) for raised intracranial pressure and disrupted CSF flow, and rarely for performance of a meningeal biopsy when a tissue diagnosis is sought (20–24). Meningeal biopsy as stated is rarely performed for NM but rather may be utilized in disorders of the meninges (e.g. CNS sarcoid) in which the diagnosis is uncertain notwithstanding laboratory investigations (21). In general, meningeal biopsies are directed at regions of anatomical abnormality defined by MRI regardless if in the intracranial or intraspinal compartments. With the increasing utility of neuraxis imaging, CSF cytology or flow cytometry and recognition of clinical syndromes compatible with NM, the need for meningeal biopsy and pathological diagnosis of NM is almost extinct.

Patients with NM often suffer from intracranial hypertension caused by CSF flow disruption that results in a communicating (most common) or non-communicating/obstructive hydrocephalus (least common) (20). Symptoms of raised intracranial pressure (headache, nausea, vomiting, visual obscurations, or gait instability) may be ameliorated by either whole-brain radiotherapy (WBRT) or alternatively placement of a VPS. Intra-CSF chemotherapy rarely palliates intracranial hypertension and may worsen symptoms or signs due to the induction of a CSF inflammatory response. The challenge following placement of a VPS is that intra-CSF chemotherapy often results in rapid transit of drug in the CSF due to CSF diversion and consequently limited exposure to chemotherapy. In patients that can tolerate an adjustable (on–off valve) VPS placed in the off position, intra-CSF chemotherapy may be administered through the VPS access port (23).

The most common utilization of surgery for NM is the placement of a VAD such as an Ommaya or Hickman reservoir (22). These devices permit either the instillation of intra-CSF chemotherapy or CSF sampling to assess response to treatment in patients with positive CSF cytology or flow cytometry. Placement of a VAD may be performed as same-day surgery or as a single-day admission. Intraoperative ultrasound is frequently utilized for guidance of the ventricular catheter to ensure proper localization in the target ventricle.

Complications of intra-CSF chemotherapy include those related to the ventricular reservoir and those related to the chemotherapy administered (24). The most frequent complications of ventricular reservoir placement are malposition (rates reported 3–12%), obstruction, and infection (usually skin flora). CSF infection occurs in 2–13% of patients receiving intraventricular chemotherapy. It commonly presents with headache, changes in neurological status, fever, and malfunction of the reservoir. CSF pleocytosis is commonly encountered. The most frequently isolated organism is *Staphylococcus epidermidis*. Treatment requires intravenous with or without oral and intraventricular antibiotics. Some authors advocate the routine removal of the ventricular reservoir, while others reserve device removal for those that do not clear with antibiotic therapy. In patients with few to no symptoms due to an iatrogenic bacterial meningitis it is reasonable to first treat medically with combined systemic and intra-CSF antibiotics. Subcutaneous CSF pooling and leakage are also serious complications when a VAD is placed in patients with intracranial hypertension due to NM.

Radiotherapy

Radiotherapy plays a central role in a number of situations in NM including when associated with macroscopically, neuroradiographically visible lesions that are inadequately treated by intra-CSF chemotherapy (e.g. NM co-associated with brain metastases), clinically symptomatic neurological deficits (e.g. presentation with a cauda equina syndrome), and in instances of CSF flow disturbance documented by radioisotope CSF flow studies (25–29). Depending on the extent of the disease, the clinical presentation, the overall performance status, as well as prior treatment, radiotherapy is administered as WBRT, or to defined regions only, so-called involved-field radiotherapy (25–29). For certain situations, radiotherapy of the complete craniospinal axis may be indicated, and modern radiation techniques may improve efficacy of craniospinal axis irradiation (CSI) while side effects may be lessened.

Whole-brain radiotherapy

With WBRT, the whole brain, generally down to the first or second cervical vertebra, is included in the irradiation fields. Prior to radiation, an individual fixation mask generally made of Aquaplast materials is manufactured for the patient to allow for precise daily repositioning during every treatment fraction. The patient should be conscious and cooperative and therefore with an overall acceptable Karnofsky performance score (KPS) prior to treatment. Treatment simulation is performed with the patient in the supine position; nowadays, virtual CT-based simulation is the standard in most institutions. In selected cases when mask fixation is not tolerated, irradiation without a head mask but with, for example, tape fixation can be considered. Parallel opposed fields are generally used, with gantry angles at 273° and 87° adjusted to beam divergence, or simple configurations such as 270° and 90°. The collimator should be chosen to parallel the inferior border of the radiation field to the inferior border of the first or second cervical vertebra, to avoid dose application should further irradiation be required below. The target point is commonly set to the inferior border of the irradiation field to minimize beam divergence to areas of the cervical spine, for the same reason. The target volume includes the whole brain, spinal canal down until the first or second cervical vertebra, 2 cm below the skull base bony region, with special caution to include the rostrum and lamina cribrosa when trying to spare the eyes and lenses from radiation. Radiotherapy is performed daily, five times per week, up to a total dose of 40 Gy in 2 Gy fractions, or 30 Gy in 3 Gy fractions, with a 6 MV linear accelerator. For patients with reduced performance status, hypofractionated regimens, such as 5 × 4 Gy, can be prescribed.

Few studies have evaluated WBRT for NM, most data or recommendations derive from summaries on different treatment schedules. The majority of studies represent retrospective analyses; however, data support radiotherapy effectiveness mainly for symptom control, but are not compelling for improvement in overall survival (mean range of survival 1.5–5 months) (25–28). A study by Gani et al. evaluated 27 patients with leptomeningeal metastases from breast or lung cancer treated with WBRT; the authors report a median survival of 8.1 weeks, with survival rates of 26% and 15% at 6 and 12 months, respectively (27). The only significant prognostic factors for survival were the absence of cranial nerve dysfunction ($P > 0.001$), KPS, and time interval of 35 months between initial diagnosis and the development of NM. In 75% of patients receiving follow-up MRI, size reduction of the enhancing lesions could be shown.

Morris et al. published a retrospective study on WBRT in 125 patients with NM from non-small cell lung cancer (28). Radiotherapy was applied at doses from 30 to 37.5 Gy in 10–15 fractions. In contrast to the positive prognostic effect of intra-CSF chemotherapy, WBRT did not impact overall survival. The indication for WBRT was based on positive CSF or radiographic lesions consistent with NM.

In spite of prospective data evaluating WBRT for NM demonstrating no or a negligible impact on survival, WBRT is the treatment of choice when NM presents with macroscopic disease as defined by neuraxis MRI (such as brain metastases) as intra-CSF chemotherapy is associated with only limited efficacy. For patients with symptomatic NM as, for example, raised intracranial pressure, WBRT can provide symptom relief and neurological stabilization. Additionally, radiotherapy can be administered to re-establish CSF flow in instances of documented CSF flow blocks (26, 27).

In general, radiotherapy is not combined with intra-CSF chemotherapy, as, especially with methotrexate, severe neurotoxicity may occur. Therefore, sequential treatment is recommended, if both intra-CSF chemotherapy and radiotherapy are indicated. With presumably less radiosensitizing intra-CSF chemotherapies such as cytarabine, chemoradiotherapy combination regimens may be applied. A German-Austrian trial, DEP 101 (NCT00854867), is evaluating WBRT followed by intra-CSF liposomal cytarabine, versus WBRT together with and followed by intra-CSF liposomal cytarabine in patients with NM.

Involved-field radiotherapy

Localized radiotherapy for macroscopically visible lesions with or without neurological deficits can be performed to prevent or palliate symptoms and is the most commonly used modality of radiotherapy in patients with NM. Treatment planning can be conventional, utilizing CT-based virtual simulation when the target is located in the spine using one posterior field. A safety margin of one vertebra above and below the target is commonly used to minimize edge recurrences. Alternatively, three-dimensional conformal radiotherapy based on CT imaging can be performed using a three-dimensional treatment planning system. In this case, the target lesion plus a safety margin depending on the technique applied is defined. Dose recommendations are determined in part by the overall performance status of the patient and are in line with the doses for WBRT (25–29).

Craniospinal axis irradiation

In very select cases of NM, for example, leukaemic and on occasion lymphomatous meningitis, CSI may be indicated. In the past, the radiation oncologist was often hesitant to employ CSI especially in the adult population due to the high risk of severe haematological toxicity due to irradiation of nearly 60% of all haematologically active bone marrow encompassed by neuraxis irradiation. However, small case studies have reported overall tolerability and efficacy of this treatment (30).

Conventional craniospinal radiation techniques usually require an immobilization cast with patients in the prone position to ensure daily reproducibility. The intracranial components including the upper two segments of the cervical spine are treated with opposed lateral fields, as used for WBRT. The spine is treated using one or two posterior fields, depending on the size of the patient. Special care must be taken that no overlapping of the fields occurs leading to addition of doses exceeding the tolerance dose of the spinal cord. Substantial haematological toxicity can be associated with CSI, since all vertebra containing haematopoietic bone marrow are irradiated. Therefore, the indication for CSI is limited to patients with multiple circumscriptive lesions along the spinal axis.

Novel radiation techniques, such as helical tomotherapy, might change the indication for CSI. With helical tomotherapy, a combination of CT-based image guidance and intensity-modulated radiotherapy was developed (30–33). Radiation is delivered using a fan beam by a linear accelerator which is built on a rotating gantry, and is modulated by a fast pneumatically driven binary slit collimator; this system is connected with an integrated megavoltage CT scanner, to enable daily position verification and the possibility of per-treatment position corrections. One main advantage of tomotherapy is the possibility to perform multitarget treatments, treatment of complex anatomies, but also the treatment of long volumes, such is the case in CSI (31, 32). The whole neuraxis can be treated in one volume, minimizing the risk of dose overlap or underdosing in the gap area. Additionally, steep dose gradients can be calculated, and sparing of ventral parts of the vertebra can be achieved to reduce haematological toxicity.

Complications of radiotherapy
Complications of treatment with WBRT include alopecia, transient worsening of neurological symptoms, fatigue, headache, nausea and vomiting, or otitis. Administering dexamethasone during WBRT can help alleviate most acute side effects of irradiation. Long-term side effects may be more pronounced, but in lieu of the overall poor prognosis of patients with NM (median survival 3 months), the risks and benefits should be weighed accordingly. Memory loss, dementia, and leucoencephalopathy manifested as a decreased ability to focus and concentrate along with other neurocognitive impairments can be attributed to WBRT. It is known that higher single doses of irradiation contribute more significantly to these side effects; therefore, in patients with overall good prognosis, dosing schemes of 2 Gy per day are commonly favoured (34).

For CSI, additional haematological side effects include thrombocytopenia and leucopenia; the risk for severe haematological toxicity increases with age. Novel treatment modalities, such as helical tomotherapy, may help prevent these side effects since doses to the vertebra in adult patients can be spared, while the CSF, spinal cord, and terminating nerve roots can be safely included into the target volume.

Chemotherapy
Two particular challenges arise with respect to the treatment of NM: determining whom to treat and if NM-directed treatment is believed to be warranted, how to treat (35–50). Patients assessed to be candidates for treatment include those with low tumour burden as reflected by independence in a performance scale and lack of major neurological deficits, no evidence of bulky CNS disease by neuroimaging, absence of CSF flow block by radioisotope imaging, expected survival greater than 3 months, and limited extraneural metastatic disease (16–18, 49, 50). Many of these parameters require laboratory investigation including the performance of neuraxis imaging (most commonly MRI with contrast) and a radioisotope CSF flow study. CSF flow studies, though recommended in guidelines, are infrequently utilized; however, they may assist in determining whether intra-CSF chemotherapy, if administered, distributes homogenously throughout the CSF or whether intra-CSF chemotherapy will likely be confined to a single CSF compartment resulting in failure to treat all sites of leptomeningeal disease as well as increasing the risk for treatment-related neurotoxicity (16–18, 49). If after clinical and laboratory assessment intra-CSF chemotherapy treatment is believed warranted, a decision is made whether to treat by lumbar administration (intrathecal) or by way of a surgically implanted subgaleal reservoir and intraventricular catheter (i.e. an Ommaya or Rickham reservoir system). Intralumbar treatment is relatively convenient but suffers from the time required to perform the procedure, patient discomfort from the procedure, frequent need for performance by interventional radiology, failure to deliver drug to the thecal sac (10–12% of intralumbar treatments do not enter the CSF compartment), limited distribution within the cranial CSF compartments when administering short half-life intra-CSF chemotherapy agents (i.e. methotrexate, cytarabine), and the apparent diminished survival in patients with NM treated by intralumbar drug administration compared to intraventricular treatment (51). Treatment by intraventricular intra-CSF chemotherapy administration results in improved drug dose and distribution in the CSF and is more convenient, especially for treatment that is often two or more times per week (Table 21.2). However, surgical implantation of a device and the risk of complications, especially iatrogenic bacterial meningitis, need to be balanced against the above-mentioned benefits of intraventricular intra-CSF drug administration.

High-dose systemic chemotherapy (in particular methotrexate and cytarabine) may obviate the need for intra-CSF chemotherapy (37, 52). High-dose therapy achieves cytotoxic CSF levels as, for example, reported in patients with lymphomatous meningitis or breast cancer-related NM. However, the majority of systemic chemotherapy agents and some targeted therapies (i.e. imatinib, rituximab, and trastuzumab) do not achieve adequate CNS penetration and consequently will not treat the CSF compartment. This statement does not imply systemic chemotherapy has no role in the treatment of NM but rather for the majority of patients with NM, systemic chemotherapy is an adjunctive treatment useful to treat extraneural disease and bulky subarachnoid disease (1, 16, 38, 46).

Intra-CSF chemotherapy in NM is based upon limited studies with comparatively small numbers of patients (38–41, 43–48) (Table 21.3). Consequently, the role of intra-CSF chemotherapy in the treatment of NM has never been established in a prospective randomized trial. Nonetheless, several statements can be made regarding intra-CSF chemotherapy. Among the three most common intra-CSF chemotherapy agents used (i.e. methotrexate, cytarabine, and thiotepa), there does not appear to be an

Table 21.2 Regional chemotherapy for leptomeningeal metastasis

Drugs (reference)	Induction regimens		Consolidation regimen		Maintenance regimen	
	Bolus regimen	Concentration × time regimen	Bolus regimen	Concentration × time regimen	Bolus regimen	Concentration × time regimen
α-Interferon (44)	1×10⁶ U 2 times weekly (total 4 weeks)		1×10⁶ U 3 times weekly every other week (total 4 weeks)		1×10⁶ U 3 times weekly 1 week per month	
Cytarabine (41)	25–100 mg 2 times weekly (total 4 weeks)	25 mg/day for 3 days weekly (total 4 weeks)	25–100 mg once weekly (total 4 weeks)	25 mg/day for 3 days every other week (total 4 weeks)	25–100 mg once a month	25 mg/day for 3 days once a month
DepoCyta (41, 42, 45)	50 mg every 2 weeks (total 8 weeks)		50 mg every 4 weeks (total 24 weeks)			
Etoposide (43)		0.5 mg/day for 5 days every other week (total 8 weeks)		0.5 mg/day for 5 days every other week (total 4 weeks)		0.5 mg/day for 5 days once a month
Methotrexate (36, 39, 40, 46)	10–15 mg twice weekly (total 4 weeks)	2 mg/day for 5 days every other week (total 8 weeks)	10–15 mg once weekly (total 4 weeks)	2 mg/day for 5 days every other week (total 4 weeks)	10–15 mg once a month	2 mg/day for 5 days once a month
Rituximab (1)	25 mg 2 times weekly (total 4 weeks)		25 mg 2 times weekly every other week (total 4 weeks)		25 mg 2 times weekly once a month	
Thiotepa (39)	10 mg 2 times weekly (total 4 weeks)	10 mg/day for 3 days weekly (total 4 weeks)	10 mg once weekly (total 4 weeks)	10 mg/day for 3 days every other week (total 4 weeks)	10 mg once a month	10 mg/day for 3 days once a month
Topotecan (48)	0.4 mg 2 times weekly (total 4 weeks)		0.4 mg 2 times weekly every other week (total 4 weeks)		0.4 mg 2 times weekly once a month	
Trastuzumab (47)	20–100 mg 1 time weekly (total 4 weeks)		20–60 mg 1 time every other week (total 4 weeks)		20–60 mg 1 time every 4 weeks	

Adapted from *Current Opinion in Oncology*, 22(6), Chamberlain MC, Leptomeningeal metastases, pp. 627–35, Copyright (2010), with permission from Wolters Kluwer Health, Inc.

advantage of one agent versus another nor does there appear to be an advantage for combining agents as is commonly prescribed for lymphomatous and leukaemic meningitis (38, 39) (Table 21.3). Liposomal cytarabine, an intra-CSF chemotherapy agent with a long half-life (approximately 140 hours), has been shown in two small randomized trials to be superior to methotrexate or cytarabine though potentially with increased neurotoxicity (40, 41) (Table 21.3). Due to increased efficacy (cytological response, time to neurological disease progression, non-neurological cause of death, and improved quality of life), an argument has been made to consider liposomal cytarabine as the agent of first choice in patients with NM unless an investigational trial is available. Small trials with alternative intra-CSF chemotherapies (i.e. topotecan, etoposide, α-interferon, and trastuzumab) have been utilized in adults with NM though the appropriate role for these agents is unclear (42–44, 47, 48). Suggestions including treatment of melanoma-related NM with α-interferon, germ cell and small cell lung cancer NM with etoposide, Her2/neu-positive breast cancer-related NM with trastuzumab, and topotecan for non-small cell lung cancer-related NM appear reasonable but unfortunately are not evidenced based. All intra-CSF chemotherapy is associated with side effects and can be ascribed to those directly related to therapy such as fatigue associated with WBRT and the induction of a chemical meningitis with intra-CSF chemotherapy. Intra-CSF chemotherapy commonly causes transient (less than 5 days) aseptic chemical meningitis that may be mitigated by administration of concurrent oral steroids (1, 2, 40, 41). The chemical meningitis often manifests as headache, nausea/vomiting, fever, photophobia, meningismus, CSF pleocytosis, and occasionally delirium. It is likely that the majority of patients manifest laboratory evidence of intra-CSF chemotherapy-related chemical meningitis; however, only a minority are symptomatic and most are easily managed with oral medications. The major differential diagnosis is with respect to iatrogenic infectious meningitis wherein skin contaminants are introduced at the time of intra-CSF chemotherapy.

Commentary on National Comprehensive Cancer Network guidelines

National Comprehensive Cancer Network (NCCN) guidelines, the most widely used and most frequently cited cancer guidelines,

Table 21.3 Randomized clinical trials

Study (reference)	Design	Response	Toxicity
Boogerd et al. (46)	N = 35 Breast cancer IT vs no IT†	IT vs no IT: Improvement or stabilization: 59% vs 67% TTP: 23 vs 24 wk Median survival: 18.3 vs 30.3 wk	IT vs no IT: Neurological complications: 47% vs 6%
Glantz et al. (41)	N = 28 Lymphoma DepoCyt® vs Ara-C	DepoCyt® vs Ara-C: TTP*: 78.5 vs 42 d OS*: 99.5 vs 63 d RR: 71% vs 15%	DepoCyt® vs Ara-C: Headache: 27% vs 2%; nausea: 9% vs 2%; fever: 8% vs 4%; pain: 5% vs 4%; confusion: 7% vs 0%; somnolence: 8% vs 4%
Glantz et al. (40)	N = 61 Solid tumours DepoCyt® vs MTX	DepoCyt® vs MTX: RR* 26% vs 20% OS* 105 vs 78 d TTP 58 vs 30 d	DepoCyt® vs MTX: Sensory/motor: 4% vs 10%; altered mental status: 5% vs 2%; headache: 4% vs 2%
Grossman et al. (39)	N = 59 Solid tumours and lymphoma (in 90%) IT MTX vs thiotepa	IT MTX vs thiotepa: Neurological improvements: none Median survival: 15.9 vs 14.1 wk	IT MTX vs thiotepa: Serious toxicities similar between groups Mucositis and neurological complications more common in MTX group
Hitchins et al. (38)	N = 44 Solid tumours and lymphomas IT MTX vs MTX + Ara-C	IT MTX vs. MTX + Ara-C: RR*: 61% vs 45% Median survival*: 12 vs 7 wk	IT MTX vs MTX + Ara-C: N/V: 36% vs 50%; septicaemia, neutropenia: 9% vs 15%; mucositis: 14% vs 10%; pancytopenia: 9% vs 10%. AEs related to reservoir: blocked Ommaya: 17% vs 0%; intracranial haemorrhage: 11% vs 0%
Shapiro et al. (45)	Solid tumours (N = 103) DepoCyt® vs MTX Lymphoma (N = 25) DepoCyt® vs Ara-C	DepoCyt® vs MTX/Ara-C: PFS*: 35 vs 43 d DepoCyt® vs MTX: PFS: 35 vs 37.5 DepoCyt® vs Ara-C: CR*: 33.3% vs 16.7% PFS: 34 vs 50 d	DepoCyt® vs MTX/Ara-C: Drug-related AEs: 48% vs 60% Serious AEs: 86% vs 77%

* No significant differences between groups.

† Appropriate systemic chemotherapy and/or radiotherapy given in both arms.

AE, adverse event; Ara-C, cytarabine; CR, complete response; d, day; IT, intra-CSF; MTX, methotrexate; N/V, nausea/vomiting; OS, overall survival; PFS, progression-free survival; RR, response rate; TTP, time to progression; wk, weeks.

Adapted from *Current Opinion in Oncology*, 22(6), Chamberlain MC, Leptomeningeal metastases, pp. 627–35, Copyright (2010), with permission from Wolters Kluwer Health, Inc.

predominantly reflect expert opinion due to a paucity of high-level evidence (mostly IIa) for the treatment and management of NM (16). Consequently, the guidelines should be viewed as expert consensus on good clinical practice. Because of limitations in the guidelines (low-level evidence, expert opinion based), it is uncertain if clinical outcomes are impacted by their use. Importantly, there is no assessment of cost-effectiveness (economic impact or comparative effectiveness). Nonetheless, the NCCN guidelines recommend a staging evaluation in patients suspected to harbour NM that includes CSF interrogation, neuraxis MRI, and, in patients being considered for intra-CSF chemotherapy, a radioisotope CSF flow study. The utility of intra-CSF chemotherapy is recognized as a standard of care treatment notwithstanding a paucity of evidence demonstrating benefit, particularly in the setting of carcinomatous meningitis (46).

Other therapy including surveillance recommendations

Symptomatic treatment of NM is directed at alleviating pain which is most often headache and secondary to raised intracranial pressure that is best managed either by CSF shunting or treatment with WBRT. Similarly, nausea and vomiting are usually related to raised intracranial pressure and are managed in a similar manner. As a general principle there is little benefit from steroid administration in managing NM-related symptoms with two exceptions. Patients with treatment-related chemical meningitis often benefit from steroid administration as mentioned previously. In addition, patients with coexisting parenchymal brain metastases also derive benefit from steroids when peritumoural oedema exists. Antiepileptic drugs are rarely indicated as less than 10%

of patients with NM manifest seizures and there is no benefit to prophylactic antiepileptic drug use. Importantly, a candid discussion regarding potential treatment side effects and expected treatment outcome is important as many patients may conclude that treatment is ineffective and consequently, decline therapy. In patients proceeding with NM-directed therapy, preparing patients and families for a neurological death and the expected sequential loss of neurological function may help to alleviate stress and provide an improved understanding of the dying process.

Current research topics

At present, there is an enormous unmet need for investigational trials of novel treatments for NM; however, there are several reasons why this is unlikely, at least for the immediate future. Neuro-oncology collaborative groups are historically focused on gliomas with limited interest in studying NM. Because of the comparatively low incidence of NM and limited survival following diagnosis, there is little economic incentive for pharmaceutical companies to invest resources in NM and lastly, a certain degree of therapeutic nihilism exists among oncologists in managing patients with NM that serves as a disincentive for development of clinical trials.

NM is a complicated disease for a variety of reasons. First, most reports concerning NM treat all subtypes as equivalent with respect to CNS staging, treatment, and outcome. However, clinical trials in oncology are based on specific tumour histology and biology. Comparing responses in patients with carcinomatous meningitis due to breast cancer to patients with non-small cell lung cancer outside of investigational new drug trials may be misleading.

A second feature of NM, which complicates therapy, is deciding whom to treat. Not all patients necessarily warrant aggressive CNS-directed therapy; however, few guidelines exist to direct the appropriate choice of therapy. Based on the prognostic variables determined clinically and by evaluation of the extent of disease, a sizable minority of patients will not be candidates for aggressive NM-directed therapy. Therefore supportive care (radiotherapy to symptomatic disease, antiemetics, and narcotics) is reasonably offered to patients with NM considered poor candidates for aggressive therapy as seen in Fig. 21.1.

Third, optimal treatment of NM remains poorly defined. Given these constraints, the treatment of NM today is palliative and rarely curative with a median patient survival of 2–3 months based on data from the six prospective randomized trials in this disease.

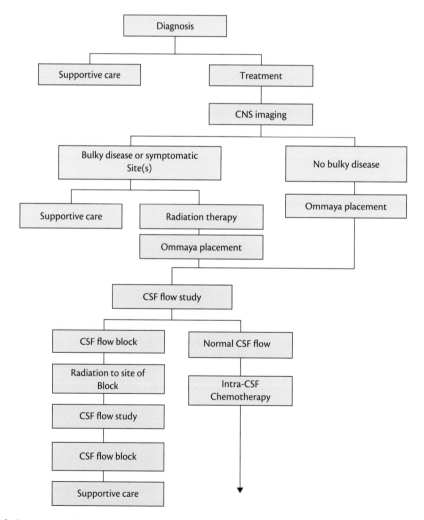

Fig. 21.1 Treatment algorithm for leptomeningeal metastases.

Adapted from *Current Opinion in Oncology*, 22(6), Chamberlain MC, Leptomeningeal metastases, pp. 627–35, Copyright (2010), with permission from Wolters Kluwer Health, Inc.

However, palliative therapy of NM often affords the patient protection from further neurological deterioration and consequently an improved neurological quality of life. No studies to date have attempted an economic assessment of the treatment of NM and therefore no information is available regarding a cost–benefit analysis as has been performed for other cancer-directed therapies.

Finally, in patients with NM, the response to treatment has been based primarily on CSF cytology or flow cytometry. Many experts would, however, argue that response to NM-directed treatment should be based on clinical outcome rather than CSF analysis. In general, only pain-related neurological symptoms improve with treatment. Neurological signs such as confusion, cranial nerve deficit(s), ataxia, and segmental weakness minimally improve or stabilize with successful treatment.

References

1. Chamberlain MC. Leptomeningeal metastases. *Curr Opin Oncol* 2010; 22:627–635.

2. Jaeckle KA. Neoplastic meningitis from systemic malignancies: diagnosis, prognosis, and treatment. *Semin Oncol* 2006; 33:312–323.

3. Pace P, Fabi A. Chemotherapy in neoplastic meningitis. *Crit Rev Oncol Hematol* 2006; 60(3):528–534.

4. Glass JP, Melamed M, Chernik NL, et al. Malignant cells in cerebrospinal fluid (CSF): the meaning of a positive CSF cytology. *Neurology* 1979; 29(10):1369–1375.

5. Gleissner B, Chamberlain MC. Clinical presentation and therapy of neoplastic meningitis. *Lancet Neurol* 2006; 5:443–452.

6. van de Langerijt B, Gijtenbeek JM, de Reus HP, et al. CSF levels of growth factors and plasminogen activators in leptomeningeal metastases. *Neurology* 2006; 67(1):114–119.

7. Brandsma D, Taphoorn MJ, de Jager W, et al. Interleukin-8 CSF levels predict survival in patients with leptomeningeal metastases. *Neurology* 2006; 66(2):243–246.

8. Brandsma D, Ulfman L, Reijneveld JC, et al. Constitutive integrin activation on tumor cells contributes to progression of leptomeningeal metastases. *Neuro Oncol* 2006; 8(2):127–136.

9. Glantz MJ, Cole BF, Glantz LK, et al. Cerebrospinal fluid cytology in patients with cancer: minimizing false-negative results. *Cancer* 1998; 82(4):733–739.

10. Chamberlain MC. Cytologically negative carcinomatous meningitis: usefulness of CSF biochemical markers. *Neurology* 1998; 50(4):1173–1175.

11. Quijano S, Lopez A, Sanchos JM, et al. Identification of leptomeningeal disease in aggressive B-cell non-Hodgkin's lymphoma: improved sensitivity of flow Cytometry. *J Clin Oncol* 2009; 27(9):1462–1469.

12. Bromberg JEC, Breems DA, Kraan J, et al. CSF flow cytometry greatly improves diagnostic accuracy in CNS hematologic malignancies. *Neurology* 2007; 66:1674–1679.

13. Hegde U, Filie A, Little RF, et al. High incidence of leptomeningeal disease detected by flow cytometry in newly diagnosed aggressive B-cell lymphoma at risk for central nervous system involvement: the role of flow cytometry versus cytology. *Blood* 2005; 105:496–502.

14. Chamberlain MC. Comparative spine imaging in leptomeningeal metastases. *J Neuro Oncol* 1995; 23(3):233–238.

15. Clarke JL, Perez HR, Jacks LM, et al. Leptomeningeal metastases in the MRI era. *Neurology* 2010; 74:1449–1454.

16. Brem SS, Bierman PJ, Black P, et al. Central nervous system cancers: clinical practice guidelines in oncology. *J Natl Compr Canc Netw* 2008; 6(5):456–504.

17. Grossman SA, Trump CL, Chen DCP, et al. Cerebrospinal flow abnormalities in patients with neoplastic meningitis. *Am J Med* 1982; 73:641–647.

18. Chamberlain MC. Radioisotope CSF flow studies in leptomeningeal metastases. *J Neuro Oncol* 1998; 38(2–3):135–140.

19. Glantz MJ, Hall WA, Cole BF, et al. Diagnosis, management, and survival of patients with leptomeningeal cancer based on cerebrospinal fluid-flow status, *Cancer* 1995; 75:2919–2931.

20. Lin N, Dunn ID, Glantz M, et al. Benefit of ventriculoperitoneal cerebrospinal fluid shunting and intrathecal chemotherapy in neoplastic meningitis: a retrospective, case controlled study. *J Neurosurg* 2011; 115:730–736.

21. Cheng TM, O'Neill BP, Scheithauer BW, et al. Chronic meningitis: the role of meningeal or cortical biopsy. *Neurosurgery* 1994; 34(4):590–595.

22. Sandberg DI, Bilsky MH, Souweidane MM, et al. Ommaya reservoirs for the treatment of leptomeningeal metastases. *Neurosurgery* 2000; 47(1):49–54.

23. Zada G, Chen TC. A novel method for administering intrathecal chemotherapy in patients with leptomeningeal metastases and shunted hydrocephalus: case report. *Neurosurgery* 2010; 67(3 Suppl Operative):onsE306–E307.

24. Chamberlain MC, Kormanik PA, Barba D. Complications associated with intraventricular chemotherapy in patients with leptomeningeal metastases. *J Neurosurgery* 1997; 87:694–699.

25. Chuang TY, Yu CJ, Shih JY, et al. Cytologically proven meningeal carcinomatosis in patients with lung cancer: clinical observation of 34 cases. *J Formos Med Assoc* 2008; 107:851–856.

26. Sause WT, Crowley J, Eyre HJ, et al. Whole brain irradiation and intrathecal methotrexate in the treatment of solid tumor leptomeningeal metastases—a Southwest Oncology Group study. *J Neurooncol* 1988; 6:107–112.

27. Gani C, Muller AC, Eckert F, et al. Outcome after whole brain radiotherapy alone in intracranial leptomeningeal carcinomatosis from solid tumors. *Strahlenther Onkol* 2012; 188:148–153.

28. Morris PG, Reiner AS, Szenberg OR, et al. Leptomeningeal metastasis from non-small cell lung cancer: survival and the impact of whole brain radiotherapy. *J Thorac Oncol* 2012; 7:382–385.

29. Taillibert S, Laigle-Donadey F, Chodkiewicz C, et al. Leptomeningeal metastases from solid malignancy: a review. *J Neurooncol* 2005; 75:85–99.

30. Hermann B, Hultenschmidt B, Sautter-Bihl ML. Radiotherapy of the neuraxis for palliative treatment of leptomeningeal carcinomatosis. *Strahlenther Onkol* 2001; 177:195–199.

31. Feyer P, Sautter-Bihl ML, Budach W, et al. Breast Cancer Expert Panel of the German Society of Radiation Oncology (DEGRO). DEGRO Practical Guidelines for palliative radiotherapy of breast cancer patients: brain metastases and leptomeningeal carcinomatosis. *Strahlenther Onkol* 2010; 186(2):63–69.

32. Combs SE, Sterzing F, Uhl M, et al. Helical tomotherapy for meningiomas of the skull base and in paraspinal regions with complex anatomy and/or multiple lesions. *Tumori* 2011; 97:484–491.

33. Stoiber EM, Giske K, Schubert K, et al. Local setup reproducibility of the spinal column when using intensity-modulated radiation therapy for craniospinal irradiation with patient in supine position. *Int J Radiat Oncol Biol Phys* 2011; 81:1552–1559.

34. DeAngelis LM, Delattre JY, Posner JB. Radiation-induced dementia in patients cured of brain metastases. *Neurology* 1989; 39:789–796.

35. Chamberlain MC. Neoplastic meningitis: deciding who to treat. *Expert Rev Neurother* 2004; 4(4):89–96.

36. Shapiro WR, Young DF, Mehta BM. Methotrexate: distribution in cerebrospinal fluid after intravenous, ventricular and lumbar injections. *N Engl J Med* 1975; 293(4):161–166.

37. Siegal T. Leptomeningeal metastases: rationale for systemic chemotherapy or what is the role of intra-CSF-chemotherapy? *J Neuro Oncol* 1998; 38(2–3):151–157.

38. Hitchins RN, Bell DR, Woods RL, et al. A prospective randomized trial of single-agent versus combination chemotherapy in meningeal carcinomatosis. *J Clin Oncol* 1987; 5(10):1655–1662.

39. Grossman SA, Finkelstein DM, Ruckdeschel JC, et al. Randomized prospective comparison of intraventricular methotrexate and thiotepa in patients with previously untreated neoplastic meningitis. *J Clin Oncol* 1993; 11:561–569.

40. Glantz MJ, Jaeckle KA, Chamberlain MC, et al. A randomized controlled trial comparing intrathecal sustained-release cytarabine (DepoCyt) to intrathecal methotrexate in patients with neoplastic meningitis from solid tumors. *Clin Cancer Res* 1999; 5(11):3394–3402.

41. Glantz MJ, LaFollette S, Jaeckle KA, et al. Randomized trial of a slow release versus a standard formulation of cytarabine for the intrathecal treatment of lymphomatous meningitis. *J Clin Oncol* 1999; 17:3110–3116.

42. Stapleton S, Blaney SM. New agents for intrathecal administration. *Cancer Invest* 2006; 24:528–534.

43. Chamberlain MC, Wei-Tao DD, Groshen S. A phase II trial of intracerebrospinal fluid etoposide in the treatment of neoplastic meningitis. *Cancer* 2006; 106(9):2021–2027.

44. Chamberlain MC. A phase II trial of intra-cerebrospinal fluid alpha interferon in the treatment of neoplastic meningitis. *Cancer* 2002; 94:2675–2680.

45. Shapiro WR, Schmid M, Glantz M, et al. A randomized phase III/IV study to determine benefit and safety of cytarabine liposome injection for treatment of neoplastic meningitis. *J Clin Oncol* 2006; 24(June 6 Suppl):1528 (abstract).

46. Boogerd W, van den Bent MJ, Koehler PJ, et al. The relevance of intraventricular chemotherapy for leptomeningeal metastasis in breast cancer: a randomized study. *Eur J Cancer* 2004; 40:2726–2733.

47. Mir O, Ropert S, Alexandre J, et al. High-dose intrathecal trastuzumab for leptomeningeal metastases secondary to HER-2 overexpressing breast cancer. *Ann Oncol* 2008; 19(11):1978–1980.

48. Groves MD, Glantz MJ, Chamberlain MC, et al. A multicenter phase II trial of intrathecal topotecan in patients with meningeal malignancies. *Neuro-Oncology* 2008; 10(2):208–215.

49. Chamberlain MC, Kormanik PA. Prognostic significance of coexistent bulky metastatic central nervous system disease in patients with leptomeningeal metastases. *Arch Neurol* 1997; 54(11):1364–1368.

50. Chamberlain MC, Johnston SK, Glantz MJ. Neoplastic meningitis-related prognostic significance of the Karnofsky performance status. *Arch Neurol* 2009; 66(1):74–78.

51. Glantz MJ, Van Horn A, Fisher R, et al. Route of intra-CSF chemotherapy administration and efficacy of therapy in neoplastic meningitis. *Cancer* 2010; 116:1947–1952.

52. Glantz MJ, Cole BF, Recht L, et al. High-dose intravenous methotrexate for patients with non-leukemic leptomeningeal cancer: is intrathecal chemotherapy necessary? *J Clin Oncol* 1998; 16(4):1561–1567.

Index

Tables, figures, and boxes are indicated by an italic *t*, *f*, and *b* following the page number.